T0314159

Brain Arteriovenous Malformations and Arteriovenous Fistulas

Aaron S. Dumont, MD, FACS, FAHA
Charles B. Wilson Professor & Chairman
Department of Neurosurgery
Director
Tulane Center for Clinical Neurosciences
Tulane University School of Medicine
New Orleans, Louisiana

Giuseppe Lanzino, MD
Professor of Neurosurgery
Department of Neurological Surgery
Mayo Clinic
Rochester, Minnesota

Jason P. Sheehan, MD, PhD
Vice Chair and Harrison Distinguished Professor of Neurological Surgery
Department of Neurosurgery, Radiation Oncology, and Neuroscience
University of Virginia
Charlottesville, Virginia

250 illustrations

Thieme
New York • Stuttgart • Delhi • Rio de Janeiro

Executive Editor: Timothy Hiscock
Managing Editor: Sarah Landis
Director, Editorial Services: Mary Jo Casey
Editorial Assistant: Nikole Connors
Production Editor: Naamah Schwartz
International Production Director: Andreas Schabert
Editorial Director: Sue Hodgson
International Marketing Director: Fiona Henderson
International Sales Director: Louisa Turrell
Director of Institutional Sales: Adam Bernacki
Senior Vice President and Chief Operating Officer: Sarah Vanderbilt
President: Brian D. Scanlan

Library of Congress Cataloging-in-Publication Data

Names: Dumont, Aaron S., editor. | Sheehan, Jason P., editor. |
    Lanzino, Giuseppe, editor.
Title: Brain arteriovenous malformations and arteriovenous
    fistulas / Aaron S. Dumont, Jason Sheehan, Giuseppe Lanzino.
Description: New York : Thieme, [2018] | Includes bibliographical
    references.
Identifiers: LCCN 2017026868| ISBN 9781626233225 (print) |
    ISBN 9781626233232 (eISBN)
Subjects: | MESH: Intracranial Arteriovenous Malformations–
    therapy | Arteriovenous Fistula–physiopathology | Cerebral
    Arteries–abnormalities
Classification: LCC RD598.5 | NLM WL 355 | DDC 611.81–dc23
    LC record available at https://lccn.loc.gov/2017026868

© 2018 Thieme Medical Publishers, Inc.
Thieme Publishers New York
333 Seventh Avenue, New York, NY 10001 USA
+1 800 782 3488, customerservice@thieme.com

Thieme Publishers Stuttgart
Rüdigerstrasse 14, 70469 Stuttgart, Germany
+49 [0]711 8931 421, customerservice@thieme.de

Thieme Publishers Delhi
A-12, Second Floor, Sector-2, Noida-201301
Uttar Pradesh, India
+91 120 45 566 00, customerservice@thieme.in

Thieme Revinter Publicações Ltda.
Rua do Matoso, 170
Rio de Janeiro, RJ, CEP 20270-135, Brasil
+55 21 2563 9700

Cover design: Thieme Publishing Group
Typesetting by Thomson Digital, India

Printed in The United States of America by King Printing
Company, Inc.   5 4 3 2 1

ISBN 978-1-62623-322-5

Also available as an e-book:
eISBN 978-1-62623-323-2

Important note: Medicine is an ever-changing science undergoing continual development. Research and clinical experience are continually expanding our knowledge, in particular our knowledge of proper treatment and drug therapy. Insofar as this book mentions any dosage or application, readers may rest assured that the authors, editors, and publishers have made every effort to ensure that such references are in accordance with **the state of knowledge at the time of production of the book.**

Nevertheless, this does not involve, imply, or express any guarantee or responsibility on the part of the publishers in respect to any dosage instructions and forms of applications stated in the book. **Every user is requested to examine carefully** the manufacturers' leaflets accompanying each drug and to check, if necessary in consultation with a physician or specialist, whether the dosage schedules mentioned therein or the contraindications stated by the manufacturers differ from the statements made in the present book. Such examination is particularly important with drugs that are either rarely used or have been newly released on the market. Every dosage schedule or every form of application used is entirely at the user's own risk and responsibility. The authors and publishers request every user to report to the publishers any discrepancies or inaccuracies noticed. If errors in this work are found after publication, errata will be posted at www.thieme.com on the product description page.

Some of the product names, patents, and registered designs referred to in this book are in fact registered trademarks or proprietary names even though specific reference to this fact is not always made in the text. Therefore, the appearance of a name without designation as proprietary is not to be construed as a representation by the publisher that it is in the public domain.

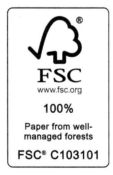

Contents

Contents

Foreword

Twenty-three years ago, when I was operating with Dr. Charles Drake as a fellow and he was struggling to achieve hemostasis with a large complex AVM, I recall him saying "Gary, AVMs are the toughest cases I deal with!" Of course, this was prior to the widespread use of embolization or radiosurgery treatment of these lesions. Now, with the incorporation of these adjuncts, increased understanding of the natural history, and advances in neuroanesthesia, electrophysiological monitoring and navigation, as well as surgical instrumentation, the treatment of brain AVMs and AVFs is much safer and more effective. However, they are still extremely challenging in other respects. Which patients with AVMs and AVFs should be treated? Which therapeutic modality or combination of modalities is best? How can we reduce complications and morbidity further?

This timely and authoritative text edited by Drs. Dumont, Lanzino, and Sheehan nicely addresses these issues and many others in 31 chapters written by experts in the field. These sections are clearly composed and enjoyable to read, with excellent figures. They appropriately discuss intracranial AVM and AVF anatomy and physiology, clinical presentation and imaging, natural history, and indications for treatment. There are chapters describing the latest surgical, endovascular, and radiosurgical management, including multidisciplinary therapy, anesthesia, intraoperative monitoring, and critical care management. Special consideration is given to residual/recurrent, pediatric, and syndromic AVMs. Surgical nuances for AVMs in different locations are elegantly conveyed.

I learned a great deal from this book and expect it to remain a definitive source related to brain AVMs and AVFs for many years.

Gary K. Steinberg, MD, PhD

Preface

During the past decade, there have been significant advances in the area of intracranial arteriovenous malformations (AVMs) and arteriovenous fistulas (AVFs). The development and physiology of these vascular malformations have become much better defined. Also, additional light has been shed on their natural history. Essential aspects of modern intervention for AVMs and AVFs are detailed in the current work. We underscore the collegial interdisciplinary approach taken to successfully treating such patients and the need for more than one strategy in the management of patients harboring complex vascular malformations.

The overriding aim of the current work is to summarize contemporary clinical knowledge and multidisciplinary approaches. To that end, contributions focus on surgical techniques, embolization, and radiosurgery, and particular emphasis is placed on the risk and benefit profile of each therapeutic strategy. We also highlight the limitations of the different treatments and situations where conservative management may be the best solution. A realistic analysis of the pros and cons of each therapy is provided herein as any clinician treating patients with AVMs or AVFs must possess a thorough understanding of complication recognition and management. The majority of the chapters also contain illustrations and tables to stress the main features of each chapter.

All of the chapters are written by widely recognized and established cerebrovascular experts. The professional editorial efforts of Thieme, including Sarah Landis and Tim Hiscock, have been essential to the completion of the work. On a personal note, we wish to express our gratitude to our families for their support throughout this endeavor. The time spent working on this project will of course be worthwhile if we help improve the care provided to patients who so courageously live with AVMs and AVFs.

Aaron S. Dumont, MD, FACS, FAHA
Giuseppe Lanzino, MD
Jason P. Sheehan, MD, PhD

Contributors

Felipe C. Albuquerque, MD
Assistant Director, Endovascular Surgery
Professor of Neurosurgery
Department of Neurosurgery
Barrow Neurological Institute
Phoenix, Arizona

João Paulo Almeida, MD
Neurosurgeon
Institute of Neurological Sciences
Sao Paulo, Brazil

Peter S. Amenta, MD
Assistant Professor of Neurosurgery
Tulane University School of Medicine
New Orleans, Louisiana

Aimee M. Aysenne, MD, MPH
Director of Neurocritical Care
Department of Clinical Neurosciences
School of Medicine
Tulane University
New Orleans, Louisiana

H. Hunt Batjer, MD, FACS, FAANS
Lois C.A. and Darwin E. Smith Professor and Chair
Department of Neurological Surgery
University of Texas Southwestern Medical School
Dallas, Texas

Edoardo Boccardi, MD
Director
Diagnostic and Interventional Neuroradiology
Niguarda Ca' Granda Hospital
Milan, Italy

Waleed Brinjikji, MD
Assistant Professor of Radiology and Neurosurgery
Mayo Clinic
Rochester, Minnesota

Federico Cagnazzo, MD
Neurosurgeon
Department of Neurosurgery
University of Pisa
Pisa, Italy

Feres Chaddad Neto, MD, PhD
Adjunct Professor
Department of Neurosurgery
Federal University of São Paolo
São Paolo, Brazil

Ameet V. Chitale, MD
Chief Resident
Department of Neurological Surgery
Thomas Jefferson University Hospital
Philadelphia, Pennsylvania

Wen-Yuh Chung, MD
Director of Functional Neurosurgery
Department of Neurology
Taipei Veterans General Hospital
Taipei, Taiwan, ROC

Aaron Cohen-Gadol, MD, MSc
Neurosurgeon
Goodman Campbell Brain and Spine
Indianapolis, Indiana

Or Cohen-Inbar, MD, PhD
Visiting Assistant Professor
Department of Neurological Surgery
University of Virginia
Charlottesville, Virginia
Attending Neurosurgeon
Department of Neurosurgery
Rambam Health Care Center
Technion – Israel Institute of Technology
Haifa, Israel

Marshall C. Cress, MD
Assistant Professor
Orlando Regional Medical Center
UF Health Neurosurgery
Orlando, Florida

Badih Daou, MD
Resident Physician
Department of Neurosurgery
University of Michigan
Ann Arbor, Michigan

Jason M. Davies, MD, PhD
Assistant Professor
Cerebrovascular and Skullbase Neurosurgery
Departments of Neurosurgery and Biomedical Informatics
Director of Cerebrovascular Microsurgery
Co-Director of Neurovascular Surgery Fellowship,
    Open Cerebrovascular
Director of Endoscopy, Kaleida Health
Research Director, Jacobs Institute
State University of New York, Buffalo
Buffalo, New York

Evandro de Oliveira, MD, PhD
Professor of Neurosurgery
Adjunct Professor of Neurological Surgery
Mayo Clinic
Jacksonville, Florida
Director
Institute of Neurological Sciences
Chief of Neurosurgery Residency Program
Hospital Beneficência Portuguesa
São Paulo, Brazil

Colin Derdeyn, MD
Krabbenhoft Professor and Chair
Department of Radiology
Professor of Neurology
Director, NeuroEndovascular Service
Director, Iowa Institute of Biomedical Imaging
University of Iowa Hospitals and Clinics
Iowa City, Iowa

Dale Ding, MD
Resident Physician
Department of Neurological Surgery
University of Virginia
Charlottesville, Virginia

Peter Dirks, MD, PhD
Neurosurgeon
Department of Neurosurgery
The Hospital for Sick Children
Toronto, Canada

Brian Drake, BESc, MB BCh BAO, FRCSC
Staff Neurosurgeon
University of Ottawa
Division of Neurosurgery
The Ottawa Hospital, Civic Campus
Ottawa, Ontario, Canada

Aaron S. Dumont, MD, FACS, FAHA
Charles B. Wilson Professor & Chairman
Department of Neurosurgery
Director
Tulane Center for Clinical Neurosciences
Tulane University School of Medicine
New Orleans, Louisiana

Andrew Faramand, MD, MSc
Research Assistant
Department of Neurosurgery
University of Pittsburgh Medical Center
Pittsburgh, Pennsylvania

Michaelangelo Fuortes, MD
Instructor
Department of Radiology
University of Iowa Hospitals and Clinics
Iowa City, Iowa

Joseph Gastala, MD
Instructor
Department of Radiology
University of Iowa Hospitals and Clinics
Iowa City, Iowa

Wan-Yuo Guo, MD, PhD
Director, Department of Radiology
Taipei Veteran General Hospital
Taipei, Taiwan, ROC

Tomoki Hashimoto, MD
Professor
Department of Anesthesia and Perioperative Care
Department of Neurological Surgery
University of California, San Francisco
San Francisco, California

Minako Hayakawa, MD
Assistant Professor
Department of Radiology
University of Iowa
Iowa City, Iowa

Jeremy J. Heit, MD, PhD
Clinical Assistant Professor of Radiology
Stanford University
Stanford, California

Benjamin K. Hendricks, MD
Resident Physician
Division of Neurological Surgery
Barrow Neurological Institute
Phoenix, Arizona

Brian Hoh, MD, FACS, FAHA, FAANS
James and Brigitte Marino Family Professor and Associate
    Chair of Neurosurgery
Chief of Cerebrovascular Surgery
University of Florida
Gainesville, Florida

Pascal Jabbour, MD
Associate Professor
Department of Neurological Surgery
Chief Division of Neurovascular Surgery and Endovascular
    Neurosurgery
Thomas Jefferson University Hospital
Philadelphia, Pennsylvania

M. Yashar S. Kalani, MD, PhD
Assistant Professor of Neurosurgery, Radiology, Anatomy
    and Neurobiology
University of Utah School of Medicine
Salt Lake City, Utah

Louis J. Kim, MD
Professor of Neurological Surgery
Department of Neurological Surgery
University of Washington School of Medicine
Seattle, Washington

Timo Krings, MD, PhD, FRCP(C)
The David Braley and Nancy Gordon Chair in Interventional
    Neuroradiology
Chief of Diagnostic and Interventional Neuroradiology
    at the Toronto Western Hospital & University
    Health Network
Professor, Departments of Radiology and Surgery
University of Toronto
Toronto, Ontario

Giuseppe Lanzino, MD
Professor of Neurosurgery
Department of Neurological Surgery
Mayo Clinic
Rochester, Minnesota

Michael T. Lawton, MD
Professor and Vice-Chairman, Neurological Surgery
Professor, Anesthesia and Perioperative Care
Chief of Vascular Neurosurgery
Tong-Po Kan Endowed Chair
Director Center for Cerebrovascular Research
University of California–San Francisco
San Francisco, California

Cheng-Chia Lee, MD
Neurosurgeon
Taipei Veteran General Hospital
Taipei, Taiwan, ROC

Elad I. Levy, MD, MBA, FACS, FAHA
L. Nelson Hopkins MD Professor of Neurosurgery
Chairman of the Department of Neurosurgery
Professor of Radiology
Jacobs School of Medicine and Biomedical Sciences
University at Buffalo
State University of New York
Buffalo, New York

Adam Liudahl, MD
Instructor
Department of Radiology
University of Iowa
Iowa City, Iowa

Joseph Lockwood, MD, MS
Resident Physician
Department of Neurosurgery
School of Medicine
Tulane University
New Orleans, Louisiana

Demetrius K. Lopes, MD
Professor of Neurosurgery
Section Chief
Cerebrovascular Neurosurgery
Rush University
Chicago, Illinois

L. Dade Lunsford, MD, FACS
Lars Leksell Professor of Neurological Surgery
Distinguished Professor of Neurological Surgery
The University of Pittsburgh
Director, Center for Image Guided Neurosurgery
Director, Neurosurgery Residency Program
Chair, Technology and Innovative Practice Committee
UPMC Presbyterian
Pittsburgh, Pennsylvania

Venkatesh S. Madhugiri, MCh
Assistant Professor of Neurosurgery
Tata Memorial Hospital
Mumbai, India

Cameron G. McDougall, MD
Medical Director
Cerebrovascular Neurosurgery
Swedish Neuroscience Institute
Seattle, Washington

Ricky Medel, MD, FAANS
Co-Director of Cerebrovascular, Endovascular,
    and Skull Base Surgery
Department of Neurological Surgery
Tulane University School of Medicine
New Orleans, Louisiana

Pietro Meneghelli, MD
Attending Neurosurgeon
Institute of Neurosurgery
University Hospital
Verona, Italy

Edward A. Monaco III, MD, PhD
Assistant Professor of Neurological Surgery
Center for Image Guided Neurosurgery
University of Pittsburgh Medical Center
Pittsburgh, Pennsylvania

Ryan P. Morton, MD
Acting Instructor and Endovascular Fellow
Department of Neurological Surgery
University of Washington
Seattle, Washington

Celene B. Mulholland, MD, MPH
Resident
Department of Neurosurgery
Barrow Neurological Institute
Phoenix, Arizona

Stephan Munich, MD
Neurosurgery
Rush University Medical Center
Chicago, Illinois

Peter Nakaji, MD
Professor of Neurosurgery
Director, Neurosurgery Residency Program
Director, Minimally Invasive Neurosurgery
Department of Neurosurgery
Barrow Neurological Institute
Phoenix, Arizona

Ajay Niranjan, MD, MBA
Professor of Neurological Surgery
University of Pittsburgh
Pittsburgh, Pennsylvania

Mohan Narayanan, MD
Neurosurgery Research Fellow
Department of Neurosurgery
Barrow Neurological Institute
Phoenix, Arizona

John D. Nerva, MD
Resident Physician
Department of Neurological Surgery
University of Washington
Seattle, Washington

David H.C. Pan, MD
Director, Functional Neurosurgery
Taipei Veteran General Hospital
Taipei, Taiwan, ROC

Alberto Pasqualin, MD
Section of Vascular Neurosurgery
University and City Hospital
Verona, Italy

Ross Puffer, MD
Neurosurgeon
Department of Neurological Surgery
Mayo Clinic
Rochester, Minnesota

Mark Quigg, MD, MSc, FANA
Professor
Department of Neurology
University of Virginia
Charlottesville, Virginia

Daniel Raper, MBBS
Department of Neurosurgery
University of Virginia
Charlottesville, Virginia

Mateus Reghin Neto, MD
Neurosurgeon
Institute of Neurological Sciences
São Paolo, Brazil

†Albert Rhoton Jr., MD
Professor
Department of Neurosurgery
University of Florida
Gainesville, Florida

Robert H. Rosenwasser, MD, MBA, FACS, FAHA
Jewell L. Osterholm, MD Professor and Chair of Neurological
    Surgery
Professor of Radiology, Neurovascular Surgery,
    Interventional Neuroradiology
President, Vickie and Jack Farber Institute for Neuroscience
Medical Director, Jefferson Neuroscience Network
Thomas Jefferson Hospital
Philadelphia, Pennsylvania

W. Caleb Rutledge, MD
Resident Physician
Department of Neurological Surgery
University of California, San Francisco
San Francisco, California

Francesco Sala, MD
Section of Neurosurgery
Department of Neurological, Biomedical and Movement Sciences
University of Verona
Verona, Italy

David M. Sawyer, BS
Medical Student
Tulane University School of Medicine
New Orleans, Louisiana

Laligam N. Sekhar, MD, FACS, FAANS
Professor and Vice Chairman
Department of Neurological Surgery
University of Washington
Seattle, Washington

Jason P. Sheehan, MD, PhD
Vice Chair and Harrison Distinguished Professor of
    Neurological Surgery
Department of Neurosurgery, Radiation Oncology,
    and Neuroscience
University of Virginia
Charlottesville, Virginia

Amit Singla, MBBS, MS
Neurosurgeon
Covenant Medical Center
Waterloo, Iowa

Lee-Anne Slater, MBBS(Hons), MBBS, FRANZCR
Interventional and Diagnostic Neuroradiologist
Monash Health
Melbourne, Victoria, Australia

Thomas J. Sorenson, BS
Research Fellow
Department of Radiology and Neurosurgery
Mayo Clinic
Rochester, Minnesota

Gary K. Steinberg, MD, PhD
Bernard and Ronni Lacroute-William Randolph Hearst
    Professor of Neurosurgery and the Neurosciences
Chairman
Department of Neurosurgery
Stanford University School of Medicine
Stanford, California

Mario Teo, MBChB(Hons), FRCS (SN)
Consultant Neurosurgeon
Department of Neurosurgery
Bristol Institute of Clinical Neuroscience
Southmead Hospital
Bristol, United Kingdom

Stavropoula I. Tjoumakaris, MD
Associate Professor
Department of Neurological Surgery
Division of Cerebrovascular Surgery and Endovascular
    Neurosurgery
Thomas Jefferson Hospital
Philadelphia, Pennsylvania

Derrick L. Umansky, MD
Resident Physician
Department of Neuroscience
Tulane University
New Orleans, Louisiana

Luca Valvassori, MD
Interventional Neuroradiologist
Ospedale Niguarda
Milano, Italy

Jonathan White, MD
Professor of Neurological Surgery
UT Southwestern Medical Center
Dallas, Texas

Max Wintermark, MD
Chief of Neuroradiology
Stanford University
Stanford, California

Hsiu-Mei Wu, MD
Neuroradiologist
Veteran General Hospital
Taipei, Taiwan, ROC

Vitor Yamaki, MD
Resident Physician
Division of Neurosurgery
University of São Paulo
São Paulo, Brazil

Huai-Che Yang
Neurosurgeon
Veteran General Hospital
Taipei, Taiwan, ROC

1 Cerebrovascular Anatomy and Implications for Arteriovenous Malformation Treatment

W. Caleb Rutledge and Michael T. Lawton

Abstract

Arteriovenous malformations (AVMs) are complex vascular lesions. The Spetzler–Martin system and Lawton–Young supplementary grading scale are used to categorize AVMs and select patients for surgery. However, organizing AVMs into types and subtypes based on their location in the brain, arterial supply, draining veins, and eloquent structures allows for a unique surgical strategy for each AVM. There are seven AVM types based on their location in the brain: frontal AVMs, temporal AVMs, parieto-occipital AVMs, ventricular or periventricular AVMs, and AVMs in the deep central core, brainstem, and cerebellum. Each type comprises four to six subtypes based on their surgical anatomy, allowing for a tailored surgical approach and resection strategy.

Keywords: arteriovenous malformation, Spetzler–Martin, supplementary

- Judicious patient selection is essential to avoid poor outcomes with arteriovenous malformation (AVM) surgery.
- Organizing AVMs into types and subtypes based on their location in the brain, arterial supply, draining veins, and eloquent structures allows for a unique surgical strategy for each AVM.
- There are seven AVM types: frontal AVMs, temporal AVMs, parieto-occipital AVMs, ventricular or periventricular AVMs, and AVMs in the deep central core, brainstem, and cerebellum.
- Each type is further divided into four to six subtypes depending on the brain surface the AVM is based (i.e., lateral, medial, basal) or other specific anatomy (i.e., midbrain, pons, medulla). Each subtype has a unique arterial supply, draining veins, eloquent structures, surgical approaches, and resection strategy.

1.1 Introduction

Brain arteriovenous malformations (AVMs) are complex vascular lesions with varying feeding arteries, draining veins, and niduses distributed throughout the brain. The Spetzler–Martin system and supplementary grading scales have long been used to categorize AVMs, as well as predict outcomes after AVM surgery and guide patient selection for surgery. However, AVM surgery requires a multitude of approaches, tailored to each AVM's unique anatomy. Other than superficial AVMs immediately apparent on the brain's surface, AVMs may require transsylvian, interhemispheric, skull base, or transtorcular approaches. Organization of AVMs into types and subtypes based on surgical anatomy allows for a unique surgical strategy for each AVM.[1]

There are seven AVM types based on their location in the brain: frontal AVMs, temporal AVMs, parieto-occipital AVMs, ventricular or periventricular AVMs, and AVMs in the deep central core, brainstem, and cerebellum. Each type is further divided into four to six subtypes depending on the brain surface the AVM is based (i.e., lateral, medial, basal) or other specific anatomy (i.e., midbrain, pons, medulla). Each subtype has a unique arterial supply, draining veins, eloquent structures, surgical approaches, and resection strategy.

1.2 Frontal Arteriovenous Malformations

The frontal lobe has four surfaces: lateral, medial, basal, and sylvian. Frontal AVMs are supplied by branches from the superior trunk of the middle cerebral artery (MCA), including the orbitofrontal, prefrontal, precentral, and central arteries, as well as branches from the anterior cerebral artery (ACA), including the orbitofrontal, frontopolar, callosomarginal, anterior internal frontal, middle internal frontal, posterior internal frontal, paracentral, and pericallosal arteries. On the lateral and medial convexity, cortical veins ascend to the superior sagittal sinus (SSS). Veins from the sylvian and basal surfaces descend to the inferior sagittal sinus (ISS) and deep sylvian veins that continue to the basal vein of Rosenthal. Eloquent structures in the frontal lobe include the motor strip and Broca's area in the dominant hemisphere.

1.2.1 Subtypes

There are five frontal AVM subtypes: the lateral frontal, medial frontal, paramedian frontal, basal frontal, and sylvian frontal. Lateral frontal AVMs are the most common subtype. These are stereotypical cone-shaped AVMs that extend toward the ventricle (▶ Fig. 1.1a). They are fed by MCA cortical branches ascending from the sylvian fissure to the inferior margin of the AVM. Venous drainage is superficial to the SSS. Lateral frontal AVMs may include eloquent structures such as the motor strip posteriorly and Broca's area in the dominant hemisphere. Lateral frontal AVMs are easily exposed with a unilateral frontal craniotomy.

Medial frontal AVMs are visible only after opening the interhemispheric fissure and may be superficially based in the superior frontal gyrus or deep in the cingulate gyrus (▶ Fig. 1.1b). ACA branches feed medial frontal AVMs. Drainage is usually ascending to the SSS, but large medial frontal AVMs or those in the cingulate gyrus may have descending drainage to the ISS. Medial frontal AVMs may involve the motor strip posteriorly. Unlike lateral frontal AVMs, medial frontal AVMs are more difficult to expose and require a bifrontal craniotomy with opening of the interhemispheric fissure and gravity retraction to expose the medial surface of the frontal lobe.

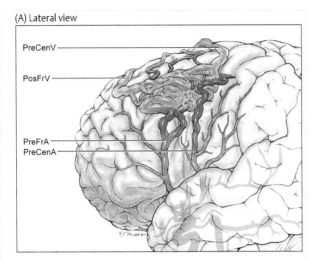

(A) Lateral view

PreCenV
PosFrV
PreFrA
PreCenA

(B) Coronal section

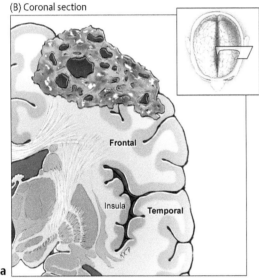

Frontal

Insula   Temporal

a

Fig. 1.1 Frontal lobe AVM subtypes (a) Lateral (A) and coronal (B) views of lateral frontal AVM (*continued*).

Paramedian frontal AVMs are a combination of lateral and medial frontal subtypes and occupy two surfaces of the frontal lobe (▶ Fig. 1.1c). Unlike other frontal subtypes, cortical branches from two arterial territories, the MCA and ACA, supply paramedian AVMs. Venous drainage is to the SSS. Similar to lateral and medial frontal AVMs, paramedian AVMs involve the motor strip when they are posteriorly located. Paramedian AVMs also require a bifrontal craniotomy to expose, but gravity retraction is avoided to preserve access to the lateral convexity.

Basal frontal AVMs are located along the anterior cranial fossa floor in the lateral orbital gyri or medially in the gyrus rectus and olfactory apparatus (▶ Fig. 1.1d). Basal frontal AVMs are fed by MCA branches posterolaterally and ACA branches anteromedially. Venous drainage is usually superficial to the SSS, but may be deep to the basal vein of Rosenthal. Basal frontal AVMs are considered noneloquent, but care should be taken to preserve the olfactory apparatus and its blood supply. Basal frontal AVMs are exposed with an orbital-pterional craniotomy.

Sylvian frontal AVMs are located in the pars orbitalis, pars triangularis, and pars opercularis of the inferior frontal gyrus

and the frontal operculum (▶ Fig. 1.1e). They are supplied by M3 branches rather than cortical MCA branches, and drained by superficial and deep sylvian veins. As they are based in the pars opercularis and pars triangularis comprising Broca's area, sylvian frontal AVMs are highly eloquent. They are exposed with a standard pterional craniotomy.

1.3 Temporal Arteriovenous Malformations

The temporal lobe also has four surfaces: lateral, basal, sylvian, and medial. Blood supply is from proximal M1 branches, the temporopolar and anterior temporal arteries coursing inferiorly to the temporal pole, and branches from the inferior trunk of the MCA, including middle temporal, posterior temporal, temporo-occipital, and angular arteries, descending from the sylvian fissure to the lateral surface of the temporal lobe. Branches from the P2 segment of the posterior cerebral artery (PCA), the hippocampal and posterior temporal arteries, supply the basal surface of the temporal lobe. Finally, the anterior choroidal artery supplies the choroid plexus of the temporal horn of the lateral ventricle. Venous drainage of the temporal lobe is complex, with drainage to the sphenoparietal sinus anteriorly, posteriorly to the vein of Labbé and transverse sinus, medially to the basal vein of Rosenthal and galenic system, and superiorly to sylvian veins and SSS. Eloquent structures in the temporal lobe include Wernicke's area in the dominant hemisphere, Heschl's gyrus, the hippocampus and parahippocampus, and optic radiations.

1.3.1 Subtypes

There are four temporal AVM subtypes: lateral temporal, basal temporal, sylvian temporal, and medial temporal. The lateral temporal subtype is the most common (▶ Fig. 1.2a). Its blood supply is from the inferior trunk of the MCA descending from the sylvian fissure to the superior border of the AVM. Feeders from the temporopolar and anterior temporal arteries may course around the temporal pole to its anterior border, while branches from the PCA occasionally feed posteriorly located lateral temporal AVMs. Drainage is usually superficial to the vein of Labbé and transverse sinus. Lateral temporal AVMs may involve Wernicke's area when they are posteriorly located in the dominant hemisphere. Like lateral frontal AVMs, lateral temporal AVMs are easy to expose using a pterional craniotomy for AVMs in front of the external auditory canal and a temporal craniotomy for those behind the external auditory canal.

Basal temporal AVMs are based in the inferior temporal gyrus, fusiform gyrus, and parahippocampal gyrus (▶ Fig. 1.2b). P2 PCA branches emanating from the crural and ambient cistern supply the AVM's medial border. MCA feeders may descend and wrap around the inferior temporal gyrus to its lateral border. Basal temporal AVMs also often have meningeal feeders from the dura of the middle fossa floor. Drainage is usually superficial, but may be deep to the basal vein of Rosenthal. There are no eloquent structures on the basal temporal surface. A temporal craniotomy is used to expose basal temporal AVMs. They are not visible on the lateral surface and require a subtemporal approach and dissection.

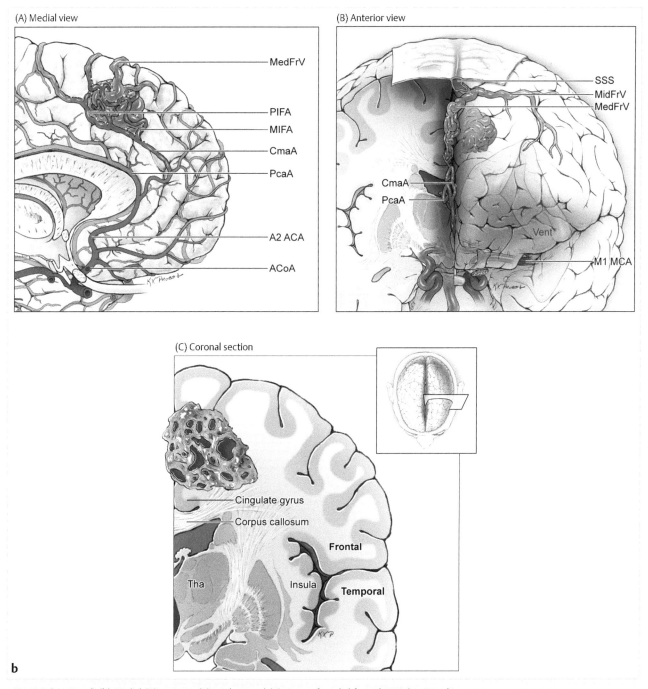

(A) Medial view

MedFrV

PIFA
MIFA
CmaA
PcaA

A2 ACA

ACoA

(B) Anterior view

SSS
MidFrV
MedFrV

CmaA
PcaA

Vent

M1 MCA

(C) Coronal section

Cingulate gyrus
Corpus callosum

Frontal

Tha   Insula   Temporal

b

Fig. 1.1 (*continued*) (**b**) Medial (A), anterior (B), and coronal (C) views of medial frontal AVM (*continued*).

Sylvian AVMs are supplied by MCA M3 opercular branches (▶ Fig. 1.2c). Additionally, the anterior choroidal artery may supply the medial margin. Venous drainage is usually superficial to sylvian veins. Sylvian AVMs may involve Heschl's gyrus or Wernicke's area when they are posteriorly located in the dominant hemisphere. Similar to sylvian frontal AVMs, temporal sylvian AVMs are exposed though a standard pterional craniotomy and transsylvian dissection.

Medial temporal AVMs involve the uncus, parahippocampal gyrus, and hippocampus (▶ Fig. 1.2d). Feeders from the anterior choroidal artery and branches of the P2 PCA supply the medial

and posterior borders. Anteriorly located medial temporal AVMs may have supply from the temporopolar and anterior temporal artery, while posteriorly located ones tend to have PCA supply. Additionally, thalamoperforators from the posterior communicating artery may contribute. Venous drainage is deep to the basal vein of Rosenthal. Medial temporal AVMs are eloquent given they involve the hippocampus and memory function. Exposure of these AVMs is challenging. An orbitozygomatic craniotomy and a deep transsylvian dissection along the anterior choroidal artery are required to mobilize the temporal lobe away from the frontal lobe and afford a limited view at

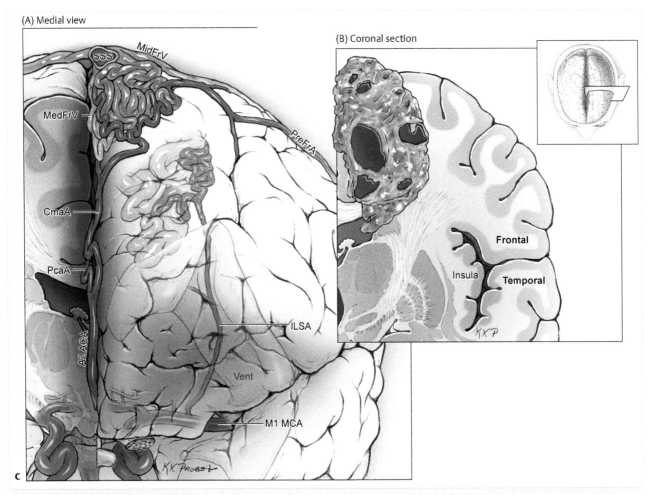

(A) Medial view

(B) Coronal section

Frontal

Insula   Temporal

Fig. 1.1 (*continued*) (**c**) Anterior (A) and coronal (B) views of paramedian frontal AVM (*continued*).

best. More posteriorly located medial temporal AVMs require a transcortical transventricular approach if the transsylvian view is inadequate.

1.4 Parieto-Occipital Arteriovenous Malformations

Unlike the frontal and temporal lobes, the parietal and occipital lobes have only three anatomic surfaces: lateral, medial, and basal. Parieto-occipital AVMs differ from frontal and temporal AVMs in that they have robust arterial supply from multiple territories: distal MCA cortical arteries exiting the sylvian fissure, including the central, anterior parietal, posterior parietal, angular, and temporo-occipital arteries; terminal ACA cortical arteries; the superior and inferior parietal arteries; and finally branches from the PCA, including the posterior temporal artery arising from the P2 PCA, and the calcarine and parieto-occipital divisions of the P3 segment. Venous drainage is from cortical veins, including the vein of Trolard, which ascends to the SSS, but also cortical veins descending to the sylvian fissure, transverse sinus, or vein of Labbé. Eloquent structures in the parieto-occipital lobe include the postcentral gyrus, supramarginal and

angular gyrus in the parietal lobe, and visual cortex at the pole of the occipital lobe.

1.4.1 Subtypes

There are four parieto-occipital subtypes: lateral parieto-occipital, medial parieto-occipital, paramedian, and basal occipital. The lateral parieto-occipital AVM is one of the most common AVMs and often has a cortical base with a tapered extension toward the ventricle (▶ Fig. 1.3a). MCA cortical arteries mainly supply them. Drainage is superficial, ascending to the SSS or descending to sylvian veins. Parieto-occipital AVMs are eloquent when located in the postcentral gyrus, visual cortex, or angular or supramarginal gyrus. They are exposed with a simple convexity craniotomy. There is no need to cross a sinus or expose the interhemispheric fissure or undersurface of the occipital lobe.

Medial parieto-occipital AVMs are based in the posterior interhemispheric fissure and are supplied mainly by PCA branches, but also have an ACA contribution (▶ Fig. 1.3b). Drainage is usually superficial, ascending to the SSS, or less commonly deep, descending to the vein of Galen. Medial parietal AVMs in the somatosensory cortex of the paracentral lobule

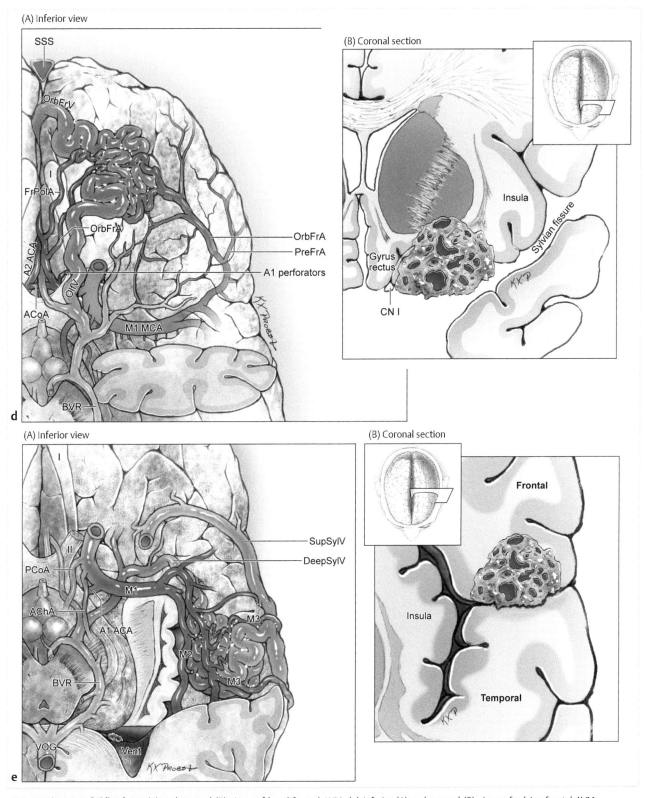

Fig. 1.1 (*continued*) **(d)** Inferior (A) and coronal (B) views of basal frontal AVM. **(e)** Inferior (A) and coronal (B) views of sylvian frontal AVM.

are eloquent, as are medial occipital AVMs around the calcarine fissure in visual cortex. These require a torcular craniotomy over the torcula, SSS, and transverse sinus to open the posterior interhemispheric fissure. The patient should be positioned laterally with the AVM on the down side to allow the occipital pole to fall away from the falx and open the fissure.

Paramedian AVMs are a combination of the medial and lateral subtypes as they reside on both surfaces (► Fig. 1.3c).

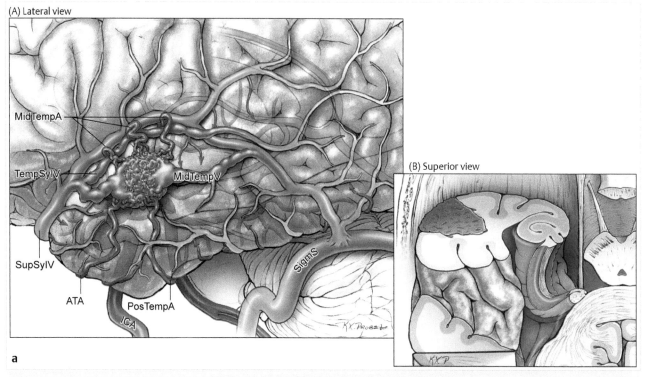

Fig. 1.2 Temporal lobe AVM subtypes. **(a)** Lateral (A) and superior (B) views of lateral temporal AVM (*continued*).

All three cerebral arteries, MCA, ACA, and PCA, supply blood. Venous drainage is predominantly superficial to the SSS. Similar to other parieto-occipital subtypes, paramedian AVMs may be located in somatosensory cortex of the postcentral gyrus or visual cortex. Exposure of both the medial and lateral surfaces of paramedian AVMs requires orienting the midline vertically for both interhemispheric and lateral convexity dissection. A biparietal or biparieto-occipital craniotomy is used for parietal AVMs, while a torcular craniotomy is used for occipital AVMs. In either case, access to the posterior interhemispheric fissure requires crossing the SSS.

Basal occipital AVMs are uncommon (▶ Fig. 1.3d). They reside on the undersurface of the occipital lobe along the tentorium. Their main blood supply is from the PCA and drainage is usually superficial to the transverse sinus. These are highly eloquent AVMs given they involve the occipital cortex and optic radiations. Medial basal occipital AVMs require a torcular craniotomy, while lateral AVMs need only an occipital-suboccipital craniotomy. In both case, the craniotomy crosses the transverse sinus to expose the undersurface of the occipital lobe.

1.5 Ventricular and Periventricular Arteriovenous Malformations

Unlike frontal, temporal, and parieto-occipital AVMs, ventricular and periventricular AVMs are not based on a cortical surface; however, they do have an ependymal surface. Ventricular and periventricular AVMs reside in choroid plexus. They are found in the body, atrium, and temporal horn of the lateral ventricle, but not the frontal and occipital horns, where choroid plexus is absent. Along with the choroid plexus and fornix, the ventricle wraps around the thalamus in a **C** shape. The caudate nucleus forms the lateral wall of the ventricle. The corpus callosum also makes up a large part of the ventricular wall. The anterior choroidal artery, arising from the lateral supraclinoid internal carotid artery, and the medial and lateral posterior choroidal arteries supply the ependyma and choroid plexus of the ventricles. The medial posterior choroidal artery arises from the PCA, usually the proximal P2 postcommunicating segment. The lateral posterior choroidal artery arises from the distal P2 PCA. The ACA and pericallosal artery supply the corpus callosum. Anastomoses connect the ACA and PCA circulations. Ventricular veins are often more obvious and orienting than the arteries during surgery. The septal veins drain the medial frontal horn and course toward the foramen of Monro, where they terminate in the internal cerebral vein (ICV). Caudate veins drain the lateral frontal horn and terminate in the thalamostriate vein near the foramen of Monro, which joins the ICVs. The paired ICVs course in the velum interpositum to the vein of Galen

1.5.1 Subtypes

Ventricular AVMs are deep and require long surgical corridors; however, unlike other deep-seated AVMs, they are floating in cerebrospinal fluid (CSF). There are four ventricular AVM subtypes: callosal, ventricular body, atrial, and temporal horn. Callosal AVMs are located in the roof of the lateral ventricles from the rostrum to splenium. Enlarged feeders from the medial and inferior surface of the ACA and pericallosal artery supply them (▶ Fig. 1.4a). Posteriorly located callosal AVMs in

(A) Inferior view

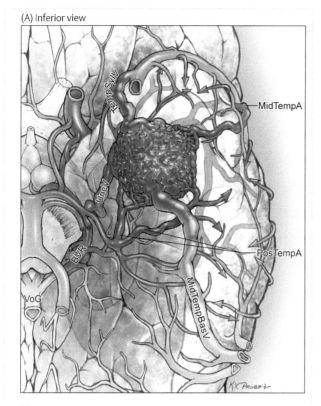

(B) Superior view

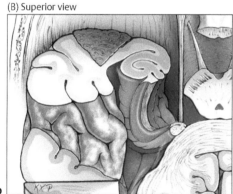

b

Fig. 1.2 (*continued*) **(b)** Inferior (A) and superior (B) views of basal temporal AVM (*continued*).

the splenium are supplied by the splenial artery from the PCA. Lenticulostriates may supply callosal AVMs that extend laterally into the frontal white matter. By definition, callosal AVMs are not in choroid and are not supplied by the choroidal arteries. Venous drainage is deep to the septal, caudate, thalamostriate, ICVs, and vein of Galen. Callosal AVMs are exposed with a bifrontal craniotomy based on the nondominant hemisphere and gravity retraction to open the anterior interhemispheric fissure. The patient is positioned supine with the head turned 90 degrees to the right. This approach preserves bridging veins on the dominant hemisphere. During resection, the pericallosal artery as well as normal branches to the cingulate gyrus and medial frontal lobe must be preserved.

Ventricular body AVMs are midline lesions involving the fornix, septum, velum interpositum, choroid plexus, or third

ventricle (AVMs in the lateral wall are considered in the basal ganglial or thalamic subtypes of deep AVMs, while lesions involving the roof of the ventricle are considered callosal AVMs) (▶ Fig. 1.4b). The medial posterior choroidal is the main arterial feeder. Drainage is to the ICV. The fornix is intimately associated with ventricular body AVMs making them highly eloquent. Ventricular body AVMs are challenging and are accessible only through the corpus callosum and choroidal fissure. Similar to the callosal subtype, ventricular body AVMs are exposed with a bifrontal craniotomy, opening of the anterior interhemispheric, and gravity retraction of the right hemisphere. A right-sided approach is used even for left-sided AVMs to protect the bridging veins of the dominant hemisphere. Division of the corpus callosum accesses the ventricle body. The foramen of Monro is enlarged posteriorly into the velum interpositum exposing the draining ICV as well as the medial posterior choroidal artery. The fornix must be carefully protected during dissection.

Unlike the midline callosal and ventricular body subtypes, atrial AVMs have laterality (▶ Fig. 1.4c). They are located posterior and lateral to the ventricle body. Blood supply is from the lateral posterior choroidal artery, as well as connections from the anterior choroidal artery. They drain to the ICV and basal vein of Rosenthal via the medial and lateral atrial veins. Atrial AVMs are exposed with a parietal craniotomy and transcortical approach through the superior parietal lobule. Opening the choroidal fissure accesses their venous drainage and arterial supply.

Temporal horn AVMs are located in the choroid plexus of the temporal horn of the lateral ventricle (▶ Fig. 1.4d). They differ from medial temporal AVMs in that they are surrounded almost entirely by ependyma. The anterior choroidal artery is the main supply, but the lateral posterior choroidal artery may also contribute. Venous drainage is to the basal vein of Rosenthal. Like medial temporal AVMs, temporal horn AVMs are exposed with a temporal craniotomy and transcortical approach through the inferior temporal gyrus. Like all ventricular AVMs, temporal horn AVMs are not strictly eloquent, but are adjacent to eloquent structures such as the thalamus, caudate, fornix, and hippocampus.

1.6 Deep Arteriovenous Malformations

Unlike ventricular AVMs that float in CSF, deep AVMs are based in parenchyma of the insula and central core of the hemisphere. The insula is composed of anterior and posterior gyri. The central sulcus of the insula separates several short anterior gyri from two posterior long gyri, coursing from the limen insulae. The central core is composed of the basal ganglia, thalamus, fornix, and internal, external, and extreme capsules. Deep AVMs are supplied by the lateral lenticulostriate perforators from the MCA and medial lenticulostriate perforators from the ACA, which pierce the anterior perforated substance on their way to the internal capsule and basal ganglia. Additionally, thalamoperforators from the posterior communicating artery and PCA, as well as peduncular, circumflex perforators, and thalamogeniculate arteries from the P1 and P2 PCA, also supply the central core and deep AVMs. Venous drainage is from anterior and posterior caudate veins and thalamostriate veins on the ventricular

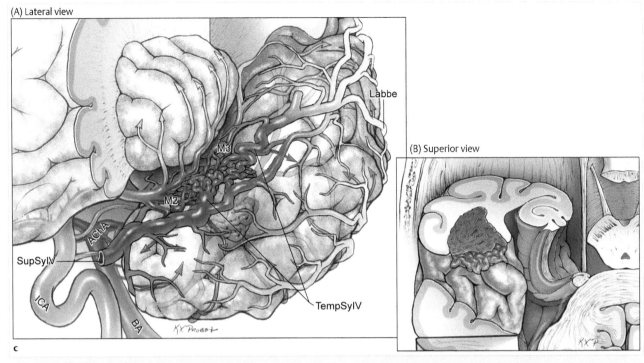

(A) Lateral view

Labbe

(B) Superior view

M3

M2

ACiA

SupSylV

ICA

BA

KX PROBST

TempSylV

c

Fig. 1.2 (*continued*) **(c)** Anterior (A) and superior (B) views of sylvian temporal AVM (*continued*).

surface of the central core, which empties into the deep venous system. The insula is drained by deep sylvian veins, which empty into the basal vein of Rosenthal.

1.6.1 Subtypes

There are four deep AVM subtypes: pure sylvian, insular, basal ganglial, and thalamic AVMs. Pure sylvian AVMs are based almost entirely in the subarachnoid space, and not in the parenchyma of the frontal, temporal, or insular cortex (▶ Fig. 1.5a). They displace the superior temporal gyrus inferiorly and the frontal operculum superiorly. MCA branches from M2 and M3 segments supply them. Venous drainage is to superficial and deep sylvian veins. Because they are based entirely in the subarachnoid space, they are considered noneloquent. Pure sylvian AVMs are exposed with a pterional craniotomy. No parenchymal transgression is needed for dissection.

Insular AVMs are based in the limen insulae, short or long gyri, but remain lateral to the claustrum and basal ganglia (▶ Fig. 1.5b). M2 MCA branches supply them, and venous drainage is to superficial and deep sylvian veins. They are considered noneloquent, although they are often adjacent and deep to Broca's and Wernicke's areas in the frontal and temporal lobes. Insular AVMs are also exposed with a pterional craniotomy and transsylvian approach.

Basal ganglial AVMs are deep to the insular cortex and lateral to the internal capsule, and involve the putamen (▶ Fig. 1.5c), globus pallidus, or caudate nucleus (▶ Fig. 1.5d). Lateral lenticulostriates supply laterally located AVMs, while medially located ones are supplied by the medial lenticulostriates. Venous drainage is to the deep venous system via deep sylvian veins, caudate veins, and thalamostriate veins. Basal ganglia AVMs are highly

eloquent. They can only be reached through a transcortical approach. Those located laterally in the putamen or medial in the caudate are favorable for resection. Lateral basal ganglial AVMs are resected through a pterional craniotomy and transsylvian-transinsular approach, while medial basal ganglia AVMs are resected through a transventricular approach, similar to ventricular body AVMs with a bifrontal craniotomy and contralateral interhemispheric dissection with gravity retraction and transcallosal approach to the ipsilateral ventricle.

The thalamus is encircled by the lateral ventricles and divided by the third ventricle. Anterior thalamoperforators from the posterior communicating artery and posterior thalamoperforators from the P1 PCA, as well as the lateral and medial posterior choroidal arteries, supply thalamic AVMs. Venous drainage is deep. Superiorly located thalamic AVMs (▶ Fig. 1.5e) drain to the ICV, while those on the medial wall drain to the basal vein of Rosenthal (▶ Fig. 1.5f). The ventricles are used to access most thalamic AVM with anterior or posterior transcallosal approaches for AVMs in the superior or posterior thalamus and a transcallosal-transchoroidal for AVMs in the medial thalamus. Transcortical approaches are useful when a hematoma has created a surgical corridor.

1.7 Brainstem Arteriovenous Malformations

The brainstem is composed of the midbrain, pons, and medulla; and the superior, middle, and inferior cerebellar peduncles connect the brainstem and cerebellum. Cerebellomesencephalic, cerebellopontine, and cerebellomedullary fissures divide brainstem and cerebellum. Blood supply is from the superior

(A) Inferior view

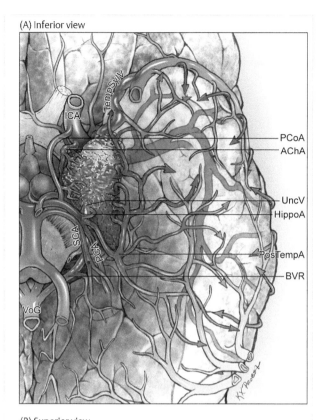

(B) Superior view

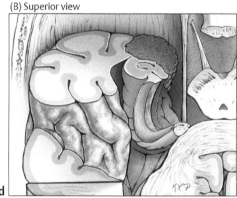

Fig. 1.2 (*continued*) **(d)** Inferior (A) and superior (B) views of medial temporal AVM.

cerebellar artery (SCA), anterior inferior cerebellar artery (AICA), and posterior inferior cerebellar artery (PICA). There are three neurovascular complexes defined by their relationship to brainstem, cranial nerves, peduncles, fissures, and cerebellar arteries. The upper complex includes the midbrain, cranial nerves III, IV, and V, superior cerebellar peduncle, cerebellomesencephalic fissure, and SCA. The middle complex includes the pons, cranial nerves VI, VII, and VIII, middle cerebellar peduncle, cerebellopontine fissure, and AICA. The lower complex includes the medulla, cranial nerves IX, X, XI, and XII, the inferior cerebellar peduncle, cerebellomedullary fissure, and PICA. Brainstem veins include longitudinal and transverse drains that ascend to basal vein of Rosenthal/vein of Galen, course laterally to the superior and inferior petrosal veins and sinuses, and cross subarachnoid spaces to dural sinuses. The

brainstem is made up of cranial nerve nuclei and tracts; thus, all brainstem AVMs are considered eloquent and have deep venous drainage.

1.7.1 Subtypes

There are six brainstem AVM subtypes: anterior midbrain AVM, posterior midbrain AVM, anterior pontine AVM, lateral pontine AVM, anterior medullary AVM, and lateral medullary AVM. The anterior midbrain AVM is in or between the cerebral peduncles and often extends into the interpeduncular cistern (▶ Fig. 1.6a). It is associated with cranial nerve III. Blood supply is from P1 PCA perforators, and venous drainage is to the basal vein of Rosenthal. Surgery for all brainstem AVMs requires avoidance of intraparenchymal transgression. Unruptured brainstems are often occluded with circumferential pial dissection and left in situ rather than resected. Rupture may create a corridor to the nidus and facilitate resection. Preservation of normal perforators is essential. Anterior midbrain AVMs are exposed with an orbitozygomatic-pterional craniotomy and transsylvian approach. The interpeduncular cistern is entered through Liliequist's membrane.

Posterior midbrain AVMs are located in the tectum or quadrigeminal plate and are associated with cranial nerve IV (▶ Fig. 1.6b). Perforators from P1 and P2 PCA, as well as branches from the cerebellomesencephalic segment of SCA, supply them. Venous drainage is to the vein of Galen. They are exposed with a torcular craniotomy and supracerebellar-infratentorial approach. Patients may be positioned sitting or prone.

Anterior pontine AVMs are medial to cranial nerve V roots and often protrude into the prepontine or cerebellopontine cisterns (▶ Fig. 1.6c). They are unilateral and do not cross midline. They are supplied by braches from SCA superiorly and AICA inferiorly, as well as perforators from the basilar artery. Venous drainage is usually to the superior petrosal vein and sinus. Anterior pontine AVMs are exposed through an extended retrosigmoid craniotomy and limited mastoidectomy. Access is limited by cranial nerve V given these AVMs are located anterior to the trigeminal nerve, leaving a supratrigeminal triangle containing descending feeders from the SCA and an infratrigeminal triangle containing ascending feeders from AICA.

Lateral pontine AVMs are located in the cerebellopontine angle (▶ Fig. 1.6d). Unlike anterior pontine AVM, they are located lateral to cranial nerve V roots. Additionally, they are supplied only by AICA, and do not receive input from SCA. The lateral pons is more forgiving of surgical transgression, making lateral pontine AVMs potentially resectable lesions. Like anterior pontine AVMs, they are exposed with an extended retrosigmoid craniotomy. Because they are lateral to cranial nerve V, access is not limited to supra- and infratrigeminal triangles. Unlike other brainstem AVMs, their superior, inferior, and lateral borders are made up of noneloquent cerebellum allowing for parenchymal circumdissection, making it the easiest brainstem AVM to resect.

Anterior medullary AVMs are anterior to the hypoglossal nerve rootlets and posteroinferior to the vertebral basilar junction (▶ Fig. 1.6e). Blood supply is from the vertebral arteries. These AVMs are difficult to access and often resectable only when a hematoma from rupture creates a corridor from the fourth ventricle. In such cases, a suboccipital craniotomy

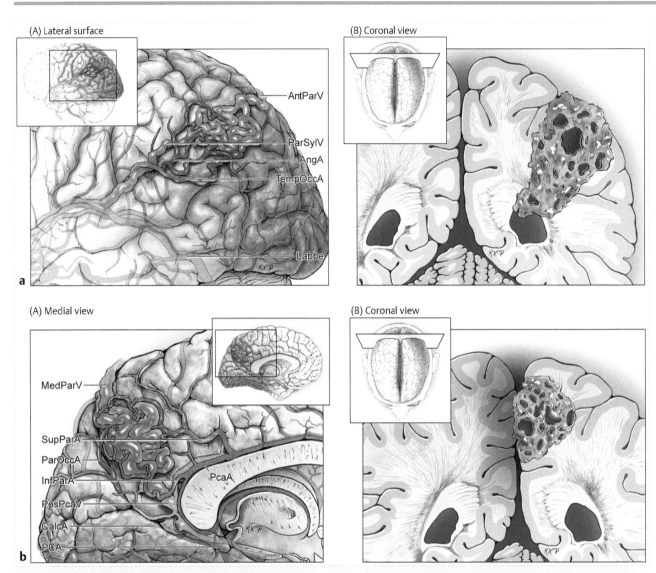

(A) Lateral surface

AntParV

ParSylV

AngA

TempOccA

Labbe

a

(B) Coronal view

(A) Medial view

MedParV

SupParA

ParOccA

InfParA

PcaA

PosPcaV

CalcA

PCA

b

(B) Coronal view

Fig. 1.3 Parieto-occipital lobe AVM subtypes. **(a)** Lateral (A) and coronal (B) views of lateral parieto-occipital AVM. **(b)** Medial (A) and coronal (B) views of medial parieto-occipital AVM (*continued*).

provides access. The hematoma is evacuated through the ventricular floor to access the anterior medulla.

Lateral medullary AVMs are posterior to hypoglossal nerve rootlets (▶ Fig. 1.6f). They are supplied by braches from the vertebral artery and PICA. Lateral medullary AVMs are exposed with a far lateral craniotomy.

1.8 Cerebellar Arteriovenous Malformations

The cerebellum is composed of the midline vermis and two hemispheres. Cerebellar AVMs are supplied by the SCA, AICA, and PICA. The SCA bifurcates into a rostral and caudal trunk in the cerebellomesencephalic fissure. The rostral trunk supplies the superior vermis, while the caudal trunk goes to the hemisphere. These trunks give rise to deep perforating precerebellar arteries that supply deep cerebellar nuclei as well as cerebellar AVMs. AICA courses through the cerebellopontine angle along with cranial nerves VII and VIII, and also bifurcates into rostral

and caudal trunks, supplying the middle cerebellar peduncle and cerebellopontine fissure, flocculus, and choroid plexus. PICA exits the cerebellomedullary fissure, and bifurcates into a trunk that supplies the inferior vermis and adjacent hemisphere and a trunk that supplies the suboccipital surface and tonsils. Superficial and deep cerebellar veins empty into the vein of Galen, torcula or tentorial sinus, and superior and inferior petrosal sinuses. Unless they extend to involve deep cerebellar nuclei, cerebellar AVMs are considered noneloquent.

1.8.1 Subtypes

There are five cerebellar AVM subtypes: suboccipital, tentorial, vermian, tonsillar, and petrosal. Suboccipital AVMs are located on the suboccipital surface below and between the transverse and sigmoid sinuses (▶ Fig. 1.7a). Blood supply is from all three cerebellar arteries (SCA, AICA, and PICA) with superficial venous drainage to the torcula or transverse sinus. Suboccipital AVMs are exposed with a lateral suboccipital craniotomy.

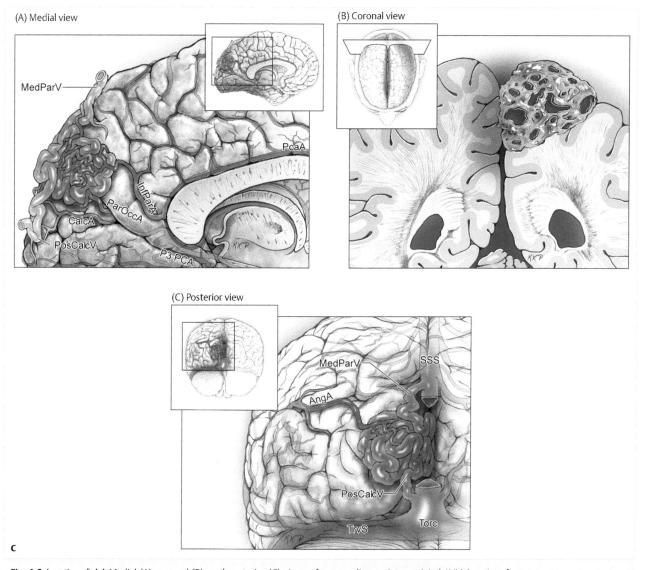

c

Fig. 1.3 (*continued*) **(c)** Medial (A), coronal (B), and posterior (C) views of paramedian parieto-occipital AVM (*continued*).

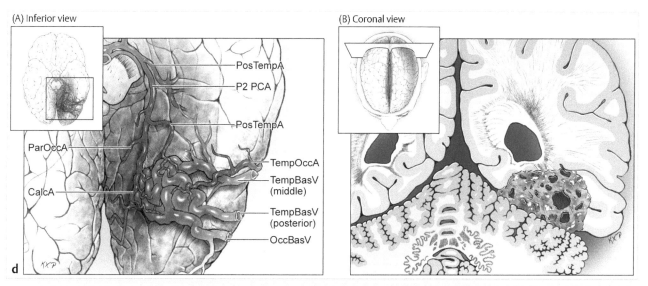

d

Fig. 1.3 (*continued*) **(d)** Inferior (A) and coronal (B) views of basal occipital AVM.

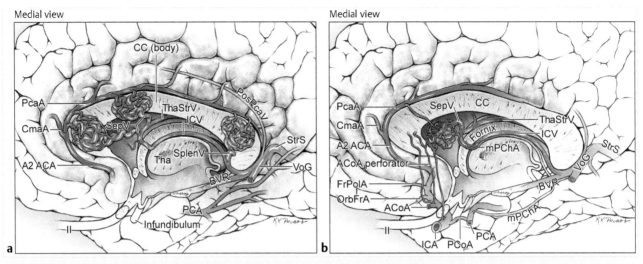

Fig. 1.4 Ventricular and periventricular AVM subtypes. **(a)** Medial view of callosal AVM. **(b)** Medial view of ventricular body AVM (*continued*).

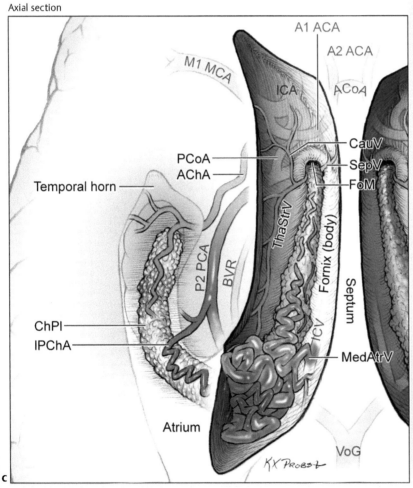

Fig. 1.4 (*continued*) **(c)** Axial view of ventricular atrium AVM (*continued*).

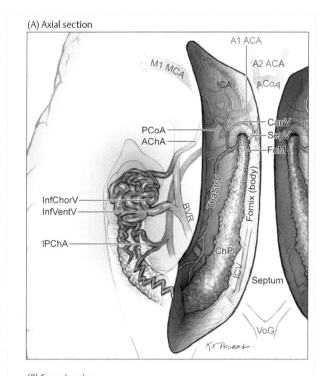

(A) Axial section

(B) Superior view

Fig. 1.4 (*continued*) **(d)** Axial (A) and superior (B) view of temporal horn AVM.

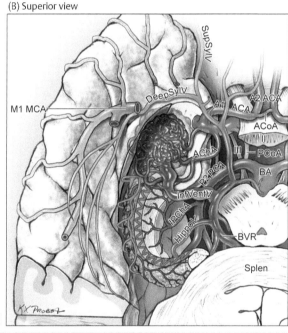

Tentorial AVMs are based on tentorial surface (▶ Fig. 1.7b). They are unilateral with blood supply from branches of SCA and venous drainage to vein of Galen anteriorly, torcula posteriorly, or straight sinus superiorly. Tentorial AVMs are exposed with torcular craniotomies.

Vermian AVMs are midline lesions in the superior or inferior vermis (▶ Fig. 1.7c). Arterial supply is usually bilateral, SCA for superior vermian lesions and PICA for AVMs in the inferior vermis. Superior vermian AVMs have deep venous drainage to vein of Galen, while inferior vermian AVMs drain superficially to the torcula. Like tentorial AVMs, vermian AVMs are also exposed with a torcular craniotomy.

Tonsillar AVMs lie in the cerebellar tonsils (▶ Fig. 1.7d). They are unilateral AVMs supplied by ipsilateral PICA. They are exposed with suboccipital craniotomy.

Petrosal cerebellar AVMs are located on the anterior cerebellum facing the petrous bone (▶ Fig. 1.7e). They are unilateral and supplied by branches from AICA with drainage to superior petrosal vein and sinus. Petrosal AVMs are exposed with an extended retrosigmoid approach and skeletonization of the sigmoid sinus to access the cerebellopontine angle.

1.9 Implications for Treatment

Judicious patient selection is essential to avoid poor outcomes with AVM surgery. The widely used Spetzler–Martin grading system and the newer supplementary system are used to predict surgical risk and select patients for AVM surgery.[2,3,4] Spetzler–Martin includes AVM size, eloquence of surrounding brain, and venous drainage patterns, while the supplementary system incorporates additional factors important to surgical selection and outcome, including patient age, hemorrhagic presentation, and compactness. A patient with a supplemented grade less than or equal to 6 is considered for surgery, while patients with grades greater than 6 are high risk for surgical complications and poor outcomes.

While modern management of AVMs is multimodal, AVM surgery remains the mainstay of treatment, as outcomes in patients with favorable grades are excellent.[5,6] Radiosurgery is a competitive alternative to surgery with excellent results for smaller AVMs, but patients remain at risk for hemorrhage during the latency period. Newer embolic agents and delivery systems have improved obliteration rates with fewer complications, but curative embolization is only in select cases.

AVM surgery follows sequential steps that include exposure, subarachnoid dissection, defining the draining vein, defining the feeding arteries, pial dissection, parenchymal dissection, ependymal or deep dissection, and finally resection. Preservation of the draining vein until the end of the resection is critical to prevent intraoperative rupture. Occluding venous outflow prematurely causes increased intranidal pressure and distension of the malformation resulting in rupture and bleeding in the surgical field. Tamponade and suction are often not effective to control the bleeding and clear the field. Feeding arteries should be disconnected as close as possible to the AVM to prevent sacrifice of normal branches and infarcts in adjacent normal brain. As the AVM is circumferentially dissected and feeding arteries disconnected, the draining vein changes color from red to blue, indicating complete dearterialization of nidus and resectability.

Organizing AVMs into types and subtypes based on surgical anatomy allows for a unique surgical strategy for each AVM. Each subtype has a unique arterial supply, draining veins, eloquent structures, surgical approaches, and resection strategy. This approach allows for safe resection of most AVMs.

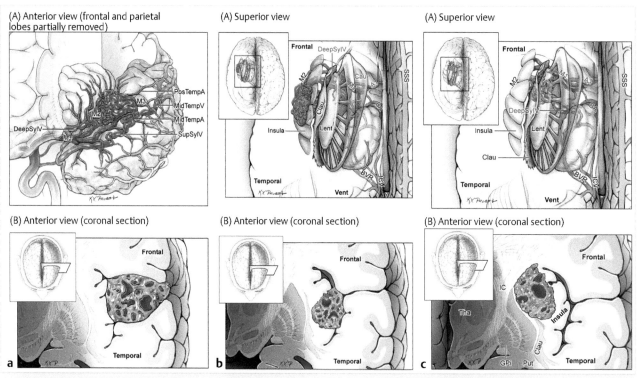

Fig. 1.5 Deep AVM subtypes. **(a)** Anterior (A) and coronal (B) views of pure sylvian AVM. **(b)** Superior (A) and coronal (B) view of insular AVM. **(c)** Superior (A) and coronal (B) views of basal ganglial AVM in putamen *(continued)*.

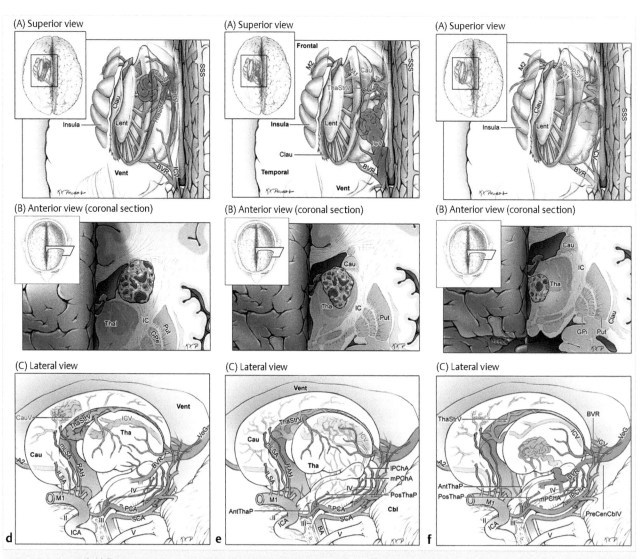

Fig. 1.5 *(continued)* **(d-f)** Superior (A), coronal (B), and lateral (C) views of basal ganglial AVM in caudate nucleus.

14

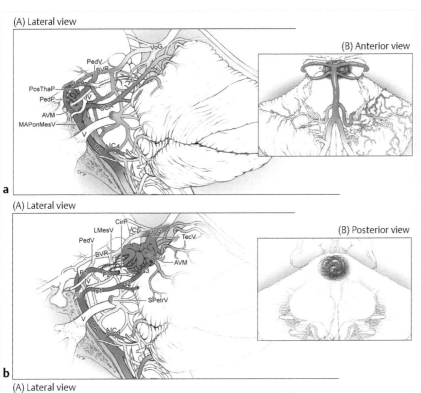

Fig. 1.6 Brainstem AVM subtypes. **(a)** Lateral (A) and anterior (B) views of anterior midbrain AVM. **(b)** Lateral (A) and posterior (B) views of posterior midbrain AVM. **(c)** Lateral (A) and anterior (B) view of anterior pontine AVM (*continued*).

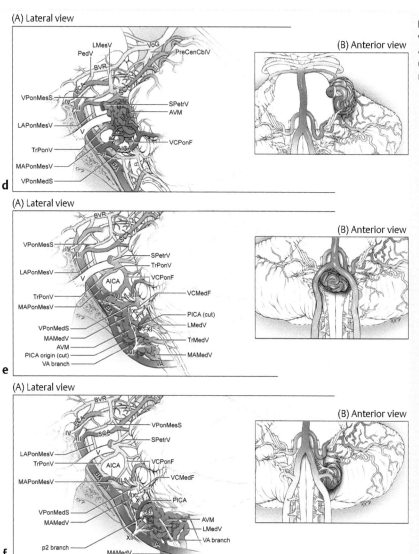

Fig. 1.6 (*continued*) **(d)** Lateral (A) and anterior (B) view of lateral pontine AVM. **(e)** Lateral (A) and anterior (B) views of anterior medullary AVM. **(f)** Lateral (A) and anterior (B) views of lateral medullary AVM.

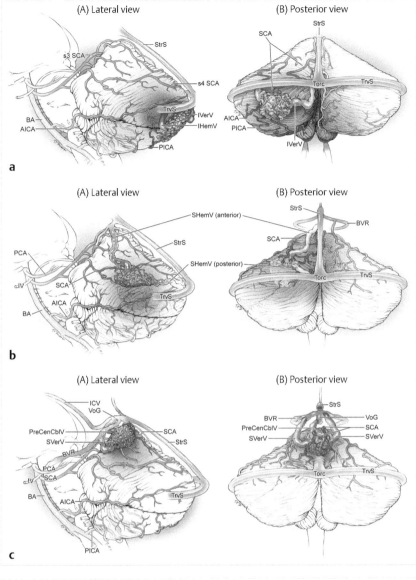

Fig. 1.7 Cerebellar AVM subtypes. **(a)** Lateral (A) and posterior (B) views of suboccipital cerebellar AVM. **(b)** Lateral (A) and posterior (B) views of tentorial cerebellar AVM. **(c)** Lateral (A) and posterior (B) views of vermian AVM (*continued*).

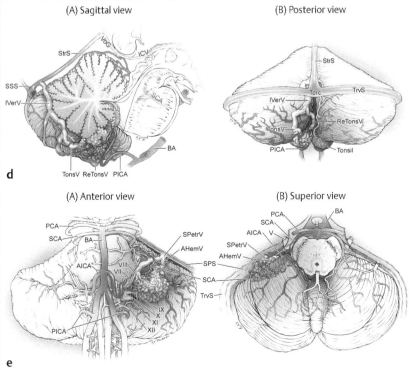

Fig. 1.7 (*continued*) **(d)** Sagittal (A) and posterior (B) views of tonsillar cerebellar AVM. **(e)** Anterior (A) and superior (B) views of petrosal cerebellar AVM.

References

[1] Lawton M. Seven AVMs: Tenets and Techniques for Resection. New York, NY: Thieme; 2014

[2] Spetzler RF, Martin NA. A proposed grading system for arteriovenous malformations. J Neurosurg. 1986; 65(4):476–483

[3] Lawton MT, Kim H, McCulloch CE, Mikhak B, Young WL. A supplementary grading scale for selecting patients with brain arteriovenous malformations for surgery. Neurosurgery. 2010; 66(4):702–713, discussion 713

[4] Kim H, Abla AA, Nelson J, et al. Validation of the supplemented Spetzler-Martin grading system for brain arteriovenous malformations in a multicenter cohort of 1009 surgical patients. Neurosurgery. 2015; 76(1): 25–31, discussion 31–32, quiz 32–33

[5] Potts MB, Lau D, Abla AA, Kim H, Young WL, Lawton MT, UCSF Brain AVM Study Project. Current surgical results with low-grade brain arteriovenous malformations. J Neurosurg. 2015; 122(4):912–920

[6] Davidson AS, Morgan MK. How safe is arteriovenous malformation surgery? A prospective, observational study of surgery as first-line treatment for brain arteriovenous malformations. Neurosurgery. 2010; 66(3):498–504, discussion 504–505

2 Development of the Cerebrovasculature and Pathogenesis of Arteriovenous Malformations and Arteriovenous Fistulas

W. Caleb Rutledge and Tomoki Hashimoto

Abstract

Arteriovenous malformations (AVMs) and arteriovenous fistulas (AVFs) are the most common cerebrovascular malformations (CVMs) and exhibit arteriovenous shunting due to abnormal connections between arteries and veins. Generally, most AVMs and AVFs occur sporadically without a clear genetic basis. Multiple AVMs are often associated with hereditary hemorrhagic telangiectasia and capillary malformation-arteriovenous malformation (CM-AVM) syndrome. The pathogenesis of AVMs and AVFs is not well understood. AVFs are usually acquired from venous hypertension and upregulated angiogenesis, while AVMs are considered congenital malformations, arising from errors during embryogenesis when primitive arteries and veins are in direct communication.

Keywords: vasculogenesis, angiogenesis, arteriovenous malformations (AVMs), arteriovenous fistulas (AVFs)

- Cerebral vascular malformations are classified functionally by the presence or absence of arteriovenous shunting.
- Arteriovenous malformations and arteriovenous fistulas are the most common cerebral vascular malformations.
- Arteriovenous malformations and arteriovenous fistulas are high-flow lesions exhibiting arteriovenous shunting.

2.1 Introduction

Arteries are thick-walled vessels capable of withstanding high pressures as they transport blood and nutrients to organs, while veins have thin walls and transmit lower pressures as they carry blood back to the heart. Arteries and veins are never in direct communication, except in the primitive vascular plexus early in embryogenesis when capillary networks organize and mature, ultimately separating arteries from veins. Arteriovenous malformations (AVMs) and arteriovenous fistulas (AVFs) are both characterized by abnormal arteriovenous connections between arteries and veins. Most AVMs occur sporadically without an identifiable genetic basis. However, multiple AVMs often occur as part of syndromes, such as hereditary hemorrhagic telangiectasia (HHT) and capillary malformation-arteriovenous malformation (CM-AVM) syndrome. These disorders provide insight into the pathogenesis of AVMs.

2.2 Development of the Cerebrovasculature

Development of the cerebrovasculature during embryogenesis involves vasculogenesis and angiogenesis.[1] During vasculogenesis, mesoderm-derived angioblasts differentiate into vascular endothelial cells and form capillarylike tubes. This primitive vascular plexus is remodeled into arteries, capillaries, and veins during angiogenesis by vascular endothelial cell proliferation and migration. Cell signaling and growth factors such as Notch pathway signaling and vascular endothelial growth factor (*VEGF*) are crucial in the development of a functional circulatory system and regulate proliferation and migration of vascular endothelial cells during angiogenesis.

Early in embryonic development, primitive arteries and veins express ephrin-B2 and ephrin-B4, respectively. *VEGF*, neuropilin-1, and Notch pathway signaling maintain arterial patterning. Activation of *VEGF* promotes differentiation of the arterial phenotype during embryogenesis through its receptors, VEGFR1 and VEGFR2. Neuropilin-1 is a *VEGF* co-receptor expressed in arterial endothelial cells and modulates its activity. Activation of *VEGF* induces Notch signaling. Transcription factors FOXC1 and FOXC2 regulate Notch signaling.[2] Notch signaling induces ephrin-B2,[3] and it also represses ephrin-B4 expression in arterial endothelium and maintains the arterial phenotype.[4]

Similarly, cell signaling and growth factors also regulate development of the venous phenotype; however, venous endothelial cells lack neuropilin-1, and Notch signaling is not activated. The retinoic acid-activated receptor COUP-transcription factor 2 (COUP-TF2) represses Notch signaling and promotes expression of ephrin-B4 to establish the venous phenotype.[5] Errors during venous and arterial patterning may result in formation of cerebrovascular malformations (CVMs)

2.3 Cerebrovascular Malformations

CVMs are classified functionally by the presence or absence of arteriovenous shunting. AVMs and AVFs shunt blood from the arterial to the venous circulation, while cavernous malformations, telangiectasias, and developmental venous anomalies are nonshunting. Patients commonly present with hemorrhage from rupture, seizures, or focal neurologic deficits from mass effect.

2.4 Arteriovenous Malformations

An AVM is a tangle of abnormal vessels, including a nidus, dilated feeding arteries, and arterialized draining veins without intervening capillaries, and forms a high-flow, low-resistance shunt. AVMs are the most common symptomatic CVM. A hallmark of hemodynamic feature of AVMs is that AVM niduses are exposed to abnormally high blood flow rates. Lacking capillary beds, AVMs act as arteriovenous shunts in the cerebral circulation. High blood flow rates can trigger vascular remodeling, the process that can further affect local hemodynamics. Presence of arteriovenous shunts in peripheral circulation results in venous hypertension in the downstream and arterial hypotension in the upstream. In patients with large, high-flow arteriovenous shunts, there may be normal brain regions in which arterial pressure is below the range of normal autoregulation. Despite significant cerebral arterial hypotension, the majority of patients are free from ischemic symptoms. Hypotensive normal brain regions can, for the most part, be demonstrated to have relatively normal rates of tissue perfusion, implying some adaptive change in total cerebrovascular resistance.[6,7] Despite their genesis (i.e., acquired or congenital), ongoing vascular remodeling presumably triggered by aberrant local hemodynamic has been considered to be a critical component of their pathophysiology.[8,9,10]

Patients commonly present in the third and fourth decade of life with hemorrhage and headaches, seizures, or focal neurologic deficits from mass effect. The overall incidence of AVMs is about 1 per 100,000 person-years. While the annual risk of hemorrhage is about 1% for unruptured AVMs, ruptured AVMs have a much higher rate of rehemorrhage.

Hemodynamic stress can trigger vascular remodeling and angiogenesis by activating endothelial and inflammatory cells. High shear stress—high blood flow—activates endothelial cells and upregulates leukocyte adhesion molecules including intercellular adhesion molecule-1 (ICAM-1) and chemokines such as monocyte chemotactic protein-1 (MCP-1).[11,12,13,14] These molecules attract circulating neutrophils and monocytes, and facilitate their invasion into the vascular wall. At the same time, shear stress can activate endothelial and smooth muscle cells and promotes their production and release of angiogenic factors and other cytokines that are critical for vascular remodeling.[15,16]

Along with activated endothelial and smooth muscle cells, these inflammatory cells secrete proteinases, including matrix metalloproteinases (MMPs) and elastases.[11] MMPs can destabilize the vascular wall and facilitate vascular remodeling by directly digesting the vascular matrix, activating other proteinases, and releasing angiogenic factors.[17,18] Various MMPs and cytokines can interact with each other to carry out physiological and pathological vascular remodeling. Among MMPs, MMP-9 has been most extensively studied, and appears to be critical for various types of vascular remodeling.[17,19]

There is a growing body of clinical and experimental evidences suggesting that AVMs undergo significant vascular remodeling and angiogenesis in adult life. The variable nature of the clinical course of AVMs, especially with respect to their propensity to growth, regression, and spontaneous hemorrhage, strongly suggests that AVMs represent unstable blood vessels that continuously undergo vascular remodeling. A study that examined interval angiography from a total of 106 patients with mean follow-up periods of 8.4 years showed that over half of the cases increased in size. Approximately one-fifth of the cases decreased in size or vanished,[8] and this suggests most AVMs undergo active remodeling processes.

Histopathological studies presented further evidence to support the notion of active vascular remodeling and angiogenesis in AVMs. Hatva et al examined the endothelial cell proliferation rates in nine adult AVM specimens using the Ki-67 index and compared them to a single control cortical sample from an 11-year-old patient.[20] The Ki-67 index of AVM endothelial cells was higher than the control brain (2.5 vs. 0.5%). A study using a much larger number of specimens (37 AVMs and 5 controls) found approximately a sevenfold increase in nonnesting endothelial cells in AVMs compared to control brain specimens.[8] This finding provided additional histopathological evidence for the presence of active vascular remodeling and angiogenesis in AVMs.

Underlying mechanisms for active vascular remodeling and angiogenesis in AVMs are under vigorous investigation. A number of angiogenic factors have been implicated in their pathophysiology. Concerted effects of key angiogenic factors may be maintaining active vascular remodeling in AVMs.[21]

MMPs, a family of proteolytic enzymes, degrade extracellular matrix proteins, cell surface molecules, and other pericellular substances.[22] By degrading vascular extracellular matrix, MMPs can create a micro-environment that facilitates angiogenesis and vascular remodeling. MMP-9 and MMP-2, having a capability of degrading gelatin, have been extensively studied in physiological and pathological angiogenesis and vascular remodeling. MMP-9, known as gelatinase B, degrades components of vascular extracellular matrices including type IV and V collagen, fibronectin, and elastin.[22] High levels of MMP-9 expression are detected in structurally unstable vasculature including cerebral aneurysms,[23,24] abdominal aortic aneurysms,[25,26,27] and atherosclerotic carotid artery.[28] Excessive degradation of the vascular matrix may contribute to the destabilization of vessels, leading to the weakening of the vessel wall and to vessel rupture.[29]

An abnormal expression pattern of MMP-9 and TIMPs (tissue inhibitors of metalloproteinases) has been observed in AVMs.[30] There is markedly increased MMP-9 activity in AVMs compared with control brain samples. MMP-9 is expressed in the endothelial cell/periendothelial cell layer of AVMs. Along with endothelial and smooth muscle cells, inflammatory cells seem to be a major contributor to the abnormally high levels of MMP-9 in AVM tissue.[31] The increased MMP-9 activity can be expected to cause degradation of the vascular matrix, impairing structural stability of AVM vessels. Interestingly, higher levels of MMP-9 were associated with clinical characteristics that were linked to AVM hemorrhage.[30]

There is an increasing interest in utilizing MMP inhibitors to treat vascular diseases including abdominal aortic aneurysms. It has been proposed that pharmacological inhibition of MMPs may stabilize the unstable blood vessels and prevent their rupture.[32] In patients with abdominal aortic aneurysm, treatment with doxycycline, a nonspecific MMP inhibitor, for 1 week prior to the repair surgery resulted in decreased MMP-9 and MMP-2 in the wall of the aneurysms.[27] Similar results have been reported in patients with atherosclerotic carotid plaques who received doxycycline for 2 to 8 weeks.[33] Doxycycline can inhibit MMP-9 activity in mouse brain, which is hyperstimulated with adenovirally transduced VEGF, an animal model developed in Core C.[34] Because MMP-9 appears highly expressed in the nidal vessels, this protease or related ones may serve as potential pharmacological targets to modify clinical behavior of AVMs. A small pilot clinical study demonstrated the feasibility for inhibiting MMP-9 by oral doxycycline in AVM patients.[35] Doxycycline or other tetracycline derivatives can be an attracting choice for clinical use because of their long safety record. However, they are not specific inhibitors of MMPs, and they exert cellular effects that are not related to MMP inhibition.

Vascular endothelial cell growth factor-A (VEGF-A) is a potent endothelial cell mitogen and morphogen, which drives vascular remodeling and angiogenesis in a wide variety of tissues and lesions. There are a number of observational studies that showed increased expression of VEGF in AVMs at both protein and mRNA levels.[21,36,37,38,39] These reports showed increased VEGF expression in the vascular wall of AVMs, suggesting increased endothelial mitogenic activity in AVMs that can maintain a higher angiogenic activity. Increased expression of VEGF seems to be associated with clinical behavior (i.e., recurrence) of AVMs. Interestingly, a higher degree of astrocytic VEGF expression was associated with recurrence of AVMs after initial resection in small case series.[40,41] Along with other angiogenic factors, abnormally high levels of VEGF may be critical for maintaining active vascular remodeling and angiogenesis in AVMs.

Angiopoietins (Ang) and their receptor, Tie2, play a critical role in regulating vascular stability.[42,43,44,45,46] Ang1, an agonist for the Tie2 receptor, promotes interaction between endothelial cells (ECs) and peri-EC support cells to stabilize vessels.[42,43] When expression of Ang-2 (antagonist) blocks the Ang-1 signal, vascular *deconstruction* ensues, e.g., loosening of the tight complex of endothelial support cells. The presence of VEGF appears to influence Ang-2 actions. If VEGF is present, the proangiogenic state is enhanced. In the absence of VEGF, however, vessels undergo involution and regression.[47]

There is an abnormal balance in the angiopoietin-Tie2 system in AVMs. In AVM tissues, Ang2 (antagonist) is markedly increased and Ang1 (agonist) is decreased.[48] In addition, AVM tissues showed markedly decreased Tie-2 expression at both mRNA and protein levels.[37,49] These findings were confirmed by another independent study using the gene microarray technique.[50] Another study using immunohistochemistry showed a similar result showing Tie-2 expression only in 2 out of 185 blood vessels from AVMs.[51]

The abnormal imbalance in angiopoietins in AVMs— decreased levels of Ang-1 along with increased levels of Ang-2 —would be expected to result in an overall decrease in Tie-2 signaling, thus leading to vascular instability. Furthermore, decreased levels of Tie-2 will further impair vascular stability in AVMs. Interestingly, there is a positive correlation between VEGF and Ang-2 levels in AVM tissues, indicating potential synergistic effects of VEGF and Ang-2 to cause vascular instability, which can result in active vascular remodeling or, in some cases, spontaneous hemorrhage.[21]

Active angiogenesis and vascular remodeling are controlled by orchestration of a number of angiogenesis-related factors.[47,52] Concerted effects of key angiogenic factors may be maintaining the angiogenic phenotype of AVMs, and thereby determining clinical course. For example, in addition to serving as a major proteolytic factor during angiogenesis, MMP-9 can initiate and sustain angiogenesis during carcinogenesis by increasing bioavailability of VEGF.[18] Angiopoietin-2 appears to increase MMP-9 expression in the presence of VEGF.[53] Increased expression of angiopoietin-2 and VEGF in AVMs may be contributing to increased MMP-9 activity, and an intricate balance among these factors may be determining an angiogenic potential of AVMs.

There have been two studies that analyzed gene expression profile of AVM samples using the gene microarray technique. Shenkar et al compared gene expression profile of AVMs with superficial temporal artery samples.[50] They found a number of genes related to angiogenesis and structural components of the vascular wall to be differentially expressed between AVMs and superficial temporal arteries. Another study compared gene expression profile between AVM and control brain samples, and confirmed main findings from the gene microarray by performing western blot and immunohistochemistry.[37] From 12,625 gene probes assayed, 1,781 gene probes showed differential expression between AVMs and controls. AVM samples had a gene expression pattern that was distinct from those of control brain samples. Although these studies were still preliminary, they clearly showed that AVM tissues present gene expression profiles that are consistent with active vascular remodeling and angiogenesis.

HHT is an autosomal dominant disorder characterized by mucocutaneous telangiectasias and AVMs of major organs, predominantly the liver, lung, and brain.[2] Patients commonly present with epistaxis from rupture of telangiectasias of the nasal mucosa, but hemorrhage of brain AVMs is an important cause of premature morbidity and mortality. HHT is caused by mutations in genes of the transforming growth factor-β (*TGF-β*) family. Mutations in genes encoding endoglin (*ENG*), a *TGF-β* co-receptor, causes HHT type 1. HHT type 2 is caused by mutations in a gene encoding activin receptorlike kinase 1 (*ALK1*), a *TGF-β* receptor that interacts with *ENG*. Polymorphisms in these genes have also been linked to sporadic AVMs.[54] Mutation in *SMAD4*, yet another member of the *TGF-β* signaling pathway, is also associated with HHT.[55]

ENG and *ALK1* are expressed in primitive vascular endothelium and are essential for vascular development during embryogenesis. *ENG* and *ALK1* knockout models form a primitive vascular plexus, but vascular remodeling is impaired. Deletion of both copies of either *ENG* or *ALK1* in mice models results is lethal in the embryo[56,57]; however, deficiency or tissue specific deletion results in thin-walled dilated vascular lesions and spontaneous hemorrhage, particularly when angiogenesis is stimulated by *VEGF* in response to injury.[58,59,60,61] In HHT, tissues most prone to damage and repair, the face, hands, and mucosa of the lips and nasal passages, are most prone to developing telangiectasias, suggesting inflammation and angiogenesis in addition to a genetic predisposition important in AVM pathogenesis.

CM-AVM syndrome is also characterized by brain AVMs and is caused by missense mutations in *RASA1* resulting in increased RAS activity.[62,63]

Candidate gene and genome-wide associations studies have identified polymorphisms associated with the more common, sporadically occurring AVMs. While mutation in *ALK1* causes HHT2, a common *ALK1* polymorphism is also associated with sporadic AVMs.[64] Polymorphisms in integrin β8 (*ITGB8*), interleukin-1β (*IL1B*), angiopoietinlike 4 (*ANGPTL4*), G-protein-coupled receptor 124 (*GPR124*), *VEGF63*, and matrix metallopeptidase 3 (*MMP3*) are also associated with sporadic, but not familial, AVMs.[65,66,67,68,69,70] While the molecular function of these polymorphisms is unknown, they may be used as risk predictors. Alterations in genes involved in arterial and venous patterning during embryogenesis, such as *EPHB4*, as well as inflammation and angiogenesis, including interleukin-6 (*IL6*), *IL1B60*, and apolipoprotein E (*APOE*), are associated with AVM hemorrhage.[71,72,73,74]

2.5 Arteriovenous Fistulas

AVFs are much less common than AVMs, but also cause premature morbidity and mortality due to intracranial hemorrhage. Like AVMs, there is an abnormal connection between arteries and veins without an intervening capillary bed, but AVFs lack a true nidus. Feeding arteries are derived from either pia or more commonly dura and shunt blood to small venules within a dural sinus. AVFs are further classified according to pattern of venous drainage using the Cognard and Borden classifications.[75,76] They may involve all of the venous sinuses, including the transverse, sigmoid, cavernous, and superior sagittal sinuses, but the most common site is the transverse sigmoid sinus junction in the skull base. Most have a benign clinical course, but patients may present with hemorrhage, a bruit, tinnitus, pulsatile proptosis, seizures, or focal neurologic deficits.

Although their pathogenesis is also not well understood, unlike AVMs, AVFs are usually acquired.[77,78] They are hypothesized to arise from upregulated angiogenesis,[10] usually in the setting of venous sinus thrombosis and venous hypertension.[79] Surgically inducing venous hypertension in rats by common carotid artery and external jugular vein anastomosis and embolization of the dural sinuses reliably induces AVF formation.[80,81] Many studies have since shown high expression of angiogenic factors, including hypoxia-inducible factor-1 (*HIF-1*) and *VEGF*, in both venous hypertensive rat models and clinical specimens from patients with AVFs, suggesting angiogenic factors mediate formation of venous hypertension induced AVFs.[9,82,83]

2.6 Conclusion

AVMs and AVFs are the most common CVMs exhibiting arteriovenous shunting. AVMs and AVFs are characterized by abnormal connections between arteries and veins. While their pathogenesis is not well understood, AVMs are often considered congenital lesions. Although most AVMs occur sporadically without a clear genetic basis, multiple AVMs occurring in HHT and CM-AVM syndrome provide some insight into their pathogenesis. Alterations in genes involved in arterial and venous patterning during development, as well as inflammation and angiogenesis, are associated with sporadic AVMs. While genetic factors may render individuals susceptible to formation of AVMs, inflammation and angiogenesis in response to injury likely influence their pathogenesis. Unlike AVMs, AVFs are acquired in response to venous hypertension and upregulated angiogenesis.

References

[1] Risau W. Mechanisms of angiogenesis. Nature. 1997; 386(6626):671–674

[2] Hayashi H, Kume T. Foxc transcription factors directly regulate Dll4 and Hey2 expression by interacting with the VEGF-Notch signaling pathways in endothelial cells. PLoS One. 2008; 3(6):e2401

[3] Gerety SS, Anderson DJ. Cardiovascular ephrinB2 function is essential for embryonic angiogenesis. Development. 2002; 129(6):1397–1410

[4] Kume T. Specification of arterial, venous, and lymphatic endothelial cells during embryonic development. Histol Histopathol. 2010; 25(5):637–646

[5] You LR, Lin FJ, Lee CT, DeMayo FJ, Tsai MJ, Tsai SY. Suppression of Notch signalling by the COUP-TFII transcription factor regulates vein identity. Nature. 2005; 435(7038):98–104

[6] Young WL, Kader A, Ornstein E, et al. The Columbia University Arteriovenous Malformation Study Project. Cerebral hyperemia after arteriovenous malformation resection is related to "breakthrough" complications but not to feeding artery pressure. Neurosurgery. 1996; 38(6):1085–1093, discussion 1093–1095

[7] Hacein-Bey L, Nour R, Pile-Spellman J, Van Heertum R, Esser PD, Young WL. Adaptive changes of autoregulation in chronic cerebral hypotension with arteriovenous malformations: an acetazolamide-enhanced single-photon emission CT study. AJNR Am J Neuroradiol. 1995; 16(9):1865–1874

[8] Hashimoto T, Mesa-Tejada R, Quick CM, et al. Evidence of increased endothelial cell turnover in brain arteriovenous malformations. Neurosurgery. 2001; 49(1):124–131, discussion 131–132

[9] Uranishi R, Nakase H, Sakaki T. Expression of angiogenic growth factors in dural arteriovenous fistula. J Neurosurg. 1999; 91(5):781–786

[10] Lawton MT, Jacobowitz R, Spetzler RF. Redefined role of angiogenesis in the pathogenesis of dural arteriovenous malformations. J Neurosurg. 1997; 87 (2):267–274

[11] Hoefer IE, van Royen N, Rectenwald JE, et al. Arteriogenesis proceeds via ICAM-1/Mac-1- mediated mechanisms. Circ Res. 2004; 94(9):1179–1185

[12] Tzima E, del Pozo MA, Shattil SJ, Chien S, Schwartz MA. Activation of integrins in endothelial cells by fluid shear stress mediates Rho-dependent cytoskeletal alignment. EMBO J. 2001; 20(17):4639–4647

[13] Shyy JY, Chien S. Role of integrins in cellular responses to mechanical stress and adhesion. Curr Opin Cell Biol. 1997; 9(5):707–713

[14] Shyy YJ, Hsieh HJ, Usami S, Chien S. Fluid shear stress induces a biphasic response of human monocyte chemotactic protein 1 gene expression in vascular endothelium. Proc Natl Acad Sci U S A. 1994; 91(11):4678–4682

[15] Chien S, Li S, Shyy YJ. Effects of mechanical forces on signal transduction and gene expression in endothelial cells. Hypertension. 1998; 31(1, Pt 2): 162–169

[16] Malek AM, Gibbons GH, Dzau VJ, Izumo S. Fluid shear stress differentially modulates expression of genes encoding basic fibroblast growth factor and platelet-derived growth factor B chain in vascular endothelium. J Clin Invest. 1993; 92(4):2013–2021

[17] Tronc F, Mallat Z, Lehoux S, Wassef M, Esposito B, Tedgui A. Role of matrix metalloproteinases in blood flow-induced arterial enlargement: interaction with NO. Arterioscler Thromb Vasc Biol. 2000; 20(12):E120–E126

[18] Bergers G, Brekken R, McMahon G, et al. Matrix metalloproteinase-9 triggers the angiogenic switch during carcinogenesis. Nat Cell Biol. 2000; 2(10):737–744

[19] Tronc F, Wassef M, Esposito B, Henrion D, Glagov S, Tedgui A. Role of NO in flow-induced remodeling of the rabbit common carotid artery. Arterioscler Thromb Vasc Biol. 1996; 16(10):1256–1262

[20] Hatva E, Jääskeläinen J, Hirvonen H, Alitalo K, Haltia M. Tie endothelial cell-specific receptor tyrosine kinase is upregulated in the vasculature of arteriovenous malformations. J Neuropathol Exp Neurol. 1996; 55(11):1124–1133

[21] Hashimoto T, Wu Y, Lawton MT, Yang GY, Barbaro NM, Young WL. Coexpression of angiogenic factors in brain arteriovenous malformations. Neurosurgery. 2005; 56(5):1058–1065, discussion 1058–1065

[22] Sternlicht M, Bergers G. Matrix metalloproteinases as emerging targets in anticancer therapy: status and prospects. Emerg Ther Targets. 2000; 4(5): 609–633

[23] Gaetani P, Rodriguez y Baena R, Tartara F, et al. Metalloproteases and intracranial vascular lesions. Neurol Res. 1999; 21(4):385–390

[24] Todor DR, Lewis I, Bruno G, Chyatte D. Identification of a serum gelatinase associated with the occurrence of cerebral aneurysms as pro-matrix metalloproteinase-2. Stroke. 1998; 29(8):1580–1583

[25] Knox JB, Sukhova GK, Whittemore AD, Libby P. Evidence for altered balance between matrix metalloproteinases and their inhibitors in human aortic diseases. Circulation. 1997; 95(1):205–212

[26] Goodall S, Crowther M, Hemingway DM, Bell PR, Thompson MM. Ubiquitous elevation of matrix metalloproteinase-2 expression in the vasculature of patients with abdominal aneurysms. Circulation. 2001; 104(3):304–309

[27] Curci JA, Mao D, Bohner DG, et al. Preoperative treatment with doxycycline reduces aortic wall expression and activation of matrix metalloproteinases in patients with abdominal aortic aneurysms. J Vasc Surg. 2000; 31(2):325–342

[28] Loftus IM, Naylor AR, Goodall S, et al. Increased matrix metalloproteinase-9 activity in unstable carotid plaques. A potential role in acute plaque disruption. Stroke. 2000; 31(1):40–47

[29] Chyatte D, Lewis I. Gelatinase activity and the occurrence of cerebral aneurysms. Stroke. 1997; 28(4):799–804

[30] Hashimoto T, Wen G, Lawton MT, et al. University of California, San Francisco BAVM Study Group. Abnormal expression of matrix metalloproteinases and tissue inhibitors of metalloproteinases in brain arteriovenous malformations. Stroke. 2003; 34(4):925–931

[31] Chen Y, Fan Y, Poon KYT, et al. MMP-9 expression is associated with leukocytic but not endothelial markers in brain arteriovenous malformations. Front Biosci. 2006; 11:3121–3128

[32] Rosenberg GA. Growth and bleeding in BAVM: another role for MMPs. Stroke. 2003; 34(4):925–931

[33] Axisa B, Loftus IM, Naylor AR, et al. Prospective, randomized, double-blind trial investigating the effect of doxycycline on matrix metalloproteinase expression within atherosclerotic carotid plaques. Stroke. 2002; 33(12):2858–2864

[34] Lee CZ, Xu B, Hashimoto T, McCulloch CE, Yang GY, Young WL. Doxycycline suppresses cerebral matrix metalloproteinase-9 and angiogenesis induced by focal hyperstimulation of vascular endothelial growth factor in a mouse model. Stroke. 2004; 35(7):1715–1719

[35] Hashimoto T, Matsumoto MM, Li JF, Lawton MT, Young WL, University of California, San Francisco, BAVM Study Group. Suppression of MMP-9 by doxycycline in brain arteriovenous malformations. BMC Neurol. 2005; 5(1):1

[36] Hashimoto T, Young WL. Roles of Angiogenesis and Vascular Remodeling in Brain Vascular Malformations. Seminars in Cerebrovascular Diseases and Stroke.. 2004; 4(4):217–225

[37] Hashimoto T, Lawton MT, Wen G, et al. Gene microarray analysis of human brain arteriovenous malformations. Neurosurgery. 2004; 54(2):410–423, discussion 423–425

[38] Rothbart D, Awad IA, Lee J, Kim J, Harbaugh R, Criscuolo GR. Expression of angiogenic factors and structural proteins in central nervous system vascular malformations. Neurosurgery. 1996; 38(5):915–924, discussion 924–925

[39] Kiliç T, Pamir MN, Küllü S, Eren F, Ozek MM, Black PM. Expression of structural proteins and angiogenic factors in cerebrovascular anomalies. Neurosurgery. 2000; 46(5):1179–1191, discussion 1191–1192

[40] Kader A, Goodrich JT, Sonstein WJ, Stein BM, Carmel PW, Michelsen WJ. Recurrent cerebral arteriovenous malformations after negative postoperative angiograms. J Neurosurg. 1996; 85(1):14–18

[41] Sonstein WJ, Kader A, Michelsen WJ, Llena JF, Hirano A, Casper D. Expression of vascular endothelial growth factor in pediatric and adult cerebral arteriovenous malformations: an immunocytochemical study. J Neurosurg. 1996; 85(5):838–845

[42] Suri C, Jones PF, Patan S, et al. Requisite role of angiopoietin-1, a ligand for the TIE2 receptor, during embryonic angiogenesis. Cell. 1996; 87(7):1171–1180

[43] Davis S, Aldrich TH, Jones PF, et al. Isolation of angiopoietin-1, a ligand for the TIE2 receptor, by secretion-trap expression cloning. Cell. 1996; 87(7):1161–1169

[44] Maisonpierre PC, Suri C, Jones PF, et al. Angiopoietin-2, a natural antagonist for Tie2 that disrupts in vivo angiogenesis. Science. 1997; 277(5322):55–60

[45] Dumont DJ, Gradwohl G, Fong G-H, et al. Dominant-negative and targeted null mutations in the endothelial receptor tyrosine kinase, tek, reveal a critical role in vasculogenesis of the embryo. Genes Dev. 1994; 8(16):1897–1909

[46] Sato TN, Tozawa Y, Deutsch U, et al. Distinct roles of the receptor tyrosine kinases Tie-1 and Tie-2 in blood vessel formation. Nature. 1995; 376(6535):70–74

[47] Hanahan D. Signaling vascular morphogenesis and maintenance. Science. 1997; 277(5322):48–50

[48] Hashimoto T, Lam T, Boudreau NJ, Bollen AW, Lawton MT, Young WL. Abnormal balance in the angiopoietin-tie2 system in human brain arteriovenous malformations. Circ Res. 2001; 89(2):111–113

[49] Hashimoto T, Emala CW, Joshi S, et al. Abnormal pattern of Tie-2 and vascular endothelial growth factor receptor expression in human cerebral arteriovenous malformations. Neurosurgery. 2000; 47(4):910–918, discussion 918–919

[50] Shenkar R, Elliott JP, Diener K, et al. Differential gene expression in human cerebrovascular malformations. Neurosurgery. 2003; 52(2):465–477, discussion 477–478

[51] Uranishi R, Baev NI, Ng PY, Kim JH, Awad IA. Expression of endothelial cell angiogenesis receptors in human cerebrovascular malformations. Neurosurgery. 2001; 48(2):359–367, discussion 367–368

[52] Bergers G, Benjamin LE. Tumorigenesis and the angiogenic switch. Nat Rev Cancer. 2003; 3(6):401–410

[53] Etoh T, Inoue H, Tanaka S, Barnard GF, Kitano S, Mori M. Angiopoietin-2 is related to tumor angiogenesis in gastric carcinoma: possible in vivo regulation via induction of proteases. Cancer Res. 2001; 61(5):2145–2153

[54] Xia C, Zhang R, Mao Y, Zhou L. Pediatric cavernous malformation in the central nervous system: report of 66 cases. Pediatr Neurosurg. 2009; 45(2):105–113

[55] Gallione CJ, Richards JA, Letteboer TG, et al. SMAD4 mutations found in unselected HHT patients. J Med Genet. 2006; 43(10):793–797

[56] Li DY, Sorensen LK, Brooke BS, et al. Defective angiogenesis in mice lacking endoglin. Science. 1999; 284(5419):1534–1537

[57] Urness LD, Sorensen LK, Li DY. Arteriovenous malformations in mice lacking activin receptor-like kinase-1. Nat Genet. 2000; 26(3):328–331

[58] Park SO, Lee YJ, Seki T, et al. ALK5- and TGFBR2-independent role of ALK1 in the pathogenesis of hereditary hemorrhagic telangiectasia type 2. Blood. 2008; 111(2):633–642

[59] Torsney E, Charlton R, Diamond AG, Burn J, Soames JV, Arthur HM. Mouse model for hereditary hemorrhagic telangiectasia has a generalized vascular abnormality. Circulation. 2003; 107(12):1653–1657

[60] Srinivasan S, Hanes MA, Dickens T, et al. A mouse model for hereditary hemorrhagic telangiectasia (HHT) type 2. Hum Mol Genet. 2003; 12(5):473–482

[61] Satomi J, Mount RJ, Toporsian M, et al. Cerebral vascular abnormalities in a murine model of hereditary hemorrhagic telangiectasia. Stroke. 2003; 34(3):783–789

[62] Eerola I, Boon LM, Mulliken JB, et al. Capillary malformation-arteriovenous malformation, a new clinical and genetic disorder caused by RASA1 mutations. Am J Hum Genet. 2003; 73(6):1240–1249

[63] Revencu N, Boon LM, Mendola A, et al. RASA1 mutations and associated phenotypes in 68 families with capillary malformation-arteriovenous malformation. Hum Mutat. 2013; 34(12):1632–1641

[64] Pawlikowska L, Tran MN, Achrol AS, et al. UCSF BAVM Study Project. Polymorphisms in transforming growth factor-beta-related genes ALK1 and ENG are associated with sporadic brain arteriovenous malformations. Stroke. 2005; 36(10):2278–2280

[65] Su H, Kim H, Pawlikowska L, et al. Reduced expression of integrin alphavbeta8 is associated with brain arteriovenous malformation pathogenesis. Am J Pathol. 2010; 176(2):1018–1027

[66] Kim H, Hysi PG, Pawlikowska L, et al. Common variants in interleukin-1-Beta gene are associated with intracranial hemorrhage and susceptibility to brain arteriovenous malformation. Cerebrovasc Dis. 2009; 27(2):176–182

[67] Mikhak B, Weinsheimer S, Pawlikowska L, et al. Angiopoietin-like 4 (ANGPTL4) gene polymorphisms and risk of brain arteriovenous malformations. Cerebrovasc Dis. 2011; 31(4):338–345

[68] Weinsheimer S, Brettman AD, Pawlikowska L, et al. G Protein-Coupled Receptor 124 (GPR124) Gene Polymorphisms and Risk of Brain Arteriovenous Malformation. Transl Stroke Res. 2012; 3(4):418–427

[69] Chen H, Gu Y, Wu W, et al. Polymorphisms of the vascular endothelial growth factor A gene and susceptibility to sporadic brain arteriovenous malformation in a Chinese population. J Clin Neurosci. 2011; 18(4):549–553

[70] Zhao Y, Li P, Fan W, et al. The rs522616 polymorphism in the matrix metalloproteinase-3 (MMP-3) gene is associated with sporadic brain arteriovenous malformation in a Chinese population. J Clin Neurosci. 2010; 17(12):1568–1572

[71] Pawlikowska L, Tran MN, Achrol AS, et al. UCSF BAVM Study Project. Polymorphisms in genes involved in inflammatory and angiogenic pathways and the risk of hemorrhagic presentation of brain arteriovenous malformations. Stroke. 2004; 35(10):2294–2300

[72] Weinsheimer S, Kim H, Pawlikowska L, et al. EPHB4 gene polymorphisms and risk of intracranial hemorrhage in patients with brain arteriovenous malformations. Circ Cardiovasc Genet. 2009; 2(5):476–482

[73] Pawlikowska L, Poon KY, Achrol AS, et al. Apolipoprotein E epsilon 2 is associated with new hemorrhage risk in brain arteriovenous malformations. Neurosurgery. 2006; 58(5):838–843, discussion 838–843

[74] Achrol AS, Kim H, Pawlikowska L, et al. Association of tumor necrosis factor-alpha-238G > A and apolipoprotein E2 polymorphisms with intracranial hemorrhage after brain arteriovenous malformation treatment. Neurosurgery. 2007; 61(4):731–739, discussion 740

[75] Cognard C, Gobin YP, Pierot L, et al. Cerebral dural arteriovenous fistulas: clinical and angiographic correlation with a revised classification of venous drainage. Radiology. 1995; 194(3):671–680

[76] Borden JA, Wu JK, Shucart WA. A proposed classification for spinal and cranial dural arteriovenous fistulous malformations and implications for treatment. J Neurosurg. 1995; 82(2):166–179

[77] Chaudhary MY, Sachdev VP, Cho SH, Weitzner I , Jr, Puljic S, Huang YP. Dural arteriovenous malformation of the major venous sinuses: an acquired lesion. AJNR Am J Neuroradiol. 1982; 3(1):13–19

[78] Cognard C, Casasco A, Toevi M, Houdart E, Chiras J, Merland JJ. Dural arteriovenous fistulas as a cause of intracranial hypertension due to impairment of cranial venous outflow. J Neurol Neurosurg Psychiatry. 1998; 65(3):308–316

[79] Tsai LK, Jeng JS, Liu HM, Wang HJ, Yip PK. Intracranial dural arteriovenous fistulas with or without cerebral sinus thrombosis: analysis of 69 patients. J Neurol Neurosurg Psychiatry. 2004; 75(11):1639–1641

[80] Terada T, Higashida RT, Halbach VV, et al. Development of acquired arteriovenous fistulas in rats due to venous hypertension. J Neurosurg. 1994; 80(5):884–889

[81] Herman JM, Spetzler RF, Bederson JB, Kurbat JM, Zabramski JM. Genesis of a dural arteriovenous malformation in a rat model. J Neurosurg. 1995; 83(3):539–545

[82] Zhu Y, Lawton MT, Du R, et al. Expression of hypoxia-inducible factor-1 and vascular endothelial growth factor in response to venous hypertension. Neurosurgery. 2006; 59(3):687–696, discussion 687–696

[83] Shin Y, Nakase H, Nakamura M, Shimada K, Konishi N, Sakaki T. Expression of angiogenic growth factor in the rat DAVF model. Neurol Res. 2007; 29(7):727–733

3 Physiology and Hemodynamics of Arteriovenous Malformations and Arteriovenous Fistulas

Mohan Narayanan and Peter Nakaji

Abstract

Most studies on arteriovenous malformations (AVMs) and dural arteriovenous fistulas (AVFs; previously often called dural AVMs in older literature) have focused on the natural history, anatomy, histopathology, treatment, and prognosis of these lesions. More recently, studies have also been published on molecular development. However, few publications clearly describe the physiology and flow hemodynamics of these lesions. This chapter focuses on a summary of the historical and current knowledge and literature on the physiology and flow dynamics of AVMs and AVFs.

Keywords: arteriovenous fistula, arteriovenous malformation, autoregulation, flow hemodynamics, physiology, steal, venous hypertension

- Arteriovenous malformations (AVMs) and arteriovenous fistulas (AVFs) are formed when an abnormally low-resistance pathway allows blood to be shunted from the arterial system to the venous system.
- In AVMs, arterial steal can cause chronic local tissue ischemia in areas surrounding the nidus due to shunting of blood through a low-resistance circuit, but this effect is not often seen in AVFs.
- In both AVMs and AVFs, venous hypertension and congestion can further contribute to surrounding tissue ischemia and increased risk of spontaneous hemorrhage or neurological dysfunction, such as seizure.
- It is theorized that normal perfusion pressure breakthrough, occlusive hyperemia, and loss of autoregulation contribute to postoperative edema and hemorrhage in patients after AVM resection.

3.1 Introduction

This chapter focuses on the physiology and hemodynamics of intracranial arteriovenous malformations (AVMs) and dural arteriovenous fistulas (AVFs, sometimes also called dural AVMs in older literature). These pathologically important lesions are characterized by direct arteriovenous (AV) shunts. AVMs are characterized by a nidus—a tangle of blood vessels in which the arteries and veins connect directly, without an intervening capillary bed. In contrast, AVFs may have many associated dilated pathological vessels, but the true pathology lies in the direct connection point or points. Until recently, few studies have been published regarding the flow and hemodynamics of cerebral AVMs and AVFs. However, in the last 10 years, there has been a significant increase in publication on this subject, leading to a better characterization of the physiology of AVMs

and AVFs that can aid in our understanding and treatment of these lesions.

3.2 Normal Flow and Physiology

3.2.1 Overview

Models of normal flow through the human circulatory system (and subsequently cerebral circulation) have been created using adaptations of Ohm's law and Poiseuille's law. Poiseuille's law applies to ideal newtonian fluids undergoing laminar flow, which occurs when blood flows at a steady rate through a long, smooth vessel, and the centermost portion of blood stays in the center of the blood vessel. Generally, these principles state that flow can be equated to the change in pressure for any given resistance, and flow rate is related to the change in pressure multiplied by πr^4 and divided by the viscosity (or resistance) of the fluid and the length of the tube. Ohm's law can be expressed by the equation

$$Q = \Delta P/R,$$

where Q is flow, ΔP is the difference in pressure between two measured points, and R is resistance. Poiseuille's law can be expressed by the equation

$$Q = \alpha \Delta P \pi r^4 / 8\eta L,$$

where Q is flow, ΔP is the difference in pressure between two measured points, r is the radius of the tube, η is the viscosity of the fluid, and L is the length of the tube.

It should be noted that even small increases in vessel radius or diameter cause corresponding exponential increases in flow.

In normal circulation, however, blood is not a newtonian fluid, blood vessels are not rigid, and blood flow is not perfectly laminar. Many conditions, such as vascular stenosis, the presence of aneurysms, and asymmetry, can lead to turbulent flow, in which blood flows in all directions in the vessel and is continually mixing, in contrast to laminar flow. The occurrence of turbulent flow increases with increasing blood flow velocity, increasing diameter of the blood vessel, and increasing blood density. With respect to AVMs and AVFs, the factors above make exact modeling difficult. However, these basic principles form the foundation for understanding their hemodynamics.

3.2.2 Vascular Reactivity

Blood vessels have the ability to change vascular resistance in response to changes in arterial pressure in order to maintain a relatively constant rate of blood flow. This process allows the autoregulation of blood flow. In normal tissue with intact autoregulation, increases in arterial pressure cause a compensatory increase in vascular resistance through activation of local control mechanisms. Similarly, a decrease in arterial pressure causes a decrease of vascular resistance in order to maintain a stable rate of blood flow.[1] In the brain, autoregulation protects tissues from experiencing ischemia or hyperemia within a range of blood pressures.[2]

The processes by which this autoregulation occurs, arterial vasodilation and vasoconstriction, have many biochemical mechanisms. In a hallmark study, Furchgott and Vanhoutte[3] reviewed the importance of endothelium-derived relaxing factor (EDRF), which stimulates a cyclic guanosine monophosphate–mediated relaxation mechanism. Increased wall shear stress, which can be observed in increased arterial pressure or turbulent flow, stimulates the release of EDRF. In laboratory studies, increased flow induces vasodilation, which is not observed when the endothelium is removed. Furchgott and Vanhoutte also showed that endothelium-derived contracting factors, such as arachidonic acid, augment arterial contractions evoked by norepinephrine, and these findings were also not observed after removal of the arterial intima.[3]

3.3 Arteriovenous Malformations

3.3.1 Overview

In AVMs, an abnormal connection exists between the arterial and venous systems that bypasses the normal intervening network of capillaries. Although a clear genetic transmission pattern has not yet been defined, the occurrence of AVMs has been associated with some genetic syndromes, in particular, hereditary hemorrhagic telangiectasia.[4] The AVM nidus is a point toward which multiple feeding arteries converge and from which an enlarged vein or veins drain.[5] AVMs may drain through either the deep or the superficial venous systems, and although there may be large or dysplastic draining veins, the drainage generally continues in an anterograde fashion into the normal venous system. Conventional angiography is the preferred method for evaluating the anatomy of AVMs. Angiography clearly defines feeding arterial vessels, nidus location, venous drainage patterns, the presence of aneurysmal dilations, venous varices, and vasculopathy. Often, AVMs with retrograde leptomeningeal venous drainage have intrinsic varices or aneurysms associated with them that affect their hemodynamic stability and risk of hemorrhage. An increased risk of hemorrhage is conferred by small AVM size, high-flow lesions with increased intraluminal pressure, deep location, and previous AVM hemorrhage. Angiographic characteristics such as intranidal aneurysm, flow-related arterial aneurysm, deep venous drainage, and venous stenosis have also been associated with an increased risk of AVM hemorrhage.[6,7] The overall annual risk of hemorrhage is approximately 2 to 4%, with higher risk for ruptured lesions than unruptured lesions.[8,9]

3.3.2 Physiology and Hemodynamics

AVMs lack a diffusing capillary bed and therefore are subject to high-flow shunting and increased wall shear stress forces through feeding arteries and intranidal vessels.[10] This shunting can initiate abnormal vascular remodeling, which leads to dilatation of vessels and aneurysm formation. The low-resistance environment of the AVM causes a sump effect, drawing flow so

that the adjacent brain tissue surrounding an AVM also experiences reductions in blood flow, which leads to a state of chronic hypoperfusion.[11] The transfer of high-pressure arterial blood to the veins through this low-resistance circuit also results in venous hypertension and can generate aneurysms and promote venous mural remodeling, which especially in the setting of impaired outflow can produce rupture.[12] An illustration of relative pressures in an AVM circuit are shown in ▶ Fig. 3.1a, with a pressure gradient that favors flow through the AVM and diverting flow from arterial territories downstream.

Uranishi et al studied the expression of smoothelin, a cytoskeletal protein found in mature smooth muscle cells used as a marker for the identification of these particular cells.[13] The authors examined vascular smooth muscle cell differentiation in various lesions, and found decreased expression of smoothelin in large AVM vessels when compared to vessels in the normal brain. They postulated that the decrease in smoothelin expression correlated with a reduced presence of mature vascular smooth muscle cells in AVMs and subsequent diminished autoregulation and contractility in AVM vasculature. The decrease in smoothelin expression was associated with increased hemodynamic stress within the AVM.[13] Gao et al have published evidence that endothelial progenitor cells are present in increased levels in AVMs and that they contribute to the continuous pathological remodeling of the lesion.[14]

The prevailing theory in growth and rupture of AVMs involves inflammation and remodeling of the extracellular matrix. Evidence suggests that proinflammatory cytokine release, increased expression of cell adhesion molecules, and inflammatory cell invasion in the vessel walls contribute to the instability of the AVM nidus.[12,15] Recent animal studies have shown a correlation between increasing wall shear stress and AVM angiogenesis.[16] In high-flow AVMs, increasing diameter and variability of nidal vessels can cause turbulent flow, as evidenced by endothelial cell turnover, focal dilatation of vessels, and platelet aggregation.[16]

Imaging Techniques Used to Characterize Hemodynamic Parameters

Real-time indocyanine green videoangiography (ICG-VA) has been used to help identify vascular architecture, flow direction, and qualitative blood flow transit speed.[11] FLOW 800 software has been applied by one group to obtain quantitative flow measurements from the operating microscope ICG-VA data.[11] The data should be interpreted as relative quantitative values because they are based on an arbitrary intensity number to denote flow.[11]

Intraoperative micro-Doppler flowmetry has been used and validated in cerebral aneurysm surgery, and more recently has been used to model flow through cerebral AVMs.[17,18] Metrics such as velocity (with direction), pulsatility index, and resistance index (RI) are useful for characterizing flow in AVMs. These metrics are obtained from arterial feeders, venous draining vessels, and relevant vessels during dissection or possible transit arteries.[17,18] RI is defined by the equation

$$RI = (systolic\ velocity - diastolic\ velocity)/(systolic\ velocity).$$

This value is calculated in real time by Doppler imaging and is used to distinguish AVM feeding arteries from normal arteries.

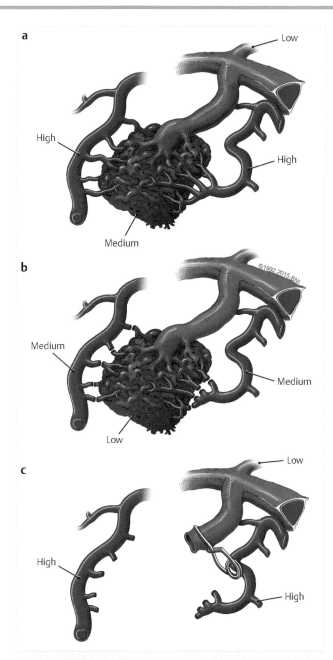

Fig. 3.1 Illustration of changes in relative pressure in AVM feeding vessels, AVM nidus, AVM draining vein, and normal veins. **(a)** At normal systemic pressure, relative pressures in arterial feeding vessels, AVM nidus, draining vein, and normal veins are high, medium, medium, and low, respectively. **(b)** Systemic pressure is decreased intraoperatively to decrease flow through the AVM. Relative pressures through arterial feeding vessels, draining vein, and normal veins are medium, low, and medium, respectively, and pressure in the AVM nidus is low because of disconnection of arterial feeders. **(c)** After the AVM nidus has been resected and the patient's systemic pressure has returned to normal, the relative pressures in the arterial feeders and normal veins are high and low, respectively. When the feeding vessels experience a return to normal perfusion pressure, it is theorized that there is a loss of the ability to autoregulate, and there may be postoperative hyperemia or hemorrhage. (These images are provided courtesy of Barrow Neurological Institute, Phoenix, Arizona.)

The lack of an intervening capillary bed causes a lower resistance circuit compared to normal vasculature, and results in a higher diastolic flow and a subsequently lower RI. Normal RI values are found to be between 0.5 and 0.7, and RI values of AVM feeding arteries are consistently below 0.5.

The RI is an important method for characterizing AVM flow intraoperatively, because it is not affected by the angulation of the Doppler probe, which reduces operator error in obtaining measurements. After surgical resection of an AVM, the RI of the feeding artery returns to values within the normal range.[19]

Flowmetry can be used to distinguish between arteries and veins by evaluating flow direction when ICG-VA is not conclusive, and it can also be used to identify multiple draining vessels and secondary draining veins. Main draining veins have a higher flow quantity, and secondary draining veins have a relatively lower flow quantity. Spetzler–Martin grade II AVMs have the highest arterial and venous flow rates. Flowmetry is of limited value for measuring small, deep vessels of AVMs because of the difficulty of positioning a probe on these vessels. Another disadvantage of using this technique is the potential for injuring fragile draining veins during the measurement process.[18]

Noninvasive quantitative magnetic resonance (MR) angiography has been used to characterize hemodynamic factors contributing to the formation of aneurysms in AVMs. The investigators examined flow, vessel diameter, and wall shear stress in AVM feeding vessels with and without aneurysms. A significantly greater degree of increased wall shear stress was seen in feeding arteries with aneurysms than in those without aneurysms.[20] The same investigators found that successful AVM embolization and resection reduced wall shear stress in feeding vessels down to normal values.[21]

Vascular Steal

Vascular steal is thought to occur in AVMs because of the relatively low resistance to flow in the AVM vasculature compared to the circulation in neighboring tissue. This disparity creates a pressure differential that causes blood flow to be shunted away from neighboring brain tissue. Supporters of this theory believe that the steal phenomenon leads to a state of chronic hypoperfusion of neighboring brain tissue, contributing to brain dysfunction and loss of vascular autoregulation.[22] Spetzler et al associated low feeding artery pressures measured in large AVMs to fluctuations in neurological deficits because of relative ischemia.[23] One proposed mechanism of seizure associated with AVMs is related to vascular steal. It is thought that AV shunting away from the downstream arterial territory causes hypoperfusion-induced remodeling of the perinidal cortex, creating a molecular environment conducive to epileptogenesis.[24] This theory is controversial, because many AVMs have low-flow states with no angiographic evidence of steal and no significant contribution of arterial supply from the internal carotid or vertebral arteries.[25] Others have produced concordant results that show no significant difference in feeding artery pressure, arterial flow velocity, or pulsatility index between patients who present with focal neurological deficits and those who present without deficits.[26] The exact pathophysiological mechanism of steal, if it exists, is unclear; however, it remains a useful concept.

CO$_2$ Reactivity

Hypercapnia causes dilation of the arterioles and increased cerebral blood flow, and the reverse is true in hypocapnia. This effect has been studied using ventilatory control as the mechanism to affect CO$_2$ regulation. Classically, in AVMs, it was thought that when hypercapnia is induced, feeding vessels show only a slight increase in flow, as measured by Doppler, and in hypocapnia feeding vessels show stable flow.[27] In a later study by De Salles and Manchola, hypocapnia was shown to significantly decrease flow velocity in both AVM feeding and nonfeeding vessels as measured by transcranial Doppler at the level of small vessels.[28] Conversely, during hypercapnia, flow volume was significantly higher in AVM feeding vessels when compared to nonfeeding vessels.[28] Of note, the definition of measured vessels was specific to this study, and transcranial Doppler is operator-dependent with regard to the validity of measurements. After resection of an AVM, a normal vasomotor response is observed, particularly in branches of vessels that supplied the AVM.[27]

Autoregulation and Normal Perfusion Pressure Breakthrough

There are conflicting reports on whether autoregulation is preserved in tissues surrounding AVMs; one group reports augmented vasodilation, but others show intact autoregulation pre- and postoperatively. Hoffman et al noted that the tissue surrounding an AVM has lower partial pressure of oxygen (Po$_2$) at baseline, with a normal partial pressure of carbon dioxide (Pco$_2$) and pH. In this study, induced hypercapnia caused an increased Po$_2$ and a decreased pH in the surrounding brain tissue with no change in Pco$_2$. Hypercapnia was thought to transiently increase cerebral blood flow and wash out local CO$_2$ in the tissues surrounding the AVM.[29]

Intraoperatively, systemic arterial pressure is decreased and arterial feeding branches are disconnected from the AVM nidus (▶ Fig. 3.1b). Spetzler et al defined the term "normal perfusion pressure breakthrough," in a theory that stated that impaired autoregulation contributes to the formation of AVMs, and to edema and hemorrhage after AVM resection (▶ Fig. 3.1c).[30] The theory stated that because of chronic hypoperfusion of the tissue surrounding an AVM, vascular CO$_2$ reactivity and autoregulation were lost. Larger AVMs have a lower flow resistance because of larger feeding vessels. After AVM resection, redirection of blood flow to chronically dilated vessels that have lost the ability to vasoconstrict at the level of resistance vessels overwhelms their capacity, resulting in edema or hemorrhage.[30] In an updated review of the literature regarding this theory, Rangel-Castilla et al found that postoperative hyperventilation, hyperoxia, and nitric oxide balance play a role in restoring normal autoregulation.[2]

Young et al showed that, in areas of normal brain supplied by AVM feeders, when systemic arterial pressure increased, there was no resultant increase in cerebral blood flow.[31] The authors postulated that chronic hypotension in areas that are supplied by AVM feeding vessels may be associated with an adaptive shift or displacement of the intact autoregulation curve to the left, but it is not associated with loss of autoregulation or "vasomotor paralysis." They also reported no instances of postoperative edema or hemorrhage; however, they stated that an increase in pressure postoperatively that exceeded the upper limit of the autoregulatory curve could cause "breakthrough" edema and hemorrhage.[31]

Schaller et al pointed out that a difficulty in measuring cerebral vascular reactivity (CVR) is that it cannot be measured quantitatively with adequate temporal and spatial resolution.[32] These authors employed the use of spectrophotometry to compare AVM-specific CVR patterns with a control group, and found no clinically significant difference between the two groups before or after surgery.[32]

Venous Hypertension

AVM draining veins are often dilated from experiencing increased blood flow from AV shunting, which can result in variceal or aneurysmal formation. Wall shear stress can play a role in rupture by promoting remodeling that causes decreased integrity of vessel walls and weakening of draining veins. However, an inverse relationship exists between the number of draining veins and venous outflow pressure; a greater number of draining vessels decreases the venous pressure in the draining system, because of more potential outflow pathways for the AV shunted blood. Increased intravascular pressure may lead to tissue hypoxia and ischemia upstream from the nidus, and venous congestion also impairs outflow from surrounding brain tissue that drains to the same venous bed as the AVM. If the draining veins are obstructed, increased pressure can open preexisting AV channels and further contribute to the growth of AVMs.[33]

Increased venous outflow caused by AV shunting can result in venous congestion and may impair microvascular autoregulation. This mechanism of venous congestion is thought to result in parenchymal irritation and subsequent epileptogenesis.[34]

A proposed mechanism termed "occlusive hyperemia" was discussed by al-Rodhan et al in 1993.[35] They described a mechanism in which stagnation of arterial flow in AVM feeding vessels, exacerbated ischemia of surrounding tissue, and obstruction of draining veins caused venous engorgement, hyperemia, and worsening stagnation of arterial flow. These factors contributed to an environment prone to hemorrhage and edema after AVM resection,[35] and can cause postoperative neurological deficits.

3.4 Arteriovenous Fistulas

3.4.1 Overview

AVFs are characterized by abnormal connections between the arterial and venous systems with no true nidus as seen in AVMs.[36] They have been associated with a history of trauma, prior surgery, and congenital abnormalities, which lead to venous sinus thrombosis and other factors that contribute to the formation and progression of AVFs (▶ Fig. 3.2).[7,37] The arterial supply of AVFs is typically recruited from dural arteries and from meningeal branches of cerebral arteries. The venous drainage occurs through dural venous sinuses or through other dural and leptomeningeal venous outflow tracts.[37] They do not contain a "nidus" in the parenchyma, but do contain one or more AV shunts with relation to the dural vasculature.[38] Intracranial AVFs are classified according to different grading scales,

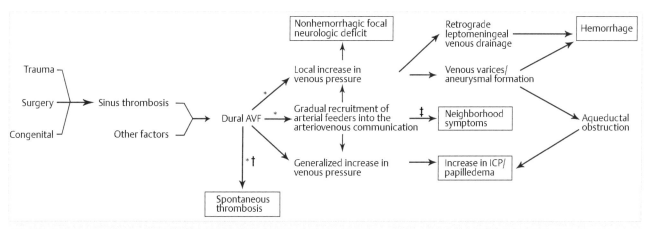

Fig. 3.2 Factors contributing to the formation and progression of dural AVFs. Trauma, surgery, and congenital factors contribute to venous sinus thrombosis, which along with other factors has been associated with dural AVF formation. Recruitment of arterial feeders into the AV communication leads to shunting (*), neighborhood symptoms such as pulsatile tinnitus and cavernous sinus syndrome (‡), and an increase in local and generalized venous pressures, resulting in nonhemorrhagic focal neurological deficit. Prolonged increase in venous pressure leads to retrograde leptomeningeal venous drainage and the formation of venous varices and aneurysms, which are prone to hemorrhage and rupture. Generalized increases in venous pressure, and additional venous varix or aneurysm formation, can cause aqueductal obstruction and further contribute to increased intracranial pressure. Most dural AVF are asymptomatic and spontaneously thrombose (†) without further recurrence. (Adapted from Awad et al.[37])

including the traditional Borden–Shucart system,[39] the Cognard system,[40] and the UCSF[41] system. These grading systems typically characterize AVFs by the type of venous drainage present in the lesion. AVFs are most often observed at the transverse, sigmoid, and cavernous sinuses.[42] As seen with AVMs, AVFs may exhibit retrograde leptomeningeal venous drainage, and additionally can be associated with varices and aneurysmal dilation which, when present, increase the risk of hemorrhage. Angiographic evidence shows that variceal or aneurysmal formation, retrograde leptomeningeal venous drainage, and galenic venous drainage are all associated with increased risk of hemorrhage.[37] Hemorrhage risk in patients with AVFs associated with retrograde leptomeningeal venous drainage is approximately 8.1%, with a mortality rate of 10.4% annually.[25]

3.4.2 Physiology and Hemodynamics

In the Borden–Shucart grading system, AVFs are classified based on the type of venous drainage. Type I lesions have venous sinus or meningeal venous drainage in the normal anterograde direction (► Fig. 3.3a). An increased rate of flow has been correlated to symptoms of pulsatile tinnitus, depending on the location of the AVF, most often along the pathway of the transverse or sigmoid sinus.

Type II lesions have venous sinus or meningeal venous outflow with retrograde leptomeningeal drainage. The venous outflow tract can become stenotic (► Fig. 3.3b) or partially thrombosed and obstructed from turbulent flow or arterialization of the veins, causing a subsequent elevation in sinus pressure. The flow in the subarachnoid veins in these lesions travels in retrograde fashion. Arterialized blood travels from the draining venous sinus into the subarachnoid leptomeningeal veins (► Fig. 3.3c). These veins then become chronically arterialized, and create collateral drainage pathways, allowing for directed ligation of the major sinus.

Type III lesions have retrograde leptomeningeal venous drainage only (► Fig. 3.3d). These lesions drain into subarachnoid

veins, and are located on the wall of dural venous sinuses. The increased blood flow with no alternative drainage route causes significant venous hypertension and can cause subsequent neurological deficits from hemorrhage, edema, or ischemia. Retrograde leptomeningeal venous drainage occurs here regardless of whether the sinus is patent or occluded. If the sinus is patent, Borden describes no communication between the arterialized vein and sinus. Type II and III lesions experience venous hypertension and can present with subsequent hemorrhage when untreated.[39]

Invasive pressure monitoring can be achieved using intraoperative venous puncture (► Fig. 3.4a, b), but longitudinal evaluation of shunt flow in AVFs has not been studied by invasive or direct quantitative measurements to date. Several studies have used MR imaging and single-photon emission computed tomography (SPECT) in an attempt to noninvasively quantify shunt volume and flow.[43,44]

In contrast to AVMs, in which CO_2 reactivity has been studied in depth, no studies have been published on the CO_2 reactivity of vessels in cerebral AVFs, although Hassler and Thron have studied vessels supplying the spinal cord in spinal AVFs.[45]

Arterial Steal

Unlike AVMs, AVFs are typically low-resistance, low-flow AV shunts that show no angiographic evidence of arterial steal. Steal phenomenon has been proposed as a mechanism to explain cranial nerve deficits in meningeal arteries,[46,47] but other studies have published results that support venous congestion and local mass effect as the major cause of cranial nerve manifestations in cavernous sinus AVFs.[25,48,49]

Retrograde Leptomeningeal Venous Drainage

If venous sinus outflow is obstructed by stenosis, thrombosis, or occlusion, sinus pressure increases. Over time, this may drive the sinus to become arterialized, which increases intravascular

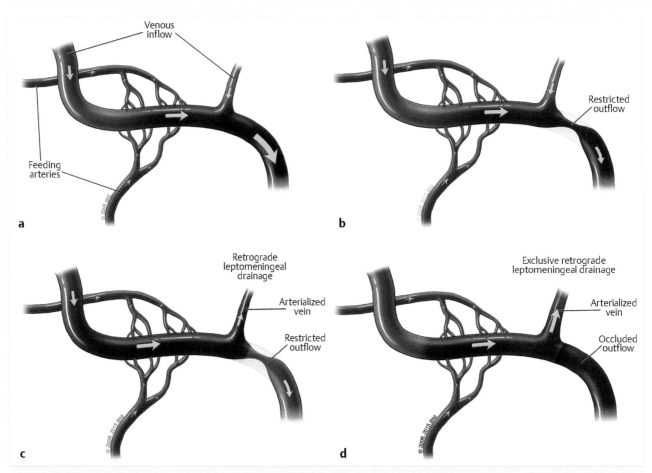

Fig. 3.3 Illustrations of cerebral dural AVF. (a) Type I lesion with anterograde flow. (b) Type I lesion with anterograde flow and restricted venous outflow from stenosis. This leads to flow diversion through leptomeningeal veins. (c) Type II lesion with venous outflow obstruction, causing reversal of flow and leptomeningeal drainage and chronic venous arterialization. (d) Type III lesion with exclusive retrograde leptomeningeal drainage. (Used with permission from Barrow Neurological Institute, Phoenix, Arizona.)

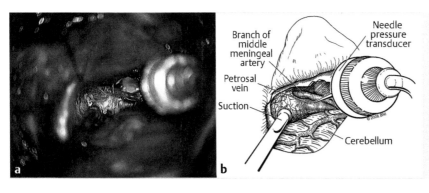

Fig. 3.4 Invasive pressure monitoring in cerebral dural AVF. (a) Actual intraoperative photograph of petrosal dural AVF, with a needle pressure transducer in the petrosal vein. (b) The same photograph, reproduced as an illustrative figure. (Used with permission from Barrow Neurological Institute, Phoenix, Arizona.)

pressure. Subarachnoid veins that normally drain into the sinus then experience arterialized retrograde blood flow, which arterializes the subarachnoid veins, and new collateral draining veins develop.[39] In AVFs that have no sinus drainage, it has been shown that venous occlusion does not exacerbate venous hypertension unless the normal venous drainage system is thrombosed.[50] AVFs with retrograde leptomeningeal venous drainage can cause venous congestive encephalopathy with

reversible and irreversible effects. Patients who are symptomatic upon presentation are likely to be more hemodynamically compromised than asymptomatic patients.[51]

Kanemaru et al prospectively studied AVFs with retrograde leptomeningeal venous drainage pre- and postoperatively using clinical examination, MR imaging, digital subtraction angiography, and ^{123}I-iodoamphetamine ([123]IMP) SPECT.[44] The SPECT imaging was used to determine CVR (with acetazolamide) and the affected-to-contralateral side asymmetry ratio (ACR). These metrics are functions of regional cerebral blood flow (rCBF) and were used to create information about relative changes in hemodynamics through AVFs with retrograde leptomeningeal venous drainage pre- and postoperatively. These metrics were also compared to T2-weighted MR images to determine any high-intensity areas that were possible areas of venous congestion, vasogenic edema, or venous infarction. In this way, ACR was calculated by the equation

$$ACR = rCBF_{affected} / rCBF_{contralateral} \times 100,$$

and CVR was calculated by the equation

$$CVR = (rCBF_{acetazolamide} - rCBF_{rest}) / rCBF_{rest} \times 100.$$

This study concluded that a reduction in the ACR corresponded to findings of venous congestive encephalopathy, while a decrease in CVR corresponded to irreversibility of the lesion.[44]

Increased Intracranial Pressure

Superior sagittal sinus (SSS) hypertension may lead to additional increases in intracranial pressure (ICP) because of decreased cerebrospinal fluid (CSF) resorption. The CSF resorption rate is calculated by the equation (CSF pressure – SSS pressure)/(resistance of outflow).[52] Sigmoid sinus thrombosis may also limit venous outflow and lead to increased ICP.[25]

Spontaneous Thrombosis

Spontaneous thrombosis of an AVF can occur if a thrombus forms within the arterial feeding vessels, venous outflow vessels, or involved dural venous sinus. Occlusion of the venous outflow tract may cause proximal engorgement and increase risk for hemorrhage, although this may not be observed in thrombosis of the fistula itself, which may lead to spontaneous resolution of AVFs. Low-flow dural-based AVFs are more likely to regress spontaneously because the blood has more time to pool and coagulate in the fistulous connection.[25]

Venous Arterialization

In one animal study, a high-flow surgical fistula was created between the external jugular vein and the common carotid artery to model AVF. This study found that blood flow increases with time through the fistula, and like other peripheral fistulas, there is arterialization of the vein after creation of the fistula.[53]

Special Situations

Vein of Galen Malformations

Vein of Galen malformations occur in predominantly pediatric patients and are characterized as high-flow lesions. The high rate of shunting causes an increase in venous drainage, which in turn causes an increase in cardiac preload, which when untreated leads to congestive heart failure. The resultant upstream venous congestion can present with symptoms of increased ICP because of the mass effect from development of venous lakes as well as hydrocephalus.[25]

Carotid Cavernous Fistulas

Carotid cavernous fistulas (CCFs) are a special type of AVF with arterial inflow from the internal carotid artery. AVFs involving the cavernous sinus may present with ophthalmoplegia, proptosis, chemosis, pain, or decreased visual acuity, which may be explained by their drainage routes because these routes often include the orbital veins.[38] Patients may experience visual deterioration resulting from a combination of decreased arterial perfusion and venous hypertension with glaucoma. Low-flow CCFs have a high rate of spontaneous resolution. There are four subtypes as classified by Barrow et al.[54] Broadly, CCFs may be direct or indirect, based largely on whether there is a direct connection or intervening vasculature. Although most of these fistulas are supplied by the internal carotid artery, one should undertake an intense angiographic search for any supply from the external carotid artery in order to plan treatment.[54] They may be treated by either transarterial or transvenous embolization, depending on the anatomy.

3.5 Other Considerations

3.5.1 Epileptogenesis in Vascular Malformations

In cavernous malformations, deposits of hemosiderin surrounding the lesion can alter the physiologic environment of certain neurotransmitters, promoting hypersynchronization and perilesional excitatory stimuli to other cortical regions.[55] It is not clear whether there is increased or decreased expression of excitatory and inhibitory neurotransmitters, receptors, and enzymes universally across vascular malformations.[24]

3.5.2 Computational Modeling

Computational flow dynamics have been used to evaluate various intracranial aneurysms; however, these studies are limited by assumptions about flow characteristics. For example, studies may assume discrete parameters for blood volume density and viscosity and that vessel walls are rigid in order to model flow. However, there is significant correlation between angiographic flow (the gold standard for subjective assessment) and computational models. The shear stress on the wall of the aneurysm has been analyzed as well, to predict vessel wall weakness and areas of potential rupture.[56] With improvements in technology, and in our understanding of the physiology and flow characteristics of AVMs and AVFs, better models in computational flow dynamics can be created. These studies have been applied to AVMs and AVFs also, but there are many limitations in our understanding about the underlying properties of these lesions for creating models that limit the usefulness of their predictions.

3.5.3 Noninvasive Imaging

New imaging modalities such as four-dimensional computed tomography angiography (4D-CTA) are being developed as noninvasive alternatives to diagnose and follow untreated AVMs.

This imaging modality offers the ability to add the variable of time resolution to conventional 3D-CTA. 4D-CTA allows qualitative flow review. This novel technique could be beneficial for patients who are hemodynamically unstable and cannot undergo invasive angiography (or in locations where angiography is not readily available) or in a situation where invasive angiography may delay definitive intervention.[57]

Noninvasive time-resolved MR angiography can also be used to quantify hemodynamic characteristics of AVM and AVF, with limitation of temporal resolution to approximately 1 second. Recent development of time-resolved, spin-labeled MR angiography has allowed the characterization of AVMs with high resolution, up to 50 to 100 ms.[58]

3.6 Conclusion

In summary, a fair amount of primary data exists to characterize the physiology and hemodynamics of AVMs and AVFs. However, much remains to be understood. At present, our limited knowledge of the physiology of these lesions only allows us to rationally direct therapy based on these principles in broad strokes. With a wealth of new imaging and computational techniques becoming available, we can anticipate that future research will yield more answers that can benefit the care of these patients.

References

[1] Hall JE. Guyton and Hall Textbook of Medical Physiology. 13th ed. Philadelphia, PA: Elsevier; 2015:169–178

[2] Rangel-Castilla L, Spetzler RF, Nakaji P. Normal perfusion pressure breakthrough theory: a reappraisal after 35 years. Neurosurg Rev. 2015; 38(3):399–404, discussion 404–405

[3] Furchgott RF, Vanhoutte PM. Endothelium-derived relaxing and contracting factors. FASEB J. 1989; 3(9):2007–2018

[4] McDonald J, Pyeritz RE. Hereditary hemorrhagic telangiectasia. In: Pagon RA, Adam MP, Ardinger HH, et al. eds. GeneReviews® [Internet]. Seattle, WA: University of Washington; 1993

[5] Doppman JL. The nidus concept of spinal cord arteriovenous malformations. A surgical recommendation based upon angiographic observations. Br J Radiol. 1971; 44(526):758–763

[6] Duong DH, Young WL, Vang MC, et al. Feeding artery pressure and venous drainage pattern are primary determinants of hemorrhage from cerebral arteriovenous malformations. Stroke. 1998; 29(6):1167–1176

[7] Mossa-Basha M, Chen J, Gandhi D. Imaging of cerebral arteriovenous malformations and dural arteriovenous fistulas. Neurosurg Clin N Am. 2012; 23(1):27–42

[8] Gross BA, Du R. Natural history of cerebral arteriovenous malformations: a meta-analysis. J Neurosurg. 2013; 118(2):437–443

[9] Kim H, Pourmohamad T, Westbroek EM, McCulloch CE, Lawton MT, Young WL. Evaluating performance of the spetzler-martin supplemented model in selecting patients with brain arteriovenous malformation for surgery. Stroke. 2012; 43(9):2497–2499

[10] Ajiboye N, Chalouhi N, Starke RM, Zanaty M, Bell R. Cerebral arteriovenous malformations: evaluation and management. Sci World J. 2014; 2014:649036

[11] Fukuda K, Kataoka H, Nakajima N, Masuoka J, Satow T, Iihara K. Efficacy of FLOW 800 with indocyanine green videoangiography for the quantitative assessment of flow dynamics in cerebral arteriovenous malformation surgery. World Neurosurg. 2015; 83(2):203–210

[12] Mouchtouris N, Jabbour PM, Starke RM, et al. Biology of cerebral arteriovenous malformations with a focus on inflammation. J Cereb Blood Flow Metab. 2015; 35(2):167–175

[13] Uranishi R, Baev NI, Kim JH, Awad IA. Vascular smooth muscle cell differentiation in human cerebral vascular malformations. Neurosurgery. 2001; 49(3):671–679, discussion 679–680

[14] Gao P, Chen Y, Lawton MT, et al. Evidence of endothelial progenitor cells in the human brain and spinal cord arteriovenous malformations. Neurosurgery. 2010; 67(4):1029–1035

[15] Rangel-Castilla L, Russin JJ, Martinez-Del-Campo E, Soriano-Baron H, Spetzler RF, Nakaji P. Molecular and cellular biology of cerebral arteriovenous malformations: a review of current concepts and future trends in treatment. Neurosurg Focus. 2014; 37(3):E1

[16] Tu J, Li Y, Hu Z. Notch1 and 4 signaling responds to an increasing vascular wall shear stress in a rat model of arteriovenous malformations. BioMed Res Int. 2014; 2014:368082

[17] Burkhardt T, Siasios G, Schmidt NO, Reitz M, Regelsberger J, Westphal M. Intraoperative Micro-Doppler in Cerebral Arteriovenous Malformations. J Neurol Surg A Cent Eur Neurosurg. 2015; 76(6):451–455

[18] Della Puppa A, Rustemi O, Scienza R. Intraoperative flow measurement by microflow probe during surgery for brain arteriovenous malformations. Neurosurgery. 2015; 11 Suppl 2:268–273

[19] Dempsey RJ, Moftakhar R, Pozniak M. Intraoperative Doppler to measure cerebrovascular resistance as a guide to complete resection of arteriovenous malformations. Neurosurgery. 2004; 55(1):155–160, discussion 160–161

[20] Shakur SF, Amin-Hanjani S, Mostafa H, Charbel FT, Alaraj A. Hemodynamic Characteristics of Cerebral Arteriovenous Malformation Feeder Vessels With and Without Aneurysms. Stroke. 2015; 46(7):1997–1999

[21] Alaraj A, Shakur SF, Amin-Hanjani S, et al. Changes in wall shear stress of cerebral arteriovenous malformation feeder arteries after embolization and surgery. Stroke. 2015; 46(5):1216–1220

[22] Spetzler RF, Zabramski JM. Surgical management of large AVMs. Acta Neurochir Suppl (Wien). 1988; 42:93–97

[23] Spetzler RF, Hargraves RW, McCormick PW, Zabramski JM, Flom RA, Zimmerman RS. Relationship of perfusion pressure and size to risk of hemorrhage from arteriovenous malformations. J Neurosurg. 1992; 76(6):918–923

[24] Kim H, Abla AA, Nelson J, et al. Validation of the supplemented Spetzler-Martin grading system for brain arteriovenous malformations in a multicenter cohort of 1009 surgical patients. Neurosurgery. 2015; 76(1):25–31, discussion 31–32, quiz 32–33

[25] Lasjaunias P, Chiu M, ter Brugge K, Tolia A, Hurth M, Bernstein M. Neurological manifestations of intracranial dural arteriovenous malformations. J Neurosurg. 1986; 64(5):724–730

[26] Choi JH, Mast H, Hartmann A, et al. Clinical and morphological determinants of focal neurological deficits in patients with unruptured brain arteriovenous malformation. J Neurol Sci. 2009; 287(1–2):126–130

[27] Hassler W, Steinmetz H. Cerebral hemodynamics in angioma patients: an intraoperative study. J Neurosurg. 1987; 67(6):822–831

[28] De Salles AA, Manchola I. CO2 reactivity in arteriovenous malformations of the brain: a transcranial Doppler ultrasound study. J Neurosurg. 1994; 80(4):624–630

[29] Hoffman WE, Charbel FT, Edelman G, Abood C. Brain tissue response to CO2 in patients with arteriovenous malformation. J Cereb Blood Flow Metab. 1996; 16(6):1383–1386

[30] Spetzler RF, Wilson CB, Weinstein P, Mehdorn M, Townsend J, Telles D. Normal perfusion pressure breakthrough theory. Clin Neurosurg. 1978; 25:651–672

[31] Young WL, Pile-Spellman J, Prohovnik I, Kader A, Stein BM, Columbia University AVM Study Project. Evidence for adaptive autoregulatory displacement in hypotense cortical territories adjacent to arteriovenous malformations. Neurosurgery. 1994; 34(4):601–610, discussion 610–611

[32] Schaller C, Schramm J, Haun D, Meyer B. Patterns of cortical oxygen saturation changes during CO2 reactivity testing in the vicinity of cerebral arteriovenous malformations. Stroke. 2003; 34(4):938–944

[33] Moftakhar P, Hauptman JS, Malkasian D, Martin NA. Cerebral arteriovenous malformations. Part 2: physiology. Neurosurg Focus. 2009; 26(5):E11

[34] Josephson CB, Rosenow F, Al-Shahi Salman R. Intracranial Vascular Malformations and Epilepsy. Semin Neurol. 2015; 35(3):223–234

[35] al-Rodhan NR, Sundt TM , Jr, Piepgras DG, Nichols DA, Rüfenacht D, Stevens LN. Occlusive hyperemia: a theory for the hemodynamic complications following resection of intracerebral arteriovenous malformations. J Neurosurg. 1993; 78(2):167–175

[36] Choudhri O, Ivan ME, Lawton MT. Transvenous Approach to Intracranial Arteriovenous Malformations: Challenging the Axioms of Arteriovenous Malformation Therapy? Neurosurgery. 2015; 77(4):644–651, discussion 652

[37] Awad IA, Little JR, Akarawi WP, Ahl J. Intracranial dural arteriovenous malformations: factors predisposing to an aggressive neurological course. J Neurosurg. 1990; 72(6):839–850

[38] Kwon BJ, Han MH, Kang HS, Chang KH. MR imaging findings of intracranial dural arteriovenous fistulas: relations with venous drainage patterns. AJNR Am J Neuroradiol. 2005; 26(10):2500–2507

[39] Borden JA, Wu JK, Shucart WA. A proposed classification for spinal and cranial dural arteriovenous fistulous malformations and implications for treatment. J Neurosurg. 1995; 82(2):166–179

[40] Cognard C, Gobin YP, Pierot L, et al. Cerebral dural arteriovenous fistulas: clinical and angiographic correlation with a revised classification of venous drainage. Radiology. 1995; 194(3):671–680

[41] Lalwani AK, Dowd CF, Halbach VV. Grading venous restrictive disease in patients with dural arteriovenous fistulas of the transverse/sigmoid sinus. J Neurosurg. 1993; 79(1):11–15

[42] Kirsch M, Liebig T, Kühne D, Henkes H. Endovascular management of dural arteriovenous fistulas of the transverse and sigmoid sinus in 150 patients. Neuroradiology. 2009; 51(7):477–483

[43] Youn SW, Kim HK, Lee HJ, Lee J. Quantification of cerebral circulation and shunt volume in a tentorial dural arteriovenous fistula using two-dimensional phase-contrast magnetic resonance imaging. Acta Radiol Short Rep. 2014; 3(5):2047981614536559

[44] Kanemaru K, Kinouchi H, Yoshioka H, et al. Cerebral hemodynamic disturbance in dural arteriovenous fistula with retrograde leptomeningeal venous drainage: a prospective study using (123)I-iodoamphetamine single photon emission computed tomography. J Neurosurg. 2015; 123(1):110–117

[45] Hassler W, Thron A. Flow velocity and pressure measurements in spinal dural arteriovenous fistulas. Neurosurg Rev. 1994; 17(1):29–36

[46] Lasjuanias P, Berenstein A. Craniofacial and Upper Cervical Arteries: Functional, Clinical and Angiographic Aspects. Baltimore, MD: Williams & Wilkins; 1983

[47] Lapresle J, Lasjaunias P. Cranial nerve ischaemic arterial syndromes. A review. Brain. 1986; 109(Pt 1):207–216

[48] Shownkeen H, Bova D, Origitano TC, Petruzzelli GJ, Leonetti JP. Carotid-cavernous fistulas: pathogenesis and routes of approach to endovascular treatment. Skull Base. 2001; 11(3):207–218

[49] Kühner A, Krastel A, Stoll W. Arteriovenous malformations of the transverse dural sinus. J Neurosurg. 1976; 45(1):12–19

[50] Collice M, D'Aliberti G, Talamonti G, et al. Surgical interruption of leptomeningeal drainage as treatment for intracranial dural arteriovenous fistulas without dural sinus drainage. J Neurosurg. 1996; 84(5):810–817

[51] Kuwayama N, Kubo M, Tsumura K, Yamamoto H, Endo S. Hemodynamic status and treatment of aggressive dural arteriovenous fistulas. Acta Neurochir Suppl (Wien). 2005; 94:123–126

[52] Cognard C, Casasco A, Toevi M, Houdart E, Chiras J, Merland JJ. Dural arteriovenous fistulas as a cause of intracranial hypertension due to impairment of cranial venous outflow. J Neurol Neurosurg Psychiatry. 1998; 65(3):308–316

[53] Kashba SR, Patel NJ, Grace M, et al. Angiographic, hemodynamic, and histological changes in an animal model of brain arteriovenous malformations treated with Gamma Knife radiosurgery. J Neurosurg. 2015; 123(4):954–960

[54] Barrow DL, Spector RH, Braun IF, Landman JA, Tindall SC, Tindall GT. Classification and treatment of spontaneous carotid-cavernous sinus fistulas. J Neurosurg. 1985; 62(2):248–256

[55] Williamson A, Patrylo PR, Lee S, Spencer DD. Physiology of human cortical neurons adjacent to cavernous malformations and tumors. Epilepsia. 2003; 44(11):1413–1419

[56] Russin J, Babiker H, Ryan J, Rangel-Castilla L, Frakes D, Nakaji P. Computational fluid dynamics to evaluate the management of a giant internal carotid artery aneurysm. World Neurosurg. 2015; 83(6):1057–1065

[57] Chandran A, Radon M, Biswas S, Das K, Puthuran M, Nahser H. Novel use of 4D-CTA in imaging of intranidal aneurysms in an acutely ruptured arteriovenous malformation: is this the way forward? J Neurointerv Surg. 2016; 8(9):e36

[58] Raoult H, Bannier E, Maurel P, et al. Hemodynamic quantification in brain arteriovenous malformations with time-resolved spin-labeled magnetic resonance angiography. Stroke. 2014; 45(8):2461–2464

4 Natural History, Clinical Presentation, and Indications for Treatment of Brain Arteriovenous Malformations

Amit Singla and Brian Hoh

Abstract

Brain arteriovenous malformations (BAVMs) are dynamic vascular lesions with blood flow characterized by high velocities and low resistances without normal cerebral hemodynamic autoregulation, with an innate propensity to rupture.

The patients harboring these can present with varied clinical presentations ranging from asymptomatic to symptoms resulting from hemorrhage or mass effect. Intracranial hemorrhage is the most common clinical presentation. Annual rupture rate of BAVMs ranges from 2 to 4%. The risk of rehemorrhage in the first year is 9 to 15%. Then the risk decreases over time to about 2 to 4% after 5 years. The presentation with hemorrhage, deep venous drainage, and deep location and the presence of associated aneurysms are more commonly agreed upon factors that increase the risk for future AVM hemorrhage.

Ruptured BAVMs need to be treated because of the high risk of rerupture; however, the management of unruptured BAVMs is still a matter of debate. AVMs often require multimodality treatment requiring a multidisciplinary team with expertise in cerebrovascular neurosurgery, endovascular intervention, and radiation therapy.

BAVM microsurgery is generally an elective procedure unless associated with life-threatening hematoma or prenidal or nidal aneurysm or unless it is a small, easily accessible AVM which can be completely treated. A Randomized Trial of Unruptured Brain Arteriovenous malformations (ARUBA) showed that medical management alone is superior to medical management with interventional therapy in patients followed up for 33 months. However, this trial has been criticized for multiple reasons. The current evidence suggests that conservative management cannot be generalized to all unruptured BAVMs and the management strategy needs to be individualized.

Keywords: brain arteriovenous malformations, ARUBA trial, radiosurgery, endovascular embolization, microsurgery

Key Points

- Brain AVM can be an incidental finding or the patient can present with symptoms resulting from hemorrhage or mass effect.
- Ruptured BAVMs need to be treated due to the high risk of rerupture; however, the management of unruptured BAVMs is still controversial.
- Patients with brain AVMs often require multimodality treatment requiring a multidisciplinary team.
- A randomized trial of Unruptured Brain Arteriovenous malformations (ARUBA) showed that medical management alone is superior to medical management with interventional therapy. The trial has been criticized for several study limitations.
- Current evidence recommends that the management strategy for unruptured brain AVMs should be individualized.

4.1 Introduction

There is a remarkable heterogeneity in the natural history studies of brain arteriovenous malformations (BAVMs) suggesting that our understanding has continued to evolve since BAVMs were first described by Steinheil in 1895. BAVMs are relatively rare, with a yearly incidence of approximately 1 per 100,000 persons and a prevalence of 18 per 100,000 persons.[1] BAVMs consist of a tangle of abnormal blood vessels (nidus) in which the feeding arteries are directly connected to a venous drainage network without interposition of a capillary bed. Blood flow in BAVMs is characterized by high velocities and low resistances without normal cerebral hemodynamic autoregulation with an innate propensity to rupture. Furthermore, because the brain and its blood vessels are formed together during embryological development, abnormal blood vessel formation is often associated with abnormal brain tissue. Studies are currently under way ranging from designing models to discern genetic and hemodynamic influences on disease inception and progression, to using already developed models to design therapeutic interventions.

4.2 Pathologic Inception

Studies of resected BAVMs show evidence for angiogenesis with increased endothelial cell turnover and inflammatory cell–mediated vascular remodeling; however, little is known about the etiology of BAVMs, which is likely multifactorial. Etiopathogenesis of BAVMs remains controversial with genetic influences on abnormal angiogenesis/vasculogenesis and inflammation-induced angiogenic stimulation appearing to play roles during BAVM development. Recent reports of familial occurrence of BAVM, along with the known association with genetic disorders (Sturge–Weber disease, Osler–Weber–Rendu disease, hereditary hemorrhagic telangiectasia), support a genetic basis for the development, growth, and clinical behaviors (such as rupture) of BAVMs.[2] Current research on the genetic pathophysiology of BAVMs involves hypothesis-driven candidate gene studies where genes are implicated based on associated disorders and expression profiling from resected BAVM tissue. These candidate genes are currently used for model systems to discern mechanisms of BAVM development and potential therapeutic intervention.[2]

Classically, BAVM research has centered on genetic involvement in abnormal angiogenesis or the budding of endothelial cells from existing vasculature to form additional abnormal vessels at the nidus, either congenitally or in response to injury. Elevated incidence rates of sporadic BAVM in patients have been associated with the loss of function of genes encoding for proteins involved in vascular remodeling and appropriate angiogenesis. For example, the polymorphisms in activin receptor–like kinase 1 (ALK1) and multiple genetic loci influencing vascular endothelial growth factor (VEGF) levels have been attributed to loss of distinct arterial and venous boundaries during arteriolization in vascular remodeling, thus increasing susceptibility to BAVM formation and rupture. Additionally, current research has shown that these same genes may also support vasculogenesis or the independent development of additional vessels from endothelial progenitor cells (EPCs). Immunohistological analysis of BAVM tissue has shown that EPCs accumulate at the edge of vessel walls at the BAVM nidus, thus also contributing to its expansion.[2,3]

Furthermore, recent genetic studies have implicated polymorphisms in the promoter regions of proinflammatory cytokines such as interleukin-1β (IL-1β), IL-6, and tumor necrosis factor α (TNF α), with an increased BAVM incidence, an initial clinical presentation of hemorrhage in patients leading to a diagnosis of BAVM, an increased incidence of hemorrhage in patients diagnosed with BAVM, and an increased risk of posttreatment hemorrhage (as reviewed in Kim et al[3]). The most notable is the contribution of IL-6, which leads to the upregulation of the additional cytokines.[4] The cytokines stimulate leukocyte recruitment, VEGF, and angiopoietin-2 (ANG-2) expression, leading to increased angiogenesis, vascular smooth muscle cell proliferation, and matrix metalloproteinase protein 9 (MMP9) expression. The level of MMP9 expression has been found to be an order of magnitude higher in BAVM tissue compared with controls. This leads to the overexpression of other proinflammatory markers associated with MMP9, such as myeloperoxidase and ILs (IL-6), which creates an environment of vascular instability at the BAVM nidus and increases susceptibility to rupture.[3] Future studies to elucidate the genetic pathophysiology of BAVM formation and progression to rupture will likely expand to include genome-wide association and high-density single nucleotide polymorphism studies.

4.3 Progression to Clinical End Points

As our understanding of the physiology of BAVMs increases, the traditional thought that these were static congenital lesions has now evolved into a more dynamic view. Through genetic and hemodynamic influences, formed BAVMs can undergo vascular remodeling and change in size, by either expanding or regressing. This, in turn, manifests into a varied range of clinical presentations from patients remaining asymptomatic to presenting with clinical symptoms associated with mass effect or intracerebral hemorrhage (ICH) due to rupture. Specific hemodynamic influences include elevated feeding artery pressures, disrupted venous drainage, the presence of a perinidal hypervascular network, and the vascular steal phenomenon.[5]

BAVMs can be monocompartmental, consisting of a single feeder vessel and one or more draining veins, or they can be multicompartmental, consisting of multiple feeder vessels and draining veins that are adjacent or separated by brain tissue. Studies have noted that smaller BAVMs (< 3 cm), though not as prone to be symptomatic due to mass effect, have significantly higher rates of rupture. This is due to increased intra-arterial resistance and pressure of the feeder vessels, which is inversely proportional to the size of the BAVM.[6,7] Coupled with elevated input pressures, hemodynamic strain on the BAVM can be exacerbated by obstruction of venous outflow. One study found that 30% of AVMs have abnormal venous drainage.[8] Furthermore, the decreased drainage may lead to hypoperfusion of surrounding brain tissue. This hypoperfusion, coupled with a vascular steal phenomenon created by the BAVM, is thought to stimulate expression of angiogenic factors, such as VEGF, resulting in the expansion of the BAVM. Additionally, decreased venous drainage may also increase intraluminal pressure to a level that opens preexisting patent arteriovenous connections, which would also contribute to growth of the BAVM. This can be seen particularly with multicompartmental BAVMs, in which "hidden compartments" of perinidal vessels that were not initially seen on angiography may abruptly fill, leading to rupture or edema (as reviewed in Moftakhar[5]).

4.4 Clinical Presentation

Often patients with BAVMs may experience no symptoms and they are discovered only incidentally, usually either at autopsy or during treatment for an unrelated disorder. The proportion of patients being diagnosed with unruptured AVMs has almost doubled in the past three decades with improved noninvasive imaging.[9] However, approximately 12% of people with AVMs will experience symptoms, varying in severity. ICH from a ruptured AVM is consistently described as the most common presenting symptom, occurring at 50% of initial presentations. Mortality for ICH as a first presentation of an AVM ranges from 10 to 30%.[10] Traditionally, an annual rupture rate of 4% has been cited for BAVMs based on a study on natural history of symptomatic BAVMs; this study also included the AVMs, which had previously ruptured.[11] A Randomized Trial of Unruptured Brain Arteriovenous Malformations (ARUBA) reported a low spontaneous rupture rate of 2.2% per year (95% confidence interval [CI] 0.9–4.5).[12] Other recent prospective studies have also reported lower bleeding rates of about 1% per year for unruptured BAVMs.[13,14]

Overall, studies have shown that the rate of rehemorrhage in patients with the initial presentation of a hemorrhage decreases over time. The highest risk is within the first year of diagnosis, from 9.65 to 15.42%. In years 2 to 5, the risk drops from 5.32 to 6.3%, and is the lowest after 5 years (1.7–3.67%).[15] Fewer studies have quantified the effect of the additional factors on the risk of hemorrhage. One study has found that deep venous drainage increases the risk by 0.9 to 2.4% per year, and that the deep or infratentorial brain region increases the risk by 0.9 to 3.1%.[14] However, these risk factors are intricately interlaced, and studies looking at them in isolation do not give a true picture of disease progression to hemorrhage.

Unruptured BAVMs can become symptomatic by mass effect due to irritation of the surrounding brain. This may result in the second most common presenting symptom, seizures, seen in approximately 30% of cases. Alternately, the third most common presenting symptom, also due to mass effect, is headache, which occurs in 5 to 14% of cases.[16,17] Additional symptoms that may occur corresponding to the location of the AVM include myasthenia, paralysis, ataxia, executive dysfunction, dizziness, visual disturbances, dysphasia, dysesthesia, memory deficits, hallucinations, and dementia.

4.5 Indications for Treatment of BAVMs

Although the management of ruptured BAVMs is less of a dilemma with the intervention recommended for most cases except the high-risk ones, the management of unruptured BAVMs is still a matter of debate. Both conservative close follow-up with medical management of the symptoms and eradication with an intervention are recognized management strategies in patients with BAVMs. The definitive treatment for BAVMs is targeted toward eliminating the risk for ICH while preserving or maximizing the functional status. When the decision has been made to pursue intervention, complete nidal obliteration should be the goal, given that subtotal obliteration does not provide protection from future hemorrhage.

4.5.1 Classification Schemes

Various classification systems have been proposed over the years in an effort to assist the treating physicians in *surgical decision making* when dealing with BAVM. In 1986, Spetzler and Martin introduced a classification system, which was based on the dimensions, location, and type of venous drainage from the BAVMs.[18] In this classification system, the higher the grade of the AVM, the higher the surgical risk. The authors recommended that small lesions in noneloquent tissue that fall under Spetzler–Martin (SM) grades I and II are primarily treated via surgical resection with or without adjunct endovascular embolization, while grade III lesions may be treated with endovascular embolization followed by surgery. Grade IV and V lesions are often considered high risk and preferentially managed medically.[18] To simplify the treatment decision, Spetzler and Ponce proposed the three-tier classification system in which the grades I and II and grades IV and V from the original classification were clubbed together in tiers A and C, respectively, and tier B corresponded to grade III. Surgery was recommended as the treatment modality for class A and multimodality treatment for class B. No treatment was recommended for class C. The high reported rates (25–30%) of morbidity associated with surgery, lack of immediate protection, and possible elevated risk of hemorrhage associated with radiation or partial embolization are cited as the reasons for recommending conservative or palliative management in patients with grade IV and V AVMs.[19]

Lawton et al proposed a simple supplementary grading system for BAVM which could be used to improve and refine patient selection for AVM surgery.[20] This was based on the authors' previous experience that factors such as hemorrhagic presentation, young age, compactness of the AVM nidus, and absence of deep perforator supply were identified as the predictors of good outcomes after microsurgical resection.[21,22] The supplementary grade may influence surgical decisions for AVM patients at the borderline between high and low risk based on SM grading system.[20]

4.6 Factors Influencing the Treatment Decision

Broadly, the factors influencing the treatment decision can be divided into AVM architecture–related and patient-related factors.

4.6.1 AVM Architecture–Related Factors

The factors mentioned in the literature as being related to increased risk of hemorrhage from BAVMs include[23,24,25,26,27]
- Presentation with hemorrhage.
- Presence of deep venous drainage.
- Associated aneurysms.
- Deep brain location.
- Smaller AVM size.
- Venous outlet restriction.
- Single draining vein.
- Diffuse AVM morphology.

The presentation with *hemorrhage, deep venous drainage, and deep location and the presence of associated aneurysms* are more commonly agreed upon factors that increase the risk for future AVM hemorrhage.[28] Previous history of rupture is probably the strongest factor related to the increased future risk of rehemorrhage from an AVM. Recent meta-analysis showed that unruptured AVMs had an overall annual risk of hemorrhage of 2.2% (95% CI, 1.7–2.7%), whereas ruptured AVMs had an overall annual rupture rate of 4.5% (95% CI, 3.7–5.5%).[28] Deep brain involvement, basal ganglia or thalamic lesions, or in the periventricular region, or the AVMs with exclusively deep venous drainage also appear to have a higher hemorrhage rate.[29,30] AVM-related aneurysms, seen in approximately 15 to 18% of patients, have been shown to independently increase the risk of future hemorrhage.[28,31] The patients having these factors are more likely to have future hemorrhage, and the treatment, if indicated, should commence sooner rather than later. It is important to highlight that the influence of these risk factors is additive.[32]

Old Hemorrhage

Abla et al stressed upon another important criterion of "old hemorrhage" in determining the "seemingly" unruptured AVMs which had silent hemorrhages before the presentation. Such AVMs with prior small hemorrhages labeled as "microhemorrhage" are clinically silent, often without even a headache. This study showed that silent intralesional microhemorrhage was a risk factor for later AVM rupture. Both evidence of old hemorrhage (odds ratio [OR], 3.97; *p* = 0.001) and hemosiderin positivity (OR, 3.64; *p* = 0.034) were highly predictive of index intracerebral AVM hemorrhage. One-third of patients have been reported to present with silent hemorrhage; they are best diagnosed with *iron-sensitive imaging protocol magnetic resonance imaging (MRI) scan*. They suggested that such AVMs are at a high risk of rupture and should be treated with intervention.[33]

AVMs with Aneurysms

AVMs with associated aneurysms deserve mention as a separate entity. Aneurysms in conjunction with BAVMs are seen in about 20 to 25% of patients with AVMs. In a recent meta-analysis, associated aneurysms were found to be a statistically significant risk factor for hemorrhage with a hazard ratio of 1.8 (95% CI, 1.6–2).[28] Hemorrhages from AVMs are classically thought to have a relatively small early rebleeding rate compared to simple intracranial aneurysms, although there are reports of early rebleeding from AVM-associated aneurysms. Such aneurysms are treated according to their location and size, preferably prior to treating the

AVM itself because of the elevated risk of rupture. The aneurysms located within the nidus or prenidal aneurysms should be treated in the setting of hemorrhage or if they are large (> 7 mm) in unruptured AVMs. Distal flow–related aneurysms often involute after treatment of the AVM nidus.[32]

Giant AVMs

Large or giant AVMs with diffuse hemispheric or bilateral cerebral involvement (SM grade IV or V) or Spetzler and Ponce tier C may not be amenable for the treatment and are managed conservatively. The patients with such AVMs can present with ischemic symptoms from the steal phenomenon; palliative care with endovascular embolization may be offered to such patients to decrease size of the lesion and for symptomatic improvement.[34]

4.6.2 Patient-Related Factors

Age

Age is one of the most important factors in determining the treatment versus conservative management and also the modality of treatment. The lifetime risk of hemorrhage from an AVM is higher in the younger patients, justifying a lower threshold for offering the treatment.

Symptomatic versus Asymptomatic

Symptomatic patients such as those presenting with seizures might benefit from treatment. Obliteration of the AVM may result in symptomatic improvement including seizures; a study showed that after treatment of symptomatic AVMs, 83% patients were seizure-free 2 years after undergoing microsurgery.[35]

Medical Status

Similarly, patients with significant medical comorbidities and limited longevity may not be good candidates for more aggressive treatment option such as surgery; however, stereotactic radiosurgery (SRS) might still be offered.

4.7 Lifetime Risk of Hemorrhage

To predict the lifetime risk of hemorrhage in a given individual, Kondziolka and colleagues[36] suggested a simple model based on life expectancy and the multiplicative law of probability. This predictive model assumes that for a particular individual in question, the risk of hemorrhage is constant over time. According to their calculations, the lifetime risk of hemorrhage can be estimated using the following formula:

$$1 - (\text{risk of no hemorrhage})^{\text{expected years of remaining life}}.$$

Using this formula, a patient with a life expectancy of 50 years and a yearly risk of hemorrhage of 4% would be predicted to have the lifetime risk of AVM bleed as follows:

$$1 - (0.96)^{50} \approx 87\%.$$

A *simpler model* assuming a constant 3% yearly risk of hemorrhage can also be used and still maintains a similar sensitivity[10]:

Lifetime risk of hemorrhage = 105 − patient age in years.

For example, a 35-year-old person with an AVM would have a lifetime risk of hemorrhage of

$$105 - 35 = 70\%.$$

4.8 Ruptured Brain Arteriovenous Malformations

Hemorrhage from a ruptured BAVM carries a 10 to 30% risk of death and a 30 to 50% chance of permanent neurologic deficits.[10] The published literature is consistent with the finding that previous rupture is the most important factor when assessing a patient's future risk of hemorrhage. BAVM rupture is associated with an increased risk of 6% rerupture in the year following the initial hemorrhage, versus 1 to 3% predicted annual risk in nonruptured lesions.[10] Fults and Kelly, in a retrospective analysis of 131 patients with AVM, discovered a tendency of increasing mortality with subsequent episodes of hemorrhage from 13.6 to 20.7 to 25%, after the first, second, and third episodes, respectively, although statistical significance was not reached.[37] In contrast, other studies have shown that recurrent hemorrhages do not have a cumulative impact on the prognosis.[38,39] Although the data on the issue of cumulative effects of each subsequent hemorrhage are conflicting, each individual hemorrhagic episode has its own associated morbidity and mortality, underscoring the importance of the fact that ruptured AVMs need to be treated. However, ruptured AVMs are classically thought to have a relatively small early rebleeding rate as compared to ruptured saccular intracranial aneurysms, justifying delay in treatment after stabilizing the patient and allowing the brain swelling to decrease. A rest period of a few weeks to months after hemorrhage is recommended before definitive treatment to allow for the brain swelling to decrease, for better delineation of the lesion and to avoid disrupting friable parenchyma.[32]

4.8.1 Timing of Surgery

Timing of AVM microsurgery is generally an elective procedure unless the patient presents with ICH or life-threatening hydrocephalus secondary to hematoma. In such emergent cases, resection at the time of clot removal is only indicated for superficial AVMs in which the anatomy can be readily elucidated. Otherwise, hemorrhage or hematoma-related complications must be resolved first, followed by postoperative rehabilitation and angiographic analysis. However, there are certain clinical and radiological features which can justify emergent/earlier surgical and/or endovascular management. These include large life-threatening hematomas causing cerebral herniation, hydrocephalus, or prenidal or nidal aneurysms, and small, easily accessible AVMs which can be completely treated.[10,32] The patients presenting with ICH and suspected of harboring a vascular malformation should be evaluated with noninvasive studies such as computed tomography angiography (CTA)/magnetic resonance angiography

(MRA) as the initial screening tools. Conventional digital subtraction angiography (DSA) remains the most sensitive and specific diagnostic modality and should be performed within the next 24 hours of presentation to evaluate the cause of hemorrhage and to identify high-risk factors.[10,32]

Aneurysms associated with AVMs are treated according to their location and size, preferably prior to treating the AVM itself because of the elevated risk of rupture. Small feeding aneurysms < 5 mm may regress after AVM treatment and thus may not require treatment prior to AVM resection; larger feeding artery aneurysms (> 7 mm) are usually treated endovascularly prior to obliteration or resection of the AVM. Once the prenidal or nidal aneurysms are treated, the definitive treatment with embolization with or without other modalities such as surgical resection and radiosurgery can be deferred until the patient and the hematoma have stabilized.[32]

4.9 Unruptured Brain Arteriovenous Malformations

In contrast to the ruptured BAVMs, the management of unruptured BAVMs remains controversial at this time, more so if they are asymptomatic. Some of the more recent studies have reported the *annual AVM rupture rate of as low as 1%*, much lower than the 4% reported in an earlier retrospective study.[13,14] Besides the lower ruptures, another reason cited for conservative management of unruptured AVMs is the *mild first hemorrhagic episode* associated with AVM rupture.[40,41] The notion that patients with incidental AVMs may have worse outcomes with the intervention as compared to those with hemorrhagic presentation, and the morbidity and mortality of hemorrhagic episodes associated with AVM rupture might have been overestimated in the literature in the past, argues for close monitoring of incidental AVMs instead of the intervention.[42] The ARUBA trial showed that medical management alone is superior to medical management with interventional therapy for prevention of death or stroke in patients followed up for 33 months. This trial was stopped prematurely because of significant benefit seen in the medically managed group. Medical management group (109 patients) in this trial had a threefold lower incidence of stroke or death (10.1 vs. 30.7%) as compared to the patients assigned to interventional therapy (114 patients). The interventions performed consisted of embolization (32%), radiosurgery (33%), embolization plus radiosurgery (16%), or surgery (18%).[12]

The ARUBA study has been criticized for multiple reasons including the fact that surgical resection as the intervention was performed for only 18 patients out of 76 patients with low-grade AVMs who were randomized to intervention.[43] Most AVMs were treated with embolization or radiosurgery, both of which have lower obliteration rates than microsurgical resection.[44,45] Thus, the higher rate of stroke or death and clinical impairment in ARUBA's interventional therapy arm reflects not only treatment-associated effects, but also complications from partially treated AVMs. Finally, ARUBA's relatively short follow-up of 33 months favors medical management, since curative effects would take longer for the any-treatment group and differences observed between the two arms might dissipate over time.[43] In contrast to the ARUBA trial, a large series of patients

from a prospectively collected database which was retrospectively analyzed showed Spetzler–Ponce class A and Spetzler–Ponce class B unruptured BAVMs treated by surgery had a better outcome than conservatively managed unruptured BAVMs within a short period of time with a high rate of cure. One of the reasons cited for the difference in the outcome is due to the fact that most patients in this study were treated with surgery alone and the rest of the patients were treated by surgery with adjunctive preoperative embolization. They concluded that the defined group of patients can be better managed with surgery than conservative management alone.[46]

Nonetheless, the literature suggests that the conservative management cannot be generalized to all unruptured BAVMs. This decision dilemma has led to the attempts to better identify/define the risk factors that significantly increase the risk of future hemorrhage making the intervention a more reasonable and better option than conservative treatment. With more diagnostic and therapeutic options available, it seems prudent to determine the future bleeding risk for an unruptured BAVM to provide adequate management strategy, either an aggressive treatment plan targeted at complete occlusion for BAVMs with risk factors for hemorrhage or supporting a more conservative approach for those at lesser risk.

4.10 Treatment Planning

Once the decision has been made to treat an AVM, the goal is directed toward complete AVM nidal obliteration. The three major treatment modalities include microsurgery, SRS, and endovascular embolization; all have been successfully used alone or in combination to treat AVMs (▶ Fig. 4.1 and ▶ Fig. 4.2).

4.10.1 Microsurgical Treatment

Microsurgical curative resection of the AVM remains the mainstay treatment modality when viable, primarily due to the fact that it provides immediate cure.[47] Microsurgery is also performed as a part of multimodal treatment planning involving a preliminary endovascular approach to reduce the nidal size and curing associated high surgical risk vascular anomalies such as aneurysms (▶ Fig. 4.1). Microsurgical resection has been reported to be able to achieve 94 to 100% angiographic cure with low morbidity rates (1–10%) in small AVMs.[48] Surgical resection of AVMs has also been credited with providing good seizure control in patients with AVMs without hemorrhage.[49,50] In a comparative study looking at seizure control with surgery resection versus radiosurgery, Wang et al reported that surgical resection may result in improved seizure control compared with radiosurgery for patients presenting with seizures. Conversely, in patients without presenting seizures, surgical resection was found to increase the risk of new-onset seizures compared with radiosurgery, primarily within the early post-treatment period.[51]

The SM grading system developed in 1986 provides risk stratification associated with surgical resection of the AVM. SM grades I and II are considered suitable for surgical resection with a low morbidity and mortality. Grade III lesions are generally treated with microsurgical resection or SRS with or without adjunctive endovascular embolization.[42] To further assist with

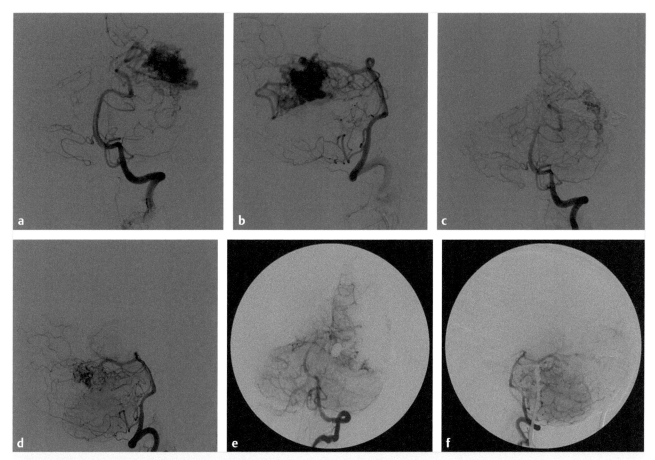

Fig. 4.1 (a,b) A 40-year-old woman presented with frequent episodes of alexia, headache, nausea, and memory loss suspicious for temporal lobe seizures. She was found to have a left posterotemporal lobe arteriovenous malformation supplied by multiple distal branches of the left posterotemporal branch of the left posterior cerebral artery, the left anterior choroidal artery, and the left temporal branch of the left middle cerebral artery. The venous drainage is via multiple superficial cortical draining veins, which drain to the transverse sinus and the superior sagittal sinus. This is a Spetzler–Martin grade II AVM (less than 3 cm, superficial venous drainage, eloquent location). **(c,d)** Two-stage Onyx embolization of the AVM was performed via a left posterotemporal branch of the left posterior cerebral artery and a left temporal branch of the left middle cerebral artery, resulting in partial obliteration of the AVM. There was still persistent supply from a small left posterior temporal branch of the left posterior cerebral artery with preserved venous drainage. **(e,f)** Surgical resection was performed for the residual AVM through left subtemporal approach. Intraoperative cerebral angiogram demonstrated 100% complete surgical obliteration of the AVM.

treatment planning in patients with SM grade III lesions, a revised classification scheme suggested that SM grade IIIA (size > 6 cm) lesions should be managed with microsurgical resection with adjunctive embolization. SM grade IIIB (venous drainage or eloquence) lesions should be managed with SRS with or without embolization.[52] For this heterogeneous group of grade III AVMs, additional modification scheme has been proposed in which grade III AVMs have been subdivided into the following four types[53]:

- S1V1E1 (small nidus size, deep venous drainage, and eloquent adjacent brain tissue).
- S2V1E0 (medium nidus size, deep venous drainage, and noneloquent adjacent brain tissue).
- S2V0E1 (medium nidus size, superficial venous drainage, and eloquent adjacent brain tissue).
- S3V0E0 (large nidus size, superficial venous drainage, and noneloquent adjacent brain tissue).

The authors concluded that small SM grade III AVMs (S1V1E1) have a surgical risk similar to that of grade I and II AVMs and

can be safely treated with microsurgical resection. Medium size/eloquent grade III AVMs (S2V0E1) have a surgical risk similar to that of high-grade AVMs and are best managed conservatively. Medium size/deep venous drainage grade III AVMs (S2V1E0) have intermediate surgical risks and careful selection for surgery is warranted. Large grade III AVMs (S3V0E0) are rare with an unclear surgical risk, although surgical resection with or without embolization can be carefully considered on an individual patient basis.[53] As discussed before, surgery is generally avoided in patients with grade IV and V AVMs because of high morbidity risk.

4.10.2 Endovascular Embolization

AVM embolization can be performed as a *curative*, *adjunctive*, or *palliative* treatment modality. Embolization is usually performed with liquid embolic agents such as *n*-butyl cyanoacrylate (Raynham, Massachusetts) or Onyx (Medtronic, Minneapolis, Minnesota).[54] The goals of the embolization procedure should be specifically and prospectively identified as they vary

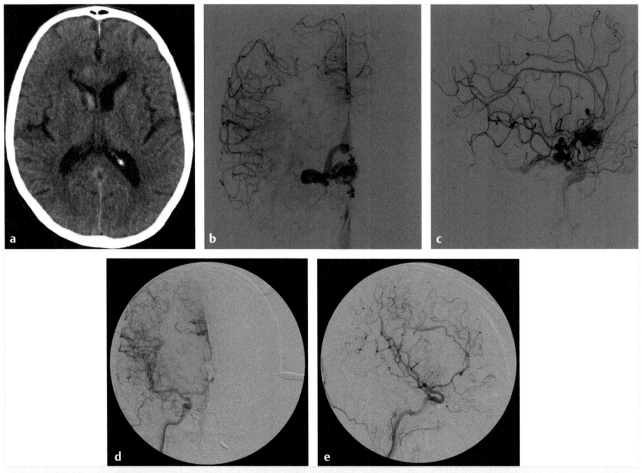

Fig. 4.2 A 64-year-old male presented with acute onset of frontal headache approximately 1 week prior. It was associated with photophobia, nausea/emesis, and neck stiffness. (a) Non-contrast head CT showing right frontal horn intraventricular hemorrhage and right frontal hyperdensity suggestive of hemorrhage from AVM. (b,c) Right internal carotid artery cerebral angiogram, anteroposterior and lateral views. Right frontal arteriovenous malformation is seen supplied by the right anterior cerebral artery. The AVM drains into the basal vein of Rosenthal. This is a Spetzler–Martin grade II AVM (less than 3 cm, noneloquent, deep venous drainage). Also seen is a 6.3 mm × 4.7 mm × 5 mm right A2–A3 aneurysm. (d,e) After unsuccessful attempted coiling of the associated aneurysm, surgical resection of the AVM with aneurysm clipping was performed. Intraoperative anteroposterior and lateral cerebral angiogram demonstrated complete clipping of the right A2–A3 aneurysm, as well as complete obliteration of the right frontal arteriovenous malformation.

with the indication of the procedure. Preoperative embolization of AVMs may not need aggressive attempts at deep nidal penetration of embolic materials as it may require for preradiosurgical or curative embolization. Complication rates of approximately 5 to 15% have been reported with AVM embolization.[55,56] A recent meta-analysis by van Beijnum et al found that complications leading to permanent neurological deficits or death occurred in 6.6% (range, 0–18%) of patients after AVM embolization.[57] Ledezma et al reported that SM grades III to V and periprocedural hemorrhage were the most important predictive factors in determining outcome after embolization.[58]

Embolization is most commonly performed as an *adjunct to microsurgical resection or SRS*. As a primary treatment modality, embolization leads to a low obliteration rate; the success rate is higher in a carefully selected group of patients.[59] As a *preoperative adjunct*, embolization is often performed to minimize blood loss, reduce operative time, and facilitate resection of larger lesions. Premicrosurgical embolization can help reduce the AVM size and eliminate the deep arterial pedicles, which can be

difficult to control surgically and can often only be accessed during the latter stages of surgical resection. Also, it helps in obliterating AVM-related aneurysms, especially if they are remote from the area of resection. Endovascular embolization has been shown to reduce operative times, decrease transfusions, and lower the morbidity and mortality.[60,61] *Preradiosurgical embolization* can be used to reduce overall nidal volume or target high-risk angiographic features of the lesion that may represent a source of hemorrhage during the latency period after SRS. Controversial outcomes on AVM obliteration rates with SRS have been reported in the literature with respect to the role of preradiosurgical embolization.[62,63,64,65] Because of these conflicting reports, the strategy of preradiosurgical embolization remains controversial at this time.

AVM cure with embolization has historically been achieved in only about 10 to 40% of cases.[34] Small AVMs with single-pedicle or few feeders, noncompartmental fistulous niduses, and no perinidal angiogenesis are some of the features of AVMs which are more amenable to complete cure with embolization alone. Frizzel and

Fisher reported a 5% cure rate for AVMs treated by endovascular embolization.[66] However, patients with angiographically "cured" AVMs may still be at risk for devastating hemorrhage if unseen feeders continue to fill a partially embolized nidus.

Palliative AVM embolization may be performed in patients with large/giant AVMs in whom the hope of cure by multimodality therapy is small. The goal of AVM embolization in such patients may include the targeted embolization of certain angioarchitectural features such as aneurysms or to provide symptomatic relief from ischemic symptoms from vascular steal. Aside from these scenarios, partial AVM embolization is not recommended, as outcomes seem to be worse than the natural history.[67]

4.10.3 Stereotactic Radiosurgery

SRS provides a less invasive management strategy for grade I or II patients who are either not good surgical candidates or unwilling to undergo surgical resection. It has also been recommended for patients with SM grade IIIB AVMs with or without adjunctive endovascular embolization. SRS is typically reserved for compact lesions < 3 cm and is highly beneficial for deep-seated lesions such as brainstem, thalamus, and basal ganglia, where surgical resection can be difficult and associated with high morbidity. SRS has been reported to be a more effective treatment modality for central lesions as compared to peripheral AVMs.[68] Limitations of SRS as a treatment modality include (1) iatrogenic morbidity and (2) latency in AVM obliteration of about 2 years from the treatment. During the latency, the risk of hemorrhage remains similar to the untreated unruptured AVMs.[69,70]

SRS is often performed as an adjunct to endovascular embolization, which is used to reduce the size of the AVM nidus prior to SRS. With the AVM volumes reduced to 10 mL or less with embolization, obliteration rates of about 80% have been reported with postembolization SRS.[63,69,70] Blackburn et al reported the AVM obliteration rate of 81% (13 of 16 cases) in patients who had follow-up catheter angiography. The maximum diameter of all AVMs in this series was > 3 cm (mean, 4.2 cm); 12 (57%) were SM grade IV or V.[62]

In contrast, some other reports suggest worse outcomes in such patients as compared to those in which SRS is used without preceding embolization.[64] A meta-analysis regarding the efficiency and safety of SRS for AVM patients with and without prior embolization showed that embolization before SRS significantly decreases the AVM obliteration rate. No significant difference was found in the risk of hemorrhage and permanent neurological deficits after SRS alone and following embolization.[65]

With SRS, complete obliteration of the AVM has been reported in about 50 to 90% of the cases.[69,70] The obliteration rate is inversely proportional to the AVM nidus size.[71,72] Complications leading to permanent neurological deficits or death are reported in 5.1% (range, 0–21%) of the cases.[68] Once considered cured after SRS, hemorrhagic events may still occur in < 1% patients.

4.11 Conclusion

AVMs often require multimodality treatment requiring a multi-disciplinary team with expertise in cerebrovascular neurosurgery, endovascular intervention, and radiation therapy in order to provide all therapeutic options and determine the most appropriate treatment regimen depending on patient characteristics and AVM morphology. Current therapeutic options include microsurgical resection, SRS, and endovascular embolization. It is critical to discuss the natural history of the AVMs as well as different treatment modalities with their risks and benefits to help patients make a well-informed decision.

References

[1] Laakso A, Hernesniemi J. Arteriovenous malformations: epidemiology and clinical presentation. Neurosurg Clin N Am. 2012; 23(1):1–6

[2] Achrol AS, Guzman R, Varga M, Adler JR, Steinberg GK, Chang SD. Pathogenesis and radiobiology of brain arteriovenous malformations: implications for risk stratification in natural history and posttreatment course. Neurosurg Focus. 2009; 26(5):E9

[3] Kim H, Su H, Weinsheimer S, Pawlikowska L, Young WL. Brain arteriovenous malformation pathogenesis: a response-to-injury paradigm. Acta Neurochir Suppl (Wien). 2011; 111:83–92

[4] Mouchtouris N, Jabbour PM, Starke RM, et al. Biology of cerebral arteriovenous malformations with a focus on inflammation. J Cereb Blood Flow Metab. 2015; 35(2):167–175

[5] Moftakhar P, Hauptman JS, Malkasian D, Martin NA. Cerebral arteriovenous malformations. Part 2: physiology. Neurosurg Focus. 2009; 26(5):E11

[6] Norris JS, Valiante TA, Wallace MC, et al. A simple relationship between radiological arteriovenous malformation hemodynamics and clinical presentation: a prospective, blinded analysis of 31 cases. J Neurosurg. 1999; 90(4):673–679

[7] Spetzler RF, Hargraves RW, McCormick PW, Zabramski JM, Flom RA, Zimmerman RS. Relationship of perfusion pressure and size to risk of hemorrhage from arteriovenous malformations. J Neurosurg. 1992; 76(6):918–923

[8] Yasargil MG. Pathological considerations. In: Yasargil MG, ed. Microneurosurgery. New York, NY: Thieme; 1987:49–211

[9] Al-Shahi R, Bhattacharya JJ, Currie DG, et al. Scottish Intracranial Vascular Malformation Study Collaborators. Prospective, population-based detection of intracranial vascular malformations in adults: the Scottish Intracranial Vascular Malformation Study (SIVMS). Stroke. 2003; 34(5):1163–1169

[10] Aoun SG, Bendok BR, Batjer HH. Acute management of ruptured arteriovenous malformations and dural arteriovenous fistulas. Neurosurg Clin N Am. 2012; 23(1):87–103

[11] Ondra SL, Troupp H, George ED, Schwab K. The natural history of symptomatic arteriovenous malformations of the brain: a 24-year follow-up assessment. J Neurosurg. 1990; 73(3):387–391

[12] Mohr JP, Parides MK, Stapf C, et al. international ARUBA investigators. Medical management with or without interventional therapy for unruptured brain arteriovenous malformations (ARUBA): a multicentre, non-blinded, randomised trial. Lancet. 2014; 383(9917):614–621

[13] Halim AX, Johnston SC, Singh V, et al. Longitudinal risk of intracranial hemorrhage in patients with arteriovenous malformation of the brain within a defined population. Stroke. 2004; 35(7):1697–1702

[14] Stapf C, Mast H, Sciacca RR, et al. Predictors of hemorrhage in patients with untreated brain arteriovenous malformation. Neurology. 2006; 66(9):1350–1355

[15] Abecassis IJ, Xu DS, Batjer HH, Bendok BR. Natural history of brain arteriovenous malformations: a systematic review. Neurosurg Focus. 2014; 37(3):E7

[16] Hofmeister C, Stapf C, Hartmann A, et al. Demographic, morphological, and clinical characteristics of 1289 patients with brain arteriovenous malformation. Stroke. 2000; 31(6):1307–1310

[17] Stapf C, Mohr JP, Pile-Spellman J, Solomon RA, Sacco RL, Connolly ES , Jr. Epidemiology and natural history of arteriovenous malformations. Neurosurg Focus. 2001; 11(5):e1

[18] Spetzler RF, Martin NA. A proposed grading system for arteriovenous malformations. J Neurosurg. 1986; 65(4):476–483

[19] Spetzler RF, Ponce FA. A 3-tier classification of cerebral arteriovenous malformations. Clinical article. J Neurosurg. 2011; 114(3):842–849

[20] Lawton MT, Kim H, McCulloch CE, Mikhak B, Young WL. A supplementary grading scale for selecting patients with brain arteriovenous malformations for surgery. Neurosurgery. 2010; 66(4):702–713, discussion 713

[21] Du R, Keyoung HM, Dowd CF, Young WL, Lawton MT. The effects of diffuseness and deep perforating artery supply on outcomes after microsurgical resection of brain arteriovenous malformations. Neurosurgery. 2007; 60(4): 638:646

[22] Lawton MT, Du R, Tran MN, et al. Effect of presenting hemorrhage on outcome after microsurgical resection of brain arteriovenous malformations. Neurosurgery. 2005; 56(3):485–493, discussion 485–493

[23] Khaw AV, Mohr JP, Sciacca RR, et al. Association of infratentorial brain arteriovenous malformations with hemorrhage at initial presentation. Stroke. 2004; 35(3):660–663

[24] Kubalek R, Moghtaderi A, Klisch J, Berlis A, Quiske A, Schumacher M. Cerebral arteriovenous malformations: influence of angioarchitecture on bleeding risk. Acta Neurochir (Wien). 2003; 145(12):1045–1052, discussion 1052

[25] Meisel HJ, Mansmann U, Alvarez H, Rodesch G, Brock M, Lasjaunias P. Cerebral arteriovenous malformations and associated aneurysms: analysis of 305 cases from a series of 662 patients. Neurosurgery. 2000; 46(4):793–800–; discussion 800–792

[26] Stapf C, Khaw AV, Sciacca RR, et al. Effect of age on clinical and morphological characteristics in patients with brain arteriovenous malformation. Stroke. 2003; 34(11):2664–2669

[27] Stefani MA, Porter PJ, terBrugge KG, Montanera W, Willinsky RA, Wallace MC. Large and deep brain arteriovenous malformations are associated with risk of future hemorrhage. Stroke. 2002; 33(5):1220–1224

[28] Gross BA, Du R. Natural history of cerebral arteriovenous malformations: a meta-analysis. J Neurosurg. 2013; 118(2):437–443

[29] Fleetwood IG, Marcellus ML, Levy RP, Marks MP, Steinberg GK. Deep arteriovenous malformations of the basal ganglia and thalamus: natural history. J Neurosurg. 2003; 98(4):747–750

[30] Stefani MA, Porter PJ, terBrugge KG, Montanera W, Willinsky RA, Wallace MC. Angioarchitectural factors present in brain arteriovenous malformations associated with hemorrhagic presentation. Stroke. 2002; 33(4):920–924

[31] Redekop G, TerBrugge K, Montanera W, Willinsky R. Arterial aneurysms associated with cerebral arteriovenous malformations: classification, incidence, and risk of hemorrhage. J Neurosurg. 1998; 89(4):539–546

[32] Zacharia BE, Vaughan KA, Jacoby A, Hickman ZL, Bodmer D, Connolly ES , Jr. Management of ruptured brain arteriovenous malformations. Curr Atheroscler Rep. 2012; 14(4):335–342

[33] Abla AA, Nelson J, Kim H, Hess CP, Tihan T, Lawton MT. Silent arteriovenous malformation hemorrhage and the recognition of "unruptured" arteriovenous malformation patients who benefit from surgical intervention. Neurosurgery. 2015; 76(5):592–600, discussion 600

[34] Barr JC, Ogilvy CS. Selection of treatment modalities or observation of arteriovenous malformations. Neurosurg Clin N Am. 2012; 23(1):63–75

[35] Piepgras DG, Sundt TM , Jr, Ragoowansi AT, Stevens L. Seizure outcome in patients with surgically treated cerebral arteriovenous malformations. J Neurosurg. 1993; 78(1):5–11

[36] Kondziolka D, McLaughlin MR, Kestle JR. Simple risk predictions for arteriovenous malformation hemorrhage. Neurosurgery. 1995; 37(5):851–855

[37] Fults D, Kelly DL , Jr. Natural history of arteriovenous malformations of the brain: a clinical study. Neurosurgery. 1984; 15(5):658–662

[38] Hartmann A, Mast H, Mohr JP, et al. Morbidity of intracranial hemorrhage in patients with cerebral arteriovenous malformation. Stroke. 1998; 29(5):931–934

[39] Tomak PR, Cloft HJ, Kaga A, Cawley CM, Dion J, Barrow DL. Evolution of the management of tentorial dural arteriovenous malformations. Neurosurgery. 2003; 52(4):750–760–; discussion 760–2

[40] Choi JH, Mast H, Sciacca RR, et al. Clinical outcome after first and recurrent hemorrhage in patients with untreated brain arteriovenous malformation. Stroke. 2006; 37(5):1243–1247

[41] van Beijnum J, Lovelock CE, Cordonnier C, Rothwell PM, Klijn CJ, Al-Shahi Salman R, SIVMS Steering Committee and the Oxford Vascular Study. Outcome after spontaneous and arteriovenous malformation-related intracerebral haemorrhage: population-based studies. Brain. 2009; 132(Pt 2):537–543

[42] Starke RM, Komotar RJ, Hwang BY, et al. Treatment guidelines for cerebral arteriovenous malformation microsurgery. Br J Neurosurg. 2009; 23(4):376–386

[43] Rutledge WC, Abla AA, Nelson J, Halbach VV, Kim H, Lawton MT. Treatment and outcomes of ARUBA-eligible patients with unruptured brain arteriovenous malformations at a single institution. Neurosurg Focus. 2014; 37(3):E8

[44] Lunsford LD, Kondziolka D, Flickinger JC, et al. Stereotactic radiosurgery for arteriovenous malformations of the brain. J Neurosurg. 1991; 75(4):512–524

[45] Pierot L, Cognard C, Herbreteau D, et al. Endovascular treatment of brain arteriovenous malformations using a liquid embolic agent: results of a prospective, multicentre study (BRAVO). Eur Radiol. 2013; 23(10):2838–2845

[46] Bervini D, Morgan MK, Ritson EA, Heller G. Surgery for unruptured arteriovenous malformations of the brain is better than conservative management for selected cases: a prospective cohort study. J Neurosurg. 2014; 121(4):878–890

[47] Hoh BL, Carter BS, Ogilvy CS. Incidence of residual intracranial AVMs after surgical resection and efficacy of immediate surgical re-exploration. Acta Neurochir (Wien). 2004; 146(1):1–7, discussion 7

[48] Fleetwood IG, Steinberg GK. Arteriovenous malformations. Lancet. 2002; 359 (9309):863–873

[49] Yeh HS, Tew JM , Jr, Gartner M. Seizure control after surgery on cerebral arteriovenous malformations. J Neurosurg. 1993; 78(1):12–18

[50] Hoh BL, Chapman PH, Loeffler JS, Carter BS, Ogilvy CS. Results of multimodality treatment for 141 patients with brain arteriovenous malformations and seizures: factors associated with seizure incidence and seizure outcomes. Neurosurgery. 2002; 51(2):303–309, discussion 309–311

[51] Wang JY, Yang W, Ye X, et al. Impact on seizure control of surgical resection or radiosurgery for cerebral arteriovenous malformations. Neurosurgery. 2013; 73(4):648–655; discussion 655–646

[52] de Oliveira E, Tedeschi H, Raso J. Multidisciplinary approach to arteriovenous malformations. Neurol Med Chir (Tokyo). 1998; 38 Suppl:177–185

[53] Lawton MT, Project UBAMS, UCSF Brain Arteriovenous Malformation Study Project. Spetzler-Martin Grade III arteriovenous malformations: surgical results and a modification of the grading scale. Neurosurgery. 2003; 52(4): 740–748, discussion 748–749

[54] Velat GJ, Reavey-Cantwell JF, Sistrom C, et al. Comparison of N-butyl cyanoacrylate and onyx for the embolization of intracranial arteriovenous malformations: analysis of fluoroscopy and procedure times. Neurosurgery. 2008; 63 1, Suppl 1:ONS73–ONS78

[55] Arteriovenous malformations of the brain in adults. N Engl J Med. 1999; 340 (23):1812–1818

[56] Friedlander RM. Clinical practice. Arteriovenous malformations of the brain. N Engl J Med. 2007; 356(26):2704–2712

[57] van Beijnum J, van der Worp HB, Buis DR, et al. Treatment of brain arteriovenous malformations: a systematic review and meta-analysis. JAMA. 2011; 306(18):2011–2019

[58] Ledezma CJ, Hoh BL, Carter BS, Pryor JC, Putman CM, Ogilvy CS. Complications of cerebral arteriovenous malformation embolization: multivariate analysis of predictive factors. Neurosurgery. 2006; 58(4):602–611, discussion 602–611

[59] Ogilvy CS, Stieg PE, Awad I, et al. Special Writing Group of the Stroke Council, American Stroke Association. AHA Scientific Statement: Recommendations for the management of intracranial arteriovenous malformations: a statement for healthcare professionals from a special writing group of the Stroke Council, American Stroke Association. Stroke. 2001; 32(6):1458–1471

[60] Jafar JJ, Davis AJ, Berenstein A, Choi IS, Kupersmith MJ. The effect of embolization with N-butyl cyanoacrylate prior to surgical resection of cerebral arteriovenous malformations. J Neurosurg. 1993; 78(1):60–69

[61] Spetzler RF, Martin NA, Carter LP, Flom RA, Raudzens PA, Wilkinson E. Surgical management of large AVM's by staged embolization and operative excision. J Neurosurg. 1987; 67(1):17–28

[62] Blackburn SL, Ashley WW , Jr, Rich KM, et al. Combined endovascular embolization and stereotactic radiosurgery in the treatment of large arteriovenous malformations. J Neurosurg. 2011; 114(6):1758–1767

[63] Crowley RW, Ducruet AF, McDougall CG, Albuquerque FC. Endovascular advances for brain arteriovenous malformations. Neurosurgery. 2014; 74 Suppl 1:S74–S82

[64] Rubin BA, Brunswick A, Riina H, Kondziolka D. Advances in radiosurgery for arteriovenous malformations of the brain. Neurosurgery. 2014; 74 Suppl 1: S50–S59

[65] Xu F, Zhong J, Ray A, Manjila S, Bambakidis NC. Stereotactic radiosurgery with and without embolization for intracranial arteriovenous malformations: a systematic review and meta-analysis. Neurosurg Focus. 2014; 37(3):E16

[66] Frizzel RT, Fisher WS , III. Cure, morbidity, and mortality associated with embolization of brain arteriovenous malformations: a review of 1246

patients in 32 series over a 35-year period. Neurosurgery. 1995; 37(6):1031–1039, discussion 1039–1040

[67] Ellis JA, Lavine SD. Role of embolization for cerebral arteriovenous malformations. Methodist DeBakey Cardiovasc J. 2014; 10(4):234–239

[68] Kato Y, Sano H, Kanaoka N, Imai F, Katada K, Kanno T. Successful resection of arteriovenous malformations in eloquent areas diagnosed by surface anatomy scanning and motor evoked potential. Neurol Med Chir (Tokyo). 1998; 38 Suppl:217–221

[69] Friedman WA. Stereotactic radiosurgery of intracranial arteriovenous malformations. Neurosurg Clin N Am. 2013; 24(4):561–574

[70] Friedman WA, Bova FJ. Radiosurgery for arteriovenous malformations. Neurol Res. 2011; 33(8):803–819

[71] Kano H, Kondziolka D, Flickinger JC, et al. Stereotactic radiosurgery for arteriovenous malformations, Part 3: outcome predictors and risks after repeat radiosurgery. J Neurosurg. 2012; 116(1):21–32

[72] Karlsson B, Lindquist C, Steiner L. Prediction of obliteration after gamma knife surgery for cerebral arteriovenous malformations. Neurosurgery. 1997; 40 (3):425–430

5 Syndromic Arteriovenous Malformations

Waleed Brinjikji and Giuseppe Lanzino

Abstract

There are a number of syndromes that have a strong association with the formation of brain arteriovenous malformation (AVM). Hereditary hemorrhagic telangiectasia (HHT) is the most common brain AVM–associated genetic syndrome affecting up to 1 in 5,000 people. Patients with HHT can present with intracranial nidal AVMs, pial arteriovenous fistulas, and capillary vascular malformations (also known as micro-AVMs). Capillary malformation-AVM (CM-AVM) syndrome, caused by a mutation in the RAS/MAPK pathway, affects 1 in 100,000 people and is associated with cutaneous capillary malformations and nidal-type brain AVMs. Parkes-Weber's syndrome, often considered a subtype of CM-AVM syndrome, is characterized by limb AVMs, which result in hypertrophy of the affected limb. Patients with these syndromes and their relatives should consider genetic testing, and AVM screening with brain magnetic resonance imaging is recommended for affected individuals and their relatives. Wyburn-Mason's syndrome, in which AVMs can affect any part of the optic apparatus extending from the orbit to the occipital lobe, is exceedingly rare and no known genetic associations have been found. Management of AVMs in these syndromes should be done on a case-by-case basis because each AVM and each individual are unique. Given our increased understanding of the genetic and pathophysiological aspects of AVM formation in these populations, more and more research is being done to identify nonsurgical therapies aimed at stemming the formation and long-term effects of AVMs in these populations.

Keywords: arteriovenous malformation, hereditary hemorrhagic telangiectasia, RASA, arteriovenous fistula, congenital

Key Points

- Syndrome-associated arteriovenous malformations (AVMs) often have specific angioarchitectural features that can help distinguish them from sporadic AVMs.
- Hereditary hemorrhagic telangiectasia is the most prevalent syndrome that is associated with brain AVMs.
- In many cases, sporadic AVMs are associated with single-nucleotide polymorphisms in genes involved in inflammation and vasculogenesis. This points to a potential genetic etiology for sporadic AVMs.

5.1 Introduction

Most arteriovenous malformations (AVMs) are sporadic and exhibit variable sizes, angioarchitectural features, and locations. The estimated prevalence of sporadic brain AVMs is 10:100,000 to 20:100,000 adults.[1] While the underlying pathophysiologic and genetic causes of these sporadic AVMs are unclear, there is increasing evidence that genetic factors do play a role in their development.[1]

Among the AVM patient population is a subset of patients who suffer from AVMs as part of a familial or genetic syndrome. The two most common syndromes associated with brain AVMs are hereditary hemorrhagic telangiectasia (HHT), which is also known as Osler–Weber–Rendu syndrome, and the capillary malformation-AVM (CM-AVM) syndrome, which is associated with the RASA mutation. Other, more rare AVM-associated syndromes include Wyburn-Mason's syndrome and Parkes-Weber's syndrome (PWS).[2]

An understanding of syndrome-associated AVMs is important for a number of reasons. First, when working with patients who have syndrome-associated AVMs, it is important for clinicians to be aware of the other systemic manifestations of these diseases to allow for appropriate coordination of care, screening, and management. Second, in many cases, secondary central nervous system (CNS) manifestations and angioarchitectural features of AVMs can provide a clue regarding whether or not the AVM is syndrome-associated. In these cases, it is possible that the neurologist, neurosurgeon, or neuroradiologist seeing the patient could be the first to suggest the possibility of an underlying syndrome as the culprit for the AVM. Lastly, findings regarding the genetics of these syndromes have provided valuable information regarding the pathophysiology of both syndrome-associated and sporadic AVMs.

The aims of this chapter are the following: (1) to introduce the clinician to some of the more common AVM-associated syndromes including their systemic manifestations and genetics, (2) to discuss the management of patients with AVM-associated syndromes, and (3) to provide an updated review of the literature regarding the role of genetics in sporadic AVMs. For the purposes of this review, we will not be covering syndromes associated with nonshunting vascular abnormalities such as those seen in Sturge–Weber syndrome and **posterior fossa malformations–hemangiomas–arterial anomalies–cardiac defects–eye abnormalities–sternal cleft and supraumbilical raphe syndrome** (PHACES syndrome).

5.2 Materials and Methods

In accumulating information for the purposes of this chapter, we searched the PubMed and Online Mendelian Inheritance in Man (OMIM) databases for information regarding the genetics of brain AVMs using the following search terms: brain AVM, arteriovenous malformation, hereditary hemorrhagic telangiectasia, RASA, single-nucleotide polymorphism, genetics, Wyburn-Mason's syndrome, and Parkes-Weber's syndrome. We retrieved all case reports, case series, review articles, and meta-analyses regarding these syndromes and the genetics of AVMs.

5.3 Results

5.3.1 AVM-Associated Syndromes

▶ Table 5.1 and ▶ Table 5.2 summarize the salient characteristics of AVM-associated syndromes found on our literature

Table 5.1 AVM-associated syndrome genetics

Syndrome	OMIM#	Mutated gene	Gene product	Molecular mechanism for AVM formation	Mode of inheritance
Hereditary hemorrhagic telangiectasia (HHT)					
HHT1	187300	ENG			Autosomal dominant
HHT2	600376	ACVRL/ALK1			
Juvenile polyposis–HHT overlap	175050	SMAD4			
Capillary malformation-arteriovenous malformation	608354	RASA1	RAS p21 protein activator	Abnormal angiogenic remodeling of primary capillary plexus	Autosomal dominant/sporadic in 30%
Parkes-Weber's syndrome	139150	RASA1	RAS p21 protein activator	Abnormal angiogenic remodeling of primary capillary plexus	Autosomal dominant/sporadic
Wyburn-Mason's syndrome	NA	NA	NA	Unknown	Sporadic

Abbreviations: AVM, arteriovenous malformation; OMIM, Online Mendelian Inheritance in Man.

review, including estimated diseases prevalence, estimates regarding the proportion of patients with AVMs (when available), other systemic and CNS manifestations of these syndromes, associated gene mutation and gene function, and typical angioarchitectural features (when available).

5.3.2 Genetics of Sporadic AVMs

▶ Table 5.3 summarizes the single-nucleotide polymorphisms (SNPs) and somatic mutations that have been associated with sporadic AVMs. Included in this table are data on the function

of the genes that are associated with these mutations and their putative role in AVM pathogenesis.

5.4 Discussion

5.4.1 Hereditary Hemorrhagic Telangiectasia

HHT is the most common of the AVM-associated syndromes affecting anywhere from 1:5,000 to 1:10,000 people worldwide. HHT is diagnosed clinically using the Curacao criteria.[3] The four

Table 5.2 AVM-associated syndrome characteristics

Syndrome	Other CNS manifestations	Systemic manifestations	Disease prevalence	AVM characteristics
Hereditary hemorrhagic telangiectasia (HHT) HHT1 HHT2 Juvenile polyposis–HHT overlap	Spinal arteriovenous malformations, ischemic stroke secondary to pulmonary AVM, cerebral abscess	Pulmonary AVMs, epistaxis, GI AVMs, hepatic AVMs, mucocutaneous telangiectasia, colon polyps in polyp-associated disease	1:5,000 to 1:10,000	Generally smaller than sporadic AVMs. AVM multiplicity an HHT marker. Capillary vascular malformation/micro-AVMs highly prevalent. Pial AVF ~10% of AVMs
Capillary malformation-arteriovenous malformation	Spinal arteriovenous malformations	Face or extremity arteriovenous malformations. Port-wine stains on the face and neck, rarely in the mucosa. Capillary lesions are multifocal. High prevalence of neoplasm	1:100,000	Nidal-type arteriovenous malformations (80%), pial AVFs (10%), and vein of Galen malformation (10%)
Parkes-Weber's syndrome	Spinal arteriovenous malformations	Face or extremity arteriovenous malformations primarily in lower extremities, port-wine stains on the face or neck. High prevalence of neoplasm	Unknown	Nidal-type arteriovenous malformations, pial AVFs, and vein of Galen malformation
Wyburn-Mason's syndrome	Occular/retinal AVMs	Facial AVMs	Rare. About 50 cases reported in literature	Vascular lesions of the orbit, optic tract, optic radiations and occipital lobe

Abbreviations: AVF, arteriovenous fistula; AVM, arteriovenous malformation; GI, gastrointestinal.

Table 5.3 Sporadic mutations and SNPs associated with AVMs

SNP	Gene	Gene product and function
rs1143627	IL-1B	Interleukin-1, involved in inflammation. Produced mainly by monocytes
rs1800795	IL-6	Inflammatory cytokine produced by endothelium
rs16944	IL-1B	Interleukin-1, involved in inflammation. Produced mainly by monocytes
rs3025010	VEGFA	Vascular endothelial growth factor. Induces angiogenesis in vivo
rs7015566	GPR124	G-protein-coupled receptor 124. Important in CNS-specific angiogenesis. Overexpression results in increased endothelial sprouting and migration
rs522616	MMP-3	Matrix metalloproteinase-3. Produced by connective tissue cells. Involved in wound repair and tissue remodeling
rs11672433	ANGPTL4	Angiopoietin-like 4. Vascular growth factor, plays role in embryonic and postnatal angiogenesis

Abbreviations: AVM, arteriovenous malformation; CNS, central nervous system; SNP, single-nucleotide polymorphisms.

Curacao criteria are (1) spontaneous and recurrent epistaxis, (2) mucocutaneous telangiectasias (lips, oral cavity, face, and fingers), (3) visceral AVMs (brain, liver, lung, etc.), and (4) diagnosis of HHT in a first-degree relative using the same criteria. Patients who meet three or more of the four criteria are labeled as "definite HHT," whereas those with two of the four criteria are labeled as "possible" or "suspected" HHT.[4] The most common clinical manifestations of HHT are epistaxis, gastrointestinal bleeding, and pulmonary AVMs.

There are at least five types of HHT. HHT1 is due to a mutation in the ENG gene, which codes for endoglin. Endoglin is a component of the transforming growth factor beta (TGF-β) complex and plays an essential role in the development and regulation of human vascular endothelium. HHT2 is secondary to a mutation in the ACVRL1 gene, which codes for an activin receptor–like kinase. This protein is also involved in the TGF-β system and plays a key role in regulating vasculogenesis. There is also a juvenile polyposis with HHT syndrome secondary to a mutation in the SMAD4 gene. This gene also plays a role in vasculogenesis.

Approximately 10 to 20% of patients with HHT have a brain AVM with a higher prevalence noted in HHT1 patients.[5] HHT-associated AVMs are classified as (1) large single-hole pial arteriovenous fistulas (AVFs), (2) AVMs with a nidus, and (3) micro-AVMs or capillary vascular malformation.[6] The large AVMs/AVFs typically manifest in young children, while small AVMs are typically discovered in older age groups.[6] AVFs represent about 10% of cerebral vascular malformations, while nidus-type AVMs represent about 50% of cerebral vascular malformations.[6] Approximately 60% of patients with cerebral vascular malformations have micro-AVMs/capillary vascular malformations.

The angioarchitecture of each of these lesions differs substantially. Pial AVFs lack a nidus between the feeding artery and draining vein (i.e., a single hole with a pouch). These lesions are usually superficially located with only a tiny minority located in the deep portions of the brain.[6] These lesions have many features that portend a poorer natural history, including arterial stenoses, feeding artery aneurysms, multiple draining veins, venous ectasia, and a pseudophlebitic pattern.[6]

Nidus-type AVMs are arteriovenous connections with an intervening nidus. About 40% of these lesions are located in eloquent areas and about 15% have deep venous drainage.[6] Over 90% of these lesions have a Spetzler–Martin score of 2 or less.[6,7,8] The angioarchitecture of these lesions is typically benign. These lesions tend to measure less than 2 cm and lack features such as arterial stenoses, associated aneurysms, multiple draining veins, venous ectasia, and venous reflux. Associated aneurysms are signs of longstanding venous hypertension.[6]

Micro-AVMs and capillary vascular malformations lack definite shunting on angiography and have no dilated feeding arteries or veins. These are characterized by a blush of abnormal vessels in the arterial phase that persists into the late arterial and capillary phase.[6] Angiographically, these lesions are distinct from both capillary telangiectasia and AVMs given that these are characterized by the presence of a capillary bed that is abnormally dilated. These lesions typically measure less than 5 mm in diameter, and 80% are superficial.[6,7,8]

There are a number of salient features of HHT-AVMs that should lead one to consider a diagnosis of HHT if one has not already been established. Micro-AVMs/capillary vascular malformations are considered an HHT-defining feature by some authors. Pial AVFs are thought to be exceedingly rare in the sporadic AVM population, but are seen in up to 10% of HHT-AVM patients; thus, the presence of these lesions should trigger an investigation for HHT.[9,10] Regarding the nidal-type AVMs, features that should trigger an investigation for HHT are lesion multiplicity, especially when seen in superficial locations. An example of a patient with multiple AVMs in the setting of HHT is provided in ▶ Fig. 5.1.

Based on the angioarchitecture of these lesions, the natural history and presentation also differs substantially. Capillary vascular malformations are often detected incidentally and are not associated with symptoms such as seizures, headache, and hemorrhage. Nidal-type AVMs are typically asymptomatic with over 60% detected either incidentally or during screening.[6,11] About 25% of AVMs in HHT patients present with hemorrhage, and in a majority of cases, the AVM was unknown or had not manifested itself until the time of hemorrhage.[6,11] Because of their size and "dangerous" angioarchitecture, pial AVFs can present with hemorrhage, seizure, bruit, or heart failure, particularly in infants.[12]

Studies of natural history of cerebral AVMs (CAVMs) in HHT patients are few and limited by the fact that the angiographic characteristics of the lesions are not generally well characterized in these studies. Willemse et al found a bleeding risk of 0.4 to 0.7% for HHT-AVMs.[13] The Brain Vascular Malformation Consortium HHT Investigator Group found an overall bleeding rate of 1% per year when considering both unruptured and ruptured AVM. When stratifying outcomes by rupture status, however, the authors found a rupture rate 0.4% per year (95% confidence interval [CI], 0.1–1.7%) for unruptured HHT-AVMs and 10% per year for ruptured HHT-AVMs (95% CI, 3.3–31.2%). Little is known regarding the natural history of single-hole pial AVFs, but they are thought to have a poor prognosis when left untreated.[12,14] Capillary vascular malformations have a benign

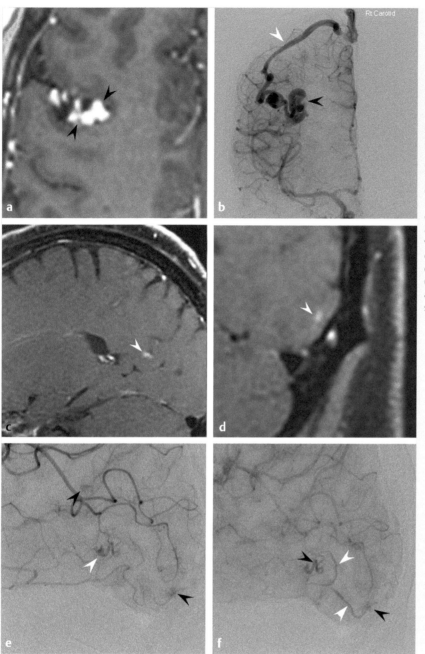

Fig. 5.1 AVMs in a young female patient with HHT. **(a)** T1 contrast-enhanced image shows an enhancing serpiginous vascular structure in the right frontal lobe consistent with a brain AVM. **(b)** Cerebral angiogram shows the right frontal AVM (*black arrowhead*) with a large superficial draining vein (*white arrowhead*). **(c)** Sagittal T1 contrast-enhanced MRI shows a superficial enhancing focus in the parietooccipital fissure. **(d)** Sagittal T1 contrast-enhanced MRI shows a second superficial enhancing focus in the occipital lobe. **(e)** Cerebral angiography during a right ICA injection demonstrates fluffy stainlike opacification of two lesions during the mid-to-late arterial phase (*black arrowheads*) consisting of capillary vascular malformations. There is also another nidus-type AVM with a small tangle of vessels (*white arrow*). **(f)** These lesions do not demonstrate rapid arteriovenous shunting as demonstrated by the fact that the draining veins (*white arrowheads*) opacify around the same time as the remainder of the cerebral venous structures

prognosis with no reports of hemorrhage or growth of these lesions to date.[6,7,9] Further studies are needed to determine the natural history of CAVMs, stratifying outcomes by type of AVM.

Precise guidelines regarding screening and management of CAVMs are not available because of lack of high-quality evidence.[15] A majority of experts (77%) agree that clinicians should screen adult patients with possible or definite HHT for cerebral vascular malformations with magnetic resonance imaging (MRI)/magnetic resonance angiography (MRA). There is less consensus regarding screening for children, with 64% of experts advocating for screening in the first 6 months of life. Those who did not agree to this recommendation cited lack of evidence for benefit of screening in children and lack of evidence of treatment efficacy for asymptomatic cerebral vascular

malformations in children. There is, however, consensus that once diagnosed with a cerebral vascular malformation, patients should be referred to centers with neurovascular expertise and that patients with hemorrhage secondary to a vascular malformation receive definitive treatment at these centers.[15] Most HHT centers do not rescreen patients after an initial negative MRI/MRA scan done in adulthood. The role of serial imaging, particularly at young ages where AVMs may be developing, has yet to be established. There is a growing body of evidence suggesting that de novo formation of AVMs can occur at any stage of life.[16]

Treatment of AVMs should be performed on a case-by-case basis with careful consideration of the angioarchitecture of the lesion, natural history, and patient comorbidities.[15] Effective treatment strategies include endovascular, microsurgical, and radiosurgical techniques. There are no studies demonstrating the superiority of one treatment over the other.[10] Treatment decisions should be guided based on local expertise. Most high-flow pial fistulas can be treated with endovascular or surgical therapy alone.[8,10] As mentioned previously, micro-AVMs are considered "do not touch" lesions. No pharmacological therapies have been shown to be effective in treatment of AVMs in humans.

5.4.2 Capillary Malformation-Arteriovenous Malformation Syndrome

CM-AVM syndrome is one of many RASopathies secondary to mutations in genes involved in the Ras/MAPK pathway. Other RASopathies include neurofibromatosis type 1, Noonan's syndrome, and cardiofaciocutaneous syndrome. The Ras/MAPK pathway is involved in vital cellular functions, including cell-cycle progression, cellular differentiation, and cellular growth. Many malignancies have somatic mutations of the Ras oncogene, which accounts for the higher rate of malignancy seen in patients with CM-AVM syndrome.[17]

Like HHT, CM-AVM syndrome is an autosomal dominant inherited disorder. The prevalence of RASA1-related syndromes is estimated at 1:100,000.[18] Patients are affected by multifocal capillary malformations (i.e., port-wine stains) and AVMs and AVFs affecting multiple tissues including muscle, bone, gastrointestinal tract, spine, and brain.[19] Approximately 10 to 15% of patients with CM-AVM syndrome suffer from various tumors, including optic gliomas, superficial basal cell carcinoma, neurofibromas, and vestibular schwannomas.[17,20] Overall, approximately 10% of patients with RASA1 mutations have CNS AVMs, 15% have systemic AVMs, and nearly 100% have capillary malformations.[20]

There is a wide variation in the types of AVMs seen in patients with CM-AVM syndrome.[18] In a review of 101 individuals with RASA mutations, Revencu et al found that 8 patients had intracerebral AVMs or AVFs, with 2 patients suffering from vein of Galen malformations.[18] In a second review of 132 individuals with RASA mutations, Revencu et al found two pial AVFs, nine nidal-type AVMs, and three vein of Galen malformations. In addition, 10 patients suffered from facial AVMs and 7 patients suffered from spinal AVMs.[20] Pial AVFs are extremely rare in the general population and are seen at a surprisingly high rate among patients with both HHT and CM-AVM syndrome. One recent review of patients with pial AVFs by Walcott et al found that two of seven patients with pial AVFs had RASA1 gene mutations, while none had mutations associated with HHT.[21] The salient feature that distinguishes AVMs associated with CM-AVM syndrome and sporadic AVMs is the presence of vascular malformations on the skin. Because these vascular malformations are difficult to distinguish from the cutaneous lesions seen in HHT patients, having patients evaluated by an experienced dermatologist is strongly recommended. An example of a CM-AVM syndrome patient with brain AVM and skin lesions is provided in ▶ Fig. 5.2.

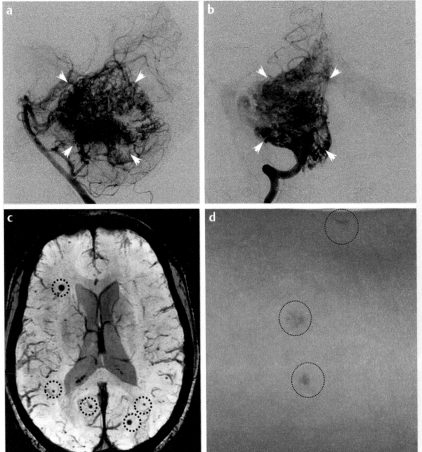

Fig. 5.2 Young female patient with CM-AVM syndrome including a brain AVM and multiple capillary malformations of the skin. The patient has a large arteriovenous malformation in the right cerebellar hemisphere, which is fed by the right superior cerebellar artery, anterior inferior cerebellar artery, and posterior inferior cerebellar artery (*arrows* in **a** and **b**). (**c**) Susceptibility-weighted MRI image demonstrates multiple tiny foci of hemosiderin deposition consistent with microhemorrhages or cavernomas (*circles*). (**d**) Three capillary malformations of the skin in the antecubital fossa (*circles*).

At this time, there are no comprehensive recommendations for the management of patients with CM-AVM syndrome. In general, AVMs are managed on a case-by-case basis depending on their angioarchitectural features and the clinical status of the patient. Some authors advocate for genetic testing of patients who present with both intracranial/facial AVMs and cutaneous capillary malformations. While no evidence-based recommendations regarding screening for brain AVMs have been published, many experts believe that brain AVM screening is important in patients with known CM-AVM syndrome or a family history of the disease.[22,23,24]

Because CM-AVM syndrome has only recently been described, many questions remain regarding the pathophysiology of the disease as well as the best management of these patients. Little is known regarding the natural history of brain AVFs and AVMs associated with RASA1 mutations. Furthermore, the mechanism by which the RASA1 gene mutation leads to the formation of vascular malformations has yet to be established. Because the Ras/MAPK pathway has been well studied in the oncological literature, there is hope that developments in small-molecule inhibition to treat Ras/MAPK-associated malignancies could help in the prevention and management of vascular abnormalities seen in patients with CM-AVM syndrome.[25]

5.4.3 Parkes-Weber's Syndrome

Like CM-AVM syndrome, PWS is also caused by mutations in the RASA1 gene, which regulates cell growth, proliferation, and differentiation.[26] There are many cases reported in the literature of autosomal dominant inheritance of PWS; however, sporadic cases have been reported as well. PWS is characterized by a cutaneous capillary malformation associated with underlying multiple AVFs and hypertrophy of the affected limb.[27] Lower extremity AVMs are the most commonly reported type of AVM in PWS. Because these AVMs are associated with overgrowth of the affected extremity, the disease is often confused with Klippel–Trénaunay–Weber syndrome (Klippel–Trénaunay–Weber syndrome consists of slow-flow malformations, while PWS consists of high-flow malformations).[28]

It is unknown what proportion of PWS patients have brain AVMs in addition to their extremity vascular malformations. However, the association is commonly reported in the literature. AVMs seen in PWS are similar to those seen in patients with CM-AVM syndrome because the mutated gene is often the same (RASA1).[18,29,30] In addition, these patients can present with spinal vascular malformations.[31,32]

Like CM-AVM syndrome, there are no evidence-based recommendations for management of these patients. In general, PWS patients should be managed at highly specialized centers because of the fact that they require high-level multidisciplinary care in managing their multiple malformations. AVMs in PWS can be managed on a case-by-case basis depending on the clinical status of the patient and angioarchitecture of the lesion. Some authors advocate screening of PWS patients at least once with a brain MRI for an intracranial vascular malformation. Genetic testing for RASA1 mutation is generally recommended.

5.4.4 Wyburn-Mason's Syndrome

Wyburn-Mason's syndrome is a neurocutaneous syndrome characterized by ipsilateral AVMs affecting the face and visual pathway including the eyes, optic nerve, optic tract, and optic radiations. The prevalence of Wyburn-Mason's syndrome is far lower than that of HHT and CM-AVM syndrome, given that only about 50 cases have been reported in the literature.[33] There is no known genetic mutation associated with the disease and most cases are sporadic. Wyburn-Mason's syndrome is thought to be the result of a developmental abnormality of the primitive vascular mesoderm of the optic cup and anterior neural tube. These structures give rise to the retinal vessels as well as the vasculature of the midbrain. The developmental insult is thought to occur within the first 7 weeks of gestation and results in persistence of primitive vascular tissue in the retina and midbrain.

Patients with Wyburn-Mason's syndrome typically present within the first three decades of life. The most common manifestation of Wyburn-Mason's syndrome is a retinal AVM resulting in loss of visual acuity and visual field deficits.[33,34] Retinal AVMs can be variable in size and are sometimes apparent on digital subtraction angiography. Outside of the retina, the most common site of AVMs in Wyburn-Mason's syndrome is the orbit, followed by the thalamus and hypothalamus, optic chiasm, optic tracts, and optic radiations. A majority of AVMs are symptomatic, presenting with retro-orbital pain and hemiparesis. About 10 to 20% of AVMs in the literature have presented with rupture.[33] Head and neck vascular malformations associated with Wyburn-Mason's syndrome are primarily located in the distribution of the trigeminal nerve and can involve the frontal or maxillary sinuses. About one-third to one-half of patients with Wyburn-Mason's syndrome present with these malformations.[33] An example of a patient with both a brain AVM and a vascular malformation in the distribution of the trigeminal nerve is provided in ▶ Fig. 5.3.

As with many syndromic AVMs, there are no current evidence-based guidelines for the management of intracranial AVMs in patients with Wyburn-Mason's syndrome. Like all brain AVMs, these lesions are typically managed on a case-by-case basis. Because of the deep-seated nature of these AVMs, surgical access can be challenging. Significant vision loss is a major risk factor in surgical treatment of AVMs located in the suprasellar regions. Because of the complexity and deep-seated nature of these lesions, some authors advocate embolization as a preferred treatment modality. Conservative management is another strategy in managing these patients.

Retinal AVMs in patients with Wyburn-Mason's syndrome are generally stable. Retinal hemorrhage can occur because of slow leaking or rupture of the AVM. There is no association between the characteristics of rupture status of retinal vascular malformations and those in the brain. Patients with Wyburn-Mason's syndrome who suffer from retinal AVMs should be managed by experienced retinal surgeons because of the complexity and rarity of these lesions.[35] There have been cases reported in the literature of retinal AVMs treated with transarterial embolization; however, this has not been shown to be a viable treatment modality.[36] Intravitreal bevacizumab has been shown to be effective in treating retinal edema.[37] Lastly, facial

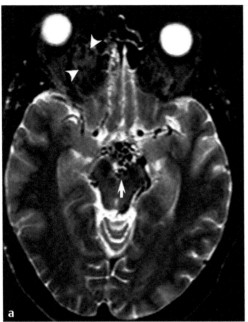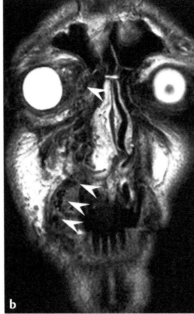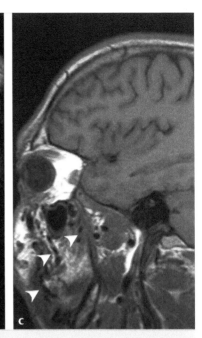

Fig. 5.3 A 40-year-old man with known Wyburn-Mason's syndrome. **(a)** T2-weighted MRI of the brain shows a small AVM in the interpeduncular and suprasellar cistern (*short arrow*). There are prominent vascular flow voids in the right orbit secondary to a large facial AVM with orbital involvement (*white arrowheads*). **(b)** Coronal T2-weighted image of the face shows multiple hypointense vascular flow voids (*white arrowheads*) extending from the right orbit to the right cheek along the distribution of the trigeminal nerve. **(c)** Sagittal T1-weighted MRI shows multiple hypointense serpiginous flow voids extending along the right side of the face with involvement of the right cheek along the distribution of the right trigeminal nerve.

AVMs are typically managed conservatively.[38,39] However, embolization is a viable treatment option.[33]

5.4.5 Sporadic AVM Genetics

SNPs are variations in a single nucleotide which occur at a specific position in the genome in which each variation is present to some appreciable degree within a population. These SNPs are thought to be a major contributing cause to each individual's susceptibility to disease. There are a number of studies that have examined the association between various SNPs in AVM patients and controls. SNPs have been found in genes involved in inflammation (interleukin-1 [IL-1] and IL-6), genes involved in embryonic and postnatal angiogenesis (vascular endothelial growth factor, angiopoietin, and G-protein-coupled receptors), and genes involved in wound repair and tissue remodeling (matrix metalloproteinase-3).[40,41] We do not understand yet how these SNPs affect gene function, their heritability, and penetrance, and what their exact role is in AVM formation. However, like the mutations seen in the genes causing HHT and the RASopathies, they do strongly point to aberrant angiogenesis and inflammation playing a role in the pathogenesis of AVMs.

5.5 Conclusion

There are a number of syndromes that have a strong association with brain AVM formation. HHT and CM-AVM syndrome are among the most common of brain AVM–associated genetic syndromes and are each associated with unique AVM characteristics. PWS, often considered a subtype of CM-AVM syndrome, is characterized by limb AVMs, which result in hypertrophy of the

affected limb. Patients with these syndromes and their relatives should consider genetic testing, and AVM screening with brain MRI is recommended for affected individuals and their relatives. Wyburn-Mason's syndrome, in which AVMs can affect any part of the optic apparatus extending from the orbit to the occipital lobe, is exceedingly rare and no known genetic associations have been found. Management of AVMs in these syndromes should be done on a case-by-case basis as each AVM and each individual are unique. Given our increased understanding of the genetic and pathophysiological aspects of AVM formation in these populations, more and more research is being done to identify nonsurgical therapies aimed at stemming the formation and long-term effects of AVMs in these populations.

References

[1] Brouillard P, Vikkula M. Genetic causes of vascular malformations. Hum Mol Genet. 2007; 16 Spec No. 2:R140–R149

[2] Frigerio A, Stevenson DA, Grimmer JF. The genetics of vascular anomalies. Curr Opin Otolaryngol Head Neck Surg. 2012; 20(6):527–532

[3] Shovlin CL, Guttmacher AE, Buscarini E, et al. Diagnostic criteria for hereditary hemorrhagic telangiectasia (Rendu-Osler-Weber syndrome). Am J Med Genet. 2000; 91(1):66–67

[4] McDonald J, Wooderchak-Donahue W, VanSant Webb C, Whitehead K, Stevenson DA, Bayrak-Toydemir P. Hereditary hemorrhagic telangiectasia: genetics and molecular diagnostics in a new era. Front Genet. 2015; 6:1

[5] Fulbright RK, Chaloupka JC, Putman CM, et al. MR of hereditary hemorrhagic telangiectasia: prevalence and spectrum of cerebrovascular malformations. AJNR Am J Neuroradiol. 1998; 19(3):477–484

[6] Krings T, Kim H, Power S, et al. Brain Vascular Malformation Consortium HHT Investigator Group. Neurovascular manifestations in hereditary hemorrhagic telangiectasia: imaging features and genotype-phenotype correlations. AJNR Am J Neuroradiol. 2015; 36(5):863–870

[7] Krings T, Ozanne A, Chng SM, Alvarez H, Rodesch G, Lasjaunias PL. Neurovascular phenotypes in hereditary haemorrhagic telangiectasia patients according to age. Review of 50 consecutive patients aged 1 day-60 years. Neuroradiology. 2005; 47(10):711–720

[8] Krings T, Ozanne A, Chng SM, Alvarez H, Rodesch G, Lasjaunias PL. Hereditary hemorrhagic telangiectasia: Neurovascular phenotypes and endovascular treatment. Clin Neuroradiol. 2006; 16(2):76–90

[9] Krings T, Chng SM, Ozanne A, Alvarez H, Rodesch G, Lasjaunias PL. Hereditary haemorrhagic telangiectasia in children. Endovascular treatment of neurovascular malformations. Results in 31 patients. Interv Neuroradiol. 2005; 11 (1):13–23

[10] Krings T, Chng SM, Ozanne A, Alvarez H, Rodesch G, Lasjaunias PL. Hereditary hemorrhagic telangiectasia in children: endovascular treatment of neurovascular malformations: results in 31 patients. Neuroradiology. 2005; 47(12): 946–954

[11] Kim H, Nelson J, Krings T, et al. Brain Vascular Malformation Consortium HHT Investigator Group. Hemorrhage rates from brain arteriovenous malformation in patients with hereditary hemorrhagic telangiectasia. Stroke. 2015; 46 (5):1362–1364

[12] Lee JS, Oh CW, Bang JS, Kwon OK, Hwang G. Intracranial pial arteriovenous fistula presenting with hemorrhage: a case report. J Cerebrovasc Endovasc Neurosurg. 2012; 14(4):305–308

[13] Willemse RB, Mager JJ, Westermann CJ, Overtoom TT, Mauser H, Wolbers JG. Bleeding risk of cerebrovascular malformations in hereditary hemorrhagic telangiectasia. J Neurosurg. 2000; 92(5):779–784

[14] Weon YC, Yoshida Y, Sachet M, et al. Supratentorial cerebral arteriovenous fistulas (AVFs) in children: review of 41 cases with 63 non choroidal single-hole AVFs. Acta Neurochir (Wien). 2005; 147(1):17–31, discussion 31

[15] Faughnan ME, Palda VA, Garcia-Tsao G, et al. HHT Foundation International - Guidelines Working Group. International guidelines for the diagnosis and management of hereditary haemorrhagic telangiectasia. J Med Genet. 2011; 48(2):73–87

[16] Du R, Hashimoto T, Tihan T, Young WL, Perry V, Lawton MT. Growth and regression of arteriovenous malformations in a patient with hereditary hemorrhagic telangiectasia. Case report. J Neurosurg. 2007; 106(3):470–477

[17] Wooderchak-Donahue W, Stevenson DA, McDonald J, Grimmer JF, Gedge F, Bayrak-Toydemir P. RASA1 analysis: clinical and molecular findings in a series of consecutive cases. Eur J Med Genet. 2012; 55(2):91–95

[18] Revencu N, Boon LM, Mulliken JB, et al. Parkes Weber syndrome, vein of Galen aneurysmal malformation, and other fast-flow vascular anomalies are caused by RASA1 mutations. Hum Mutat. 2008; 29(7):959–965

[19] Thiex R, Mulliken JB, Revencu N, et al. A novel association between RASA1 mutations and spinal arteriovenous anomalies. AJNR Am J Neuroradiol. 2010; 31(4):775–779

[20] Revencu N, Boon LM, Mendola A, et al. RASA1 mutations and associated phenotypes in 68 families with capillary malformation-arteriovenous malformation. Hum Mutat. 2013; 34(12):1632–1641

[21] Walcott BP, Smith ER, Scott RM, Orbach DB. Pial arteriovenous fistulae in pediatric patients: associated syndromes and treatment outcome. J Neurointerv Surg. 2013; 5(1):10–14

[22] Grillner P, Soderman M, Holmin S, Rodesch G. A spectrum of intracranial vascular high-flow arteriovenous shunts in RASA1 mutations. Childs Nerv Syst. 2016; 32(4):709–715

[23] Larralde M, Abad ME, Luna PC, Hoffner MV. Capillary malformation-arteriovenous malformation: a clinical review of 45 patients. Int J Dermatol. 2014; 53(4):458–461

[24] Aoki Y, Niihori T, Inoue SI, Matsubara Y. Recent advances in RASopathies. J Hum Genet. 2016; 61(1):33–39

[25] Rauen KA. The RASopathies. Annu Rev Genomics Hum Genet. 2013; 14:355–369

[26] Bayrak-Toydemir P, Stevenson D. RASA1-related disorders. In: Pagon RA, Adam MP, Ardinger HH, et al., eds. GeneReviews. Seattle, WA: University of Washington; 1993

[27] Gray AM. Haemangiectatic hypertrophy (Parkes Weber). Proc R Soc Med. 1928; 21(8):1431–1432

[28] Roebuck DJ. Klippel-Trénaunay and Parkes-Weber syndromes. AJR Am J Roentgenol. 1997; 169(1):311–312

[29] Boon LM, Mulliken JB, Vikkula M. RASA1: variable phenotype with capillary and arteriovenous malformations. Curr Opin Genet Dev. 2005; 15(3):265–269

[30] Namba K, Nemoto S. Parkes Weber syndrome and spinal arteriovenous malformations. AJNR Am J Neuroradiol. 2013; 34(9):E110–E112

[31] Matsumaru Y, Pongpech S, Laothamas J, Alvarez H, Rodesch G, Lasjaunias P. Multifocal and metameric spinal cord arteriovenous malformations. Interv Neuroradiol. 1999; 5(1):27–34

[32] Niimi Y, Ito U, Tone O, Yoshida K, Sato S, Berenstein A. Multiple spinal perimedullary arteriovenous fistulae associated with the parkes-weber syndrome. A case report. Interv Neuroradiol. 1998; 4(2):151–157

[33] Dayani PN, Sadun AA. A case report of Wyburn-Mason syndrome and review of the literature. Neuroradiology. 2007; 49(5):445–456

[34] Rasalkar DD, Paunipagar BK. Wyburn-Mason syndrome. Pediatr Radiol. 2010; 40 Suppl 1:S122

[35] Reck SD, Zacks DN, Eibschitz-Tsimhoni M. Retinal and intracranial arteriovenous malformations: Wyburn-Mason syndrome. J Neuroophthalmol. 2005; 25(3):205–208

[36] Matsuo T, Yanai H, Sugiu K, Tominaga S, Kimata Y. Orbital exenteration after transarterial embolization in a patient with Wyburn-Mason syndrome: pathological findings. Jpn J Ophthalmol. 2008; 52(4):308–313

[37] Callahan AB, Skondra D, Krzystolik M, Yonekawa Y, Eliott D. Wyburn-Mason syndrome associated with cutaneous reactive angiomatosis and central retinal vein occlusion. Ophthalmic Surg Lasers Imaging Retina. 2015; 46(7): 760–762

[38] Schmidt D, Agostini H, Schumacher M. Twenty-seven years follow-up of a patient with congenital retinocephalofacial vascular malformation syndrome and additional congenital malformations (Bonnet-Dechaume-Blanc syndrome or Wyburn-Mason syndrome). Eur J Med Res. 2010; 15(2):89–91

[39] Luo CB, Lasjaunias P, Bhattacharya J. Craniofacial vascular malformations in Wyburn-Mason syndrome. J Chin Med Assoc. 2006; 69(12):575–580

[40] Kremer PH, Koeleman BP, Rinkel GJ, et al. Susceptibility loci for sporadic brain arteriovenous malformation; a replication study and meta-analysis. J Neurol Neurosurg Psychiatry. 2016; 87(7):693–696

[41] Kremer PH, Koeleman BP, Pawlikowska L, et al. Evaluation of genetic risk loci for intracranial aneurysms in sporadic arteriovenous malformations of the brain. J Neurol Neurosurg Psychiatry. 2015; 86(5):524–529

6 Natural History of Arteriovenous Fistulas, Clinical Presentation, and Indications for Treatment

John D. Nerva, Ryan P. Morton, Laligam N. Sekhar, and Louis J. Kim

Abstract

Dural arteriovenous fistulas (dAVFs) are direct shunts between dural arteries and a dural venous sinus or cortical veins. dAVFs present with a variety of symptoms dependent on location and venous drainage patterns. The Borden and Cognard classification systems are commonly used to categorize and risk-stratify dAVFs. The natural history of dAVFs depends primarily on the presence or absence of cortical venous drainage (CVD) coupled with clinical symptoms and location. In the absence of CVD, patients rarely present with neurological deficit or hemorrhage. The presence of CVD leads to a higher risk of future neurological deficit and intracranial hemorrhage. For Borden type II dAVFs, the annual rate of hemorrhage is 6%. For Borden III dAVFs, the annual rate of hemorrhage is 10%. Combining Borden type II and III dAVFs, the annual rate of hemorrhage is 2% for asymptomatic patients, 10% for patients with nonhemorrhagic neurological deficits, and 46% for patients with a history of hemorrhage. Immediate endovascular or surgical treatment of dAVFs with symptomatic CVD is always warranted, while treatment for dAVFs with asymptomatic CVD is nearly always justifiable. Treatment is also reasonable for dAVFs without CVD but with debilitating symptoms.

Keywords: dural arteriovenous fistula, natural history, intracranial hemorrhage

Key Points

- Dural arteriovenous fistulas (dAVFs) may present with a variety of symptoms dependent on location and venous drainage patterns.
- The Borden and Cognard classification systems are commonly used to categorize and risk-stratify dAVFs.
- The natural history of dAVFs depends primarily on the presence or absence of cortical venous drainage (CVD) coupled with clinical symptoms and location.
- The presence of CVD leads to a higher risk of future neurological deficit and potentially fatal intracranial hemorrhage.
- Immediate endovascular or surgical treatment of dAVFs with symptomatic CVD is always warranted, while treatment for dAVFs with asymptomatic CVD is nearly always justifiable. Treatment is also reasonable for dAVFs without CVD but with debilitating symptoms.

6.1 Introduction

Cranial dural arteriovenous fistulas (dAVFs) are complex vascular lesions that involve direct shunts between dural arteries and a dural venous sinus or cortical veins. The etiology of most dAVFs is idiopathic, although they can occur after trauma, tumor invasion of sinus, infection, and postcraniotomy.[1] The presenting signs and symptoms depend largely on dAVF location and type of venous drainage patterns. While some dAVFs are discovered incidentally, many present with symptoms such as headache, pulsatile tinnitus, orbital symptoms, neurological deficit, and intracranial hemorrhage (ICH).[2] The natural history and subsequent risk of neurological deficit or ICH highly depend on the presence or absence of cortical venous drainage (CVD).[1,2,3,4,5,6,7,8,9,10,11] The symptomatology at presentation and knowledge of the natural history of a patient's dAVF can help guide clinical decision making.

The aim of this chapter is to review the literature on the natural history of different subtypes of dAVFs, focusing chiefly on the risk of neurological deficit and ICH to aid in the therapeutic decision-making process.

6.2 Materials and Methods

Published peer-reviewed literature regarding the natural history of dAVFs, including those specifically describing the effects of presentation, location, and venous drainage patterns on the risk of nonhemorrhagic neurological deficit (NHND) and ICH, was reviewed. The Borden and Cognard classification systems were primarily used to frame this discussion.[4,5] Lastly, illustrative cases were used to highlight the presenting symptoms and classification systems.

6.3 Results

6.3.1 Classification Systems

The Borden and Cognard classification systems stratify dAVFs on angiographic findings based on the venous drainage patterns and risk of ICH over time (▶ Table 6.1).[4,5] In the Borden system, classifications are based on the location of venous drainage and presence of CVD.[4] Borden type I dAVFs drain directly into a dural venous sinus without CVD, Borden type II dAVFs drain into a dural venous sinus and have cortical venous reflux, and Borden type III dAVFs have direct CVD. Subtypes in the Borden classification are subtype A (single fistula) and subtype B (multiple fistulas).

In the Cognard system, classifications are based on the direction of dural sinus flow, presence of CVD, and venous architecture.[5] Cognard type I dAVFs drain into a dural venous sinus with antegrade flow and without CVD. Cognard type IIa dAVFs drain into a dural venous sinus with retrograde sinus flow but without CVD. Cognard type IIb dAVFs drain into a dural venous sinus with antegrade flow but with CVD, while Cognard type IIa + b dAVFs drain into a dural venous sinus with retrograde flow and CVD. Cognard type III dAVFs have direct CVD (similar to Borden type III), while Cognard type IV dAVFs have direct CVD and venous ectasia. Lastly, Cognard type V dAVFs have direct CVD into spinal perimedullary veins.

Table 6.1 Classification systems for dAVFs

Borden[4]		Cognard[5]	
I	Drainage into dural venous sinus without CVD	I	Drainage into dural venous sinus with antegrade flow
		IIa	Drainage into dural venous sinus with retrograde flow
II	Drainage into dural venous sinus with cortical venous reflux	IIb	Drainage into dural venous sinus with antegrade flow and cortical venous reflux
		IIa + b	Drainage into dural venous sinus with retrograde flow and cortical venous reflux
III	Direct CVD	III	Direct CVD
		IV	Direct CVD with venous ectasia
		V	Direct drainage into spinal perimedullary veins

Abbreviation: CVD, cortical venous drainage.

A third classification system warrants discussion as it describes a specific type of dAVFs of the cavernous sinus (CS). Barrow et al stratified carotid-cavernous fistulas (CCFs) by fistulous vessels.[12] Type A CCFs are direct, high-flow fistulas between the internal carotid artery (ICA) and CS, type B CCFs are indirect, low-flow fistulas between dural branches of the ICA and the CS, type C CCFs are indirect, low-flow fistulas between dural branches of the external carotid artery (ECA) and CS, and type D CCFs are indirect fistulas between dural branches of both the ICA and ECA and the CS.

Borden type I and Cognard type I and IIa are frequently combined in the literature because of the absence of CVD (► Fig. 6.1 and ► Fig. 6.2). Similarly, Borden type II and Cognard type IIb and type IIa + b (► Fig. 6.3) as well as Borden type III and Cognard types III–V (► Fig. 6.4, ► Fig. 6.5, ► Fig. 6.6) are combined because of the presence of CVD.

6.3.2 Clinical Presentation and Natural History Based on Location

The mean age of presentation for all dAVFs is between 50 and 60 years, with Borden type I dAVFs usually presenting at slightly younger age.[1,6,8,9,10,11,13,14] Symptoms often precede the clinical presentation, but dAVFs are also discovered incidentally, ranging from 2 to 30% in studies focused on dAVFs without CVD.[8,13] The clinical symptoms of patients with dAVFs are highly variable and depend on location and venous drainage patterns.

Pulsatile tinnitus is a frequent presenting symptom and commonly occurs with dAVFs with drainage via the transverse and sigmoid sinuses. This finding is speculated to be due to their proximity to the auditory bone conduction system.[3,10,13]

dAVFs involving the CS (like CCFs) may present with orbit/ocular symptoms including chemosis, proptosis, diplopia, retro-orbital headache, and decreased visual acuity. dAVF location in the anterior cranial fossa, i.e., ethmoidal, may also present with a host of orbital symptoms.[12,15]

ICH and NHND—such as seizures, cognitive dysfunction, and focal neurological deficits—may arise from CVD.[2] ICH is likely from rupture of cortical veins/varices under high pressure from CVD, while NHND likely results from venous congestion and subsequent ischemia.[2,16] Ethmoidal, tentorial, cranial-cervical junction, and transverse-sigmoid dAVFs appear more likely to present with NHND or ICH than dAVFs at other locations.[1,14,17] CS dAVFs rarely present with NHND or ICH.[1] Cranial-cervical junction (i.e., foramen magnum) dAVFs also can present with lower cranial nerve palsy.[14] dAVFs along the superior sagittal sinus (SSS) may uniquely present with symptoms of global venous hypertension and encephalopathy, including hydrocephalus, seizures, and dementia.[14,18]

Gross and Du combined their cohort with findings from Satomi et al for dAVFs without CVD.[8,11] In these series, 63% patients had tinnitus, 35% had orbital symptoms, 32% had headache, and 7% were asymptomatic. The most common locations were transverse/sigmoid (51%), cavernous (38%), SSS (4%), and other locations (7%). Gross and Du also combined their cohort with Bulters et al, Söderman et al, Strom et al, and van Dijk et al to evaluate dAVFs with CVD.[7,9,10,11,19] The most common locations were transverse/sigmoid (31%), tentorial (17%), petrosal (9%), ethmoidal (8%), SSS (7%), cavernous (5%), and other locations (24%). Transverse-sigmoid dAVFs had a more diverse venous drainage patterns with 57 and 43% having no CVD and CVD, respectively. Cavernous dAVFs were the most homogeneous with 84% presenting without CVD but with often debilitating ocular symptoms, including visual loss. One hundred percent of tentorial, 94% of petrosal, 90% of ethmoidal, 86% of torcular, and 65% of SSS dAVFs had CVD, portending a more

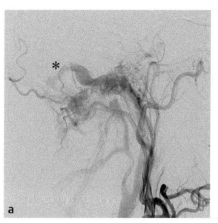
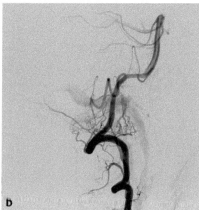

Fig. 6.1 This 60-year-old man presented with occipital headaches and right-sided pulsatile tinnitus. Cerebral angiography revealed a Borden type I, Cognard type IIa dAVF of the right sigmoid sinus and jugular bulb with supply from the ECA **(a)**, occipital artery, ascending pharyngeal artery, and vertebral artery dural branches **(b)**. Retrograde dural venous sinus drainage was observed (*); however, there was no evidence of CVD. The patient's symptoms were not debilitating, and he was managed medically.

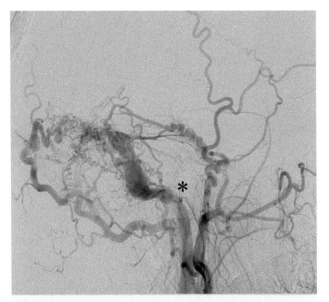

Fig. 6.2 This 43-year-old man presented with chronic debilitating left pulsatile tinnitus and history of deep venous thrombosis. Cerebral angiography revealed a Borden type I, Cognard type I left transverse-sigmoid dAVF with multiple ECA feeding arteries. There was no retrograde venous drainage or CVD; however, relatively a high grade stenosis (*) of the left sigmoid sinus and proximal jugular vein and high flow through the fistula created venous congestion. The patient was treated and radiographically cured via staged transarterial embolization with Onyx and transvenous embolization with Onyx and coils. His tinnitus completely resolved immediately after treatment.

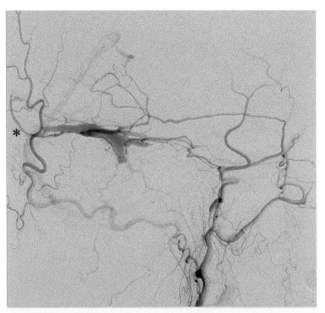

Fig. 6.3 This 70-year-old patient presented cognitive decline and seizures. Cerebral angiography revealed a Borden type II, Cognard type IIa + b right transverse-sigmoid dAVF fed by the right occipital and middle meningeal arteries with evidence of cortical venous reflux (*). The patient underwent transarterial embolization with Onyx through a branch of middle meningeal artery with occlusion of the dAVF resulting in no additional cognitive decline or seizures at follow-up.

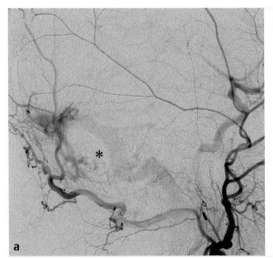
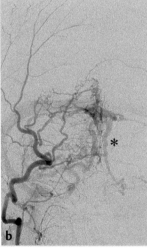

Fig. 6.4 This 68-year-old patient presented with headaches and intermittent bilateral pulsatile tinnitus. Cerebral angiography demonstrated a Borden and Cognard type III torcular dAVF with arterial feeders from bilateral occipital arteries, bilateral middle meningeal arteries, left posterior meningeal artery, and right meningohypophyseal trunk **(a,b)**. CVD (*) occurred through the inferior vermian and right superior and inferior hemispheric cerebellar veins emptying into the straight sinus (major) and right transverse sinus (minor). Transarterial embolization with Onyx was performed via two right occipital artery branches in a single session with successful occlusion of the dAVF restoring normal venous drainage. At 18-month follow-up, there was no recurrence and the patient's symptoms had resolved.

dangerous natural history in regard to ICH for these locations. ▶ Table 6.2 lists the common locations of dAVFs stratified by Borden type.

6.3.3 Natural History of dAVFs without CVD

Borden type I and Cognard types I and IIa dAVFs are often grouped together in studies due to the absence of CVD. The likelihood of NHND and ICH at presentation is low, with no patients presenting with either in several studies (▶ Table 6.3).[1,8,11] The combined cohorts Gross and Du and Satomi et al had 409 years of follow-up, and no ICH or NHND occurred in patients who did not progress to a more aggressive lesion (▶ Table 6.3).[11] However, two patients in the Satomi et al series developed CVD from spontaneous venous thrombosis, resulting in one ICH for an overall rate of conversion to higher grade in 1.4% patients.[11] Shah et al found a 1% annual rate of conversion to dAVFs with CVD, which was identified by changes in symptoms.[13]

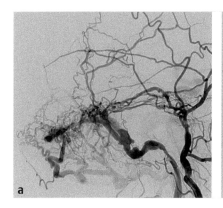

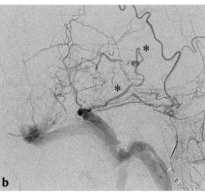

Fig. 6.5 This 67-year-old patient presented with transient word-finding difficulty and pulsatile tinnitus. Cerebral angiography revealed a Borden and Cognard type III left transverse-sigmoid sinus dAVF. Arterial supply occurred via the posterior auricular, middle meningeal, and occipital arteries (a) and evidence of CVD in the posterior temporal area (b,*). The patient underwent transvenous embolization of the isolated venous pouch with resolution of CVD and symptoms at follow-up.

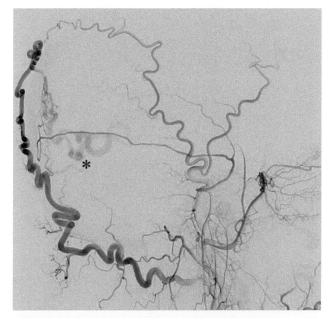

Fig. 6.6 This 44-year-old patient presented with transient left homonymous hemianopsia and occipital headaches. Cerebral angiography demonstrated a Borden and Cognard type III posterior SSS dAVF with arterial supply from bilateral occipital, superficial temporal, and middle meningeal arteries and direct CVD into right medial occipital veins (*asterisk*), which refluxed into the inferior sagittal sinus. Transarterial embolization with Onyx was performed via the right middle meningeal artery with resolution of the CVD.

6.3.4 Natural History of dAVFs with CVD

Borden types II and III and Cognard types IIb, IIa + b, and III–V are often grouped together in studies due to the presence of CVD. These types frequently present with ICH or NHND.[1,4,5,6,7,9,11] Duffau et al studied 20 patients with CVD who presented with ICH and found a 35% risk of rebleeding within 2 weeks of presentation resulting in worse deficits than the initial bleed.[6] These authors advocated "complete and early treatment" of dAVFs with CVD presenting with ICH.

Gross and Du combined their cohort with Bulters et al, Söderman et al, Strom et al, and van Dijk et al and evaluated the annual risks of NHND or ICH.[7,9,10,11,19] The adjusted rates of NHND or ICH at presentation were both 30%.[11] In this study of 254 patients, 42% were Borden type II (91 lesions in 89 patients) and 58% (163 lesions in 162 patients) were Borden type III. There were 14 NHNDs and 25 ICHs in 397.8 patient-years of follow-up. The annual rate of NHND was 4% (resultant annual mortality rate 1%) and the annual rate of ICH was 6% (resultant annual mortality rate 3%).

In the same study by Gross and Du, the majority of Borden type II lesions were female (0.7:1 male:female ratio), and locations were transverse-sigmoid (61%), cavernous (10%), tentorial (7%), SSS (6%), petrosal (4%), and torcular (4%).[11] ICH at presentation occurred in 18% patients, and the annual ICH rate was 6% (▶ Table 6.3). Borden type III dAVF patients were more often male (1.9:1 ratio), and lesions were tentorial (28%), petrosal (13%), transverse-sigmoid (9%), ethmoidal (8%), SSS (7%), cavernous (3%), and torcular (3%). The rate of ICH at presentation was 34%, and the annual rate of ICH was 10% (▶ Table 6.3). For 43 Borden type III lesions with venous ectasia, i.e., Cognard type IV, the annual rate of ICH was 21% (▶ Table 6.3).

Gross and Du also evaluated the mode of presentation for Borden type II and III dAVFs on the future risk of NHND and ICH

Table 6.2 Common locations of dAVFs by Borden type

Location	N	Type I (%)	Type II (%)	Type III (%)
Transverse-sigmoid	125	57	35	8
Cavernous	63	84	11	5
Tentorial	35	0	14	86
Petrosal	18	6	17	78
Superior sagittal sinus	17	35	24	41
Ethmoidal	10	10	0	90
Torcular	7	14	43	43

Source: Adapted from Gross et al.[11]

Table 6.3 dAVF ICH rates stratified by Borden type

Type	N	ICH at presentation (%)	Annual rate of ICH (%)
I	141	0	0
II	91	18	6
III	163	34	10
III + venous ectasia	43	26	21

Source: Adapted from Gross et al.[11]

Table 6.4 Annual NHND and ICH rates for Borden type II and III dAVFs based on presentation

Presentation	N	Annual rate of new NHND (%)	Annual rate of ICH (%)
No prior ICH	153	7	3
No prior ICH, minimal or no symptoms	63	0	2
NHND, no prior ICH	37	20	10
Prior ICH	81	0	46

Source: Adapted from Gross et al.[11]

(▶ Table 6.4).[11] For asymptomatic or minimally symptomatic (e.g., tinnitus) type II or III dAVFs, the annual ICH rate was 2%, and annual rate of NHND was 0% in 86.5 lesion-years. In patients presenting with NHNDs, the annual rate of additional NHNDs was 20%, and the annual rate of ICH was 10% in 25.1 and 29.6 lesion-years, respectively. The annual rehemorrhage rate was 46% in 74.6 lesion-years.

6.4 Discussion

The importance of CVD in dAVFs as a risk factor for neurological deficit and ICH at presentation has long been known.[2,3] This angiographic finding was the foundation of the classification systems of Borden and Cognard, which were initially evaluated by Davies et al.[1,4,5] Since then, numerous natural history studies have stratified the risks of subsequent NHND and ICH based on the presence or absence of CVD.[6,7,8,9,10,19] The study by Gross and Du reviewed their cohort and these natural history studies.[11] For dAVFs without CVD, no patients presented with NHND or ICH, and the risk of ICH and NHND appears exceedingly low. For Borden type II dAVFs, ICH at presentation occurred in 18% patients, and the annual rate of ICH was 6%. For Borden type III dAVFs, ICH at presentation occurred in 34% patients, and the annual rate of ICH was 10%. Asymptomatic or minimally symptomatic Borden type II and III dAVFs appear to have a much lower risk of NHND or ICH than patients presenting with NIND or ICH.

Lesion location, in particular ethmoidal and tentorial dAVFs, has been associated with a more aggressive course; however, these findings may be confounded by the higher likelihood of CVD at these locations. Venous drainage into the deep venous system for tentorial dAVFs and regional venous patterns mandating CVD for ethmoidal dAVFs can place these lesions at higher risk.[1,20,21] However, a higher percentage of these lesions are found to be Borden type III dAVFs, and after controlling for the location, there may be no statistical difference based on location alone.[1,11]

dAVFs without CVD need close follow-up because patients can progress to have CVD, at a rate of approximately 1% per year.[8,13] In these patients, any change in symptoms or a deterioration in clinical status deserves repeat radiographic evaluation. Upfront treatment of these lesions is controversial and must be weighed against the overall complication rate, found to be 2.5% for all dAVFs in a recent meta-analysis.[22] Treatment can be considered in otherwise healthy patients with debilitating symptoms, such as headaches, visual changes, and pulsatile tinnitus. Patients with dAVFs with asymptomatic CVD have lower risks of NHND and ICH than patients with symptomatic CVD. Treatment of these dAVFs is usually warranted in the appropriate clinical setting to prevent ICH, given the risk of subsequent events over the course of the lifetime of the patient.[16] Furthermore, angiographic findings seen at presentation or follow-up, such as venous ectasia, venous congestion, and dural sinus stenosis, can be associated with more aggressive courses and may necessitate treatment in the absence of symptomatic CVD.[23,24]

dAVFs with symptomatic CVD require immediate treatment with endovascular or surgical therapy in the majority of cases due to high risk of early, recurrent ICH and NHND. The delay of cure with stereotactic radiosurgery is not tolerable unless the medical condition of the patient or complexity of the lesion and the immediate procedural risk of endovascular or surgical therapy argue against aggressive treatment. For most dAVFs, an endovascular-first approach is used for treatment at many centers, with surgical ligation being offered after endovascular therapy has been exhausted or if the anatomy of the dAVFs portends a high endovascular procedural risk, as may be the case with certain ethmoidal, tentorial, and cranial-cervical junction dAVFs.

6.4.1 Limitations and Future Directions

The available literature regarding the natural history of dAVFs is limited by the heterogeneous nature of individual series and biases of retrospective case series and systematic literature reviews. The external validity of these studies is also limited, as asymptomatic lesions are likely more common than described. Future prospective studies evaluating long-term follow-up of asymptomatic dAVFs without and with CVD as well as the potential influences of other angiographic findings such as location, dural venous stenosis, and angiographic change over time are warranted.

6.5 Conclusion

The risk of ICH and NHND is stratified by dAVF location and the presence or absence of CVD according to the Borden and Cognard classification systems and can be further stratified by the presence or absence of symptoms at presentation. The presence of CVD leads to a higher risk of future NHND and ICH. Immediate endovascular or surgical treatment of dAVFs with symptomatic CVD is always warranted, while treatment for dAVFs with asymptomatic CVD is nearly always justifiable. Treatment is also reasonable for dAVFs without CVD but with debilitating symptoms.

References

[1] Davies MA, TerBrugge K, Willinsky R, Coyne T, Saleh J, Wallace MC. The validity of classification for the clinical presentation of intracranial dural arteriovenous fistulas. J Neurosurg. 1996; 85(5):830–837

[2] Lasjaunias P, Chiu M, ter Brugge K, Tolia A, Hurth M, Bernstein M. Neurological manifestations of intracranial dural arteriovenous malformations. J Neurosurg. 1986; 64(5):724–730

[3] Awad IA, Little JR, Akarawi WP, Ahl J. Intracranial dural arteriovenous malformations: factors predisposing to an aggressive neurological course. J Neurosurg. 1990; 72(6):839–850

[4] Borden JA, Wu JK, Shucart WA. A proposed classification for spinal and cranial dural arteriovenous fistulous malformations and implications for treatment. J Neurosurg. 1995; 82(2):166–179

[5] Cognard C, Gobin YP, Pierot L, et al. Cerebral dural arteriovenous fistulas: clinical and angiographic correlation with a revised classification of venous drainage. Radiology. 1995; 194(3):671–680

[6] Duffau H, Lopes M, Janosevic V, et al. Early rebleeding from intracranial dural arteriovenous fistulas: report of 20 cases and review of the literature. J Neurosurg. 1999; 90(1):78–84

[7] van Dijk JM, terBrugge KG, Willinsky RA, Wallace MC. Clinical course of cranial dural arteriovenous fistulas with long-term persistent cortical venous reflux. Stroke. 2002; 33(5):1233–1236

[8] Satomi J, van Dijk JM, Terbrugge KG, Willinsky RA, Wallace MC. Benign cranial dural arteriovenous fistulas: outcome of conservative management based on the natural history of the lesion. J Neurosurg. 2002; 97(4):767–770

[9] Söderman M, Pavic L, Edner G, Holmin S, Andersson T. Natural history of dural arteriovenous shunts. Stroke. 2008; 39(6):1735–1739

[10] Strom RG, Botros JA, Refai D, et al. Cranial dural arteriovenous fistulae: asymptomatic cortical venous drainage portends less aggressive clinical course. Neurosurgery. 2009; 64(2):241–247, discussion 247–248

[11] Gross BA, Du R. The natural history of cerebral dural arteriovenous fistulae. Neurosurgery. 2012; 71(3):594–602, discussion 602–603

[12] Barrow DL, Spector RH, Braun IF, Landman JA, Tindall SC, Tindall GT. Classification and treatment of spontaneous carotid-cavernous sinus fistulas. J Neurosurg. 1985; 62(2):248–256

[13] Shah MN, Botros JA, Pilgram TK, et al. Borden-Shucart Type I dural arteriovenous fistulas: clinical course including risk of conversion to higher-grade fistulas. J Neurosurg. 2012; 117(3):539–545

[14] Kim MS, Han DH, Kwon OK, Oh CW, Han MH. Clinical characteristics of dural arteriovenous fistula. J Clin Neurosci. 2002; 9(2):147–155

[15] Meyers PM, Halbach VV, Dowd CF, et al. Dural carotid cavernous fistula: definitive endovascular management and long-term follow-up. Am J Ophthalmol. 2002; 134(1):85–92

[16] Zipfel GJ, Shah MN, Refai D, Dacey RG , Jr, Derdeyn CP. Cranial dural arteriovenous fistulas: modification of angiographic classification scales based on new natural history data. Neurosurg Focus. 2009; 26(5):E14

[17] Kiyosue H, Hori Y, Okahara M, et al. Treatment of intracranial dural arteriovenous fistulas: current strategies based on location and hemodynamics, and alternative techniques of transcatheter embolization. Radiographics. 2004; 24(6):1637–1653

[18] Hurst RW, Bagley LJ, Galetta S, et al. Dementia resulting from dural arteriovenous fistulas: the pathologic findings of venous hypertensive encephalopathy. AJNR Am J Neuroradiol. 1998; 19(7):1267–1273

[19] Bulters DO, Mathad N, Culliford D, Millar J, Sparrow OC. The natural history of cranial dural arteriovenous fistulae with cortical venous reflux–the significance of venous ectasia. Neurosurgery. 2012; 70(2):312–318, discussion 318–319

[20] Lawton MT, Sanchez-Mejia RO, Pham D, Tan J, Halbach VV. Tentorial dural arteriovenous fistulae: operative strategies and microsurgical results for six types. Neurosurgery. 2008; 62(3) Suppl 1:110–124, discussion 124–125

[21] Lawton MT, Chun J, Wilson CB, Halbach VV. Ethmoidal dural arteriovenous fistulae: an assessment of surgical and endovascular management. Neurosurgery. 1999; 45(4):805–810, discussion 810–811

[22] Kobayashi A, Al-Shahi Salman R. Prognosis and treatment of intracranial dural arteriovenous fistulae: a systematic review and meta-analysis. Int J Stroke. 2014; 9(6):670–677

[23] Cognard C, Houdart E, Casasco A, Gabrillargues J, Chiras J, Merland JJ. Long-term changes in intracranial dural arteriovenous fistulae leading to worsening in the type of venous drainage. Neuroradiology. 1997; 39(1):59–66

[24] Lanzino G, Jensen ME, Kongable GL, Kassell NF. Angiographic characteristics of dural arteriovenous malformations that present with intracranial hemorrhage. Acta Neurochir (Wien). 1994; 129(3–4):140–145

7 Management of Unruptured Brain Arteriovenous Malformations

Thomas J. Sorenson and Giuseppe Lanzino

Abstract

The management of unruptured arteriovenous malformations (AVMs) is controversial. Whereas the average risk of rupture is approximately 2% per year, hemorrhage from ruptured AVM carries a significant morbidity and mortality. However, treatment of brain AVMs is not without the risk of severe complications. In the past few years, the publication of the ARUBA study has further increased the controversy surrounding the best treatment strategy for unruptured AVMs. The ARUBA trial notwithstanding, we feel that invasive treatment is indicated for young patients if the risk of treatment is acceptably low. In this chapter, we review current knowledge on the natural history of unruptured AVMs, the results of the ARUBA study, and our current approach to a patient with an unbled AVM.

Keywords: arteriovenous malformations, natural history, ARUBA study, hemorrhage, stereotactic radiosurgery, microsurgery, embolization

---

Key Points

- The publishing of ARUBA has reinvigorated the discussion about the conservative management of AVMs versus interventional treatments.
- ARUBA has shown that treatment of AVMs has clinically important complications that are higher than otherwise suggested in single-center, usually retrospective studies.
- Selection of patients with unruptured AVMs is key and if treatment is undertaken, the risk of complications must be acceptably low.
- ARUBA also provided objective data to justify conservative management in some patients, due to high risk or decreased life expectancy. These data show that short-term outlook of conservative management is acceptable, but that these benefits might be lost in the long term.
- There have been numerous criticisms of the study, but no additional large, multicenter, prospective studies, showing how difficult it is to run a study of this magnitude, and the ARUBA authors should be credited for that.

7.1 Introduction

Brain arteriovenous malformations (AVMs) are relatively uncommon vascular lesions that have traditionally been detected after hemorrhage, with notable long-term morbidity and case fatality. However, with widespread utilization of neuroimaging, AVMs are increasingly diagnosed incidentally or in the presence of minor neurological symptoms without hemorrhage.[1] This has created a paradigm shift and, today, most patients evaluated with an AVM do not have clinical history of hemorrhage. In such cases, the treating physician is faced with the dilemma of submitting the patients to the risk of invasive

treatment or submitting the patients to a small, definite risk of hemorrhage but leaving the AVM untreated, subjected to natural history. In recent years, the controversy about the best therapeutic modality in patients with unruptured AVMs has been heightened by the results of A Randomized Trial of Unruptured Brain Arteriovenous Malformations (ARUBA) study. In this chapter, we will review current knowledge on the natural history of untreated, unruptured AVMs, the results of the ARUBA study, the results of further investigations, and life after ARUBA.

7.2 Natural History of Unruptured AVMs

Sound data about the natural history of untreated, unruptured AVMs are limited and, for the majority, based on retrospective, clinical series. The main challenge in obtaining high-quality data to base clinical decision upon is the low incidence of the end point (rupture), the need for long-term (several years) follow-up, and the fact that unruptured AVMs are a very heterogeneous group in relation to their location, mode of presentation, size, and angioarchitecture. The issue is further complicated by the observation that an important subset of patients without a clinical history of hemorrhage demonstrates either radiological or histological findings consistent with prior clinically silent hemorrhage.[2]

For a long time, the best data available on the natural history of AVMs were based on a large, single-center Finnish cohort, initially analyzed by Ondra et al[3] and more recently updated by Hernesniemi et al.[4] Of 631 AVM patients admitted at Helsinki University Central Hospital between 1942 and 2005, 238 were medically managed and considered for analysis. Preadmission AVM rupture occurred in 139 patients. Average follow-up time was 13.5 years (range, 1 month to 53.1 years). A total of 77 patients experienced AVM hemorrhage during 3,222 person-years, which represents a 2.4% annual rupture rate.

The main strength of this cohort is related to the long-term follow-up and the fact that the Finnish population was very stable during the period under study, making possible to account for every patient, even many years after the initial diagnosis. The limitations of this cohort are that patients with prior history of hemorrhage are not excluded when calculating the hemorrhage rate, which could be slightly misleading. We were also not able to recalculate the hemorrhage rate as the natural history exclusively of patients who did present with hemorrhage was not defined. Additionally, limitations are related to the fact that the cohort under study spanned many years, during which there have been dramatic changes in diagnostic tools and therapeutic approach to these lesions. These limitations notwithstanding, data from this cohort suggested that the yearly risk of hemorrhage was 2.4% per patient per year. More definitive and contemporary data on the natural history of patients with unruptured AVMs come from the ARUBA study, which showed that for all-comers with unruptured AVMs, the annual rate of bleeding was similar, at 2% per year.

7.3 Outcome after First Hemorrhage

Another important issue in assessing the risk of treatment versus the natural history is to understand the clinical outcome after first hemorrhage of an AVM. After an AVM-associated hemorrhage (AVM-ICH), 72% of patients with AVM have a good functional outcome (mRS < 2).[5] The outcome from hemorrhage in a patient with an AVM is much more favorable than patients who suffer a spontaneous ICH (not secondary to AVM rupture). Patients with AVM-ICH are younger and have lower blood pressure and better Glasgow Coma Scores than patients with spontaneous hemorrhage (sICH).[6] Case fatality at 1 month was 11% for those with AVM-ICH.

However, recent population studies have shown that overall prognosis after AVM rupture, though better than sICH, is not quite as benign as single-center studies had suggested. In the Scottish study, the case fatality rate after AVM-ICH was 11% at 1 month and 13% at 2 years. The percentage of patients who were dead or dependent (mRS > 3) at 1 year was 40%. Case fatality rate is age dependent and was 9.2% at 1 month in patients younger than 60 years and 21% in those older than 60 years.[7]

To select those patients at higher risk of hemorrhage from an originally unruptured AVM, several publications have analyzed factors predictive of higher risk of hemorrhage. The main limitations of these studies are that these are usually retrospective and the analysis of the risk factors (especially those related to angioarchitecture) is retrospective in patients who have already presented with hemorrhage, which does not always allow for an accurate understanding of prehemorrhage angioarchitecture. Considering these important methodological limitations, there are still some factors that are likely associated with a higher risk of bleeding. Most of these factors are related to the angioarchitecture and include (1) presence of venous varices and evidence of outflow obstruction of the drainage pathways; (2) presence of intranidal aneurysms, which indicate areas of hemodynamic stress within the nidus; and (3) presence of feeding pedicle aneurysms.

Though controversy exists about the predictive ability of size, location, and patient age to increased risk of rupture, it is our feeling that mode and symptoms of presentation are most important in trying to understand if a patient might bleed. In other words, there are some situations where the onset of symptoms might indicate that hemodynamic factors might have acutely changed in an AVM, thus causing the symptoms. Therefore, we think that it is not only important to analyze patient symptoms and reason of AVM diagnoses, but also important to make careful analysis of risk factors associated with AVM in question. It is also our belief that for unruptured AVMs, the risk of rupture is highest soon after diagnosis, and then starts decreasing if no hemorrhage occurs during a period of a few years. This observation is corroborated by the Finnish cohort in which it was observed that the risk of bleeding was much higher during the first 5 years after diagnosis than thereafter.

As mentioned above, anecdotal observations and recent data have suggested that an important subset of patients without clinical history of hemorrhage has radiological or histological findings consistent with a silent bleed. Whether these patients are at increased risk of bleeding than patients without such history is a matter of debate. Like other asymptomatic, often prevalent cerebrovascular disorders, such as intracranial aneurysms, cavernous malformations, and carotid stenosis, not all unruptured AVMs are similar, and it will be important in the future to try to identify those patients at higher risk of bleeding who might be more likely to benefit from treatment and for whom the risk of invasive treatment might be justified.

7.4 ARUBA (A Randomized Trial of Unruptured Brain Arteriovenous Malformations) Results and Critiques

ARUBA was the first randomized trial that attempted to determine the best approach for management of unruptured brain AVMs, specifically whether the medical management or interventional therapy posed a greater risk to the patient. Given the risks associated with invasive treatment, the ARUBA investigators aimed to answer the questions of whether invasive treatment of unruptured AVMs is indeed better than conservative management in patients with unruptured AVMs.

The primary end point measured in the trial was time to death or symptomatic stroke. Symptomatic stroke was defined as onset of neurological deficit or headache with corresponding neuroimaging of new hemorrhage or infarction. The secondary end point measured was clinical impairment at 5 years (mRS score ≥ 2).

The authors screened 1,514 patients across 39 active clinical sites in 9 countries and found 1,014 patients ineligible, 323 refusing participation, and 42 unable to participate. In total, 226 patients were randomized into two cohorts: interventional therapy (n = 116) or conservative management (n = 110). Based on modern clinical practice, three interventional therapies were utilized alone or in a multimodal approach: neurosurgery alone (n = 5), embolization alone (n = 30), stereotactic radiosurgery alone (n = 31), embolization and neurosurgery (n = 12), embolization and radiosurgery (n = 15), or embolization, neurosurgery, and radiosurgery (n = 1). Following randomization, median time to first intervention was 76 days. There were no statistically significant differences between the two cohort characteristics at randomization or treatment. Seven patients crossed over from conservative management to interventional therapy, while three patients assigned to interventional therapy suffered an outcome event between randomization and intervention and crossed over to conservative management. Seven patients discontinued their participation in the trial at follow-up (average: 33 months). At randomization, all patients had Spetzler–Martin (SM) grade scores < 4 and most (62%) were ≤ 2 and all patients had mRS score ≤ 1. Patient enrollment was halted by the NINDS/NIH at the recommendation of the data and monitoring board.

During follow-up, a primary event occurred in 10 (8%) patients in the conservative management cohort versus 36 (36.7%) patients in the interventional therapy cohort (▶ Table 7.1). This significant difference between cohorts held true for the secondary event (clinical impairment) as well, with 8 (15.1%) patients from conservative management cohort versus 24 (46.2%) patients from interventional therapy cohort having an mRS score ≥ 2 at 30 weeks' follow-up.[8]

Table 7.1 Primary outcome (stroke or mortality) in ARUBA

	Interventional therapy (n = 114)	Medical management (n = 109)
Death or stroke	36 (36.7%)	10 (8.0%)
Death (any cause)	3 (2.6%)	2 (1.8%)
Death (AVM-related)	2 (1.8%)	0
First stroke (all)	35 (35.7%)	8 (6.4%)
First stroke (hemorrhagic)	24 (24.5%)	7 (5.6%)
First stroke (ischemic)	11 (11.2%)	1 (0.8%)

Source: Adapted from Mohr et al.[8]

7.5 ARUBA Critiques

Publication of ARUBA sparked heated debate on treatment of unruptured AVMs. Many authors criticized the approach taken by ARUBA and believed that the separation of treatment into two groups was a drastic oversimplification.[9,10,11,12] While conservative management can be performed with little clinical variability, the interventional cohort included three different interventions: neurosurgery, embolization, and radiosurgery, which can hardly all be grouped to make an accurate general conclusion between the two treatment options.[12] Additionally, grouping multiple treatment options into a single "arm" without randomization removes the ability to compare results between treatment options within the arm.[13]

Authors also highly criticized the end points in the refuting literature. Many questions were raised about the interpretation of findings[9,10,12,14,15] and the high number of patients who reached primary end point, along with the low number of total patients.[10,16,17]

Additionally, authors believed that the choice of outcome measures was not appropriate based on the different optimal outcomes of each treatment technique. For example, the optimal outcome of surgical AVM treatment is complete obliteration, but endovascular techniques rarely achieve this goal and radiosurgery requires years to obliterate most of the AVM.[18] Thus, for most patients, treatment conclusions were not evaluated based on each technique's accepted end point.

7.6 Life after ARUBA

A prospective, population-based cohort study of 114 adults published by Wedderburn et al corroborates the ARUBA data. The authors compared the baseline characteristics and 3-year outcome of adults who received intervention (n = 63) and those who did not (n = 51) and reported no difference in progression to Oxford Handicap Scale (OHS) score of 2 to 6 or 3 to 6. In a multivariable Cox proportional hazards analysis, the authors determined that the risk of poor outcome (OHS, 2 to 6) was greater in patients of interventional cohort (hazard ratio [HR], 2.5) and in patients with larger AVM nidus (HR, 1.3). However, the cohorts did not differ in time to OHS score ≥ 2 that was sustained until the end of follow-up, so long-term effects of intervention are unclear.[19]

Al-Shahi Salman et al published another cohort study that corroborated ARUBA and revealed that conservative management of unruptured AVMs compared to intervention was associated with better clinical outcomes for up to 12 years. A total of 438 patients were identified as having first-in-lifetime unruptured AVM diagnosis between 1999–2003 and 2006–2010. Of these 438 patients, 234 were excluded for previous intracranial hemorrhage or death. The remaining 204 were eligible for analysis. A total of 103 patients had undergone intervention for their AVM, and 101 patients had undergone conservative management. Follow-up occurred for a median of 6.9 years (range, 4–11 years) and 1,479 person-years. During the first 4 years of follow-up when the proportional hazards assumption was met, the rate of progression to primary outcome (death or nonfatal handicap) was lower during conservative management than after intervention (36 vs. 39 events; adjusted HR, 0.59). When the subsequent periods were analyzed separately, the rates were not so different (for 4–8 years, 8 vs. 8 events; adjusted HR: 1.07; for 8–12 years, 5 vs. 1 events; adjusted HR: 4.70). The death rate was higher overall for the conservative management cohort, but this was attributable to deaths from other causes and these differences disappeared after age adjustment. The proportional hazards assumption for the secondary outcome (intracranial hemorrhage) was met for all 12 years of follow-up, and rate of progression to secondary outcome was lower with conservative management than after intervention (14 vs. 38 events; adjusted HR, 0.37). The authors report that this is largely due to symptomatic strokes from intervention.[20]

7.7 Intervention for Unruptured AVM

Following the publication of the ARUBA study, several single-center series have focused on the results of neurosurgery (with or without embolization) or radiosurgery for "ARUBA-eligible" patients.[21,22,23,24] These series have suggested that surgery in low-grade AVMs (SM grade I and II) is associated with a complication rate much lower than the one observed in observational arm of ARUBA study and therefore is justified in such cases. Similarly, radiosurgery series have reported similar observations. The problem with these studies is that these are single-center series without prospective, third-party assessment of outcome.

Based on current evidence and personal opinions, we think that despite the ARUBA study, treatment should be offered to young patients with unruptured AVMs, provided the risk of treatment is acceptably low. We currently recommend surgery or radiosurgery for unruptured SM grade I and II AVMs. The decisions to perform surgery or radiosurgery is based on patient symptomatology, perceived risk of bleeding over the latency period, and patient preference. For SM grade III unruptured AVMs, we prefer radiosurgery in most cases, if possible. Surgery or staged Gamma Knife is considered only judiciously in selected patients with SM grade IV AVMs. Observation is reserved to all unruptured SM grade V AVMs and several patients with SM grade IV AVMs, especially if older than 50 years.

7.8 Summary

The publishing of ARUBA has reinvigorated the discussion about the conservative management of AVMs versus interventional treatments. While ARUBA is not conclusive in its results, it provides several important lessons and merits. First, treatment of AVMs has clinically important complications that are higher than otherwise suggested in single-center, usually retrospective studies. We feel that the ARUBA study, like ISUIA, has hopefully resulted in improvement in treatment of patients with AVMs in that physicians should be much more careful and realize that if treatment is undertaken, it must be done with very low morbidity. ARUBA also provided objective data to justify conservative management in some patients, due to high risk or decreased life expectancy. These data show that short-term outlook of conservative management is acceptable, but that these benefits might be lost in the long term. There have been numerous criticisms of the study but no additional large, multicenter, prospective studies, showing how difficult it is to run a study of this magnitude, and the ARUBA authors should be credited for that.

References

[1] Stapf C, Mohr JP. Unruptured brain arteriovenous malformations should be treated conservatively: yes. Stroke. 2007; 38(12):3308–3309

[2] Abla AA, Nelson J, Kim H, Hess CP, Tihan T, Lawton MT. Silent arteriovenous malformation hemorrhage and the recognition of "unruptured" arteriovenous malformation patients who benefit from surgical intervention. Neurosurgery. 2015; 76(5):592–600, discussion 600

[3] Ondra SL, Troupp H, George ED, Schwab K. The natural history of symptomatic arteriovenous malformations of the brain: a 24-year follow-up assessment. J Neurosurg. 1990; 73(3):387–391

[4] Hernesniemi JA, Dashti R, Juvela S, Väärt K, Niemelä M, Laakso A. Natural history of brain arteriovenous malformations: a long-term follow-up study of risk of hemorrhage in 238 patients. Neurosurgery. 2008; 63(5):823–829, discussion 829–831

[5] Choi JH, Mast H, Sciacca RR, et al. Clinical outcome after first and recurrent hemorrhage in patients with untreated brain arteriovenous malformation. Stroke. 2006; 37(5):1243–1247

[6] van Beijnum J, Lovelock CE, Cordonnier C, Rothwell PM, Klijn CJ, Al-Shahi Salman R, SIVMS Steering Committee and the Oxford Vascular Study. Outcome after spontaneous and arteriovenous malformation-related intracerebral haemorrhage: population-based studies. Brain. 2009; 132(Pt 2):537–543

[7] Al-Shahi R, Bhattacharya JJ, Currie DG, et al. Scottish Intracranial Vascular Malformation Study Collaborators. Prospective, population-based detection of intracranial vascular malformations in adults: the Scottish Intracranial Vascular Malformation Study (SIVMS). Stroke. 2003; 34(5):1163–1169

[8] Mohr JP, Parides MK, Stapf C, et al. international ARUBA investigators. Medical management with or without interventional therapy for unruptured brain arteriovenous malformations (ARUBA): a multicentre, non-blinded, randomised trial. Lancet. 2014; 383(9917):614–621

[9] Amin-Hanjani S. ARUBA results are not applicable to all patients with arteriovenous malformation. Stroke. 2014; 45(5):1539–1540

[10] Bambakidis NC, Cockroft K, Connolly ES, et al. Preliminary results of the ARUBA study. Neurosurgery. 2013; 73(2):E379–E381

[11] Cockroft KM, Jayaraman MV, Amin-Hanjani S, Derdeyn CP, McDougall CG, Wilson JA. A perfect storm: how a randomized trial of unruptured brain arteriovenous malformations' (ARUBA's) trial design challenges notions of external validity. Stroke. 2012; 43(7):1979–1981

[12] Day AL, Dannenbaum M, Jung S. A randomized trial of unruptured brain arteriovenous malformations trial: an editorial review. Stroke. 2014; 45(10): 3147–3148

[13] Magro E, Gentric JC, Darsaut TE, et al. Responses to ARUBA: a systematic review and critical analysis for the design of future arteriovenous malformation trials. J Neurosurg. 2017; 126(2):486–494

[14] Elhammady MS, Heros RC. Editorial: surgical management of unruptured cerebral arteriovenous malformations. J Neurosurg. 2014; 121(4):875–876

[15] Grasso G. The ARUBA study: what is the evidence? World Neurosurg. 2014; 82(3–4):e576

[16] Knopman J, Stieg PE. Management of unruptured brain arteriovenous malformations. Lancet. 2014; 383(9917):581–583

[17] Lawton MT, Abla AA. Management of brain arteriovenous malformations. Lancet. 2014; 383(9929):1634–1635

[18] Hartmann A, Mast H, Mohr JP, et al. Determinants of staged endovascular and surgical treatment outcome of brain arteriovenous malformations. Stroke. 2005; 36(11):2431–2435

[19] Wedderburn CJ, van Beijnum J, Bhattacharya JJ, et al. SIVMS Collaborators. Outcome after interventional or conservative management of unruptured brain arteriovenous malformations: a prospective, population-based cohort study. Lancet Neurol. 2008; 7(3):223–230

[20] Al-Shahi Salman R, White PM, Counsell CE, et al. Scottish Audit of Intracranial Vascular Malformations Collaborators. Outcome after conservative management or intervention for unruptured brain arteriovenous malformations. JAMA. 2014; 311(16):1661–1669

[21] Rutledge WC, Abla AA, Nelson J, Halbach VV, Kim H, Lawton MT. Treatment and outcomes of ARUBA-eligible patients with unruptured brain arteriovenous malformations at a single institution. Neurosurg Focus. 2014; 37(3):E8

[22] Schramm J, Schaller K, Esche J, Boström A. Microsurgery for cerebral arteriovenous malformations: subgroup outcomes in a consecutive series of 288 cases. J Neurosurg. 2017; 126(4):1056–1063

[23] Steiger HJ, Fischer I, Rohn B, Turowski B, Etminan N, Hänggi D. Microsurgical resection of Spetzler-Martin grades 1 and 2 unruptured brain arteriovenous malformations results in lower long-term morbidity and loss of quality-adjusted life-years (QALY) than conservative management–results of a single group series. Acta Neurochir (Wien). 2015; 157(8):1279–1287

[24] Wong J, Slomovic A, Ibrahim G, Radovanovic I, Tymianski M. Microsurgery for ARUBA Trial (A Randomized Trial of Unruptured Brain Arteriovenous Malformation)-Eligible Unruptured Brain Arteriovenous Malformations. Stroke. 2017; 48(1):136–144

8 Preoperative and Postoperative Imaging Evaluation of Arteriovenous Malformations

Michaelangelo Fuortes, Joseph Gastala, Adam Liudahl, Minako Hayakawa, and Colin Derdeyn

Abstract

Imaging features of brain arteriovenous malformations (AVMs) are critical for pretreatment planning and posttreatment decision-making. This chapter will describe the important, clinically relevant imaging features of brain AVMs as well as the relative advantages and disadvantages of the widely available imaging modalities: computed tomography (CT), magnetic resonance imaging (MRI), and digital subtraction angiography (DSA). These techniques often yield complementary information. Critical features include the size, location, and pattern of venous drainage, as well as the presence of intranidal or flow-related aneurysms. Imaging is critical for confirming cure of these lesions, particularly after stereotactic radiosurgery. Finally, we will review new and emerging applications of imaging for patients with brain AVMs, including the assessment of microhemorrhage as an indicator of increased bleeding risk for clinically asymptomatic brain AVMs.

Keywords: computed tomography, magnetic resonance imaging, digital subtraction angiography, hemorrhage, aneurysms, nidus

Key Point

- Imaging evaluation of arteriovenous malformations.
- Preoperative planning.
- Postoperative imaging of complications.

8.1 Introduction

A brain arteriovenous malformation (AVM) is a cerebrovascular pathology composed of afferent arteries and draining veins connected by a nidus of arteriovenous fistulas without an intervening capillary bed.[1,2] Management of brain AVMs is complex and requires a multidisciplinary approach, with treatment options including surgical resection, endovascular embolization, stereotactic radiosurgery, or various combinations thereof. Treatment decisions are based on risk estimates of rupture and studies of outcomes of invasive treatment. Diagnostic imaging plays a critical role in the identification, pretreatment classification, and posttreatment follow-up of brain AVMs.

8.2 Materials and Methods

A Medline search was performed utilizing PubMed for original research publications, meta-analyses, guidelines, and consensus statements discussing clinical diagnosis, imaging, and clinical management of AVMs. The search employed various combinations of the following keywords: arteriovenous malformation (AVM), digital subtraction angiography (DSA), computed tomography angiography (CTA), magnetic resonance angiography (MRA). The review was limited to English-language literature and human studies. Additional articles were selected by reviewing the reference lists of pertinent publications with identification of relevant authors. The authors performed a critical review of the identified article titles and abstracts followed by review of the full text in relevant articles. The senior authors' personal experience contributed to multiple topics covered in this chapter, more specifically regarding those topics that are sparsely covered in other resources.

8.3 Results

8.3.1 Imaging Diagnosis

The clinical scenario influences the role of diagnostic imaging in the evaluation of brain AVMs with the focus varying from primary diagnosis to clinical follow-up of a known lesion. The initial diagnosis of a brain AVM most commonly occurs in one of three clinical settings: (1) diagnostic work-up of an intracranial hemorrhage; (2) diagnostic work-up for a neurological symptom (e.g., headache, seizure, focal neurological deficit); or (3) imaging evaluation for an unrelated clinical presentation with incidental discovery of a brain AVM. The distinctions between unruptured brain AVMs and those diagnosed following a hemorrhagic episode have important potential clinical implications. The established literature has frequently reported that around 50% of brain AVMs are identified on diagnostic work-up following presentation with intracranial hemorrhage. The increasing utilization of advanced medical imaging in the emergency and outpatient clinical settings may lead to a greater proportion of incidentally discovered brain AVMs in future practice.

In the setting of nontraumatic intracranial hemorrhage, the recommended initial imaging evaluation is a noncontrast head CT. An initial CT study is quick, widely available, and can provide rapid assessment of an intracranial hemorrhage. This diagnostic approach is well validated by the literature, which demonstrates > 90% sensitivity of noncontrast CT for detection of acute subarachnoid hemorrhage.[3] Additional findings on the noncontrast head CT that may suggest an underlying vascular etiology include dilated and/or calcified vessels adjacent to the hemorrhage, hyperdense foci suggesting a vascular nidus, and atypical location of an intraparenchymal hemorrhage suggesting a secondary cause such as a vascular malformation rather than a primary hypertensive hemorrhage (▶ Fig. 8.1).[4] There may be localized brain atrophy surrounding an AVM, or the adjacent brain parenchyma may be hypodense on CT reflecting ischemic changes or gliosis.

CT angiography (CTA), magnetic resonance imaging (MRI), and MRA are frequently used in the initial work-up of AVMs and provide valuable anatomical information. The diagnostic imaging approach varies among individuals and institutions, with some advocating starting with CTA and others proposing MRI and MRA as the initial examinations. Both CTA and MRI/MRA are noninvasive alternatives to catheter angiography and likely provide safety benefits as the initial diagnostic tests.

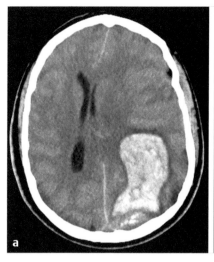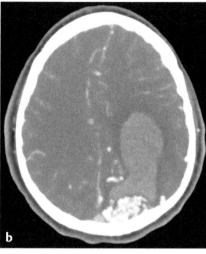

Fig. 8.1 **(a)** Noncontrasted head CT showing large acute parietal hemorrhage with abnormal calcification posteriorly. The lobar location and the calcification suggest an underlying vascular malformation. **(b)** Source image from the CTA showing a tangle of abnormal vessels consistent with a brain AVM.

CTA is widely available and commonly used in the emergency setting for assessment of intracranial hemorrhage for multiple reasons. CTA is fast, minimally invasive, and has high spatial resolution that can provide rapid diagnosis of an underlying vascular malformation in the setting of intracranial hemorrhage, including AVMs.[5] CTA may provide valuable diagnostic information about an AVM, including characterization of the angioarchitecture, localization, and presence of associated aneurysms.[6] Comparative studies of CTA versus DSA in the diagnosis of cerebral vascular disease demonstrate high sensitivity and specificity for both imaging modalities. The main drawbacks to CTA are radiation exposure and administration of intravenous contrast agents which are associated with side effects, albeit relatively infrequently.

MRI and MRA are diagnostic techniques that do not expose the patient to ionizing radiation. Various MRI and MRA techniques may provide information about surrounding brain parenchyma and allow for noninvasive characterization of the AVM. In particular, MRI/MRA provides information about the size of the nidus and number and location of feeding arteries and draining veins. Susceptibility-weighted imaging aids in the detection of hemosiderin that suggests prior episodes of bleeding. There is recent evidence supporting the superiority of initial diagnostic evaluation with MRI and MRA compared with CTA. A Cochrane review and meta-analysis of studies investigating the diagnostic work-up of nontraumatic intracranial hemorrhage for underlying vascular causes reported estimates for CTA of 95% sensitivity and 99% specificity, as compared to 98% sensitivity and 99% specificity for MRA.[7]

The gold standard for the diagnosis of AVMs and other cerebral vascular disease is DSA, which has superior spatial and time resolution to other imaging modalities. DSA has the added benefit of providing both diagnostic information and facilitating treatment of vascular lesions. The main drawbacks of DSA are that it is invasive, time-consuming, and has associated morbidity.

Recent advances in both CTA and MRI/MRA techniques are introducing the potential for noninvasive imaging studies with functional, hemodynamic, and physiologic information rivaling DSA. Four-dimensional CTA (4D CTA) and 4D MRA protocols are being developed, which provide time-resolved angiographic information allowing for more specific lesion characterization

and potential information about perfusion, early draining veins, and shunting similar to DSA. Advances have also been made in catheter angiography techniques, with a recent study reporting the development of a time-resolved 4D DSA protocol which provides detailed information about the angioarchitecture of an AVM.[8] Currently, even with the newest imaging techniques, DSA continues to demonstrate superior temporal and spatial resolution compared to CTA and MRA.

8.3.2 AVM Grading

An important factor to consider when planning treatment of brain AVMs is the estimated risk of treatment for that patient. For surgical treatment of brain AVMs, Spetzler and Martin developed a grading system to predict the risk of surgical morbidity and mortality for individual patients. The three components of the original grading system are lesion size, pattern of venous drainage, and neurological eloquence of the brain tissue (▶ Table 8.1). The brain AVM size is divided into small (<3 cm), medium (3–6 cm), and large (>6 cm). The larger the lesion is, the higher is the score. The pattern of venous drainage is related to ease of resectability. Superficial drainage is defined as AVM drainage in the cortical venous system and cerebellar hemispheric veins into the straight sinus or transverse sinus. Deep drainage is defined as a venous drainage pattern involving the deep veins such as internal cerebral veins, basal veins, or precentral cerebellar vein. Eloquence identifies the functional importance of the brain tissue near the brain AVM. If this brain tissue is injured, the eloquence factor addresses how disabling the injury would be to the patient. This area is susceptible to dissection, retraction, and postoperative hemorrhage or edema.

Table 8.1 Spetzler–Martin scale

Parameter		
Size (cm)	<3 cm (1 point)	3–6 cm (2 points) >6 cm (3 points)
Eloquence	Noneloquent (0 points)	Eloquent (1 point)
Venous drainage	Superficial (0 points)	Deep (1 point)

Total = size + eloquence + venous drainage

Table 8.2 Virginia Radiosurgical Scoring System (VRAS)

Variable	Points
AVM volume (cm^3)	
< 2	0
2–4	1
> 4	2
AVM in eloquent location	1
History of hemorrhage	1

Note: Favorable outcome (define as AVM obliteration or no posttreatment hemorrhage or permanent SRS symptoms) was 83% for VRAS = 0, 79% for VRAS = 1, 70% for VRAS = 2, 48% for VRAS = 3, and 39% for VRAS = 4.

Table 8.3 Radiosurgical Based Scoring System (RBAS)

Parameter		
Volume (cm^3)	Factor (0.1)	Volume, not size
Location	Factor (0.3)	Deep versus hemispheric
Age	Factor (0.2)	Younger age better outcome

Score = 0.1 (volume) + 0.2 (age) + 0.3 (location)

The regions considered as eloquent are the sensorimotor, language cortex, visual cortex, basal ganglia, hypothalamus, thalamus, internal capsule, brainstem, cerebellar peduncles, and deep cerebellar nuclei.[9,10] Examples of noneloquent regions are anterior frontal lobes, anterior temporal lobes, and the cerebellar cortex. The grade is the sum of these three scores. Grades I to V correlate with the operative results, respectively. A grade VI is allocated to inoperable brain AVMs such as large size in eloquent areas or a nidus in the hypothalamus or brainstem.[9] Those brain AVMs determined to be grade I or II (low-grade AVMs) are associated with low morbidity rates and frequently managed surgically. Management of grade III AVMs is not widely agreed upon.[11] Grade IV or V AVMs (high-grade AVMs) are associated with high morbidity rates, so these lesions are frequently monitored.

The Spetzler–Martin grading system was derived as a prognostic system for surgical intervention.[9,12] Other scoring systems were developed to predict outcomes of AVM radiosurgery, including the Virginia Radiosurgical Scoring System (VRAS)[13] and the Radiosurgical Based Scoring System (RBAS). These systems use volume (cm^3) instead of size, patient age (years), prior hemorrhage, and AVM location (▶ Table 8.2 and ▶ Table 8.3). Location is separated into three categories. The frontotemporal regions are assigned zero. Parietal, occipital, intraventricular, corpus callosum, and cerebellar regions are designated 1. Lastly, for RBAS, the basal ganglia, thalamus, and brainstem are assigned 2.[12] The VRAS score is a simple to use yet reliable integer scoring system similar to the Spetzler–Martin one in design, whereas the RBAS requires computation of a multitermed equation.

Many angiographic features associated with brain AVMs have been recognized as increased risk factors for future hemorrhage. These are important to identify as intracranial hemorrhage is a dreaded complication and its risk is influential in clinical management decisions. Three risk factors that are most commonly agreed upon in the literature are hemorrhage at initial presentation, deep venous drainage, and associated aneurysms (i.e., intranidal aneurysms) (▶ Fig. 8.2).[14] The strongest predictor for subsequent intracranial hemorrhage is hemorrhage at initial presentation.[15] Intranidal aneurysms and deep venous drainage are considered angioarchitectural weak points within a brain AVM.[16] Other reported factors contributing to future hemorrhage risk include venous stasis, location, size, male gender, and age.

8.3.3 Planning for Stereotactic Radiosurgery

Targeting for stereotactic radiosurgery can involve any or all of the three modalities described above. There are complementary aspects of each that may be useful in any given patient. For example, patients who have undergone embolization with ethyl vinyl alcohol or n-butyl cyanoacrylate cannot generally have treatment plans based on CT owing to the density of the embolic agents relative to brain. MRI is a much better option for these patients.[17] DSA is useful in patients with a diffuse nidus or ambiguity between nidus and angiomatous changes in collateral vessels.

8.3.4 Posttreatment Imaging

Following surgical resection, imaging follow-up is performed a few weeks to months after the procedure to evaluate for complete occlusion or for residual AVM and need for further therapy. Recurrence of AVMs has been documented with pediatric patients following surgical resection in the literature and, due to the significant risk of recurrence, follow-up imaging has been recommended by some authors in 6 months to 1 year in these patients.[18,19] Following radiosurgery, obliteration of the AVM typically occurs after 2 to 5 years and follow-up imaging should be obtained over this time period to evaluate resolution or the need for additional treatment.[20,21,22]

As with pretreatment imaging, DSA is the reference standard to evaluate AVMs after treatment. The excellent spatial and temporal resolution allows accurate assessment of potential residual nidus and residual venous drainage, as well as allows immediate therapeutic intervention. However, the invasiveness, radiation exposure, and potential complications factor into the greater than ideal risk for routine follow-up with DSA.

The noninvasiveness and absence of ionizing radiation of MRI and MRA lead to the appeal of these modalities as alternative techniques for posttreatment follow-up. Three-dimensional time-of-flight (3D TOF) MRA and 3D contrast-enhanced MRA have both been proposed for assessment and follow-up of AVMs.[22,23,24] These techniques, however, are limited by poor temporal and spatial resolution and do not provide sufficient analysis of angioarchitecture and hemodynamics needed to supplant DSA. Particularly, both contrast-enhanced and TOF MRA techniques do not have the spatial resolution to detect a

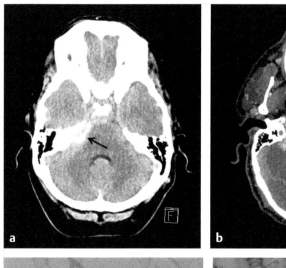
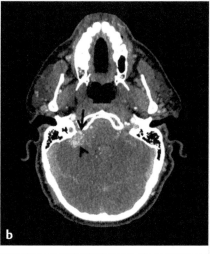

Fig. 8.2 **(a)** Noncontrast head CT showing diffuse subarachnoid hemorrhage, unusual for a typical brain AVM, and a dense focus of thrombus near the cerebellopontine angle (*black arrow*). **(b)** CTA showing a tangle of abnormal vascularity consistent with a brain AVM (*arrowhead*) and a focal contrast collection (*arrow*) suggesting an intranidal aneurysm. **(c)** Early arterial phase catheter angiogram in a right anteroposterior oblique projection showing an enlarged anterior cerebellar artery (*large black arrows*) and a feeding artery aneurysm, rather than a nidal aneurysm (*long black arrow*). **(d)** Later phase in the same projection shows the nidus (*star*) and early draining vein (*black arrow*).

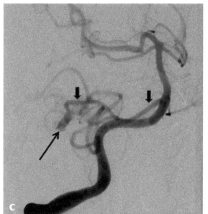
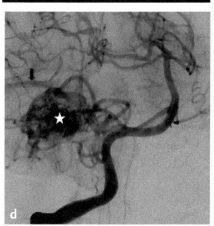

small residual nidus or the temporal resolution to distinguish some draining veins or arterial feeders.[23,24] Although an imperfect technique, MRA has been shown in some studies to have high enough sensitivity and specificity to be used for follow-up if subsequent DSA is performed for confirmation of either AVM obliteration or for the need for additional treatment.[21,25] Additionally, MRI can provide additional anatomic detail not obtained with DSA.[25]

4D MRA is a newer time-resolved MRA technique that allows even better evaluation of hemodynamics and angioarchitecture compared with the static images of 3D TOF MRA. Earlier preliminary examinations with 4D MRA were not efficient enough in acquisition, but newer techniques such as parallel imaging and intelligent sampling of k-space have allowed for sufficient acquisition time and temporal resolution to better characterize AVMs.[26] More recent studies with 4D MRA have been promising and have shown reliable diagnostic accuracy, although the temporal and spatial resolution could still be improved if they are to be considered as a replacement for DSA.[27,28,29]

Acute complications occurring within 30 days following AVM treatment include intracranial hemorrhage, ischemic stroke, intracranial infection, or hydrocephalus.[30] Late complications occurring after 30 days posttreatment typically include complications of radiosurgery, including radiation edema, necrosis, or cyst formation.[30]

8.4 Discussion

Imaging is critical for the diagnosis, treatment planning, and follow-up of patients with brain AVMs. Several recent trends in the evaluation of brain AVM patients deserve some comment. Regarding diagnosis, the incorporation of CTA into emergent stroke patient evaluation has pushed vascular imaging into the very early evaluation of patients with hemorrhagic stroke and allowed early diagnosis of many patients with underlying brain AVMs. Some small AVMs will not be evident on CTA or MRA and will require catheter angiography. The selection of these patients is based on clinical and imaging features, including age and hemorrhage location.

Several aspects of treatment planning have also seen some recent changes and development. The identification of micro or asymptomatic hemorrhage on MRI may allow identification of a subgroup of asymptomatic patients with higher risk for future hemorrhage. New 4D (time-resolved) MRA and CTA techniques provide some of the temporal resolution of DSA and allow the identification of early venous drainage. This is sometimes the only visible feature of an AVM. One very useful application of these emerging techniques will be for follow-up of treated lesions after radiosurgery. Finally, similar to brain tumors, the use of functional MRI data (mapping, functional connectivity, and fiber track mapping) may have value in guiding surgical resection.

The level of evidence for the uses of imaging described above is limited. Brain AVMs are relatively rare lesions, and the scientific evidence for different treatment options, and the imaging paradigms used for them, is limited to large case series. Nevertheless, there are some data regarding imaging in general which is relevant. CT and CTA have high sensitivity and specificity for diagnosis of brain AVMs presenting with intracranial hemorrhage. Posttreatment following excision or obliteration of brain AVM, imaging evaluation with MRI/MRA and DSA is recommended.

Areas of particular interest for future research include the importance of asymptomatic hemorrhage for future hemorrhage risk and the sensitivity/risk/benefit of DSA over 4D MRA for the follow-up of treated lesions.

8.5 Conclusion

Imaging is involved in nearly all the major decisions regarding treatment of patients with brain AVMs. The past decade has seen great advances in CTA for patients with acute hemorrhage and time-resolved MRI for the detection of early venous drainage.

References

[1] Choi JH, Mohr JP. Brain arteriovenous malformations in adults. Lancet Neurol. 2005; 4(5):299–308

[2] Fiehler J, Illies T, Piening M, et al. Territorial and microvascular perfusion impairment in brain arteriovenous malformations. AJNR Am J Neuroradiol. 2009; 30(2):356–361

[3] McCormack RF, Hutson A. Can computed tomography angiography of the brain replace lumbar puncture in the evaluation of acute-onset headache after a negative noncontrast cranial computed tomography scan? Acad Emerg Med. 2010; 17(4):444–451

[4] Delgado Almandoz JE, Schaefer PW, Forero NP, Falla JR, Gonzalez RG, Romero JM. Diagnostic accuracy and yield of multidetector CT angiography in the evaluation of spontaneous intraparenchymal cerebral hemorrhage. AJNR Am J Neuroradiol. 2009; 30(6):1213–1221

[5] Prestigiacomo CJ, Sabit A, He W, Jethwa P, Gandhi C, Russin J. Three dimensional CT angiography versus digital subtraction angiography in the detection of intracranial aneurysms in subarachnoid hemorrhage. J Neurointerv Surg. 2010; 2(4):385–389

[6] Sanelli PC, Mifsud MJ, Stieg PE. Role of CT angiography in guiding management decisions of newly diagnosed and residual arteriovenous malformations. AJR Am J Roentgenol. 2004; 183(4):1123–1126

[7] Josephson CB, White PM, Krishan A, Al-Shahi Salman R. Computed tomography angiography or magnetic resonance angiography for detection of intracranial vascular malformations in patients with intracerebral haemorrhage. Cochrane Database Syst Rev. 2014(9):CD009372

[8] Sandoval-Garcia C, Royalty K, Yang P, et al. 4D DSA a new technique for arteriovenous malformation evaluation: a feasibility study. J Neurointerv Surg. 2016; 8(3):300–304

[9] Spetzler RF, Martin NA. A proposed grading system for arteriovenous malformations. J Neurosurg. 1986; 65(4):476–483

[10] Atkinson RP, Awad IA, Batjer HH, et al. Joint Writing Group of the Technology Assessment Committee American Society of Interventional and Therapeutic Neuroradiology; Joint Section on Cerebrovascular Neurosurgery a Section of the American Association of Neurological Surgeons and Congress of Neurological Surgeons; Section of Stroke and the Section of Interventional Neurology of the American Academy of Neurology. Reporting terminology for brain arteriovenous malformation clinical and radiographic features for use in clinical trials. Stroke. 2001; 32(6):1430–1442

[11] Lawton MT, Project UBAMS, UCSF Brain Arteriovenous Malformation Study Project. Spetzler-Martin Grade III arteriovenous malformations: surgical results and a modification of the grading scale. Neurosurgery. 2003; 52(4): 740–748, discussion 748–749

[12] Pollock BE, Flickinger JC. A proposed radiosurgery-based grading system for arteriovenous malformations. J Neurosurg. 2002; 96(1):79–85

[13] Starke RM, Yen CP, Ding D, Sheehan JP. A practical grading scale for predicting outcome after radiosurgery for arteriovenous malformations: analysis of 1012 treated patients. J Neurosurg. 2013; 119(4):981–987

[14] da Costa L, Wallace MC, Ter Brugge KG, O'Kelly C, Willinsky RA, Tymianski M. The natural history and predictive features of hemorrhage from brain arteriovenous malformations. Stroke. 2009; 40(1):100–105

[15] Stapf C, Mast H, Sciacca RR, et al. Predictors of hemorrhage in patients with untreated brain arteriovenous malformation. Neurology. 2006; 66(9):1350–1355

[16] Geibprasert S, Pongpech S, Jiarakongmun P, Shroff MM, Armstrong DC, Krings T. Radiologic assessment of brain arteriovenous malformations: what clinicians need to know. Radiographics. 2010; 30(2):483–501

[17] Mamalui-Hunter M, Jiang T, Rich KM, Derdeyn CP, Drzymala RE. Effect of liquid embolic agents on Gamma Knife surgery dosimetry for arteriovenous malformations. Clinical article. J Neurosurg. 2011; 115(2):364–370

[18] Kader A, Goodrich JT, Sonstein WJ, Stein BM, Carmel PW, Michelsen WJ. Recurrent cerebral arteriovenous malformations after negative postoperative angiograms. J Neurosurg. 1996; 85(1):14–18

[19] Lang SS, Beslow LA, Bailey RL, et al. Follow-up imaging to detect recurrence of surgically treated pediatric arteriovenous malformations. J Neurosurg Pediatr. 2012; 9(5):497–504

[20] Steiner L, Lindquist C, Adler JR, Torner JC, Alves W, Steiner M. Clinical outcome of radiosurgery for cerebral arteriovenous malformations. J Neurosurg. 1992; 77(1):1–8

[21] Lee CC, Reardon MA, Ball BZ, et al. The predictive value of magnetic resonance imaging in evaluating intracranial arteriovenous malformation obliteration after stereotactic radiosurgery. J Neurosurg. 2015; 123(1):136–144

[22] Pollock BE, Kondziolka D, Flickinger JC, Patel AK, Bissonette DJ, Lunsford LD. Magnetic resonance imaging: an accurate method to evaluate arteriovenous malformations after stereotactic radiosurgery. J Neurosurg. 1996; 85(6): 1044–1049

[23] Lee KE, Choi CG, Choi JW, et al. Detection of residual brain arteriovenous malformations after radiosurgery: diagnostic accuracy of contrast-enhanced three-dimensional time of flight MR angiography at 3.0 Tesla. Korean J Radiol. 2009; 10(4):333–339

[24] Unlu E, Temizoz O, Albayram S, et al. Contrast-enhanced MR 3D angiography in the assessment of brain AVMs. Eur J Radiol. 2006; 60(3):367–378

[25] Khandanpour N, Griffiths P, Warren D, Hoggard N. Prospective comparison of late 3 T MRI with conventional angiography in evaluating the patency of cerebral arteriovenous malformations treated with stereotactic radiosurgery. Neuroradiology. 2013; 55(6):683–687

[26] Taschner CA, Gieseke J, Le Thuc V, et al. Intracranial arteriovenous malformation: time-resolved contrast-enhanced MR angiography with combination of parallel imaging, keyhole acquisition, and k-space sampling techniques at 1.5 T. Radiology. 2008; 246(3):871–879

[27] Soize S, Bouquigny F, Kadziolka K, Portefaix C, Pierot L. Value of 4D MR angiography at 3 T compared with DSA for the follow-up of treated brain arteriovenous malformation. AJNR Am J Neuroradiol. 2014; 35(10):1903–1909

[28] Hadizadeh DR, Kukuk GM, Steck DT, et al. Noninvasive evaluation of cerebral arteriovenous malformations by 4D-MRA for preoperative planning and postoperative follow-up in 56 patients: comparison with DSA and intraoperative findings. AJNR Am J Neuroradiol. 2012; 33(6):1095–1101

[29] Lim HK, Choi CG, Kim SM, et al. Detection of residual brain arteriovenous malformations after radiosurgery: diagnostic accuracy of contrast-enhanced four-dimensional MR angiography at 3.0 T. Br J Radiol. 2012; 85(1016):1064–1069

[30] van Beijnum J, van der Worp HB, Buis DR, et al. Treatment of brain arteriovenous malformations: a systematic review and meta-analysis. JAMA. 2011; 306(18):2011–2019

9 Intraoperative Imaging for Arteriovenous Malformations and Dural Arteriovenous Fistulas

Max Wintermark and Jeremy J. Heit

Abstract

The routine use of intraoperative imaging during the surgical treatment of cerebral arteriovenous malformations (AVMs) and dural arteriovenous fistulas (dAVFs) may identify unsuspected residual arteriovenous shunting (AVS) and maximize the odds of complete treatment of the target lesion. The most commonly performing imaging modalities include (1) indocyanine green (ICG) videoangiography, (2) intraoperative digital subtraction angiography (DSA), (3) intraoperative ultrasound, (4) intraoperative flat panel rotational angiography, and (5) intraoperative magnetic resonance imaging (MRI). These different intraoperative imaging modalities are discussed in this chapter.

Keywords: intraoperative angiography, intraoperative magnetic resonance imaging, intraoperative computed tomography, intraoperative ICG, intraoperative ultrasound, arteriovenous malformation, dural arteriovenous fistula

Points

- Intraoperative imaging during surgical treatment of arteriovenous malformation (AVM) and dural arteriovenous fistula (dAVF) helps verify complete treatment of the lesion and reduces the subsequent risk of intracranial hemorrhage and additional surgery.
- Intraoperative digital subtraction angiography (DSA) offers the greatest sensitivity for residual arteriovenous shunting after surgical treatment and is the gold standard for intraoperative imaging during cerebrovascular surgery.
- Intraoperative indocyanine green (ICG) videoangiography, ultrasound, flat panel rotational angiography, and magnetic resonance imaging (MRI) may also be used during the surgical treatment of AVMs and dAVFs.

9.1 Introduction

9.1.1 Cerebral Vascular Lesions with Abnormal Arteriovenous Shunting

Cerebral Arteriovenous Malformations

Cerebral arteriovenous malformations (AVMs) are uncommon vascular lesions characterized by abnormal arteriovenous shunting (AVS) between cerebral arteries and veins. The angioarchitecture of AVMs is characterized by the absence of a normal capillary bed between cerebral arteries and veins and the presence of a nidus, which is a complex of channels connecting arteries and veins within the AVM.[1,2] AVMs are thought to develop secondary to errors in vascular development and morphogenesis, and these lesions are typically identified in children or young adults.[1,2] Due to the high risk of cerebral AVM

rupture, significant effort is employed to characterize the AVM angioarchitecture, which in turn guides AVM treatment.[3,4,5]

The imaging evaluation of cerebral AVMs seeks to identify the arterial supply to the AVM, the size and location of the AVM nidus, the venous drainage of the AVM, the presence of a flow-related or nidal aneurysm, and the presence of a stenosis in the venous outflow of the AVM, all of which have treatment implications. Currently, digital subtraction angiography (DSA) remains the gold standard in the imaging evaluation of cerebral AVMs given its excellent spatial and temporal resolution with respect to these features. The identification of abnormal AVS is the most sensitive imaging feature for the presence of a cerebral AVM. AVS is therefore the most important clue as to the presence of an otherwise imaging-occult AVM, and the intraoperative imaging of AVMs seeks to identify AVS with a high sensitivity.

Computed tomography angiography (CTA) and magnetic resonance imaging (MRI) with magnetic resonance angiography (MRA) may also be used to evaluate cerebral AVMs. However, these studies lack the temporal resolution of DSA, which limits their sensitivity for AVS. Advanced MRI sequences, such as arterial spin labeling (ASL) and susceptibility-weighted imaging (SWI), may offer a high sensitivity for AVS, although these technique have not been deployed for intraoperative imaging to date.[6,7] Nevertheless, CTA and MRI are important adjuncts in the surgical treatment of cerebral AVMs, as they demonstrate the relationship of the AVM to the brain anatomy and may be used for intraoperative navigation.

Dural Arteriovenous Fistulas

Dural arteriovenous fistulas (dAVFs) are characterized by abnormal AVS between arteries and veins within the dura and account for approximately 10% of intracranial vascular lesions.[8,9,10] In contrast to AVMs, the AVS in dAVF most commonly arises from branches of the external carotid arteries and meningeal arteries. These arteries directly connect to the dural sinuses or cerebral veins without an intervening capillary bed, which results in a fistula with associated abnormal AVS.[11] The pathogenesis of dAVFs is poorly understood, but these lesions are thought to be acquired following trauma or venous sinus thrombosis and are most commonly identified in adults older than 50 years.[10,11] Presenting symptoms of dAVFs include intracranial hemorrhage, tinnitus, headache, or symptoms of increased intracranial pressure.[10,11,12,13] Intracranial hemorrhage occurs in up to 18% of patients with dAVF, and the pattern of venous drainage is the most important predictor of hemorrhage risk.[10,14]

The imaging evaluation of dAVFs must identify the fistula location, the arteries supplying the fistula, the direction of venous drainage into a dural sinus, and retrograde filling of cortical veins. The identification of a direct connection to a cortical vein or reflux from a dural sinus into a cortical vein secondary to high pressure induced by the dAVF is critical because these features best predict the risk of dAVF rupture.[10,14] Similar to cerebral AVMs, DSA is the gold standard in the imaging evaluation of dAVFs, given its high spatial and temporal resolution and superior ability to detect retrograde blood flow into a cortical vein.[11,15]

CTA and MRI with MRA are increasingly used for noninvasive imaging of dAVFs. These studies may demonstrate arterial prominence near the fistula site, engorgement of cortical veins, associated venous sinus thrombosis, and the sequela of dAVFs, including cerebral edema, hydrocephalus, flattening of the optic discs, or proptosis. In addition, there are emerging data regarding the utility of advanced MRI sequences, such as ASL and SWI, and time-resolved MRA and CTA in the diagnosis and characterization of dAVFs.[5,6,7,16,17,18] Although these techniques are currently largely investigational, they are expected to play an increasing role in the imaging evaluation of dAVFs in the near future.

9.1.2 Surgical Treatment of Cerebral AVMs and dAVFs

Surgical Treatment of Cerebral AVMs: Intraoperative Imaging Principals

Surgical resection of cerebral AVMs is effective, offers the possibility of an immediate cure of the lesion, and has a low complication rate.[19,20,21] For these reasons, surgical resection of cerebral AVMs is often considered the most optimal treatment when anatomically and technically feasible.[19] The goal of surgical treatment of cerebral AVMs is complete resection of the AVM nidus with preservation of the normal arterial and venous anatomy and brain parenchyma.[22] If the AVM nidus can be resected in its entirety, then the risk of AVM-related intracranial hemorrhage or AVM recurrence is very low. However, incomplete resection of a cerebral AVM does not reduce the subsequent risk of hemorrhage, and it may increase this risk.[23]

Intraoperative imaging may be performed during cerebral AVM resection using a variety of imaging modalities, such as indocyanine green (ICG) videoangiography, DSA, ultrasound, flat panel rotational angiography, MRI, or a combination of these modalities. The goals of intraoperative imaging are to determine the presence of any residual AVM nidus, to localize a suspected residual AVM nidus, and to assess for an operative complication. Intraoperative imaging may demonstrate unsuspected residual AVM nidus after resection in 10 to 20% of patients.[24,25,26,27,28,29] Therefore, the routine use of imaging to identify residual AVM nidus may increase the likelihood of a complete resection in a single operative session and reduce the need for repeat procedures.

Intraoperative imaging during cerebral AVM resection must have a high sensitivity for residual AVS, which is the most sensitive feature for the presence of a residual nidus. Depending on the imaging modality used in the operating room, demonstration of a residual nidus may be challenging. The most commonly used intraoperative imaging modalities are described below.

Surgical Treatment of Cerebral dAVFs and Intraoperative Imaging Principals

Endovascular embolization is the most common treatment for dAVFs. However, a subset of dAVFs are not amenable to endovascular embolization because of difficult vascular access or arterial supply arising from an anatomically important artery that cannot be embolized safely.[30,31,32] In such situations, surgical treatment of dAVFs may be performed.

In contrast to cerebral AVMs, dAVFs lack a compact vascular nidus and are composed of fistulas between arteries and a dural venous sinus or cortical vein. A dAVF may comprise a single fistula, but more commonly numerous small fistulas exist between multiple small arteries that supply the dAVF and the venous sinus or vein that drains the fistula. These anatomic differences make the surgical treatment of dAVFs different from that of AVMs. dAVFs may be treated by a combination of techniques, including surgical packing of the affected sinus, cauterization or surgical ligation of arteries feeding the dAVFs, skeletonization of the affected sinus, and cauterization or surgical ligation of cortical veins draining the dAVFs.[33,34,35] More recently, surgical disconnection of the draining veins from the dAVFs has been shown to be an effective treatment for dAVFs with a low complication rate.[36,37]

Intraoperative imaging during surgical treatment of dAVFs is less well described than in the treatment of cerebral AVMs.[24,38,39] Intraoperative imaging during dAVF treatment must identify residual AVS and retrograde filling of a cortical vein with a high sensitivity. Residual AVS and retrograde filling of a cortical vein indicate incomplete surgical treatment of the dAVF, which continues to place the patient at risk for intracranial hemorrhage. The imaging modalities used during intraoperative dAVF imaging are described in detail in the following section.[39,40,41,42,43]

9.2 Materials and Methods

PubMed searches were performed for intraoperative imaging, cerebral arteriovenous malformation, dural arteriovenous fistula, magnetic resonance imaging, computed tomography, digital subtraction angiography, indocyanine green, and ultrasound. Pertinent articles were reviewed. Additional articles were identified from the reviewed articles in some circumstances.

9.3 Results

9.3.1 Intraoperative Imaging Techniques

The most commonly used intraoperative imaging modalities during surgical treatment of cerebral AVMs and dAVFs include ICG videoangiography, DSA, ultrasound, flat panel rotational angiography, and MRI. Intraoperative MRI and flat panel rotational angiography have been described during cerebral AVM resection, but these techniques have not yet been reported during dAVF surgery, to our knowledge. In this section, we describe these imaging modalities during surgical treatment of cerebral AVMs and dAVFs.

Intraoperative Indocyanine Green

ICG is a cyanine dye that binds with a high affinity to blood-borne proteins, and it may therefore be used as a blood pool imaging agent. ICG is administered by intravenous injection and imaged within cerebral blood vessels with a high temporal

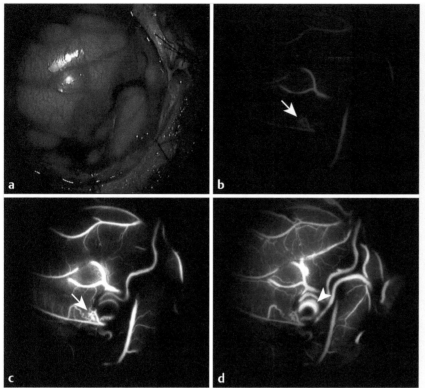

Fig. 9.1 ICG videoangiography during ruptured AVM resection. A young patient presented with intraparenchymal hemorrhage (**a**) and was taken to the operating room for hematoma evacuation. Intraoperative ICG angiography demonstrates an AVM nidus (*arrows*) in the frontal opercula in the early (**b**) and late (**c**) arterial phase (**b**). An early draining vein (*arrowhead*) is present in the early parenchymal phase (**d**). (These images are provided courtesy of Johnny Wong, MD, PhD, Sydney, Australia.)

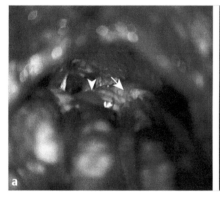
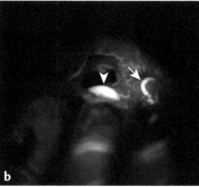

Fig. 9.2 ICG videoangiography during dAVF ligation. Intraoperative ICG angiography during treatment of a superior petrosal sinus dAVF demonstrates engorged cortical veins (**a**, *arrow and arrowhead*) with associated venous reflux in the early arterial phase following ICG injection (**b**, *arrow and arrowhead*). (These images are provided courtesy of Johnny Wong, MD, PhD, Sydney, Australia.)

and spatial resolution using near-infrared spectroscopy that is integrated with the operative microscope. Early identification of ICG fluorescence within a vein draining an AVM or dAVF indicates AVS, and the neurosurgeon may use this information to guide AVM (▶ Fig. 9.1) or dAVF (▶ Fig. 9.2) resection. For these reasons, ICG videoangiography has become a common tool in cerebrovascular surgery.

ICG videoangiography has several distinct advantages during AVM and dAVF surgery. It is easy to use multiple times during a surgery due to its short half-life of 3 to 4 minutes, and it provides real-time identification of AVS within the cerebral vasculature.[44] ICG videoangiography also minimizes interruptions during the surgery by allowing the surgical microscope to be maintained in position with continuous visualization of the operative bed. In most instances, ICG videoangiography may be performed in 5 minutes or fewer, which may translate into a significant cost savings with respect to procedural times

compared to other intraoperative imaging studies.[40] However, these advantages of ICG videoangiography must be balanced with several limitations of the technique.

The field of view during ICG videoangiography is confined to what may be seen through the surgical microscope (see ▶ Fig. 9.1 and ▶ Fig. 9.2), which may therefore limit the detection of AVS outside of the operative field. The limited visualization of ICG is exacerbated when the neurosurgeon is working deeply within the brain or in an anatomically confined operative bed.[45] For these reasons, ICG videoangiography may fail to identify residual AVS during AVM resection in up to 20 to 75% of procedures.[29,45] However, other studies have demonstrated a more favorable sensitivity of ICG videoangiography with false-negative rate of 9% or less during surgical treatment of cerebral AVMs and dAVFs.[40,42]

Although intraoperative ICG videoangiography has been more widely used during cerebral AVM resection, there are relatively few papers describing this technique during the surgical treatment of dAVFs (▶ Fig. 9.2).[40,43] However, the largest series describing the use of ICG videoangiography during surgical treatment of dAVFs in 47 procedures noted a 8.7% false-negative rate, which is similar to the reported false-negative rate of intraoperative DSA.[40] To date, there has not been a prospectively designed study to compare intraoperative ICG videoangiography and intraoperative DSA, but such a study would be of interest to undertake.

Intraoperative Digital Subtraction Angiography

Intraoperative angiography was first described in the 1960s, and today intraoperative DSA remains the gold standard for intraoperative cerebral vascular imaging.[46,47] Intraoperative DSA offers excellent temporal and spatial resolution, which allows for sensitive detection of AVS, reflux into small cortical veins, and the presence of a small residual nidus after partial AVM or dAVF resection.[24,25,26,27,28,39,48] Furthermore, intraoperative DSA performed during parenchymal hematoma after AVM rupture may identify an occult cause of hemorrhage, such as a nidal or perinidal aneurysm that was previously compressed by the hematoma.[49]

Intraoperative DSA may be performed in a standard operating suite with a portable C-arm fluoroscopic unit or in a hybrid endovascular-surgical suite with biplane angiography equipment. Typically, the patient is placed under general anesthesia, and then arterial access in the common femoral artery, radial artery, or brachial artery is obtained with or without ultrasound guidance. The sheath is then secured to the patient with a suture and connected to a continuous heparinized saline flush to present thrombus forming within the sheath or near the sheath tip. The patient is then placed in position for the surgery and placed in a radiolucent Mayfield skull clamp to facilitate subsequent DSA.

Intraoperative DSA may be performed before the surgical procedure if localization of the cerebral AVM or dAVF is required. More typically, however, the location of the AVM or dAVF has been determined based on preoperative conventional angiography, MRI, or CTA, as this information is useful in determining patient positioning in the operative suite. Furthermore, a preoperative high-quality DSA is important to understand completely the vascular anatomy of the lesion being treated. After the neurosurgeon has completed what he or she feels is a complete resection of the AVM (▶ Fig. 9.3) or obliteration of the dAVF (▶ Fig. 9.4), intraoperative DSA may be performed to exclude unsuspected AVS. The operative microscope is

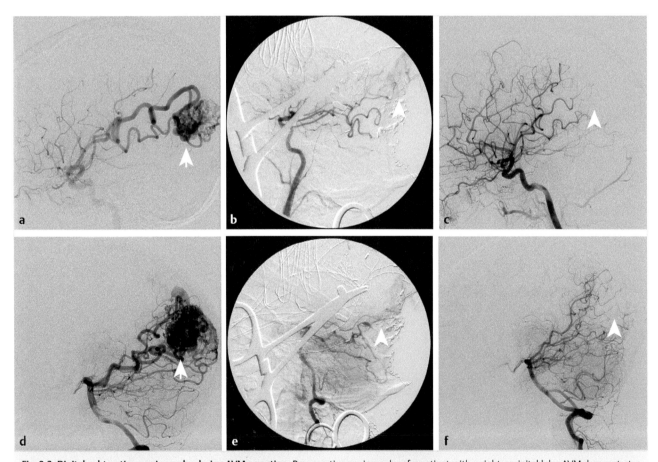

Fig. 9.3 Digital subtraction angiography during AVM resection. Preoperative angiography of a patient with a right occipital lobe AVM demonstrates arterial supply from the right middle cerebral artery (*arrow*, **a**) and the right posterior cerebral artery (*arrow*, **d**) with superficial venous drainage. Intraoperative (**b,e**) and postoperative (**c,f**) angiography demonstrates no residual AVM nidus or early draining vein (*arrowheads*, **b,c,e,f**) after injection of the right internal carotid artery (**b,c**) and the right vertebral artery (**e,f**), consistent with successful resection.

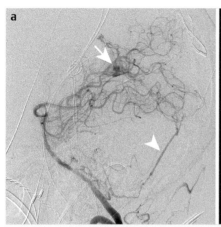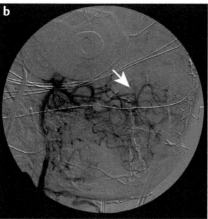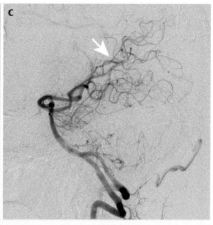

Fig. 9.4 Digital subtraction angiography during galenic dAVF resection. A patient presented with increased intracranial pressure due to a galenic dAVF. Partial embolization was performed, but residual arterial supply to the dAVF (**a**, *arrow*) arising from a posterior meningeal artery (**a**, *arrowhead*) remained. This small vessel was deemed unsafe for endovascular embolization, so surgical ligation of the arterial supply to the dAVF was performed. Intraoperative (**b**) and postoperative DSA (**c**) shows no residual filling of the vein of Galen in the arterial phase (**b,c**, *arrows*), consistent with cure of the fistula.

removed, and a portable C-arm fluoroscopic unit or a biplane fluoroscopy unit is brought into position. The neurointerventionalist then introduces a catheter through the sheath and selects the arteries known to supply the AVM or dAVF using fluoroscopic guidance. A DSA is then performed following contrast injection through the catheter. Multiple cervical vessels may be selected to ensure complete interrogation of all vessels previously shown to supply the AVM or dAVF based on the information from the preoperative DSA. The images are carefully reviewed by the neurointerventionalist and the neurosurgeon to assess for any remaining AVS with a draining vein or dural sinus or evidence of a residual nidus.

Intraoperative DSA after cerebral AVM or dAVF treatment demonstrates unexpected AVS in 9 to 20% of patients, which prompts additional surgical exploration, resection, or ligation in most patients.[24,25,26,27,28,39,48] Intraoperative DSA may be performed multiple times as needed during the surgery. For these reasons, intraoperative DSA may result in a higher operative cure rate and a decreased need for an additional surgery. However, intraoperative DSA has a false-negative rate of 5 to 11%, which may be reduced by using a hybrid endovascular-surgical suite.[26,39,48,49]

Although intraoperative DSA is very sensitive for the detection of a residual cerebral AVM or dAVF, there are disadvantages to this technique. First, intraoperative DSA is time-consuming and often challenging to deploy in the operative suite. Removing the operating microscope and introducing the fluoroscopic equipment typically takes 20 to 30 minutes. The angiographic portion of study may take 10 to 30 minutes, and, if necessary, the reintroduction of the operating microscope may take an additional 10 to 20 minutes. Therefore, an intraoperative DSA may require 30 minutes or more to complete, which may lead to a significant time delay during the surgery. Second, translation of the angiographic anatomy to the operative bed anatomy may be challenging given the discordant fields of view. Next, the need for an indwelling groin, brachial, or radial sheath may limit surgical positioning. An indwelling sheath in the absence of systemic heparinization may also lead to a complication, such

as arterial thrombosis at the access site. Lastly, intraoperative DSA has a complication rate of 1 to 5%, which is significantly higher than conventional DSA.[22,24,25,38,39,50]

Intraoperative DSA during surgical treatment of dAVFs is less well established in the literature. Pandey and colleagues published the largest series of intraoperative DSA during dAVF resection in 29 patients and 34 surgeries.[39] They found unexpected residual dAVF in 38% of patients and a false-negative rate of 11%. Therefore, the use of intraoperative DSA during dAVF surgery is recommended in these relatively uncommon surgeries.

Intraoperative Ultrasound

Intraoperative ultrasound is less commonly used when compared to ICG angiography or DSA. However, there are multiple reports describing the utility of ultrasound during the surgical treatment of cerebral AVMs and dAVFs.[51,52,53,54,55,56,57,58,59] In particular, these studies demonstrate that Doppler ultrasound may be used to localize an AVM nidus, to identify AVS in cortical veins, to differentiate hemorrhage from AVM nidus, or to verify complete excision of the AVM nidus or dAVF.[53,54,55,57,58] Intraoperative ultrasound may be particularly useful to localize an AVM nidus in situations when the navigation software misregisters the AVM location in the setting of encephalomalacia with intraoperative relaxation of the brain.[54] Intraoperative ultrasound may also be easily integrated with ICG angiography or intraoperative DSA, which further assists with achieving complete resection of a cerebral AVM.[55]

Intraoperative ultrasound is performed following sterile ultrasound probe introduction into the surgical field. The neurosurgeon manipulates the direction of the ultrasound to localize arteries feeding the AVM, the AVM nidus, or veins draining the AVM. The direction of blood flow in these vessels may be determined using Doppler ultrasound, which facilitates accurate mapping of the AVM angioarchitecture.[51,53,54,55,56,57] The images generated by intraoperative ultrasound imaging are visualized through heads-up display units or on monitors that are also integrated with the operative microscope. Importantly, intraoperative ultrasound does not require removing the microscope, which minimizes interruption of the surgery.

It is difficult to determine the sensitivity of intraoperative ultrasound for the presence of residual AVS or residual AVM nidus given the small size of most series and the paucity of prospectively designed studies. A single-center prospective study investigating the use of intraoperative ultrasound during cerebral AVM resection found the false-negative rate of this technique to be 5%, which is similar or better than the false-negative rates of intraoperative ICG videoangiography or DSA.[56] It would be of interest to determine how intraoperative ultrasound compares to intraoperative ICG videoangiography and DSA in a larger, multicenter prospective study given this reported favorable sensitivity.

The disadvantages of intraoperative ultrasound include its limited use in the evaluation of deep lesions, the necessary high level of operator expertise and comfort in interpreting Doppler ultrasound images as they relate to the vascular anatomy of the AVM in the operative field, and the limited field of view. Despite these limitations, intraoperative ultrasound, particularly with Doppler, is a useful adjunct during the surgical resection of AVMs.

Intraoperative ultrasound during surgical treatment of dAVF is much less commonly performed and sparsely described in the literature.[51,59] Eide and colleagues described their experience with intraoperative ultrasound in 12 patients undergoing dAVF ligation.[51] They found ultrasound to be most useful in identifying retrograde blood flow in cortical veins or in the deep venous sinuses, identifying unexpected arterial feeders to the dAVF, and verifying complete treatment of the fistula. The sensitivity of intraoperative ultrasound in verifying complete closure of the dAVF in this series was not reported. It would be of interest to test the utility of intraoperative ultrasound in prospective series during the surgical treatment of dAVF given the reported utility of this technique in the treatment of cerebral AVMs.

Intraoperative Flat Panel Rotational Angiography

There is no significant role for portable CT or CTA for intraoperative imaging during cerebral AVM or dAVF surgery given the small bore of portable CT scanners that do not permit scanning a patient with a Mayfield head clamp in place. However, there are reports of merging conventional CT scanners with intra-arterial contrast injection in the operative suite to localize cerebral AVMs and dAVF.[41] The main utility of this technique was found to be accurate localization of the vascular lesion being treated, but the utility of this technique to identify residual AVS was not described.[41]

By contrast, flat panel rotational angiography is emerging as a useful tool during cerebral AVM surgery.[60,61] Flat panel rotational angiography uses high-resolution flat panel detectors that are found in modern hybrid endovascular-surgical suites. The patient is placed under general anesthesia and positioned in the Mayfield head clamp. Next, arterial access is obtained, and the cervical vessel (or vessels) supplying the AVM is catheterized using fluoroscopic guidance. Once the catheter is in position, a three-dimensional image acquisition is obtained by rotating the flat panel detector around the patient's head. Next, this three-dimensional image acquisition is repeated with concomitant arterial injection into the cervical internal carotid artery or vertebral artery. The images obtained from these maneuvers may be processed in two ways. First, high-resolution images that elegantly depict the vascular anatomy of the AVM are generated by subtracting the "mask" images of the first rotation from the second rotation. These high-resolution vascular images are helpful in understanding the angiographic architecture of the AVM, which is helpful in plotting the surgical approach. Second, processing the second image acquisition without subtraction of the first acquisition may be used to generate a CT-like image that includes bone, soft tissue, and vascular information. These second images may be integrated with surgical navigation software to guide the subsequent craniotomy during AVM resection.[60]

It will be of interest to determine the most efficient use of hybrid endovascular-surgical suites as more centers are building these ultramodern rooms. There is a clear trend toward efficient and elegant integration of endovascular and open surgical procedures, which is made possible in a streamlined way with these modern suites. It will also be of interest to determine how these techniques are adapted to the surgical treatment of dAVF, which, to our knowledge, has not been reported to date. We expect to see additional advances in image-guided vascular neurosurgery as more of these hybrid suites are utilized around the world.

Intraoperative Magnetic Resonance Imaging

Intraoperative MRI was first described during cerebral AVM surgery over 15 years ago, and to date this technique has not been described during the surgical treatment of dAVF.[62] MRI provides detailed information regarding the anatomy of the brain parenchyma as it relates to the cerebral AVM being treated, and a preoperative MRI is often used for navigation during cerebral AVM resection. However, shifting of the brain parenchyma after the durotomy in the operative suite may lead to misregistration of the navigation software that may frustrate the operating neurosurgeon and adversely affect the surgical outcome.

By contrast, intraoperative MRI may be used to precisely localize a cerebral AVM after the craniotomy has been performed with excellent spatial resolution.[62,63,64] Furthermore, intraoperative MR angiography has been fused with intraoperative brain MRI to offer excellent colocalization of the arterial and venous anatomy of the AVM with the adjacent normal brain parenchyma.[63] A time-resolved imaging of contrast kinetics (TRICKS) sequence has also been used to study arterial blood flow during intraoperative MRI, and the TRICKS sequence verified successful AVM resection in a single case report.[64]

The benefits of intraoperative MRI are not limited to the excellent anatomic information about the AVM and the adjacent brain parenchyma. Intraoperative MRI performed during other nonvascular neurosurgical procedures, such as tumor resection, has been shown to be sensitive to surgical complications in the operating suite.[65] Moreover, the use of MRI in the operating suite is less invasive than DSA, which would be expected to minimize the risk of procedural-related complications. These realized and perceived advantages of intraoperative MRI must be balanced with several significant drawbacks of the technique.

There are several disadvantages of intraoperative MRI. First, performing MRI during a neurosurgical procedure is disruptive to the surgical workflow. The patient must be sterilely draped, and either the patient or the MRI must be moved into position to perform the imaging. The imaging must be interpreted and the patient repositioned for additional surgical resection if needed; these maneuvers may quickly add up to more than an hour of increased procedural time. Furthermore, in order to safely perform intraoperative MRI, all equipment being used in the operative suite and near the MRI magnet must be nonferromagnetic. This requirement places strict limits on the surgical tools and equipment within the operative suite, which may be limiting to the operative workflow. However, neurosurgeons who routinely use intraoperative MRI find it to be an asset in the treatment of their patients.

The lack of widespread use of intraoperative MRI leaves many unanswered questions at the current time. The optimal MRI sequences to localize the AVM nidus in the operating suite have not been determined to date. Moreover, the sensitivity of intraoperative MRI for residual AVS after AVM resection has not been described. It will be of interest to determine if intraoperative arterial spin label imaging may be used to detect an unsuspected residual AVM nidus given its excellent sensitivity for AVS.[6]

9.4 Conclusion

Intraoperative imaging is routine in cerebrovascular neurosurgical practice, and it plays a central role in the surgical treatment of patients with AVMs and dAVFs. Neurosurgeons may have preferences with respect to the imaging modality being used in the operative suite, but there are data demonstrating the effectiveness in identifying residual AVS after AVM and dAVF surgical treatment for almost all modalities.

At this time, intraoperative DSA remains the gold standard during AVM resection or dAVF ligation. This technique offers the highest sensitivity as to the presence of residual AVS, which, if identified, prompts additional surgical exploration in order to decrease the risk of hemorrhage related to incomplete surgical treatment and the need for a second surgery. It will be of interest to determine if the more widespread adoption of hybrid endovascular-surgical suites leads to further improvements in intraoperative DSA sensitivity. It will also be of interest to determine additional ways in which intraoperative flat panel rotational angiography might be used in these combined operative suites during the treatment of AVMs and dAVFs.

The sensitivity of other intraoperative imaging modalities, including ICG videoangiography, ultrasound, and MRI, rivals that of intraoperative DSA in some studies, and these modalities have clear utility during the surgical treatment of cerebral AVMs and dAVFs. To date, there has not been a prospectively designed study to compare the sensitivity of these different intraoperative imaging modalities. Although such a study would be difficult to perform, it would be of interest to undertake.

Intraoperative imaging during neurosurgical treatment of cerebral AVMs and dAVFs increases the likelihood of complete resection, decreases the risk of hemorrhage related to incomplete AVM or dAVF resection, and minimizes the chances of a second surgery to complete a cure of the lesion being treated. DSA is the gold-standard intraoperative imaging technique given that it offers the highest sensitivity for residual AVS after AVM or dAVF resection. Intraoperative ICG videoangiography, ultrasound, flat panel rotational angiography, and MRI are also useful intraoperative imaging modalities, although the sensitivity for residual AVS is lower than DSA.

References

[1] Laakso A, Hernesniemi J. Arteriovenous malformations: epidemiology and clinical presentation. Neurosurg Clin N Am. 2012; 23(1):1–6

[2] Friedlander RM. Clinical practice. Arteriovenous malformations of the brain. N Engl J Med. 2007; 356(26):2704–2712

[3] Crawford PM, West CR, Chadwick DW, Shaw MD. Arteriovenous malformations of the brain: natural history in unoperated patients. J Neurol Neurosurg Psychiatry. 1986; 49(1):1–10

[4] Fults D, Kelly DL, Jr. Natural history of arteriovenous malformations of the brain: a clinical study. Neurosurgery. 1984; 15(5):658–662

[5] Yamada S, Takagi Y, Nozaki K, Kikuta K, Hashimoto N. Risk factors for subsequent hemorrhage in patients with cerebral arteriovenous malformations. J Neurosurg. 2007; 107(5):965–972

[6] Le TT, Fischbein NJ, André JB, Wijman C, Rosenberg J, Zaharchuk G. Identification of venous signal on arterial spin labeling improves diagnosis of dural arteriovenous fistulas and small arteriovenous malformations. AJNR Am J Neuroradiol. 2012; 33(1):61–68

[7] Jagadeesan BD, Delgado Almandoz JE, Moran CJ, Benzinger TL. Accuracy of susceptibility-weighted imaging for the detection of arteriovenous shunting in vascular malformations of the brain. Stroke. 2011; 42(1):87–92

[8] Kajita Y, Miyachi S, Wakabayashi T, Inao S, Yoshida J. A dural arteriovenous fistula of the tentorium successfully treated by intravascular embolization. Surg Neurol. 1999; 52(3):294–298

[9] Al-Shahi R, Bhattacharya JJ, Currie DG, et al. Scottish Intracranial Vascular Malformation Study Collaborators. Prospective, population-based detection of intracranial vascular malformations in adults: the Scottish Intracranial Vascular Malformation Study (SIVMS). Stroke. 2003; 34(5):1163–1169

[10] Cognard C, Gobin YP, Pierot L, et al. Cerebral dural arteriovenous fistulas: clinical and angiographic correlation with a revised classification of venous drainage. Radiology. 1995; 194(3):671–680

[11] Hacein-Bey L, Konstas AA, Pile-Spellman J. Natural history, current concepts, classification, factors impacting endovascular therapy, and pathophysiology of cerebral and spinal dural arteriovenous fistulas. Clin Neurol Neurosurg. 2014; 121:64–75

[12] Cognard C, Casasco A, Toevi M, Houdart E, Chiras J, Merland JJ. Dural arteriovenous fistulas as a cause of intracranial hypertension due to impairment of cranial venous outflow. J Neurol Neurosurg Psychiatry. 1998; 65(3):308–316

[13] Satomi J, van Dijk JM, Terbrugge KG, Willinsky RA, Wallace MC. Benign cranial dural arteriovenous fistulas: outcome of conservative management based on the natural history of the lesion. J Neurosurg. 2002; 97(4):767–770

[14] Borden JA, Wu JK, Shucart WA. A proposed classification for spinal and cranial dural arteriovenous fistulous malformations and implications for treatment. J Neurosurg. 1995; 82(2):166–179

[15] Kuwayama N. Classification and diagnosis of intracranial dural arteriovenous fistulas [in Japanese]. Brain Nerve. 2008; 60(8):887–895

[16] Farb RI, Agid R, Willinsky RA, Johnstone DM, Terbrugge KG. Cranial dural arteriovenous fistula: diagnosis and classification with time-resolved MR angiography at 3 T. AJNR Am J Neuroradiol. 2009; 30(8):1546–1551

[17] Nishimura S, Hirai T, Sasao A, et al. Evaluation of dural arteriovenous fistulas with 4D contrast-enhanced MR angiography at 3 T. AJNR Am J Neuroradiol. 2010; 31(1):80–85

[18] Willems PW, Brouwer PA, Barfett JJ, terBrugge KG, Krings T. Detection and classification of cranial dural arteriovenous fistulas using 4D-CT angiography: initial experience. AJNR Am J Neuroradiol. 2011; 32(1):49–53

[19] Potts MB, Lau D, Abla AA, Kim H, Young WL, Lawton MT, UCSF Brain AVM Study Project. Current surgical results with low-grade brain arteriovenous malformations. J Neurosurg. 2015; 122(4):912–920

[20] Morgan MK, Rochford AM, Tsahtsarlis A, Little N, Faulder KC. Surgical risks associated with the management of Grade I and II brain arteriovenous malformations. Neurosurgery. 2004; 54(4):832–837, discussion 837–839

[21] Pandey P, Marks MP, Harraher CD, et al. Multimodality management of Spetzler-Martin Grade III arteriovenous malformations. J Neurosurg. 2012; 116 (6):1279–1288

[22] Gaballah M, Storm PB, Rabinowitz D, et al. Intraoperative cerebral angiography in arteriovenous malformation resection in children: a single institutional experience. J Neurosurg Pediatr. 2014; 13(2):222–228

[23] Miyamoto S, Hashimoto N, Nagata I, et al. Posttreatment sequelae of palliatively treated cerebral arteriovenous malformations. Neurosurgery. 2000; 46(3):589–594, discussion 594–595

[24] Barrow DL, Boyer KL, Joseph GJ. Intraoperative angiography in the management of neurovascular disorders. Neurosurgery. 1992; 30(2):153–159

[25] Martin NA, Bentson J, Viñuela F, et al. Intraoperative digital subtraction angiography and the surgical treatment of intracranial aneurysms and vascular malformations. J Neurosurg. 1990; 73(4):526–533

[26] Vitaz TW, Gaskill-Shipley M, Tomsick T, Tew JM , Jr. Utility, safety, and accuracy of intraoperative angiography in the surgical treatment of aneurysms and arteriovenous malformations. AJNR Am J Neuroradiol. 1999; 20(8):1457–1461

[27] Yuan G, Zhao JZ, Wang S, Xu J, Xin Y. Intraoperative angiography in the surgery of brain arteriovenous malformations [in Chinese]. Beijing Da Xue Xue Bao. 2007; 39(4):412–415

[28] Yanaka K, Matsumaru Y, Okazaki M, et al. Intraoperative angiography in the surgical treatment of cerebral arteriovenous malformations and fistulas. Acta Neurochir (Wien). 2003; 145(5):377–382, discussion 382–383

[29] Killory BD, Nakaji P, Gonzales LF, Ponce FA, Wait SD, Spetzler RF. Prospective evaluation of surgical microscope-integrated intraoperative near-infrared indocyanine green angiography during cerebral arteriovenous malformation surgery. Neurosurgery. 2009; 65(3):456–462, discussion 462

[30] Kakarla UK, Deshmukh VR, Zabramski JM, Albuquerque FC, McDougall CG, Spetzler RF. Surgical treatment of high-risk intracranial dural arteriovenous fistulae: clinical outcomes and avoidance of complications. Neurosurgery. 2007; 61(3):447–457, discussion 457–459

[31] Afshar JK, Doppman JL, Oldfield EH. Surgical interruption of intradural draining vein as curative treatment of spinal dural arteriovenous fistulas. J Neurosurg. 1995; 82(2):196–200

[32] Kattner KA, Roth TC, Giannotta SL. Cranial base approaches for the surgical treatment of aggressive posterior fossa dural arteriovenous fistulae with leptomeningeal drainage: report of four technical cases. Neurosurgery. 2002; 50(5):1156–1160, discussion 1160–1161

[33] Collice M, D'Aliberti G, Talamonti G, et al. Surgical interruption of leptomeningeal drainage as treatment for intracranial dural arteriovenous fistulas without dural sinus drainage. J Neurosurg. 1996; 84(5):810–817

[34] Lucas CP, De Oliveira E, Tedeschi H, et al. Sinus skeletonization: a treatment for dural arteriovenous malformations of the tentorial apex. Report of two cases. J Neurosurg. 1996; 84(3):514–517

[35] Liu JK, Dogan A, Ellegala DB, et al. The role of surgery for high-grade intracranial dural arteriovenous fistulas: importance of obliteration of venous outflow. J Neurosurg. 2009; 110(5):913–920

[36] Collice M, D'Aliberti G, Arena O, Solaini C, Fontana RA, Talamonti G. Surgical treatment of intracranial dural arteriovenous fistulae: role of venous drainage. Neurosurgery. 2000; 47(1):56–66, discussion 66–67

[37] Hoh BL, Choudhri TF, Connolly ES , Jr, Solomon RA. Surgical management of high-grade intracranial dural arteriovenous fistulas: leptomeningeal venous disruption without nidus excision. Neurosurgery. 1998; 42(4):796–804, discussion 804–805

[38] Derdeyn CP, Moran CJ, Cross DT, Grubb RL , Jr, Dacey RG , Jr. Intraoperative digital subtraction angiography: a review of 112 consecutive examinations. AJNR Am J Neuroradiol. 1995; 16(2):307–318

[39] Pandey P, Steinberg GK, Westbroek EM, Dodd R, Do HM, Marks MP. Intraoperative angiography for cranial dural arteriovenous fistula. AJNR Am J Neuroradiol. 2011; 32(6):1091–1095

[40] Thind H, Hardesty DA, Zabramski JM, Spetzler RF, Nakaji P. The role of microscope-integrated near-infrared indocyanine green videoangiography in the surgical treatment of intracranial dural arteriovenous fistulas. J Neurosurg. 2015; 122(4):876–882

[41] Raza SM, Papadimitriou K, Gandhi D, Radvany M, Olivi A, Huang J. Intra-arterial intraoperative computed tomography angiography guided navigation: a new technique for localization of vascular pathology. Neurosurgery. 2012; 71(2) Suppl Operative:ons240–ons252, discussion ons252

[42] Hänggi D, Etminan N, Steiger HJ. The impact of microscope-integrated intraoperative near-infrared indocyanine green videoangiography on surgery of arteriovenous malformations and dural arteriovenous fistulae. Neurosurgery. 2010; 67(4):1094–1103, discussion 1103–1104

[43] Schuette AJ, Cawley CM, Barrow DL. Indocyanine green videoangiography in the management of dural arteriovenous fistulae. Neurosurgery. 2010; 67(3):658–662, discussion 662

[44] Kato N, Tanaka T, Suzuki Y, et al. Multistage indocyanine green videoangiography for the convexity dural arteriovenous fistula with angiographically occult pial fistula. J Stroke Cerebrovasc Dis. 2012; 21(8):918.e1–918.e5

[45] Bilbao CJ, Bhalla T, Dalal S, Patel H, Dehdashti AR. Comparison of indocyanine green fluorescent angiography to digital subtraction angiography in brain arteriovenous malformation surgery. Acta Neurochir (Wien). 2015; 157(3):351–359

[46] Loop JW, Foltz EL. Applications of angiography during intracranial operation. Acta Radiol Diagn (Stockh). 1966; 5:363–367

[47] Allcock JM, Drake CG. Postoperative angiography in cases of ruptured intracranial aneurysm. J Neurosurg. 1963; 20:752–759

[48] Munshi I, Macdonald RL, Weir BK. Intraoperative angiography of brain arteriovenous malformations. Neurosurgery. 1999; 45(3):491–497, discussion 497–499

[49] Kotowski M, Sarrafzadeh A, Schatlo B, et al. Intraoperative angiography reloaded: a new hybrid operating theater for combined endovascular and surgical treatment of cerebral arteriovenous malformations: a pilot study on 25 patients. Acta Neurochir (Wien). 2013; 155(11):2071–2078

[50] Ghosh S, Levy ML, Stanley P, Nelson M, Giannotta SL, McComb JG. Intraoperative angiography in the management of pediatric vascular disorders. Pediatr Neurosurg. 1999; 30(1):16–22

[51] Eide PK, Sorteberg AG, Meling TR, Sorteberg W. Directional intraoperative Doppler ultrasonography during surgery on cranial dural arteriovenous fistulas. Neurosurgery. 2013; 73(2) Suppl Operative:ons211–ons222, discussion ons222–ons223

[52] Fu B, Zhao JZ, Yu LB. The application of ultrasound in the management of cerebral arteriovenous malformation. Neurosci Bull. 2008; 24(6):387–394

[53] Rubin JM, Hatfield MK, Chandler WF, Black KL, DiPietro MA. Intracerebral arteriovenous malformations: intraoperative color Doppler flow imaging. Radiology. 1989; 170(1 Pt 1):219–222

[54] Walkden JS, Zador Z, Herwadkar A, Kamaly-Asl ID. Use of intraoperative Doppler ultrasound with neuronavigation to guide arteriovenous malformation resection: a pediatric case series. J Neurosurg Pediatr. 2015; 15(3):291–300

[55] Wang H, Ye ZP, Huang ZC, Luo L, Chen C, Guo Y. Intraoperative ultrasonography combined with indocyanine green video-angiography in patients with cerebral arteriovenous malformations. J Neuroimaging. 2015; 25(6):916–921

[56] Woydt M, Perez J, Meixensberger J, Krone A, Soerensen N, Roosen K. Intraoperative colour-duplex-sonography in the surgical management of cerebral AV-malformations. Acta Neurochir (Wien). 1998; 140(7):689–698

[57] Black KL, Rubin JM, Chandler WF, McGillicuddy JE. Intraoperative color-flow Doppler imaging of AVM's and aneurysms. J Neurosurg. 1988; 68(4):635–639

[58] Westra SJ, Curran JG, Duckwiler GR, et al. Pediatric intracranial vascular malformations: evaluation of treatment results with color Doppler US. Work in progress. Radiology. 1993; 186(3):775–783

[59] Fujita A, Tamaki N, Nakamura M, Yasuo K, Morikawa M. A tentorial dural arteriovenous fistula successfully treated with interruption of leptomeningeal venous drainage using microvascular Doppler sonography: case report. Surg Neurol. 2001; 56(1):56–61

[60] Srinivasan VM, Schafer S, Ghali MG, Arthur A, Duckworth EA. Cone-beam CT angiography (Dyna CT) for intraoperative localization of cerebral arteriovenous malformations. J Neurointerv Surg. 2016; 8(1):69–74

[61] Dehdashti AR, Thines L, Da Costa LB, et al. Intraoperative biplanar rotational angiography during neurovascular surgery. Technical note. J Neurosurg. 2009; 111(1):188–192

[62] Schwartz RB, Hsu L, Wong TZ, et al. Intraoperative MR imaging guidance for intracranial neurosurgery: experience with the first 200 cases. Radiology. 1999; 211(2):477–488

[63] Bekelis K, Missios S, Desai A, Eskey C, Erkmen K. Magnetic resonance imaging/magnetic resonance angiography fusion technique for intraoperative navigation during microsurgical resection of cerebral arteriovenous malformations. Neurosurg Focus. 2012; 32(5):E7

[64] Sakurada K, Kuge A, Takemura S, et al. Intraoperative magnetic resonance imaging in the successful surgical treatment of an arteriovenous malformation–case report. Neurol Med Chir (Tokyo). 2011; 51(7):512–514

[65] Liu H, Hall WA, Martin AJ, Maxwell RE, Truwit CL. MR-guided and MR-monitored neurosurgical procedures at 1.5 T. J Comput Assist Tomogr. 2000; 24(6):909–918

10 Intraoperative Neurophysiological Monitoring during Surgical and Endovascular Treatment of Cerebral Arteriovenous Malformations

Pietro Meneghelli, Alberto Pasqualin, and Francesco Sala

Abstract

Intraoperative neurophysiological monitoring (IONM) has emerged over the past two decades as a valuable technique to promptly identify an impending injury to the nervous system, in time for corrective measures to be taken and, therefore, avoid or minimize post-operative neurological deficits. In cerebrovascular surgery, IONM provides a continuous assessment of the functional integrity of various neural pathways, including motor, sensory, auditory and visual, by monitoring evoked potentials.

The treatment of cerebral AVMs can be either surgical or endovascular. Both these treatments expose to the risk of neurological injury and IONM has been increasingly used to prevent, rather than merely predict, brain ischemia during the dissection of the AVM and temporary arterial occlusion. Depending on the location of the AVM and the degree of involvement of cortical and subcortical vascular territories, IONM techniques may include motor evoked potentials, somatosensory evoked potentials, visual evoked potentials, and brainstem auditory evoked potentials. Furthermore, mapping techniques in asleep patients may assist the surgeon to localize the motor cortex and subcortical motor pathways whenever these cannot be identified anatomically, while awake surgery allows to extend neurophysiological mapping to speech and other cognitive areas.

The use of IONM has been applied also during endovascular embolization of AVMs in general anesthesia, when associated with provocative tests. A superselective injection of short-acting barbiturates and/or local anesthetics is done before the embolization of the feeder in order to mimic the effects of the embolization. Based on the results of the provocative test, embolization can either proceed or be abandoned.

This chapter will provide a review of different neurophysiologic monitoring and cortical/subcortical mapping techniques as well as a critical review of the state-of-the art in the use of these techniques in intracranial vascular neurosurgery.

Keywords: cerebral arterio-venous malformations, endovascular embolization, intraoperative neurophysiological monitoring, motor evoked potentials, provocative tests

- IONM strategies during the surgical treatment of brain AVMs should be tailored to the location of the AVM and the vascular territories involved. A combination of upper and/or lower extremity MEPs and/or SSEPs, as well as the use of VEPs and BAERs should be considered for each specific case.
- While Penfield's technique has been the standard method for cortical mapping for several decades, currently the so-called motor evoked potential short-train technique offers several advantages for both cortical and subcortical motor mapping.
- The use of pharmacological provocative tests associated with MEP and SSEP monitoring is a valuable tool for a safe endovascular treatment of brain AVMs in sensorimotor areas under general anesthesia.
- The relationship between the duration of vascular temporary clipping and neurophysiological changes, as well as that between the duration of IONM changes and clinical outcome remains unclear, yet pivotal in understanding how long IONM changes can be tolerated before ischemia progresses to infarction.

10.1 Introduction

Surgical treatment of cerebral arteriovenous malformations (AVMs) is highly demanding, in terms of both operative technique and deep knowledge of anatomy. Furthermore, a high confidence with digital subtraction angiography (DSA) is required. The key point of cerebrovascular surgery, especially in AVM surgery, is to exclude the lesion from the vascular tree and at the same time to preserve the cerebral blood flow (CBF) in the locoregional structures. Arteries feeding the AVM often supply eloquent areas such as the sensory-motor cortex and the corticospinal tracts (CSTs), and a careful evaluation of "en passage" arteries must be performed. Direct visualization of these vessels before and after surgical excision is not enough since hidden perforators can go undetected by surgical inspection alone. In recent years, various techniques have become available to obtain a direct or indirect evaluation of CBF and perfusion. Imaging methods such as intraoperative angiography and, more recently, indocyanine green video angiography provide a real-time evaluation of the vessel patency. Moreover, intraoperative microflow probe[1] and Doppler ultrasound provide real-time evaluation of the flow in the insonated vessels. These direct techniques provide qualitative and quantitative assessment of CBF, but they do not provide feedback about the functional consequence of reduced CBF.

Intraoperative neurophysiological monitoring (IONM) allows assessment of the functional integrity of neural pathways during surgery. In cerebrovascular surgery, IONM indirectly provides an assessment of CBF and often allows detection of an impending injury to cortical and subcortical areas. In the recent past, IONM has become a very useful tool in the management of cerebrovascular lesions, especially aneurysms.[2,3,4,5,6,7,8,9] Neurophysiologic monitoring includes various techniques with different characteristics: electroencephalography (EEG) monitoring is useful to detect impending ischemia due to major vessels occlusion and to titrate anesthesia during temporary clipping in aneurysm surgery; somatosensory evoked potentials (SSEPs)

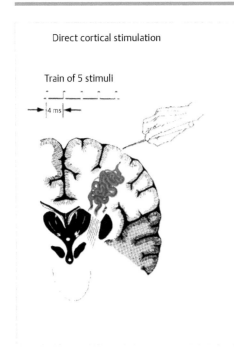

Direct cortical stimulation

Train of 5 stimuli

4 ms

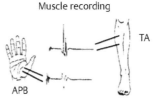

Muscle recording

TA

APB

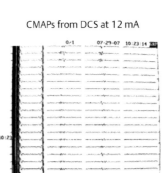

CMAPs from DCS at 12 mA

Fig. 10.1 Schematic illustration of cortical mapping during surgery for brain AVMs. Left-hand panel: direct cortical stimulation (DCS) is performed using a hand-held monopolar probe that delivers a short train of five stimuli (0.5 ms duration each; interstimulus interval, 4 ms; repetition rate, 1 Hz; maximum Intensity, 20 mA). Compound muscle action potentials (CMAPs) are recorded from the contralateral muscles. In this example, CMAPs from the left extensor digitorum (LE) and left abductor pollicis brevis (LA) muscles are recorded following DCS at 12 mA. No response is recorded from the left lower facial (LL) and the left tibialis anterior (LT) muscles.

provide an evaluation of the dorsal column pathways and their ability to transduce a peripheral stimulus and convey it to the brain; brainstem auditory evoked potentials (BAERs) evaluate the transduction of an auditory stimulus along the auditory pathways (auditory nerve, cochlear nucleus, superior olive, inferior colliculus), from the periphery to the cortex; motor evoked potentials (MEPs) provide an evaluation of the CST and other descending motor pathways, from the cortex to the muscles.

The treatment of cerebral AVMs can be either surgical or endovascular. Both these treatments expose to the risk of neurological injury, and IONM has been increasingly used to prevent, rather than merely predict, brain ischemia.

This chapter will provide a review of different neurophysiologic monitoring (SSEP, BAER, MEP) and cortical/subcortical mapping techniques as well as a critical review of the state of the art in the use of these techniques in intracranial vascular neurosurgery.

10.2 Intraoperative Neurophysiology Techniques

IONM can be essentially divided in two categories: mapping and monitoring techniques. The former provides functional identification of ambiguous neural structures such as the identification of the primary motor area in the case of a deformed functional anatomy due to the presence of a rolandic AVM. However, cortical/subcortical mapping provides only information at a given point in time, but does not allow continuous assessment of the functional integrity of a neural pathway. This latter can be achieved by using monitoring techniques such as SSEP, BAERs, and MEPs.

Unlike tumor surgery, mapping techniques are rarely needed in vascular neurosurgery. On the other hand, monitoring techniques can be used and provide valuable information.

Monitoring of SSEPs has been used since the 1980s in aneurysm surgery.[2,10,11] Other authors have used a combined SSEP– BAERs protocol,[5,12] while MEPs were introduced more recently.[6,8,9,13,14]

10.2.1 Mapping Techniques
Cortical Mapping (▶ Fig. 10.1)

For cortical and subcortical mapping, the bipolar 60-Hz stimulation technique, which is essentially based on the original Penfield technique, is still widely used in the neurosurgical community.[15] A constant-current stimulator generating biphasic square wave pulses with a 60-Hz (50 Hz in Europe) stimulating rate and 1-ms single-phase duration is used. A bipolar electrode with 5-mm spacing between the contact points is used to directly stimulate the cortex for 2 to 3 seconds. Under general anesthesia, starting current intensity is around 4 mA, and is then increased in 2-mA increments up to the point where a motor response is recorded from contralateral muscles. In an awake patient, the threshold is usually lower and movements can be elicited with current as low as 1 to 2 mA.[16,17] Visual observation of the muscle activity has been substituted by multichannel electromyography, which appears to be more sensitive.[18] In the asleep patient, if at the intensity of 16 to 20 mA no muscle contraction is obtained, the cortical area under investigation is declared not eloquent for motor function, although some patients may have higher thresholds for stimulation. During the application of this technique, it is highly recommended to predispose electrocorticography (ECoG) due to the risk of eliciting clinical or subclinical seizurelike activities (afterdischarge), which may compromise any further neurophysiological assessment. In the case of an intraoperative seizure, cortical irrigation with cold ringer lactate usually stops this activity within 20 to 30 seconds.[19]

Penfield's technique, however, has several limitations, which include a higher risk of inducing intraoperative seizures,[20] the unfeasibility to perform continuous MEP monitoring due to the prolonged stimulation of the cortex, and a low success rate in children likely due to the immaturity of the motor cortex and pathways.[21]

With the advent of the MEP monitoring technique developed by Taniguchi et al and Pechstein et al in the mid-1990s, a new strategy became possible to map the motor cortex.[22,23] This technique is used to elicit MEPs through transcranial electrical stimulation (TES) but, during cranial surgery where the motor cortex is exposed, it can be used also for performing MEP monitoring directly from a strip electrode on the motor cortex and to perform cortical mapping. The technique accounts for 500-μs square wave impulses in train of five to seven stimuli, a 4-ms interstimulus interval, and constant current intensities up to 200 mA for TES and up to 20 mA for cortical MEP monitoring and motor mapping.

In adults, threshold intensities up to 20 mA are usually considered safe for mapping the motor cortex through monopolar stimulation. Although the risk of inducing intraoperative seizures using the MEP short-train technique is considerably lower than using Penfield's technique,[20] to minimize this risk we still recommend the use of ECoG while setting the intensity for cortical mapping and direct cortical stimulation (DCS) for continuous MEP monitoring. This allows detecting any afterdischarge, which may affect the results of mapping, providing false-positive results. Unfortunately, the threshold for positive cortical mapping is sometimes higher than the threshold for afterdischarges and there is high variability across the cortex within the same subject.[24]

For a successful cortical/subcortical motor mapping and MEP monitoring, the selection of appropriate muscles to record from is critical. The small hand muscles (e.g., abductor pollicis brevis) as well as the long forearm flexors or extensors have been shown to be good options for upper extremities, due to their richer innervation with CST fibers than more proximal muscles. Similarly, for the lower extremities, the abductor hallucis brevis (AHB) is the optimal muscle because of its dominant CST innervation.[25] The tibialis anterior (TA) muscle is an alternative to the AHB. Our standard electrode montage for monitoring mMEPs is the AHB and TA muscle for the lower and the ABP and forearm flexors or extensors for the upper limbs. Finally, it is important to always monitor a muscle that cannot be affected by surgery (typically, in brain surgery, any ipsilateral muscle) as a control modality to exclude changes in evoked potentials not induced by surgery but by anesthesia or technical issues.

During surgery for brain AVMs, the choice of the appropriate muscle recordings is essential, and it should be made based on the functional anatomy of the cortical and subcortical areas related to the AVM nidus and to its angioarchitecture.

Subcortical Mapping

Subcortical mapping provides the identification of the white matter fiber tracts with the aim to preserve them during surgery. Again, either the MEP short-train or Penfield's technique can be used for subcortical mapping, but some preliminary data[26] suggest that the short-train technique delivered through a monopolar probe is the most efficient technique. The CST has received the larger attention in terms of subcortical mapping and correlation with tractography. The lower the intensity of stimulation necessary to localize the CST and elicit a muscle response, the closer the CST. A safety distance between the mapping site and the CST has not been yet unequivocally determined; however, the rule of thumb suggests that each mA of stimulation intensity corresponds to roughly 1 mm of distance from the tracts.[27,28] If so, stimulation intensities between 2 and 5 mA correspond to a distance of 2 to 5 mm from the tracts, and are reliable cut-off values for a safe distance from the CST.[21,27,29]

SSEP Phase Reversal

SSEP phase reversal is a technique that permits to identify the central sulcus and therefore, indirectly, the motor area. A subdural strip electrode is placed over the central region and then SSEPs are elicited through the stimulation of the contralateral median nerve or posterior tibial nerve (up to 40-mA intensity, 0.2-ms duration, 4.3-Hz repetition rate). Recordings are performed from the scalp at Cz-Fz (legs) and C3/C4-Cz (arms). This technique is based on the principle that an SSEP elicited by median nerve stimulation at the wrist can be recorded from the primary sensory cortex and its mirror image waveform can be recorded if the recording electrode is placed on the opposite side of the central sulcus, on the primary motor cortex.[30,31] The amplitude of the cortical response recorded at the precentral gyrus is typically positive at around 25 ms (P25), whereas the response visible at the postcentral gyrus is negative at 20 ms (N20).

10.2.2 Monitoring Techniques

MEP Monitoring (▶ Fig. 10.2)

Unlikely from motor cortical and subcortical mapping, continuous MEP monitoring provides an on-line assessment of the functional integrity of descending tracts, rather than their identification at one point in time.

MEP monitoring is used to assess the integrity of the corticospinal pathway. Two different techniques are available: TES and DCS. The former is used in cases in which the motor strip is not exposed with the craniotomy; the latter is preferred in the case of surgical exposure of the motor strip.

TES of the motor cortex is usually applied using corkscrew electrodes, which guarantee low impedance.[32] We routinely place six electrodes (C1, C2, C3, C4, Cz−1 cm, and Cz+6 cm) according to the 10/20 International Electroencephalography system. Using different montages of stimulating electrodes provides flexibility to optimize elicitation of mMEPs without muscle twitching, which can interfere with surgery. In most cases, C1/C2 is a better electrode montage for eliciting mMEPs in all contralateral limbs. Occasionally, the montage Cz−1 cm versus Cz+6 cm can better elicit mMEPs from lower extremities, offering also the advantage of less intense muscle twitching than other montages. In the case of surgical incision around the central region, leads should be displaced either in front or posterior to the skin flap, but this can require higher current to obtain MEP response with subsequent higher muscle twitches and discomfort for the surgeon.

In the DCS technique, a multicontact strip electrode is placed under the dura over the central gyrus. An electrode at the Fpz serves as cathode. The electrode with the lowest stimulation threshold to elicit a contralateral muscle response is chosen for

Continuous MEP monitoring

Train of 5 stimuli

4 ms

Muscle recording

TA

APB

MEP from strip electrode #3, at 12 mA

09:29

09:30

09:26

APB   TA

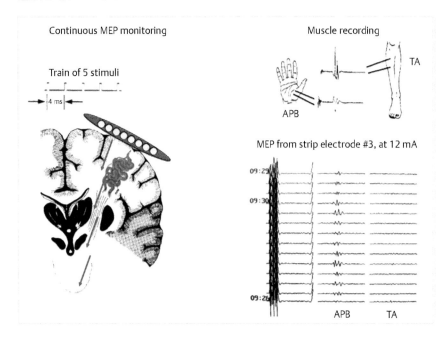

Fig. 10.2 Schematic illustration of continuous MEP monitoring during surgery for brain AVMs. Left-hand panel: MEP monitoring is performed using an eight-contact strip electrode placed on the primary motor area. The electrode with the lowest threshold to elicit contralateral mMEPs is used for monitoring. Nearby electrodes can be used to obtain mMEPs from other muscles, if needed. The selected electrode (*in yellow*) delivers short trains of five stimuli (0.5 ms duration each; interstimulus interval, 4 ms; repetition rate, 1 Hz; maximum intensity, 20 mA), which travel along the corticospinal tract (*red arrows*) and elicit mMEPs from the contralateral muscles. In this example, a response from the abductor pollicis brevis (APB) muscle is recorded following stimulation from electrode no. 3 at 12 mA. No response is recorded from the tibialis anterior (TA) muscle.

continuous MEP monitoring. MEP recording is obtained from muscle of the upper and lower extremities using pairs of needle electrodes.[33] Muscle twitches following DCS are minimized by the much lower current intensity (up to 20mA) applied to the motor cortex, as compared to transcranial MEPs (up to 200mA).

Stimulation intensity immediately above threshold is chosen for stimulation in order to avoid unnecessary charge load. MEP amplitude and latency should be evaluated in comparison with baseline values and through a standard step-by-step protocol in order to exclude anesthesiological or technical abnormalities as possible causes of changes in the evoked potentials. Although there is still an ongoing debate on what is considered a "significant" MEP change, there is agreement on the fact that changes in amplitude are more relevant than changes in latency and that any amplitude drop, which exceeds 50% of baseline values, should be reported to the surgeon as it may predict an impending injury to motor pathways.[6,27,34,35] Transcranial MEPs suffer from intrinsic variability so that threshold criteria per se are of limited value, but—at least in brain tumor surgery—there is evidence that irreversible changes in MEP amplitude correlate with some degree of postoperative motor deficit. Complete loss of MEPs correlate with a permanent paresis and postoperative evidence, at the neuroimaging, of subcortical ischemia.[35] No changes in MEPs usually predict a good motor outcome from early after surgery. In between these black and white scenarios, there is a gray zone where robust criteria to interpret MEP changes are still not well defined. This degree of uncertainty is larger in vascular neurosurgery due to the paucity of clinical studies when compared to brain tumor surgery and, in particular for AVMs, there is little amount of data in the literature.

Overall, TES is considered a safe method, and there are no major contraindications to its use in the clinical setting.[36] However, if too high intensity is used, there is a potential risk of distal activation of the CST as far as the brainstem.[37] In this case, the point of activation may be distal to the level of a subcortical injury (for example, due to an ischemic event) and this may produce a false-negative result (meaning, the patient wakes up

hemiparetic in spite of present mMEPs). To avoid this, during intracranial surgery, the use of DCS, whenever feasible, should always be preferred over TES for mMEP monitoring because the intensity required to elicit a response is about 10 times lower (1–20 vs. 30–200 mA), and this minimizes the risk of distal activation of the CST.

MEPs are generally more suitable to monitor subcortical areas, while SSEPs are more sensitive to ischemic derangements at the cortical level. Therefore, SSEP recording seems inadequate to monitor function in vascular territories supplied by perforating arteries, while it is certainly indicated when cortical ischemia represents the main risk of surgery.

From a methodological standpoint, it should be kept in mind that evoked potentials recording should be tailored to the location of the AVM and, therefore, to the territory at risk for ischemia. For example, an AVM fed mainly from an anterior communicating artery, anterior cerebral artery, or basilar artery branch would be better monitored using a bilateral tibial nerve SSEPs and bilateral MEP recordings, while for AVMs fed mainly by middle cerebral artery (MCA) branches contralateral recordings may suffice.

TES MEP monitoring is a valuable method also during the endovascular treatment of cerebral AVMs, as it provides continuous assessment of the functional integrity of motor pathways during the embolization procedure. Provocative tests can be used to mimic the effect of the embolization, as it will be discussed later in this chapter.

SSEP Monitoring

SSEPs are used to monitor the dorsal column pathway, from the periphery to cerebral cortex. The median nerve and the posterior tibial nerve are normally used, respectively, for upper extremities and lower extremities SSEP monitoring. It has to be kept in mind that upper and lower extremity SSEPs should be monitored separately because of the different somatotopy of these tracts and different vascular territories involved in the cortical generators of these potentials. So, median nerve SSEP would better assess the MCA territory and tibial nerve SSEP the anterior cerebral artery territory.

Upper extremities monitoring starts with the depolarization of the median nerve by electrical stimulation in order to produce a synchronous action potential volley through the sensory fibers of the dorsal root that reach the fasciculus cuneatus (above T6). Then the action potential travels through the nucleus cuneatus, decussate (internal arcuate fibers), reach the contralateral medial lemniscus, and terminate in the ventral posterolateral (VPL) nucleus of the thalamus. Lower extremities monitoring starts with the depolarization of the posterior tibial nerve. The action potentials travel through the fasciculus gracilis to the nucleus gracilis; then, second-order neurons decussate, travel through the contralateral medial lemniscus, and terminate in the VPL nucleus of thalamus. Third-order neurons project to the somatosensory area and parietal association fields and are processed by scalp leads. Scalp leads are placed at CP3 and CP4 with a forehead reference (Fpz or Fz). Parameters monitored are the SSEP amplitude, latency, and central conduction time (CCT), which refers to the transit time from the dorsal column nuclei to the cortex.

Baseline values are recorded prior to incision, at the craniotomy and at the beginning of the intracranial manipulation. A standard protocol has then to be used for decision-making in case of decrease of SSEP amplitude > 50%, latency delay > 10%, and CCT > 1.0 ms.

BAER Monitoring

BAER monitoring provides data on the ascending auditory pathway. Bilateral ear transducers create alternate compression and rarefaction square wave clicks with duration of 100 to 200 ms and intensity of 70 dB. The stimulation provides a seven-peak wave; peaks are related to the specific sequence of synapses along the auditory pathway: cochlear nerve (I peak), cochlear nuclei (II peak), contralateral superior olivary complex (III peak), lateral lemniscus (IV peak), inferior colliculi (V peak), medial geniculate body (VI peak), and acoustic radiation (VII peak).

Brainstem auditory-evoked potentials can provide useful information on the general well-being of the brainstem, especially during those procedures in which a significant surgical manipulation of the brainstem and/or of the cerebellum is expected. When interpreting brainstem auditory-evoked potential recordings, a thoughtful analysis of the waveform and of their correlation with neural generators provides useful information about the level of the brainstem where EP changes may occur. In summary, dysfunction of the eighth nerve proximal to its cochlear end will cause a prolongation of the I–III interpeak interval, attenuation of waves III and V, or both. The latencies of waves III and V increase in parallel, while the III–V interpeak interval remains almost unchanged as long as the auditory pathways within the brainstem are not affected.

A disappearance of wave I only may also be indicative of cochlear ischemia secondary to the compromise of the internal auditory artery. Vice versa, if the cochlea is not injured and the damage to the eighth nerve occurs in the cerebellopontine angle, wave I may persist even if the eighth nerve is completely transected. Damage to the lower pons, around the area of the cochlear nucleus or the superior olivary complex, will also

affect waves III and V with delay in latency and drop in amplitude. Damage to the brainstem at the level of the midbrain will affect waves IV–V, but not waves I or III.

VEP Monitoring

Visual evoked potential (VEP) monitoring is used to assess the function of the visual pathway in order to prevent postoperative visual deterioration. A light-stimulating device is placed on closed eyelids; flashing light intensity can be adjusted with an electric current ranging from 0 to 20 mA by a bath amplifier. Each eye is stimulated separately and averaged VEP waveforms are then obtained. Overall, 40 to 100 flashes are recorded to obtain each averaged VEP waveform, with a stimulus average of one flash (40 ms) per second. Recording montage requires five channels, with electrodes placed on the bilateral earlobes (A+) and the left occiput, occipital midline (Oz), and the right occiput. A small negative potential and a large positive potential around 100 ms are recorded, and the amplitude of the VEP is defined as the voltage difference between these two potentials. In order to verify the arrival of the light at the retina, needle electrodes are inserted subcutaneously at the lateral canthi for electroretinogram (ERG) recording. It is useful to record at least two consecutive ERG and VEP in order to confirm the reproducibility of the ERG and VEP waveforms after setup and before surgery.[38] Although many attempts have been made in order to improve the reproducibility of VEPs, stable recordings are difficult to obtain and consequently a clear clinical usefulness remains unclear. However, as previously described, the use of ERG permits the distinction between technical and clinical problems, such as light goggles displacement or preexisting visual dysfunction and VEPs disappearance.

10.2.3 Cognitive Mapping during Awake Surgery

Unlikely from sensorimotor, auditory, and visual function, cognitive functions such as language, memory, and others require the collaboration of the patient and the presence of a neuropsychologist in the operating room. Awake surgery is nowadays very popular and has revolutionized the operative management of brain gliomas, especially low-grade gliomas. As much as the use of awake craniotomy during surgery for brain AVMs is of limited use, still this can be valuable in selected patients.

For cortical and subcortical mapping in awake patients, Penfield's technique—as described above for motor mapping—is considered the standard of care given that it is considered that a prolonged cortical stimulation is necessary to interfere with cognitive processing.

Berger and Ojemann et al[17,39] have developed a classic stimulation paradigm for language mapping. Since the majority of aphasias involve a naming deficit, stimulation evoked anomia (or dysnomia) is considered significant for a language site. In order to confirm localization of Broca's area, it is then mandatory to check movements of the mouth or pharynx to rule out the possibility of a speech arrest secondary to motor activation of facial, tongue, and laryngeal muscles rather than to specific stimulation of Broca's site. As a rule, a wide exposure of the cerebral cortex increases the possibility of obtaining positive mapping results and, on average, 20 or more cortical sites need to be mapped to achieve a positive response. Every site is tested three separate times, and two errors out of three are significant for a language site, which should be preserved with a margin of at least 10 mm. Besides language, a number of other cognitive functions can nowadays be tested in the operating room, but this exceeds the goal of this chapter. It should be emphasized, nevertheless, that regardless of the specific functions going to be tested, the use of ECoG is strongly recommended to detect subclinical epileptiform activity, which may be a source of misleading results given that the falsely "positive" cortical mapping is due to the results of afterdischarges rather than the activation of truly eloquent cortex.

10.2.4 Considerations in Pediatric Neurosurgery

Corkscrew electrodes for TES and recordings should be cautiously used in infants with open fontanels and in children with shunt systems to avoid injury due to misplacement of the screw.

In children, higher intensities for either TES or DCS MEP monitoring may be needed, especially in those younger than 5 to 6 years, due to the immaturity of their motor cortex and pathways.[21,40] In young children, two opposite factors may affect the threshold to elicit mMEP after TES. The immaturity of the motor cortex and subcortical motor pathways may increase stimulating thresholds. However, this variable is counterbalanced by the thinner thickness of the skull, which should facilitate motor cortex activation at lower intensities because of lower impedance.

With regard to cortical mapping, preliminary data suggest that in children the MEP short-train technique is by far more effective than Penfield's technique in eliciting a motor response.[41]

10.2.5 Anesthesia for Neurophysiological Monitoring

The success of IONM is highly related to the anesthesiological management of the procedure. The common inhalational agents such as isoflurane, sevoflurane, and desflurane may affect the reliability of IONM by blocking neural transmission at the synaptic level. Halogenated anesthetics elevate muscle MEP stimulus thresholds and block muscle MEPs in a dose-dependent fashion, and therefore should be avoided.

Total intravenous anesthesia (TIVA) is a preferable choice in the management of anesthesia during IONM. Anesthesia is therefore maintained with a constant infusion of propofol (100–150 µg/kg/min) and fentanyl (usually around 1 µg/kg/h). Nitrous oxide not exceeding 50% can be used. Bolus injections of both intravenous agents should be avoided because this temporarily disrupts SSEPs and MEPs recordings.

Short-acting muscle relaxants are given for intubation but not thereafter, because with full relaxation muscle MEP monitoring and cortical/subcortical mapping are unfeasible. We also try to avoid any partial relaxation because a physiologic variability in the mMEP amplitude across repetitive trials and in the compound muscle action potential response already exists, so that any muscle relaxation would add another variable to the interpretation of motor responses.

10.3 IONM during Surgical Procedures

Surgical resection of brain AVMs is technically challenging. The key point is to cauterize and cut arteries that directly feed the AVM and to spare those that supply the normal brain tissue, especially in eloquent areas. During the surgical procedure, additional radiological details provided by intraoperative angiography may help the surgeon to distinguish between normal brain tissue arteries and pathologic AVM suppliers.[42] More recently, indocyanine green videoangiography has been reported as useful tool also in detecting residual nidus during AVM surgery.[43] However, intraoperative angiographic studies provide only anatomical data and in some cases it might be still difficult to differentiate between AVM feeders and passing arteries. This is even more crucial when dealing with AVMs in eloquent areas.

The principle of "eloquence" in surgery for brain AVM includes cortical and subcortical areas which can be monitored under general anesthesia and others which require cognitive mapping and, therefore, awake surgery. We will focus on IONM strategies during surgical procedures under general anesthesia as these represent, by far, the most common application of IONM. Some aspects related to IONM in awake patients will be discussed thereafter.

10.3.1 IONM during AVM Surgery under General Anesthesia

IONM in cerebrovascular surgery permits the early recognition of two main problems: impending ischemia due to inadvertent occlusion of vessels or perforators and direct damage to eloquent cortical or subcortical areas. Dissection of cerebral AVMs requires various surgical maneuvers: brain retraction, dissection of brain tissue, temporary artery occlusion. All these steps could possibly induce changes in the evoked potentials. Moreover, inadvertent occlusion of perforating arteries and vasospasm secondary to manipulation of vessels during subarachnoid dissection are other causes of evoked potential alterations. The role of IONM during the resection of eloquent AVMs therefore becomes substantial. The coupling of temporary clipping of the feeding arteries and the indirect evaluation of the perfusion around the AVM with IONM helps in reducing the risk of cerebral infarction.

Various combinations of the aforementioned IONM techniques have been used to preserve function during surgery for brain AVMs. Chang et al reported the usefulness of SSEP and BAERs in the surgical management of 53 patients (54 procedures) with cerebral AVMs.[12] SSEP changes have been reported in five patients (four transient and one permanent): in the four cases with transient SSEP alteration, three patients showed new—but transient—postoperative deficits, and one did not develop any clinical postoperative deficit; the latter patient with permanent SSEP changes developed a prolonged transient hemiparesis lasting 3 weeks. During the surgical procedure, all of the transient SSEP changes were reverted with the removal or adjustment of the temporary clip on feeding arteries or by elevating mean arterial pressure (MAP). One of the 17 patients (6%) monitored with BAERs showed a permanent alteration in

BAERs and developed a new permanent neurological deficit after surgery. The authors reported 86% sensitivity for SSEP and BAERs in the prediction of new postoperative transient or permanent deficit, and 98% specificity.

Ichikawa et al have recently described the use of MEP monitoring in AVM surgery in 21 patients.[44] In order to address a specific potential risk to motor pathways, the patients were divided in three groups. In the first group, the feeding arteries supplied the CST; the second group included patients at risk of direct injury to the CST due to surgical maneuvers, and the third group had the potential of motor pathways shift due to the AVM location. The surgeon received a warning in case of MEP disappearance or decreasing in amplitude to less than 50% of the baseline level in the course of three or more consecutive recordings. During the surgical procedure, five patients showed MEP changes. Of these, four patients were in group I. In the first patient, MEP disappeared after the occlusion of a draining vein and did not reappear; the patient developed hemiparesis due to a venous infarction of the thalamus and the internal capsule. The other three patients showed transient MEP changes related to temporary clipping in two patients and to bleeding from the nidus in the last one. Only two of the three patients with transient MEP changes developed transient postoperative hemiparesis, which resolved in 2 days; the last patient did not show any postoperative deficits. One patient in group II showed transient MEP decreased amplitude (80%) due to coagulation of fragile vessels around the nidus. In group III, there were no changes during MEP recordings.

Continuous evaluation of the functional activity of the brain in eloquent areas also includes inspection of the visual cortex. Intraoperative monitoring of VEPs may contribute to the preservation of visual function after surgery of the optic pathways (from the optic nerve to the lateral geniculate body). In 1973, Wright et al described the use of VEP monitoring during surgery of intraorbital tumors in order to prevent postoperative visual deficits.[45] However, difficulties in obtaining stable VEP recordings rendered their clinical usefulness unclear.[46,47,48] Recently, Sasaki et al reported three technical ameliorations of the technique in order to improve the reliability of the method: the introduction of a new light-stimulating device to guarantee retinal stimulation even when the scalp is reflected; the use of electroretinography in order to avoid VEPs false positive related to technical problem (light-stimulating device displacement) or preexisting visual dysfunction; and the use of TIVA to avoid the effects of inhalation anesthesia.[49] These authors reported the application of this technique in five AVMs surgeries (three temporal, one parietal, and one occipital AVMs) out of a total of 100 patients (200 eyes); the criterion for amplitude changes was defined as 50% decrease or increase compared with the control level. The VEP amplitude decreased without recovery to 50% of the control level in 14 eyes and all of these developed postoperative deficits; this group comprehended a patient treated for an occipital AVM who developed hemianopia after surgery. Of 169 eyes without VEP changes in amplitude during surgery, two eyes showed a slight visual defect in both eyes after surgery. San-Juan et al reported a case of occipital AVM surgically resected using cortical VEP monitoring.[50] The authors used an intracranial electrode grid (5 × 4) placed over the occipital lobe and, initially, over the AVM to register flash cortical VEPs obtained through binocular stimulation (flash frequencies starting from 1 to 5.1 Hz with a total duration of 10 s); the photic driving was registered on channels 1–2 and 2–3 of the ECoG and correlated with the average of the VEPs. The cortical resection was tailored to avoid those areas from which photic driving could be obtained and the patient did not experience postoperative visual defects.

In eloquent AVM surgery, the role of IONM is related not only to its capability to detect impending ischemia but also to help the surgeon in defining the localization of eloquent cortex. In facts, an AVM located in or adjacent to regions such as sensorimotor, language, and visual cortex can result in the translocation of these functions to neighboring cortical areas. Kombos et al reported the case of a left sensorimotor cortex AVM, in which intraoperative mapping showed an unexcitability of the precentral gyrus, while stimulation of the cortex anterior to the primary motor cortex elicited motor responses.[51] During surgery, the central sulcus was identified by phase reversal of the SSEPs and the motor cortex was mapped by direct high-frequency (500 Hz) monopolar anodal stimulation. Thus, stimulation of the primary motor cortex induced no motor response, whereas a motor response was elicited only by stimulation of the cortex anterior to the precentral gyrus. There was no postoperative deterioration of motor function.

10.3.2 IONM during Awake Craniotomy for AVM Surgery

The use of awake craniotomy for AVM surgery remains anecdotal. Recently, Gamble et al[52] described the use of subcortical mapping during awake resection of four AVMs in the speech area. A complete speech arrest was noted during mapping of the perimalformation zone in one case; in a second patient, a speech deficit was noted during the resection of the nidus with subcortical mapping. In all four cases, the AVMs were completely removed without permanent postoperative deficits. The patient who presented a speech deficit during subcortical mapping experienced a mild and transient dysphasia that improved in 6 weeks.

Gabarrós et al[53] furthermore emphasized the role of cortical mapping for motor and language areas as an invaluable tool in identifying the eloquent cortex, guiding the dissection to the AVM beneath the cortical surface through the identification of safe sulci. In his study, neurophysiological mapping significantly impacted the decision to completely resect the AVM. These authors reported 12 cases of AVMs in eloquent areas, 5 of which were in speech-related areas and 7 in motor areas. The five patients with tumors in speech-related areas were treated with awake craniotomy. Overall, brain mapping influenced the resection in four patients: in two cases, the AVM nidus was too intimately associated with the eloquent cortex to consent safe resection; in the other two cases, the deep extension of the nidus in proximity with the internal capsule and deep supply from lenticulostriate arteries led to halting the dissection. In these cases of incomplete resection, the nidus were left dearterialized and with preserved draining vein, and directed to radiosurgery. Finally, the authors stated that indications for intraoperative mapping include: preoperative imaging suggestive for language/sensorimotor cortex nearby the AVM; larger AVM with high Spetzler–Martin grade; and patient with unruptured AVM without deficits.

10.3.3 Presurgical Functional Imaging as an Alternative to Awake Surgery for Brain AVMs in language and other cognitive-related areas

Overall, preoperative functional imaging is still of much larger use than awake craniotomies in treating AVM located in cognitively eloquent areas. Nowadays, neuroradiological imaging can detect shifts in functional localization with functional magnetic resonance imaging (fMRI), magnetoencephalography (MEG), magnetic source imaging (MSI), positron emission tomography (PET), Wada testing, and, last but not least, transcranial magnetic stimulation (TMS).[54,55]

However, it should be considered that both fMRI and PET provide preoperative functional data that are essentially based on metabolic information. This does not necessarily correlate with the neurophysiological information offered by IONM, and vascular cases are typically those where a discrepancy between preoperative fMRI and intraoperative neurophysiological mapping may occur.[56] Moreover, as suggested by Ozdoba et al,[57] flow abnormalities such as those detected in "high-flow malformations" make it no longer possible to use a task-related increase of blood flow (related to the blood oxygen level dependent—BOLD—response in fMRI), given the reserve capacity of adjacent vessels might already be exhausted.

The reliability of preoperative functional neuroimaging is certainly higher for the localization of motor rather than cognitive, and especially language-related, areas. Lehéricy et al demonstrated that fMRI incorrectly quantified contralateral language reorganization in AVMs with significant flow abnormalities.[58] Thus, although preoperative functional imaging serves as a screening test for major reorganization of the eloquent cortex, intraoperative neurophysiology remains the gold standard in the identification of highly eloquent cortex, such as sensorimotor and language areas. Cannestra et al,[59] for example, showed that in spite of fMRI findings, suggesting feasible resection for central region AVMs, in two cases intraoperative cortical stimulation showed eloquent cortex involving the nidus, thus halting the resection.

Navigated TMS is a promising technique that has already showed great reliability in the presurgical planning of brain tumor surgery. Its role in surgery of brain AVMs remains undetermined but preliminary results are encouraging.[55]

Finally, the interest for tractography is increasing also in AVM surgery, following the much larger experience in brain tumor surgery. Although this technique does not provide any functional information but only an anatomical information on the displacement and orientation of white matter tracts, its role in AVM surgery near the CSTs has been documented by some preliminary reports.[60,61]

10.4 IONM during Endovascular Procedures

In the comprehensive management of cerebral AVMs, the development and refinement of endovascular techniques has progressively changed the treatment algorithm and their utilization prior to surgical resection has been widely accepted, especially in high-grade Spetzler–Martin AVMs.[62,63,64] However, the risk and benefits of this modality has to be incorporated into the overall risk profile for the treatment of AVMs.[65] In case of an AVM in eloquent area, a provocative test is a useful tool that enables the surgeon to distinguish between AVM direct feeders and normal brain arteries. A provocative test is based on the superselective injection of sodium amytal—a short-acting barbiturate—or similar in the AVM feeders followed by a clinical examination of the patient. If a new neurological deficit appears, the test is positive and it means that the vessel injected has a functional role and cannot be safely embolized. Rauch et al showed that the amytal test is a good predictor of neurological sequelae after embolization, even if superselective angiogram does not show supply of the normal parenchymal from the vessel(s) tested.[66] The authors reviewed their experience in 147 AVM embolization procedures for which 30 patients were submitted to preoperative amytal test with EEG monitoring and clinical examination. There were 23 positive results: 18 of them did not undergo embolization, whereas 5 patients did. Among these five patients, two (40%) developed postoperative deficits. However, the authors underlined that many patients developed EEG changes in absence of clinical symptoms. In fact, in a different article by the same group, out of a total 109 amytal test, 23 produced positive results; however, only 12 positive results were detected by clinical examination, which means that almost one-half were missed without EEG monitoring.[67] Furthermore, Paiva et al confirmed the relationship between focal or diffuse low-frequency EEG abnormalities and poor clinical outcome in patients submitted to cyanoacrylate AVM embolization.[68] In order to improve the utility and efficacy of the provocative test, Paulsen et al reported their experience during the treatment of 17 patients with rolandic AVMs.[69] In this series, in 16 of 17 patients, SSEPs were also registered in order to augment the physical examination. A total of 23 embolizations were performed in 17 patients. In two patients, the embolization was aborted based on the positive amytal test: the first patient showed a greater than 50% amplitude reduction of the cortical SSEP and physical examination showed a transient new neurological deficit; the second one was treated under general anesthesia (pediatric patient) and the result of the provocative test was the significant amplitude reduction of the cortical SSEPs. There were no permanent postoperative deficits and four minor transient deficits. Moo et al proposed an evaluation of the provocative test based on neurologic and cognitive testing customized to AVM size and location.[70] Out of a total of 29 provocative test, 27 yielded no clinical deficits, whereas in 2 cases the amytal injection caused cognitive deficits that were neuroanatomically attributable to the eloquent cortex in the region of the AVM. In these two patients, the embolization was aborted and the patients did not experience new postprocedure cognitive deficits.

Provocative tests can also be applied to the evaluation of visual fields during embolization of occipital AMVs. Tawk et al reported their experience on 13 patients with occipital AVMs who underwent 39 Wada test before embolization.[71] Patients were treated under conscious sedation. Provocative test induced neurological deficit in six patients; the positive result of the test led the authors to abort the procedure in four cases, whereas the advancement of the catheter tip more distally allowed them to proceed with embolization in the remaining

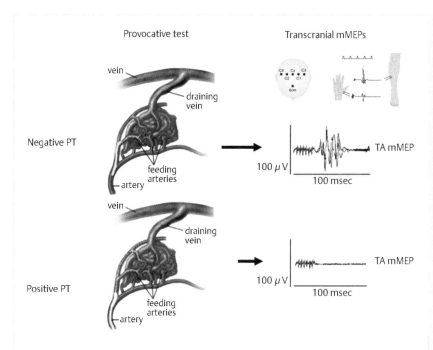

Fig. 10.3 Pharmacological provocative test (PT) during endovascular embolization for brain AVMs. A schematic illustration of a brain AVM is presented (left-hand panels) together with the result of the provocative test (right panels). Negative PT. Left-hand upper panel: The microcatheter (*in yellow*) is advanced into a feeder of the AVM nidus. Before the embolization, a pharmacological provocative test with either amytal and/or lidocaine is performed. If the microcatheter is selectively advanced into an artery feeding only the nidus and not eloquent cortex or subcortical white matter tracts, the drug (*green dots*) will diffuse only into the AVM and no changes in the evoked potentials (either SSEPs or MEPs) will occur. Accordingly, mMEPs are unchanged (right-hand upper panel). Positive PT. Left-hand lower panel: The microcatheter (*in yellow*) is not superselectively advanced into a feeder of the AVM nidus. In this situation, the drug (*green dots*) will diffuse not only into the AVM but also to either eloquent cortex or subcortical white matter tracts. Accordingly, either SSEPs and/or MEPs changes will occur (right lower panel).

two patients. Despite passing the provocative test, one patient developed a permanent visual deficit few hours after the endovascular procedure. No other patient presented alteration of the visual field after the procedure.

Endovascular management of AVMs may often require general anesthesia, either because the patient is not collaborative (e.g., pediatric patients) or because of operator preference. In such a situation, clinical examination is not possible and the only way to assess functional integrity of the sensory and motor pathways is IONM unless a wake-up test is performed. Under these circumstances, the combination of provocative tests and IONM can be used to predict the effect of embolization (▶ Fig. 10.3). Besides the use of Amytal, which selectively blocks the gray matter, a local anesthetic such as lidocaine is used to selectively blocks the white matter.[72] Thus, the combination of these two provocative agents allows testing both neuronal and axonal transmission, and its use has been well documented during endovascular procedures for spinal cord AVMs, while there is limited experience for brain AVMs.[73] A positive provocative test is usually considered as a 50% decrease of SSEP amplitude and/or MEP disappearance. A positive test indicates that the vessel distal to the microcatheter is functionally relevant and cannot be embolized. Whenever a provocative test is positive, embolization is not performed from that specific catheter position. Instead, superselective catheterization or embolization through a different feeder are preferred. If the test is negative (no IONM changes), embolization can proceed. This strategy (evoked potentials and provocative tests) has proved to be very sensitive: almost invariably, patients with negative provocative tests followed by embolization have a good outcome without new neurological deficits.[74] Unfortunately, the specificity of this technique has not been tested given that embolization is considered too risky in case of positive provocative tests.

We have combined IONM and pharmacological provocative tests during embolization of brain AVMs.[74] Overall, 11 patients

with cerebral AVMs (3 prerolandic, 6 rolandic, and 2 postrolandic AVMs) underwent 21 embolization procedure. Superselective injection of lidocaine resulted in either MEPs and/or SSEPs drop in 9 of 58 catheterized feeders with an overall incidence of positive provocative tests of 15.5%. No embolization was performed from that specific catheter position and either a more selective catheterization or embolization from a different feeder was used. Conversely, in the 49 AVM feeders where the provocative tests were negative, embolization proceeded and no patients showed changes of MEPs and SSEP during embolization. Among the patients with negative provocative tests, three showed mild and transient sensory-motor deficits after embolization: lower limb paresthesia in one case, facial weakness in another case, and arm paresthesia and weakness in the last one, all with complete resolution within one week. No instances of severe transient or permanent treatment-related morbidity were observed (▶ Fig. 10.4 and ▶ Fig. 10.5).

Li et al reported two cases of cerebral AVMs embolized under TIVA and IONM with SSEP, MEP, and EEG.[75] The first case was a parieto-occipital AVM that was fed mainly by the right posterior cerebral artery (PCA); the provocative test resulted in loss of left lower extremity MEPs, but no change in SSEP or EEG and the procedure was finally aborted. The other case was a left frontoparietal AVM that was fed mainly by M4 branches of left MCA; the provocative test was done in the two M4 branches (superior and inferior) and the superior one produced complete loss of MEP in the right hand. Finally, only the inferior branch was embolized.

10.5 Unanswered Questions and Future Directions

What is not extensively addressed in the literature is the temporal correlation between the onset of IONM changes and the

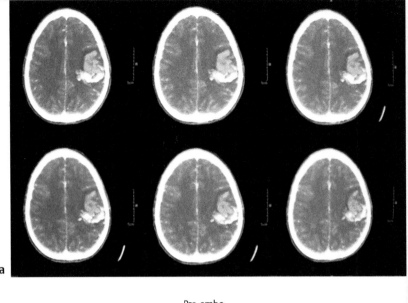

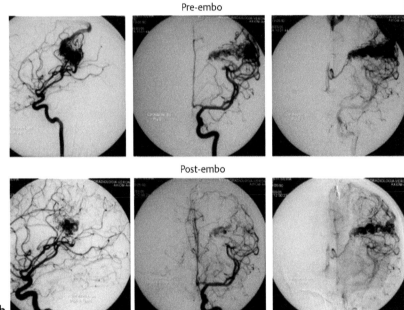

Pre-embo

Post-embo

Fig. 10.4 (a) Brain CT scan of a 12-year-old right-handed girl who was admitted for headache and right moderate hemiparesis following bleeding of a rolandic AVM. (b) Pre- (upper panels) and postembolization (lower panels) angiogram of the AVM. From left to right: laterolateral, early anteroposterior, and late anteroposterior phase of the DSA (*continued*).

risk of developing postoperative neurological deficits, and most of the available data are related to temporary clipping during aneurysm rather than during AVM surgery.

Mizoi and Yoshimoto[76] reported that postoperative sequelae do not occur if flow is reestablished within 10 minutes after SSEP attenuation. In this study, the shortest temporary occlusion time with resulting new deficit was 6 minutes. SSEP disappeared during temporary occlusion in 42 of 97 patients and in all but three it eventually returned to baseline after recirculation, with no sequelae. On average, SSEPs disappear 8.6 minutes after occlusion. The three patients in whom SSEP did not recover after recirculation experienced all neurological sequelae. In another study on 76 patients undergoing aneurysm surgery by Schick et al,[7] the sensitivity of SSEPs in determining permanent neurological deficits was 57% and the specificity

88%. The extent of recovery of SSEPs and the duration of SSEP changes strongly correlated with postoperative deficits. With regard to MEPs, Szelényi et al[14] reported that temporary clipping was performed more often and it was of longer duration in patients with MEP changes (11.8 vs. 5 minutes). Overall, the disappearance of MEPs for more than 10 minutes was likely to be followed by a postoperative motor deficit. In Horiuchi et al's study,[4] the interval between surgical maneuvers which could have induced MEP changes and the actual changes ranged between 20 seconds and 7 minutes and between 2 to 6 minutes for SSEPs. So, MEP changes tend to occur earlier than SSEP changes.

The relationship between duration of temporary clipping and neurophysiological changes, as well as the relationship between duration of IONM changes and outcome, needs to be further

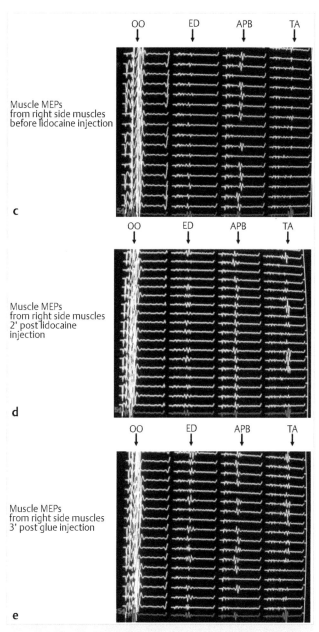

Muscle MEPs
from right side muscles
before lidocaine injection

c

Muscle MEPs
from right side muscles
2' post lidocaine
injection

d

Muscle MEPs
from right side muscles
3' post glue injection

e

Fig. 10.4 (*continued*) **(c–e)** Screenshots from muscle MEP monitoring during the provocative test. Recording from the following muscles are shown: orbicularis oris (OO), extensor digitorum (ED), abductor pollicis brevis (APB), tibialis anterior (TA). **(c)** Before lidocaine injection, all muscle responses are present. **(d)** No changes in the mMEPs occurred 2 minutes following lidocaine injection. The provocative test is therefore considered "negative" and embolization can proceed. **(e)** Glue is therefore injected and, again, no changes in mMEPs occurred. The patient woke up with no additional neurologic deficit. The AVM nidus was significantly reduced **(b)** and the patient was then sent for radiosurgery with Gamma Knife.

elucidated by future studies. These will be of paramount importance to understand how long IONM changes can be tolerated before ischemia progresses to infarction.

10.6 Conclusion

IONM is a valuable tool during surgical resection of sensorimotor, deep, and occipital AVMs. The continuous feedback provided by IONM helps the surgeon during both steps of feeders cauterization and nidus dissection. Furthermore, IONM helps in defining the location of primary sensorimotor cortex in cases of AVM located in such areas.

The role of awake surgery in AVM management is controversial and scarcely reported in the literature. In fact, the length of the surgical procedure and its technically demanding nature often limit the feasibility of awake craniotomies in AVMs localized in the speech area. The use of fMRI, MEG, and tractography can be helpful in the management of such lesions.

Provocative test during embolization of AVMs is a reliable test which allows real-time evaluation of the feeders, preventing the need of awake embolization procedure that can be troublesome, especially in young patients.

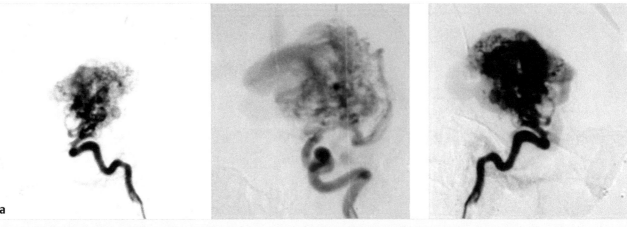

Fig. 10.5 (a) Preembolization DSA of a 30-year-old right-handed woman with a left basal ganglia AVM (*continued*).

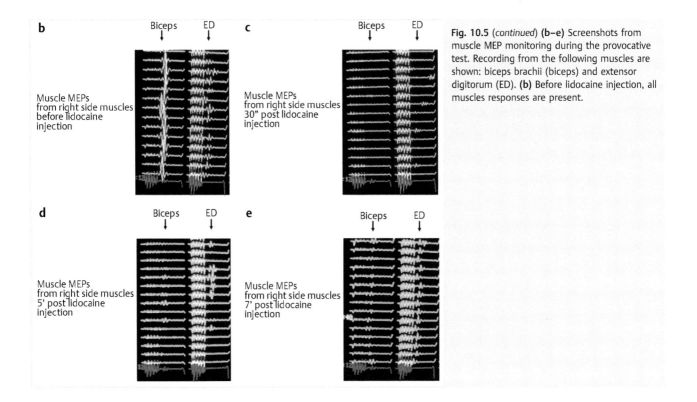

Fig. 10.5 (*continued*) **(b–e)** Screenshots from muscle MEP monitoring during the provocative test. Recording from the following muscles are shown: biceps brachii (biceps) and extensor digitorum (ED). **(b)** Before lidocaine injection, all muscles responses are present.

References

[1] Charbel FT, Hoffman WE, Misra M, Ostergren L. Ultrasonic perivascular flow probe: technique and application in neurosurgery. Neurol Res. 1998; 20(5): 439–442

[2] Friedman WA, Kaplan BL, Day AL, Sypert GW, Curran MT. Evoked potential monitoring during aneurysm operation: observations after fifty cases. Neurosurgery. 1987; 20(5):678–687

[3] Holland NR. Subcortical strokes from intracranial aneurysm surgery: implications for intraoperative neuromonitoring. J Clin Neurophysiol. 1998; 15(5): 439–446

[4] Horiuchi K, Suzuki K, Sasaki T, et al. Intraoperative monitoring of blood flow insufficiency during surgery of middle cerebral artery aneurysms. J Neurosurg. 2005; 103(2):275–283

[5] Lopéz JR, Chang SD, Steinberg GK. The use of electrophysiological monitoring in the intraoperative management of intracranial aneurysms. J Neurol Neurosurg Psychiatry. 1999; 66(2):189–196

[6] Neuloh G, Pechstein U, Cedzich C, Schramm J. Motor evoked potential monitoring with supratentorial surgery. Neurosurgery. 2004; 54(5):1061–1070, discussion 1070–1072

[7] Schick U, Döhnert J, Meyer JJ, Vitzthum HE. Effects of temporary clips on somatosensory evoked potentials in aneurysm surgery. Neurocrit Care. 2005; 2 (2):141–149

[8] Suzuki K, Kodama N, Sasaki T, et al. Intraoperative monitoring of blood flow insufficiency in the anterior choroidal artery during aneurysm surgery. J Neurosurg. 2003; 98(3):507–514

[9] Szelényi A, Kothbauer K, de Camargo AB, Langer D, Flamm ES, Deletis V. Motor evoked potential monitoring during cerebral aneurysm surgery: technical aspects and comparison of transcranial and direct cortical stimulation. Neurosurgery. 2005; 57(4) Suppl:331–338, discussion 331–338

[10] Symon L, Wang AD, Costa e Silva IE, Gentili F. Perioperative use of somatosensory evoked responses in aneurysm surgery. J Neurosurg. 1984; 60(2):269–275

[11] Schramm J, Koht A, Schmidt G, Pechstein U, Taniguchi M, Fahlbusch R. Surgical and electrophysiological observations during clipping of 134

aneurysms with evoked potential monitoring. Neurosurgery. 1990; 26(1): 61–70

[12] Chang SD, Lopez JR, Steinberg GK. The usefulness of electrophysiological monitoring during resection of central nervous system vascular malformations. J Stroke Cerebrovasc Dis. 1999; 8(6):412–422

[13] Quiñones-Hinojosa A, Alam M, Lyon R, Yingling CD, Lawton MT. Transcranial motor evoked potentials during basilar artery aneurysm surgery: technique application for 30 consecutive patients. Neurosurgery. 2004; 54(4):916–924, discussion 924

[14] Szelényi A, Langer D, Kothbauer K, De Camargo AB, Flamm ES, Deletis V. Monitoring of muscle motor evoked potentials during cerebral aneurysm surgery: intraoperative changes and postoperative outcome. J Neurosurg. 2006; 105 (5):675–681

[15] Penfield W, Boldrey E. Somatic motor and sensory representation in the cerebral cortex of man as studied by electrical stimulation. Brain. 1937; 60: 389–443

[16] Berger MS. Surgery of low-grade gliomas–technical aspects. Clin Neurosurg. 1997; 44:161–180

[17] Berger MS. Techniques for functional brain mapping during glioma surgery. In: Berger MS, Wilson CB, eds. The Gliomas. Philadelphia, PA: Saunders; 1999:421–435

[18] Yingling CD, Ojemann S, Dodson B, Harrington MJ, Berger MS. Identification of motor pathways during tumor surgery facilitated by multichannel electromyographic recording. J Neurosurg. 1999; 91(6):922–927

[19] Sartorius CJ, Berger MS. Rapid termination of intraoperative stimulation-evoked seizures with application of cold Ringer's lactate to the cortex. Technical note. J Neurosurg. 1998; 88(2):349–351

[20] Szelényi A, Joksimovic B, Seifert V. Intraoperative risk of seizures associated with transient direct cortical stimulation in patients with symptomatic epilepsy. J Clin Neurophysiol. 2007; 24(1):39–43

[21] Sala F, Manganotti P, Grossauer S, Tramontano V, Mazza C, Gerosa M. Intraoperative neurophysiology of the motor system in children: a tailored approach. Childs Nerv Syst. 2010; 26(4):473–490

[22] Taniguchi M, Cedzich C, Schramm J. Modification of cortical stimulation for motor evoked potentials under general anesthesia: technical description. Neurosurgery. 1993; 32(2):219–226

[23] Pechstein U, Cedzich C, Nadstawek J, Schramm J. Transcranial high-frequency repetitive electrical stimulation for recording myogenic motor evoked potentials with the patient under general anesthesia. Neurosurgery. 1996; 39(2): 335–343, discussion 343–344

[24] Pouratian N, Cannestra AF, Bookheimer SY, Martin NA, Toga AW. Variability of intraoperative electrocortical stimulation mapping parameters across and within individuals. J Neurosurg. 2004; 101(3):458–466

[25] Jankowska E, Padel Y, Tanaka R. Projections of pyramidal tract cells to alpha-motoneurones innervating hind-limb muscles in the monkey. J Physiol. 1975; 249(3):637–667

[26] Szelényi A, Senft C, Jardan M, et al. Intra-operative subcortical electrical stimulation: a comparison of two methods. Clin Neurophysiol. 2011; 122(7): 1470–1475

[27] Nossek E, Korn A, Shahar T, et al. Intraoperative mapping and monitoring of the corticospinal tracts with neurophysiological assessment and 3-dimensional ultrasonography-based navigation. Clinical article. J Neurosurg. 2011; 114(3):738–746

[28] Ohue S, Kohno S, Inoue A, et al. Accuracy of diffusion tensor magnetic resonance imaging-based tractography for surgery of gliomas near the pyramidal tract: a significant correlation between subcortical electrical stimulation and postoperative tractography. Neurosurgery. 2012; 70(2):283–293, discussion 294

[29] Seidel K, Beck J, Stieglitz L, Schucht P, Raabe A. The warning-sign hierarchy between quantitative subcortical motor mapping and continuous motor evoked potential monitoring during resection of supratentorial brain tumors. J Neurosurg. 2013; 118(2):287–296

[30] Cedzich C, Taniguchi M, Schäfer S, Schramm J. Somatosensory evoked potential phase reversal and direct motor cortex stimulation during surgery in and around the central region. Neurosurgery. 1996; 38(5):962–970

[31] Romstöck J, Fahlbusch R, Ganslandt O, Nimsky C, Strauss C. Localisation of the sensorimotor cortex during surgery for brain tumours: feasibility and waveform patterns of somatosensory evoked potentials. J Neurol Neurosurg Psychiatry. 2002; 72(2):221–229

[32] Journée HL, Polak HE, de Kleuver M. Influence of electrode impedance on threshold voltage for transcranial electrical stimulation in motor evoked potential monitoring. Med Biol Eng Comput. 2004; 42(4):557–561

[33] Ringel F, Sala F. Intraoperative mapping and monitoring in supratentorial tumor surgery. J Neurosurg Sci. 2015; 59(2):129–139

[34] Krieg SM, Schäffner M, Shiban E, et al. Reliability of intraoperative neurophysiological monitoring using motor evoked potentials during resection of metastases in motor-eloquent brain regions: clinical article. J Neurosurg. 2013; 118(6):1269–1278

[35] Szelényi A, Hattingen E, Weidauer S, Seifert V, Ziemann U. Intraoperative motor evoked potential alteration in intracranial tumor surgery and its relation to signal alteration in postoperative magnetic resonance imaging. Neurosurgery. 2010; 67(2):302–313

[36] MacDonald DB. Safety of intraoperative transcranial electrical stimulation motor evoked potential monitoring. J Clin Neurophysiol. 2002; 19(5):416–429

[37] Rothwell JC, Thompson PD, Day BL, Boyd S, Marsden CD. Stimulation of the human motor cortex through the scalp. Exp Physiol. 1991; 76(2):159–200

[38] Kodama K, Goto T, Sato A, Sakai K, Tanaka Y, Hongo K. Standard and limitation of intraoperative monitoring of the visual evoked potential. Acta Neurochir (Wien). 2010; 152(4):643–648

[39] Ojemann G, Ojemann J, Lettich E, Berger M. Cortical language localization in left, dominant hemisphere. An electrical stimulation mapping investigation in 117 patients. 1989. J Neurosurg. 2008; 108(2):411–421

[40] Sala F, Coppola A, Tramontano V, Babini M, Pinna G. Intraoperative neurophysiological monitoring for the resection of brain tumors in pediatric patients. J Neurosurg Sci. 2015; 59(4):373–382

[41] Korn ACS. Intraoperative neurophysiological monitoring and mapping in pediatric supratentorial surgery. Childs Nerv Syst. 2010; 26:545

[42] Pietilä TA, Stendel R, Jansons J, Schilling A, Koch HC, Brock M. The value of intraoperative angiography for surgical treatment of cerebral arteriovenous malformations in eloquent brain areas. Acta Neurochir (Wien). 1998; 140 (11):1161–1165

[43] Takagi Y, Kikuta K, Nozaki K, Sawamura K, Hashimoto N. Detection of a residual nidus by surgical microscope-integrated intraoperative near-infrared indocyanine green videoangiography in a child with a cerebral arteriovenous malformation. J Neurosurg. 2007; 107(5) Suppl:416–418

[44] Ichikawa T, Suzuki K, Sasaki T, et al. Utility and the limit of motor evoked potential monitoring for preventing complications in surgery for cerebral arteriovenous malformation. Neurosurgery. 2010; 67(3) Suppl Operative: ons222–ons228, discussion ons228

[45] Wright JE, Arden G, Jones BR. Continuous monitoring of the visually evoked response during intra-orbital surgery. Trans Ophthalmol Soc U K. 1973; 93 (0):311–314

[46] Cedzich C, Schramm J, Fahlbusch R. Are flash-evoked visual potentials useful for intraoperative monitoring of visual pathway function? Neurosurgery. 1987; 21(5):709–715

[47] Wiedemayer H, Fauser B, Armbruster W, Gasser T, Stolke D. Visual evoked potentials for intraoperative neurophysiologic monitoring using total intravenous anesthesia. J Neurosurg Anesthesiol. 2003; 15(1):19–24

[48] Wiedemayer H, Fauser B, Sandalcioglu IE, Armbruster W, Stolke D. Observations on intraoperative monitoring of visual pathways using steady-state visual evoked potentials. Eur J Anaesthesiol. 2004; 21(6):429–433

[49] Sasaki T, Itakura T, Suzuki K, et al. Intraoperative monitoring of visual evoked potential: introduction of a clinically useful method. J Neurosurg. 2010; 112 (2):273–284

[50] San-Juan D, de Dios Del Castillo Calcáneo J, Villegas TG, Elizondo DL, Torrontegui JA, Anschel DJ. Visual intraoperative monitoring of occipital arteriovenous malformation surgery. Clin Neurol Neurosurg. 2011; 113(8):680–682

[51] Kombos T, Pietilä T, Kern BC, Kopetsch O, Brock M. Demonstration of cerebral plasticity by intra-operative neurophysiological monitoring: report of an uncommon case. Acta Neurochir (Wien). 1999; 141(8):885–889

[52] Gamble AJ, Schaffer SG, Nardi DJ, Chalif DJ, Katz J, Dehdashti AR. Awake Craniotomy in Arteriovenous Malformation Surgery: The Usefulness of Cortical and Subcortical Mapping of Language Function in Selected Patients. World Neurosurg. 2015; 84(5):1394–1401

[53] Gabarrós A, Young WL, McDermott MW, Lawton MT. Language and motor mapping during resection of brain arteriovenous malformations: indications, feasibility, and utility. Neurosurgery. 2011; 68(3):744–752

[54] Kronenburg A, van Doormaal T, van Eijsden P, van der Zwan A, Leijten F, Han KS. Surgery for a giant arteriovenous malformation without motor deterioration: preoperative transcranial magnetic stimulation in a non-cooperative patient. J Neurosurg Pediatr. 2014; 14(1):38–42

[55] Kato N, Schilt S, Schneider H, et al. Functional brain mapping of patients with arteriovenous malformations using navigated transcranial magnetic

stimulation: first experience in ten patients. Acta Neurochir (Wien). 2014; 156(5):885–895

[56] Juenger H, Ressel V, Braun C, et al. Misleading functional magnetic resonance imaging mapping of the cortical hand representation in a 4-year-old boy with an arteriovenous malformation of the central region. J Neurosurg Pediatr. 2009; 4(4):333–338

[57] Ozdoba C, Nirkko AC, Remonda L, Lövblad KO, Schroth G. Whole-brain functional magnetic resonance imaging of cerebral arteriovenous malformations involving the motor pathways. Neuroradiology. 2002; 44 (1):1–10

[58] Lehéricy S, Biondi A, Sourour N, et al. Arteriovenous brain malformations: is functional MR imaging reliable for studying language reorganization in patients? Initial observations. Radiology. 2002; 223(3):672–682

[59] Cannestra AF, Pouratian N, Forage J, Bookheimer SY, Martin NA, Toga AW. Functional magnetic resonance imaging and optical imaging for dominant-hemisphere perisylvian arteriovenous malformations. Neurosurgery. 2004; 55(4):804–812, discussion 812–814

[60] Kikuta K, Takagi Y, Nozaki K, Hashimoto N. Introduction to tractography-guided navigation: using 3-tesla magnetic resonance tractography in surgery for cerebral arteriovenous malformations. Acta Neurochir Suppl (Wien). 2008; 103:11–14

[61] Ellis MJ, Rutka JT, Kulkarni AV, Dirks PB, Widjaja E. Corticospinal tract mapping in children with ruptured arteriovenous malformations using functionally guided diffusion-tensor imaging. J Neurosurg Pediatr. 2012; 9(5): 505–510

[62] Natarajan SK, Ghodke B, Britz GW, Born DE, Sekhar LN. Multimodality treatment of brain arteriovenous malformations with microsurgery after embolization with onyx: single-center experience and technical nuances. Neurosurgery. 2008; 62(6):1213–1225, discussion 1225–1226

[63] Pasqualin A, Zampieri P, Nicolato A, Meneghelli P, Cozzi F, Beltramello A. Surgery after embolization of cerebral arterio-venous malformation: experience of 123 cases. Acta Neurochir Suppl (Wien). 2014; 119:105–111

[64] Moon K, Levitt MR, Almefty RO, et al. Safety and efficacy of surgical resection of unruptured low-grade arteriovenous malformations from the modern decade. Neurosurgery. 2015; 77(6):948–952, discussion 952–953

[65] Crowley RW, Ducruet AF, Kalani MY, Kim LJ, Albuquerque FC, McDougall CG. Neurological morbidity and mortality associated with the endovascular treatment of cerebral arteriovenous malformations before and during the Onyx era. J Neurosurg. 2015; 122(6):1492–1497

[66] Rauch RA, Vinuela F, Dion J, et al. Preembolization functional evaluation in brain arteriovenous malformations: the ability of superselective Amytal test to predict neurologic dysfunction before embolization. AJNR Am J Neuroradiol. 1992; 13(1):309–314

[67] Rauch RA, Vinuela F, Dion J, et al. Preembolization functional evaluation in brain arteriovenous malformations: the superselective Amytal test. AJNR Am J Neuroradiol. 1992; 13(1):303–308

[68] Paiva T, Campos J, Baeta E, Gomes LB, Martins IP, Parreira E. EEG monitoring during endovascular embolization of cerebral arteriovenous malformations. Electroencephalogr Clin Neurophysiol. 1995; 95(1):3–13

[69] Paulsen RD, Steinberg GK, Norbash AM, Marcellus ML, Lopez JR, Marks MP. Embolization of rolandic cortex arteriovenous malformations. Neurosurgery. 1999; 44(3):479–484, discussion 484–486

[70] Moo LR, Murphy KJ, Gailloud P, Tesoro M, Hart J. Tailored cognitive testing with provocative amobarbital injection preceding AVM embolization. AJNR Am J Neuroradiol. 2002; 23(3):416–421

[71] Tawk RG, Tummala RP, Memon MZ, Siddiqui AH, Hopkins LN, Levy EI. Utility of pharmacologic provocative neurological testing before embolization of occipital lobe arteriovenous malformations. World Neurosurg. 2011; 76(3–4):276–281

[72] Tanaka K, Yamasaki M. Blocking of cortical inhibitory synapses by intravenous lidocaine. Nature. 1966; 209(5019):207–208

[73] Sala FNY. Neurophysiological monitoring during endovascular procedures on the spine and the spinal cord. In: Deletis VSJ, ed. Neurophysiology in Neurosurgery: A Modern Intraoperative Approach. San Diego, CA: Acedamic Press; 2002:119–151

[74] Sala F, Beltramello A, Gerosa M. Neuroprotective role of neurophysiological monitoring during endovascular procedures in the brain and spinal cord. Neurophysiol Clin. 2007; 37(6):415–421

[75] Li F, Deshaies E, Allott G, Gorji R. Transcranial motor evoked potential changes induced by provocative testing during embolization of cerebral arteriovenous malformations in patients under total intravenous anesthesia. Am J Electroneurodiagn Technol. 2011; 51(4):264–273

[76] Mizoi K, Yoshimoto T. Permissible temporary occlusion time in aneurysm surgery as evaluated by evoked potential monitoring. Neurosurgery. 1993; 33 (3):434–440, discussion 440

11 Critical Care and Neuroanesthetic Considerations for Arteriovenous Malformation and Arteriovenous Fistula Surgery

Joseph Lockwood, Peter S. Amenta, Ricky Medel, and Aimee M. Aysenne

Abstract

Critical care and anesthetic management are essential components of a multidisciplinary approach to the treatment of arteriovenous malformations (AVMs). Presenting symptoms of AVMs include hemorrhage, seizure, headache, and focal neurological deficits and will predict the most important first steps. Hemorrhage is the most common presenting event and requires cautious and rapid blood pressure control. Timing of surgical correction is debatable, with risk and benefits to both ultra-early resection and delayed treatment after rupture. Seizures are the most common presenting symptoms in unruptured AVMs and are treated with standard antiepileptic medications. While AVMs are a rare cause of headaches, most patients with AVMs have headaches. The least common presenting symptom is focal neurologic deficit. During open or endovascular repair, optimal control of blood pressure, intracranial pressure, ventilation, and oxygenation and monitoring are critical for the prevention of secondary brain injury, and assist the surgeon to optimize outcomes for these patients. Because of abnormal vasculature, cerebral tissues around the AVM are often underperfused and are at risk of further ischemia in the setting of hypotension. Many anesthetics including inhaled medications can increase intracranial pressure and should be avoided. Additional brain relaxation can be accomplished with hyperosmotic therapy. Intraoperative monitoring with neurophysiologists can be complementary to anesthetic and surgical planning; short-acting paralytic agents are preferred if neuromonitoring will be utilized. Occasionally, awake craniotomies can be performed to preserve eloquent areas in appropriately selected patients. With careful alignment of the management of medical and surgical care, superior patient care can be achieved.

Keywords: critical care, anesthesia, hemorrhage, ischemia, intracranial hypertension, seizure, neuromonitoring, ruptured arteriovenous malformation

- Common clinical presentations of arteriovenous malformations include hemorrhage, seizures, headaches, and focal neurological deficits.
- Acute medical therapy of arteriovenous malformations and arteriovenous fistulas is critical in multidisciplinary care of patients harboring these lesions in the neurointensive care unit, particularly for patients presenting with hemorrhage but also for patients undergoing surgical and/or endovascular interventions.
- Anesthesia is crucial for successful execution of surgical and endovascular procedures for arteriovenous malformations and arteriovenous fistulas.

11.1 Introduction

While the goals of surgical and endovascular techniques are to maximize neurological function and minimize disability and death caused by arteriovenous malformations (AVMs), the medical and anesthetic management of these patients is critical to the concurrent care while in the operating room or endovascular suite and throughout their hospital course. Cerebral AVMs can present with several distinct clinical scenarios dictating the most urgent concern, often prior to surgical or endovascular procedures, and influencing the next steps of care. The most common initial clinical presentation is hemorrhage. Over 50% of the presentations involve rupture and hemorrhage. Another 30% present with seizures.[1] Less commonly, patients can present with headaches or focal neurologic deficits. Due to more frequent imaging, currently approximately 1.2% of AVMs are asymptomatic incidental radiographic findings.[2] Patients will most commonly present between the ages of 20 and 39 years, but it is not uncommon to present in the second or fifth decades of life.[3] The location of the lesion influences clinical presentation. Most AVMs are located in lobar areas of the cerebrum, with an even distribution among AVMs found in the frontal, parietal, occipital, and temporal lobes.[4] Less commonly, AVMs are located in deep brain or infratentorially. During procedures, caution must be used to prevent rapid changes in blood flow or intracranial pressure (ICP) from medication administered from anesthesia colleagues.

11.2 Materials and Methods

Materials used in this chapter were based on literature searches from PubMed with the focus on cerebral AVMs with supplementation from literature reviews for anesthetic and medial management. Images are taken from the clinical experiences of the authors.

11.3 Presenting Symptom

11.3.1 Hemorrhage

The overall reported risk for rupture of a cerebral AVM is 2 to 4% per year. While the natural history of AVMs can vary greatly, the overarching goal of treatment is to prevent rupture and hemorrhage while minimizing risks of other complications. Lesions that present with hemorrhage have the highest risk of future hemorrhage, especially in the first year. Additionally, the risk for second hemorrhage in the first year after a rupture is between 6 and 15%, and is suspected to be higher than quoted in previous studies.[5] AVMs with a larger nidus, greater than 5 cm, are most likely to rupture, but AVMs with a smaller nidus (< 3 cm) are more likely to present initially as a hemorrhage.

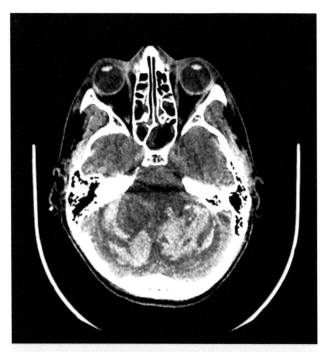

Fig. 11.1 Noncontrasted head CT. 14-year-old male who presented with coma from cerebellar AVM hemorrhage.

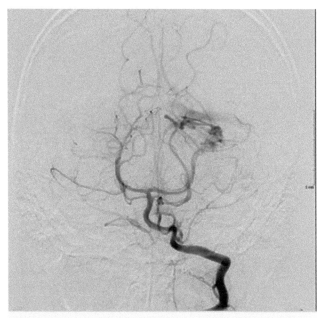

Fig. 11.2 Angiography. 14-year-old male who presented with coma from cerebellar AVM hemorrhage.

Smaller AVMs are less likely to cause other symptoms such as seizures, headaches, and neurological deficits before hemorrhage.[1] Other significant risk factors for rupture include deep or infratentorial location, exclusively deep venous drainage, and associated aneurysms.[5] ▶ Fig. 11.1 is an example of an AVM presenting as a cerebellar hemorrhage on noncontrasted head computed tomography (CT) in a 14-year-old who presented with acute loss of consciousness. ▶ Fig. 11.2 represents his cerebral angiogram.

Intracerebral hemorrhages (ICHs) caused by AVMs have better prognosis for recovery than spontaneous ICHs, with over a 20-fold decrease in mortality for hemorrhages caused by AVM rupture.[6] This highlights the prognostic importance of appropriate imaging used to identify the underlying cause of the hemorrhage before prognosticating for neurologic outcome. Bleeding patterns and patient demographics can also be important in outcome and should be considered in discussions with patients and families. Some studies have shown that parenchymal bleeding appears to be associated with a lower Glasgow Coma Score (GCS) on presentation; however, nonparenchymal hemorrhages, especially basal cistern subarachnoid hemorrhage (SAH), are associated with worse overall outcomes in patients.[7] Other studies have found parenchymal bleeding to be associated with unfavorable outcomes, along with higher patient age and patients who undergo hematoma evacuation.[8] The ICH score is used to predict outcomes in patient functionality and mortality for nontraumatic ICH. Components include GCS on presentation, ICH volume, presence of intraventricular hemorrhage (IVH), supratentorial or infratentorial location, and age of the patient. It is also accurate in predicting functional outcomes for risk stratification in patients with ICH due to a ruptured AVM, but is less reliable predicting mortality because ICHs due to AVM rupture have a much lower risk of death than other types of spontaneous ICHs.[9]

The timing of interventional treatments after hemorrhage can play an important role in critical care decisions. The most common neurosurgical interventions include microsurgical resection, embolization, and stereotactic radiosurgery. In conservatively treated ruptured AVMs, there are a significant number of patients who suffer an early rerupture within the first few weeks. Perinidal and perihematomal edema on follow-up imaging 2 weeks after rupture indicates a higher risk for early rebleed and should be treated more aggressively.[10] Periprocedural rupture rates after endovascular occlusion of the AVM have been reported to be between 4 and 16%.[11] It is important to closely monitor the neurological exam post embolization and obtain prompt imaging with significant changes. Periprocedural bleeding after endovascular occlusion should especially be considered if the patient has an intranidal aneurysm or draining vein occlusion or if any complications were reported during the procedure.[11]

About 25% of patients with cerebral AVMs also have a cerebral arterial aneurysm, with the majority occurring in the feeding artery of the AVM, and the rest either intranidal or not closely associated with the AVM.[12] There is a significantly elevated risk of hemorrhage with associated aneurysms, especially in aneurysms greater than 5 mm in diameter.[13] While most patients present with ICH or IVH, patients with feeding artery aneurysms are also at risk of SAH and subsequent complications associated with it.[12]

Medical management of ruptured AVMs is best implemented with a multidisciplinary team including neurosurgical, neurointerventional, and neurocritical care teams. Initial diagnostic testing should include basic medical work-up with complete blood counts, prothrombin time, partial thromboplastin time, imaging, and accurate GCS and ICH scores.[14] Some patients may require intubation for failure to protect the airway during coma or seizure. Diagnostic evaluations begin with a noncontrast CT to initially evaluate the location and extent of any potential hemorrhage. Noninvasive vascular imaging such as CT angiography can be helpful to look for an underlying vascular malformation including AVMs, cavernous malformations, and aneurysms, to plan the next phase of treatment, or to identify active bleeding.[14] Magnetic resonance imaging (MRI) is also often obtained to help delineate lesion and hemorrhage location within the brain more accurately. Catheter cerebral angiography is the final diagnostic step and can be performed if the patient has stabilized and does not require emergent decompressive surgery. Digital subtraction angiography is the gold standard for identifying and classifying underlying vascular malformation.

There are limited data for the medical management for AVMs, as surgeries aimed at prevention of rebleeding, both open and endovascular, are treatments of choice; however, pathophysiology and treatment are based on studies in all ICH patients and expert opinion for management of acutely neurologically injured patients. Blood pressure management is crucial in patients with ICH from ruptured AVMs, as it is with ICH without underlying structural lesions. Evidence shows that when systolic blood pressure of less than 140 mm Hg is achieved and consistently controlled, patients have better functional outcomes and are safe, especially when kept between 130 and 139 mm Hg.[15] The titration of intravenous short-acting antihypertensives is recommended to reduce the risk of hypotension and blood pressure variability.[14] All anticoagulation and antiplatelet medications should be stopped and reversed if taken recently. Blood glucose should be kept below 185 g/dL, as continuously elevated blood glucose levels have been associated with worse outcomes.[16] Acute antiepileptic treatment is often started in the intensive care unit (ICU), especially in lobar and cortical hemorrhages, but has not been proven to change outcomes.[16] Continuous electroencephalography can help detect seizures including nonconvulsive status epilepticus in unresponsive patients.[17]

Unlike with a ruptured aneurysm, where most of the complications are attributable to hydrocephalus and less likely due to local mass effect from intraparenchymal hemorrhage, both are equally important to consider in the pathology of AVM rupture.[18] Perinidal edema and hematoma volume expansion can occur with ICH caused by ruptured AVMs. The surrounding edema is caused by a complex web including vasogenic edema from plasma protein extravasation and clot retraction, inflammatory cascades, and other factors.[19] Intracranial hypertension is managed with standard practices including osmotic therapy (hypertonic saline or mannitol), sedation, or decompressive surgery for more severe cases or for failed medical management.[20] Forty-four percent of patients with ruptured AVMs require early external ventricular drain (EVD) placement, with 18% becoming shunt dependent, requiring ventriculoperitoneal shunting.[18] Placement of external ventriculostomy is based on specific patient factors. Criteria often used to perform ventriculostomy include GCS < 9, evidence of herniation and/or increased ICP, significant IVH, or hydrocephalus.[21] IVH, low GCS scores, and the presence of an associated aneurysm are risk factors for both EVD placement and shunt dependence.[18]

While acute neurological decline due to mass effect is an indication for emergent surgery, current practice, often, is to perform AVM resection surgery electively, after a period of 1 to 4 weeks, to allow for patient recovery from the initial ictus and to allow swelling to subside and associated clot to liquefy.

Recommendations for emergent clot evacuation include a decreased level of consciousness due to ICH, a hematoma volume greater than 30 mL in the temporal lobe or posterior fossa, or a hematoma volume greater than 60 mL in the cerebral hemispheres.[17] Recently, some neurosurgeons performed early resection of lower grade AVMs over delayed treatment. One study showed a mortality of 7.4% for low-grade AVMs microsurgically resected within the first day compared to 23 to 29% from natural history data with delayed resection.[22] This technique may prevent "ultra-early" rebleeds, which occur within the first 24 hours of hemorrhage, the riskiest time in the first year after event.[22] The outcomes for early resection are best predicted by severity upon admission, and are less related to location, ICH size, and grade of the AVM.[23] This is discussed further in other chapters.

Postoperatively, patients are at risk of neurological changes because of edema and postoperative bleeding. The first and oldest of the two theories to explain such events is called normal perfusion pressure breakthrough. Theoretically, the parenchyma around the AVM is in a chronically hypoperfused state and, therefore, has decreased autoregulation of local blood flow compared to normal vessels.[24] When there is more blood flow, the vessels without the ability to autoregulate will rupture. A newer theory called occlusive hyperemia postulates that stagnant blood flow in former feeding arteries leads to hypoperfusion and ischemia in surrounding tissue; simultaneously, venous outflow of surrounding parenchyma is obstructed, leading to passive hyperemia.[24] Progressive ischemia and hyperemia combine for edema and postoperative bleeding. The true answer could lie on a spectrum between the two theories, with currently unknown factors involved. Another factor, discussed elsewhere, to explain postoperative hemorrhage is potential residual nidus. Most surgeons perform intraoperative angiography or immediate postoperative angiography to reduce any potential chance of residual nidus. Regardless, progressive edema and bleeding should be closely monitored after open resection and treated swiftly.

Vasospasm after AVM rupture is extremely rare, even with blood in the subarachnoid space. Multiple case reports have been published detailing delayed cerebral ischemia from angiographically confirmed vasospasm, especially in the presence of intraventricular blood.[25,26] Of the 20 cases of delayed ischemia from vasospasm in the literature, only 56% had SAH, but interestingly, all cases involved IVH.[27] Only 6.3% of patients with SAH from AVMs developed vasospasm detected on angiography compared to approximately 70% of aneurysmal SAH patients developing angiographically visible vasospasm.[27] Vasospasm should be considered in patients with delayed neurologic deficits after a ruptured AVM, especially in the setting of associated SAH or IVH.[25] Empiric delayed angiography to assess for vasospasm is probably unnecessary,[27] although treatment principles for delayed cerebral ischemia secondary to vasospasm in the setting of completely resected AVM (or secured AVM-associated aneurysm) would be analogous to those followed in the setting of aneurysmal SAH including induced hypertension, hypervolemia, and possibly endovascular therapy.

11.3.2 Seizures

Seizures are the most common presentation for unruptured AVMs. Most of these patients presenting with seizures harbor cortical

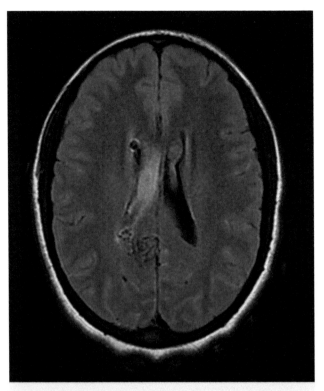

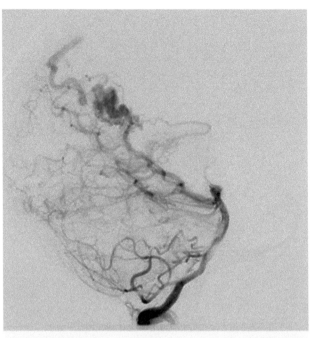

Fig. 11.4 Angiography. 17-year-old female who presented with seizure and headache due to cortical AVM and intraventricular rupture.

Fig. 11.3 T2 FLAIR MRI. 17-year-old female who presented with seizure and headache due to cortical AVM and intraventricular rupture.

AVMs. The locations have equal distribution with the exception of occipital AVMs, which have lower seizure rates. Larger nidus is a strong predictor of seizure presentation.[28] The exact etiology for the association of AVMs and seizures has not been completely determined, but several mechanisms have been proposed. These include neuronal destruction and degeneration, changes in glial structure and physiology, and formation of reactive oxygen species.[29] There has been no distinction of seizure semiology specifically associated with AVMs. ▶ Fig. 11.3 demonstrates a cortical AVM that presented with seizures on fluid-attenuated inversion recovery (FLAIR) sequence MRI. ▶ Fig. 11.4 represents the angiogram demonstrating the AVM.

Antiepileptic medications continue to be standard for patients with seizures due to AVMs. Seizures increase the metabolic demand of brain parenchyma and subsequently cerebral blood flow and ICP. Recurrent seizures and status epilepticus are especially important to treat in the ICU, as prolonged times of elevated ICPs increase the risk of rupture. Pharmacologically, seizures associated with AVMs are treated similarly to those from other pathologies, weighing the risks and benefits of each antiepileptic drug for the individual patient. Identifying AVMs and AVM rupture as the cause of initial seizure is important for ongoing management of the patient. Even smaller hemorrhages can cause seizures. In cases of drug-resistant epilepsy, video electroencephalogram and other newer imaging modalities can play an important role in localizing the symptomatic lesion. Interventional treatments including open resection and radiosurgery may reduce the incidence of posttreatment seizures in patients presenting with seizures.[30,31,32,33]

11.3.3 Headaches

Although not the most common cause of headaches, patients with unruptured cerebral AVMs commonly experience headaches. AVMs located in the occipital lobe carry the highest risk for headache and can be associated with visual disturbances.[34] A commonly proposed mechanism includes activation of the trigeminovascular system via elevated ICP, steal phenomenon, and spreading cortical depression.[35] There are no significant studies at this time on pharmacotherapies specific to headaches caused by cerebral AVMs. Medications for other types of headaches including antiepileptics such as topiramate and valproic acid, β-blockers such as propranolol, antidepressants including tricyclic antidepressants, and calcium channel blockers such as verapamil are frequently used for chronic headaches that these patients can experience. More than half of the patients with headaches that are caused by the cerebral AVM will have complete resolution or significant improvement after surgical resection.[35] ▶ Fig. 11.5 is a contrasted CT of a 34-year-old woman who presented with headache, nausea, and vomiting. ▶ Fig. 11.6 is her angiogram.

Radiologic evidence of cerebral edema is rare with unruptured cerebral AVMs, occurring in around 4% in most series. There appears to be a strong correlation with brain edema and venous congestion in unruptured AVMs. A cerebral AVM with associated edema should be considered to have an elevated risk of hemorrhage or nonhemorrhagic neurologic deficits, especially if there is evidence of venous congestion.[36] Treatment should be considered in such instances.

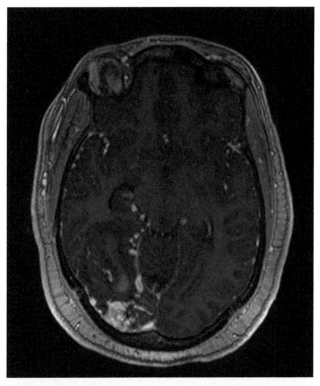

Fig. 11.5 Contrasted CT, 34-year-old woman who presented with headache, nausea, and vomiting.

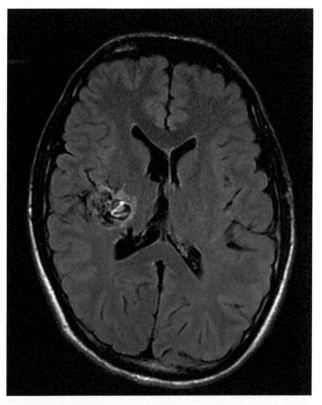

Fig. 11.7 T2 FLAIR MRI, 36-year-old man who presented with focal neurological deficit consisting of progressive left-side ataxia.

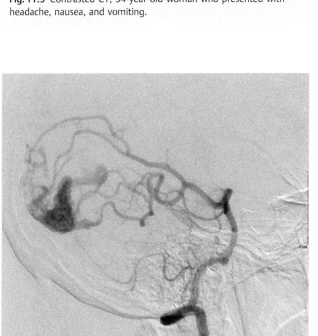

Fig. 11.6 Angiography, 34-year-old woman who presented with headache, nausea and vomiting.

11.3.4 Focal Neurologic Deficits

Neurologic deficits without hemorrhage represent fewer than 8% of patients with cerebral AVMs. The most common presenting deficit is hemiplegia and hemianopsia. Patients presenting with nonhemorrhagic neurological deficits tend to be female, have deep location of the AVM, with size larger than 3 cm, varices in venous drainage, and greater than three arterial feeders.[37] Many of the possible mechanisms previously discussed for symptomatic AVMs are proposed for the neurologic deficits, including steal phenomenon, mass effect, arterial hypotension, and venous hypertension. ▶ Fig. 11.7 shows T2 FLAIR MRI of a 36-year-old man who presented with focal neurological deficit consisting of progressive left side ataxia. ▶ Fig. 11.8 is his angiogram, which demonstrates a large nidus, varices, and multiple arterial feeders.

11.4 Anesthetic Considerations

Anesthetic management is critical in the successful treatment of patients harboring vascular malformations. Effective communication is essential between the surgical and anesthesia team as well as with other team members including neurophysiologists when neuromonitoring is used. The anesthetic plan will be different if an awake craniotomy, cortical mapping, or motor evoked potentials are to be performed, for instance. Important anesthetic considerations include blood pressure management, promotion of brain relaxation and management of ICP, anesthesia administration to allow intraoperative

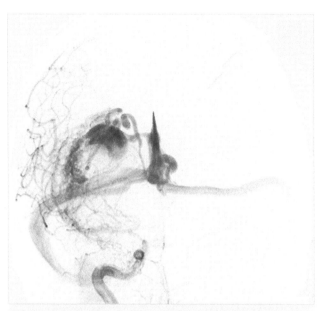

Fig. 11.8 Angiography, 36-year-old man who presented with focal neurological deficit consisting of progressive left-side ataxia.

neurophysiological monitoring and postoperative neurological examination (when appropriate), fluid and blood product management, and successful transition to the team providing postoperative care.

11.4.1 Blood Pressure Management

Cerebral AVMs have low resistance within their nidus, because of a lack of capillary beds. The surrounding parenchyma is chronically deprived of normal blood flow.[17] Perinidal capillaries lack gap junctions and are dilated, leading to a breakdown in the blood–brain barrier.[38] Cerebral blood flow is controlled by autoregulatory signals that keep mean arterial pressures (MAPs) between 50 and 150 mm Hg. In the condition of chronic hypoperfusion, the lower limit of the autoregulatory pressure range will drop below normal, and pressures below this limit can cause ischemia with even small drops in pressure.[39] These are lesions that require a watchful eye from the side of anesthesia. Many of the principles for a ruptured AVM surgery anesthesia management are the same for most craniotomies for spontaneous ICH. This section will highlight the important points and some of the special considerations for AVMs specifically.

While purposeful hypotension may be used in other types of intracranial surgeries to lessen the blood loss, this should be used with extreme caution in AVM resection. The shunt effect of the AVM causes constant arterial hypotension in the vascular supply of the surrounding normal brain tissue closest to the AVM. This hypotensive effect is even more profound as the size and number of arterial feeders grow. Rather than a loss of autoregulation in this chronically hypotensive territory, there is a shift to the left in the autoregulatory curve of cerebral blood flow where it can be maintained at a lower range of MAPs.[40] Although the lower limit of the autoregulatory curve is lower in the territories surrounding the AVM compared to normal tissue, a further drop in arterial pressure can cause the tissue to become ischemic.[39]

For many of the patients going to surgery for ruptured AVMs, intracranial hypertension can be of utmost concern. Intravenous agents may be better for induction than inhaled anesthetics, as inhaled anesthetics at higher concentrations can increase ICP and brain swelling.[39] Increases in ICP after ICH have been associated with elevated morbidity and mortality, so careful control in emergent cases is important.[16] Some drugs vasodilate cerebral vasculature, which elevates the ICP, and these should generally be avoided in elective AVM microsurgical resections. Preferred antihypertensives include nicardipine, labetalol, and esmolol. If the patient needs vasopressors, alpha agonists such as phenylephrine and norepinephrine are preferred because they do not alter cerebral blood flow.[39]

Given the prevalence of hypertension, it is important to consider the blood pressure control of chronically hypertensive patients with AVMs preoperatively and intraoperatively. In patients with chronic hypertension, the autoregulatory curve of cerebral blood pressure is shifted to the right. Lowering intraoperative blood pressures to decrease blood loss can drop below the level of autoregulation and cause ischemia. Conversely, the benefits of lowering the MAPs include reduced surgical bleeding, less hyperemia, and less chance of hyperperfusion syndrome.[39] Avoiding the extremes of both hypertension and hypotension in microsurgical AVM resections is crucial. To keep within their baseline pressures, patients should take their antihypertensive medications on the day of surgery (if elective). β-blockers and α2 agonists should especially be taken on the day of surgery, given that withdrawal can cause rebound hypertension.[39]

In general, patients are maintained in a normotensive state during induction and the resection stage of the procedure. It is important to avoid sudden, significant increases in blood pressure such as those that may occur in an inadequately anesthetized patient when the skull pins and fixation device are applied. Communication between the surgeon performing the pinning and the anesthesia team is important to avoid an abrupt spike in blood pressure, which could precipitate AVM rupture and intracranial hypertension.

11.4.2 Promotion of Brain Relaxation and Management of Intracranial Hypertension

Attention is paid to promoting brain relaxation and control of raised ICP during AVM surgery. Mannitol is typically administered as an osmotic diuretic (typically 0.5–1 g/kg intravenous). Positioning is undertaken to promote venous drainage (e.g., avoiding kinking of jugular venous outflow) and the head is typically raised above the heart with reverse Trendelenburg or the head of the bed raised. Additionally, mild hyperventilation is maintained during the early phases of surgery when necessary to promote brain relaxation. The anesthesia team is also in contact with the surgical team to drain cerebrospinal fluid when requested if an EVD or lumbar drain is in place. Collectively, such measures are designed to reduce ICP and promote a more relaxed surgical field.

11.4.3 Anesthetic Plan

Standard monitoring equipment is placed/utilized, including a pulse oximeter, temperature probe, Foley catheter, electrocardiography, oxygen sensor, end-tidal CO_2 monitor, and noninvasive blood pressure cuff. An arterial line is placed to closely monitor blood pressure and maintain blood pressure control within the desired range as well as to draw arterial samples including blood gases, blood counts, chemistries, and coagulation studies. Peripheral intravenous access is obtained with large-bore catheters, and a central line is utilized when significant blood loss is anticipated such as with larger lesions.

Intraoperative monitoring of brain tissue oxygenation can be useful for AVM microsurgery to minimize cerebral injury and its clinical impact postoperatively. Microsurgical resection can cause a drop in the regional cerebral blood flow around the AVM that can be symptomatic. Brain tissue oxygenation ($brptiO_2$) monitoring is a direct way to monitor the oxygen status of surrounding tissue, but the ratio of brain tissue oxygenation to the partial pressure of oxygen in arterial blood ($brptiO_2$/PaO_2) has become the preferred method of oxygenation monitoring.[41] In the perinidal area, 63.6% had a $brptio_2$/Pao_2 considered hypoxic, and in the more distant ipsilateral area, 43.8% were considered hypoxic.[42] Both areas showed significant improvement of the oxygenation status postoperatively.[42] Intraoperative monitoring of oxygenation status may help guide the hemodynamic management and detect impending or current hypoxia to help guide the surgeon and anesthetic management, although this has not become routine practice at this time.

The goals of anesthesia induction include control of the airway, maintenance of hemodynamic stability, and adequate ventilation and oxygenation. Oftentimes, the anesthetic plan will include total intravenous anesthesia if motor evoked potentials and/or cortical mapping (with evoked EMGs under anesthesia). Inhalational agents that may increase ICP are avoided in the setting of raised ICP. Additionally, muscle relaxants are avoided if motor evoked potentials are being monitored (or only short-acting agents are used at induction, which will not interfere with monitoring during the intradural stage).

Anesthesia is maintained to allow safe surgical resection while continuing to promote brain relaxation, allowing strict blood pressure control, facilitating neurophysiological monitoring, and also allowing rapid neurological assessment under strict blood pressure control at the completion of the procedure (when desired by the surgical team). A total intravenous anesthesia technique can be utilized (short-acting opioid infusion plus propofol) or subminimum alveolar concentration values of inhalational agent can be utilized.

Awake craniotomies are sometimes necessary for the resection of AVMs in eloquent areas. Skull blocks, infiltration of local anesthetic into the dura, and sedation during the exposure and craniotomy are useful prior to awakening the patient for the critical mapping stage. Following the mapping and positioning, the patient is needed to be awake to safely resect the lesion; the patient can be resedated if desired. We have found dexmedetomidine to be effective for sedation with less respiratory depression, but others find combinations such as propofol-remifentanil to be effective.

Postoperative blood pressure control is critical, and initial management in the operating room and on the way to ICU typically utilizes intravenous nicardipine. Communication with the surgical team to clearly decide upon the target blood pressure goal is important to avoid postoperative complications including hemorrhage.

11.4.4 Intraoperative Fluid and Blood Product Management

Generally, normal saline is administered in the operating room for maintenance of fluid, with the goal of maintenance of adequate intravascular volume and stable hemodynamics. Electrolytes are monitored, and shifts may occur with osmotic diuretics. Normoglycemia is typically maintained during the surgery.

Blood product administration is another consideration in the management of patients with AVMs. In a ruptured AVM, the caretakers need a threshold past which they will transfuse the patient. In one study, a hemoglobin level of 10 g/dL was used as the threshold for when their patients were transfused with red blood cells and these patients showed significant increases in cerebral oxygen delivery, especially in areas at highest risk of ischemia.[43] While this study was on patients with SAH, the heightened benefit in high-risk ischemic areas with maximally dilated vasculature would theoretically be beneficial for the perinidal area of similar environment. A hemoglobin level of 10 g/dL can be used as a threshold for when transfusion can be considered.

During surgery with significant blood loss, packed red blood cell (PRBC) transfusions are administered to keep pace. With significant blood loss, fresh frozen plasma (FFP) can also be administered (typically one unit for every four to five units of PRBCs). Platelets and FFP may also be given in the setting of urgent surgery and use of anticoagulants and antiplatelet agents. Furthermore, platelets may also need to be given with large transfusion volumes. Cryoprecipitate may be given in the setting of massive transfusion, especially if the fibrinogen level falls below 100 mg/dL.

11.5 Conclusion

Vascular malformations of the brain, including AVMs and arteriovenous fistulas, commonly present with hemorrhage, seizures, headaches, or focal neurological deficits or are found incidentally on noninvasive imaging studies. The presentation, in part, dictates the acute management of patients harboring these lesions. In the neurocritical care unit, management of raised ICP, blood pressure management, and medical stabilization of the acutely ill patient are paramount. Such considerations are also important in patients undergoing AVM treatment to avoid perioperative complications. Finally, anesthetic management allows for the successful treatment of patients harboring vascular malformations where treatment is undertaken with surgical and/or endovascular techniques.

References

[1] Abecassis IJ, Xu DS, Batjer HH, Bendok BR. Natural history of brain arteriovenous malformations: a systematic review. Neurosurg Focus. 2014; 37(3):E7

[2] Tong X, Wu J, Lin F, et al. The effect of age, sex, and lesion location on initial presentation in patients with brain arteriovenous malformations. World Neurosurg. 2016; 87:598–606

[3] Laakso A, Hernesniemi J. Arteriovenous malformations: epidemiology and clinical presentation. Neurosurg Clin N Am. 2012; 23(1):1–6

[4] Santos ML, Demartini Júnior Z, Matos LA, et al. Angioarchitecture and clinical presentation of brain arteriovenous malformations. Arq Neuropsiquiatr. 2009; 67 2A:316–321

[5] Gross BA, Du R. Natural history of cerebral arteriovenous malformations: a meta-analysis. J Neurosurg. 2013; 118(2):437–443

[6] van Beijnum J, Lovelock CE, Cordonnier C, Rothwell PM, Klijn CJ, Al-Shahi Salman R, SIVMS Steering Committee and the Oxford Vascular Study. Outcome after spontaneous and arteriovenous malformation-related intracerebral haemorrhage: population-based studies. Brain. 2009; 132(Pt 2):537–543

[7] Sturiale CL, Puca A, Calandrelli R, et al. Relevance of bleeding pattern on clinical appearance and outcome in patients with hemorrhagic brain arteriovenous malformations. J Neurol Sci. 2013; 324(1)(–)(2):118–123

[8] Lv X, Liu J, Hu X, Li Y. Patient age, hemorrhage patterns, and outcomes of arteriovenous malformation. World Neurosurg. 2015; 84(4):1039–1044

[9] Appelboom G, Hwang BY, Bruce SS, et al. Predicting outcome after arteriovenous malformation-associated intracerebral hemorrhage with the original ICH score. World Neurosurg. 2012; 78(6):646–650

[10] Rahme R, Weil AG, Bojanowski MW. Early rerupture of cerebral arteriovenous malformations: beware the progressive hemispheric swelling. Med Hypotheses. 2011; 76(4):570–573

[11] Liu L, Jiang C, He H, Li Y, Wu Z. Periprocedural bleeding complications of brain AVM embolization with Onyx. Interv Neuroradiol. 2010; 16(1):47–57

[12] Stapf C, Mohr JP, Pile-Spellman J, et al. Concurrent arterial aneurysms in brain arteriovenous malformations with haemorrhagic presentation. J Neurol Neurosurg Psychiatry. 2002; 73(3):294–298

[13] Stein KP, Wanke I, Forsting M, et al. Associated aneurysms in supratentorial arteriovenous malformations: impact of aneurysm size on haemorrhage. Cerebrovasc Dis. 2015; 39(2):122–129

[14] Morawo AO, Gilmore EJ. Critical care management of intracerebral hemorrhage. Semin Neurol. 2016; 36(3):225–232

[15] Lattanzi S, Silvestrini M. Optimal achieved blood pressure in acute intracerebral hemorrhage: INTERACT2. Neurology. 2015; 85(6):557–558

[16] Aoun SG, Bendok BR, Batjer HH. Acute management of ruptured arteriovenous malformations and dural arteriovenous fistulas. Neurosurg Clin N Am. 2012; 23(1):87–103

[17] Martinez JL, Macdonald RL. Surgical strategies for acutely ruptured arteriovenous malformations. Front Neurol Neurosci. 2015; 37:166–181

[18] Gross BA, Lai PM, Du R. Hydrocephalus after arteriovenous malformation rupture. Neurosurg Focus. 2013; 34(5):E11

[19] Zheng H, Chen C, Zhang J, Hu Z. Mechanism and therapy of brain edema after intracerebral hemorrhage. Cerebrovasc Dis. 2016; 42(3)(–)(4):155–169

[20] Freeman WD. Management of intracranial pressure. Continuum (Minneap Minn). 2015; 21 5 Neurocritical Care:1299–1323

[21] Hemphill JC , III, Greenberg SM, Anderson CS, et al. American Heart Association Stroke Council, Council on Cardiovascular and Stroke Nursing, Council on Clinical Cardiology. Guidelines for the management of spontaneous intracerebral hemorrhage: a guideline for healthcare professionals from the American Heart Association/American Stroke Association. Stroke. 2015; 46(7):2032–2060

[22] Pavesi G, Rustemi O, Berlucchi S, Frigo AC, Gerunda V, Scienza R. Acute surgical removal of low-grade (Spetzler-Martin I-II) bleeding arteriovenous malformations. Surg Neurol. 2009; 72(6):662–667

[23] Kuhmonen J, Piippo A, Väärt K, et al. Early surgery for ruptured cerebral arteriovenous malformations. Acta Neurochir Suppl (Wien). 2005; 94:111–114

[24] Zacharia BE, Bruce S, Appelboom G, Connolly ES , Jr. Occlusive hyperemia versus normal perfusion pressure breakthrough after treatment of cranial arteriovenous malformations. Neurosurg Clin N Am. 2012; 23(1):147–151

[25] Tseng WL, Tsai YH. Vasospasm after intraventricular hemorrhage caused by arteriovenous malformation. Asian J Neurosurg. 2015; 10(2):114–116

[26] Maeda K, Kurita H, Nakamura T, et al. Occurrence of severe vasospasm following intraventricular hemorrhage from an arteriovenous malformation. Report of two cases. J Neurosurg. 1997; 87(3):436–439

[27] Gross BA, Du R. Vasospasm after arteriovenous malformation rupture. World Neurosurg. 2012; 78(3)(–)(4):300–305

[28] Ding D, Starke RM, Quigg M, et al. Cerebral arteriovenous malformations and epilepsy, part 1: predictors of seizure presentation. World Neurosurg. 2015; 84(3):645–652

[29] Kraemer DL, Awad IA. Vascular malformations and epilepsy: clinical considerations and basic mechanisms. Epilepsia. 1994; 35 Suppl 6:S30–S43

[30] Chen CJ, Chivukula S, Ding D, et al. Seizure outcomes following radiosurgery for cerebral arteriovenous malformations. Neurosurg Focus. 2014; 37(3):E17

[31] Englot DJ, Young WL, Han SJ, McCulloch CE, Chang EF, Lawton MT. Seizure predictors and control after microsurgical resection of supratentorial arteriovenous malformations in 440 patients. Neurosurgery. 2012; 71(3):572–580, discussion 580

[32] Przybylowski CJ, Ding D, Starke RM, et al. Seizure and anticonvulsant outcomes following stereotactic radiosurgery for intracranial arteriovenous malformations. J Neurosurg. 2015; 122(6):1299–1305

[33] Rohn B, Hänggi D, Etminan N, Turowski B, Steiger HJ. Relief of epilepsy and headache and quality of life after microsurgical treatment of unruptured brain AVM-audit of a single-center series and comprehensive review of the literature. Neurosurg Rev. 2017; 40(1):59–65

[34] Dehdashti AR, Thines L, Willinsky RA, et al. Multidisciplinary care of occipital arteriovenous malformations: effect on nonhemorrhagic headache, vision, and outcome in a series of 135 patients. Clinical article. J Neurosurg. 2010; 113(4):742–748

[35] Ellis JA, Mejia Munne JC, Lavine SD, Meyers PM, Connolly ES , Jr, Solomon RA. Arteriovenous malformations and headache. J Clin Neurosci. 2016; 23:38–43

[36] Kim BS, Sarma D, Lee SK, terBrugge KG. Brain edema associated with unruptured brain arteriovenous malformations. Neuroradiology. 2009; 51(5):327–335

[37] Lv X, Li Y, Yang X, Jiang C, Wu Z. Characteristics of brain arteriovenous malformations in patients presenting with nonhemorrhagic neurologic deficits. World Neurosurg. 2013; 79(3–4):484–488

[38] Tu J, Stoodley MA, Morgan MK, Storer KP. Ultrastructure of perinidal capillaries in cerebral arteriovenous malformations. Neurosurgery. 2006; 58(5):961–970, discussion 961–970

[39] Miller C, Mirski M. Anesthesia considerations and intraoperative monitoring during surgery for arteriovenous malformations and dural arteriovenous fistulas. Neurosurg Clin N Am. 2012; 23(1):153–164

[40] Rangel-Castilla L, Spetzler RF, Nakaji P. Normal perfusion pressure breakthrough theory: a reappraisal after 35 years. Neurosurg Rev. 2015; 38(3):399–404, discussion 404–405

[41] Badenes R, García-Pérez ML, Bilotta F. Intraoperative monitoring of cerebral oximetry and depth of anaesthesia during neuroanesthesia procedures. Curr Opin Anaesthesiol. 2016; 29(5):576–581

[42] Arikan F, Vilalta J, Noguer M, Olive M, Vidal-Jorge M, Sahuquillo J. Intraoperative monitoring of brain tissue oxygenation during arteriovenous malformation resection. J Neurosurg Anesthesiol. 2014; 26(4):328–341

[43] Dhar R, Zazulia AR, Videen TO, Zipfel GJ, Derdeyn CP, Diringer MN. Red blood cell transfusion increases cerebral oxygen delivery in anemic patients with subarachnoid hemorrhage. Stroke. 2009; 40(9):3039–3044

12 Classification of Brain Arteriovenous Malformations and Fistulas

Derrick L. Umansky, Ricky Medel, and Peter S. Amenta

Abstract

The proper classification of brain arteriovenous malformations (AVMs) and dural arteriovenous fistulas (dAVFs) is critical to clinical decision making and assessment of treatment risk. The Spetzler–Martin grade is the most commonly cited and rigorously tested system when evaluating outcomes following resection. Multiple additions and supplements have been made over the past two decades. The evolution of endovascular and radiosurgical therapy has driven the need for additional classifications that capture the outcomes and risks associated with these modalities. dAVFs are a diverse group of lesions with complex angioarchitecture. The Borden and Cognard systems are currently the most referenced in the classification of dAVFs. This chapter presents a review of the systems currently used to classify intracranial AVMs and dAVFs. Microsurgical, endovascular, and radiosurgical classification schemes are discussed. Special attention is paid to the most referenced systems, particularly the Spetzler–Martin grading scale for AVMs and the Borden and Cognard systems for dAVFs.

Keywords: arteriovenous malformation, dural arteriovenous fistula, classification systems, Spetzler–Martin, Borden, Cognard, Barrow, Buffalo score, radiosurgical score

Key Points

- The Spetzler–Martin grading system of arteriovenous malformations (AVMs) remains the standard in the assessment of risk of surgical resection.
- Multiple grading systems for surgical, endovascular, and radiosurgical treatment of AVMs are currently in use.
- Dural arteriovenous fistulas (dAVFs) are a heterogeneous group of lesions with complex and variable angioarchitecture.
- The Cognard and Borden systems are the most commonly referenced classification schemes for dAVFs.

12.1 Introduction

Arteriovenous malformations (AVMs) and dural arteriovenous fistulas (dAVFs) represent challenging clinical entities that are associated with significant morbidity and mortality. Much of the difficulty in managing these malformations is derived from the great diversity that exists between individual lesions. Both AVMs and dAVFs possess complex angioarchitecture and may have relationships to critical functional anatomy. Clinical presentations range from incidental findings or minimally symptomatic to catastrophic life-threatening hemorrhage. Management decisions must weigh the risks and benefits of intervention against the natural history of the disease. Treatment planning must account for multiple variables, including patient age, symptomatology,

history of intracranial hemorrhage, and the vascular anatomy of the lesion. Multiple classification systems have been proposed to capture the key elements of an individual lesion and assess the risk of intervention. These systems have the goal of creating a reliable, easily applicable, and accurate assessment that is of clinical utility. The development of these schemes is initially rooted in the microsurgical approach to vascular disease, given that intervention was only possible via this route prior to the modern era. Treatment of these lesions has undergone a transformation in recent years, and traditional microsurgical management is now frequently supplemented or even replaced by endovascular embolization and radiosurgery. As a result, modification and supplementation of the original systems has become necessary to capture the outcomes, challenges, and complications unique to these additional modes of therapy. This chapter presents a review of the systems currently used to classify intracranial AVMs and dAVFs. Microsurgical, endovascular, and radiosurgical classification schemes are discussed. Special attention is paid to the most referenced systems, particularly the Spetzler–Martin grading system for AVMs and the Borden and Cognard systems for dAVFs.

12.2 Materials and Methods

A wide range of materials were used in the composition of this chapter. For a historical perspective, many of the original papers pertaining to the classification of AVMs and dAVFs have been included. The reviews of the established grading systems are based on the landmark papers that defined their methodology and statistical significance. Multiple contemporary sources are cited in the explanation of the additions and supplements to these systems over the past two decades. The tables are adapted from the original papers to provide a resource for the trainee searching for a useful and rapid reference. Images are taken from the institutional experience in the neurosurgical department at the Tulane Medical Center.

12.3 The Classification of Arteriovenous Malformations

12.3.1 AVM Classification and Microsurgical Resection

Spetzler–Martin Grading System

The primary goal of surgical resection of intracranial AVMs is the removal of the risk of intracranial hemorrhage and its associated morbidity and mortality. Complete removal may also benefit patients suffering from seizures, vascular steal phenomena, headaches, and other less severe but often debilitating sequelae. However, particularly in terms of intracranial hemorrhage, the risk of future rupture can only be predicted and, in

Table 12.1 Spetzler–Martin grading system

Graded feature	
Size of AVM	
Small (< 3 cm)	1
Medium (3–6 cm)	2
Large (> 6 cm)	3
Eloquence of adjacent brain	
Noneloquent	0
Eloquent	1
Pattern of venous drainage	
Superficial only	0
Deep	1

Note: In the Spetzler–Martin grading system, the grade = size + eloquence + venous drainage. AVMs with drainage into superficial veins are assigned 0 points, while those with drainage into deep veins are assigned 1 point. AVMs located in eloquent areas are assigned 1 point, while those in noneloquent areas are assigned 0 points. For instance, an AVM that is < 2 cm in an eloquent area with deep venous drainage would have a grade of I + I + I = III.

Source: Spetzler and Martin.[1]

fact, may never occur. To justify surgical intervention, one must be able to understand the potential risk of rupture, as well as the immediate morbidity and mortality of surgical resection.[1] In 1986, Spetzler and Martin proposed a grading system by which to predict the morbidity and mortality associated with open surgical resection of intracranial AVMs[1] (▶ Table 12.1). Taking into account the wide variability in angioarchitecture and anatomic location of these lesions, the authors composed a system that relied on three key features to simplify grading: AVM size, pattern of venous drainage, and relationship to eloquent tissue.

Nidus size, as measured with angiography, is considered small (< 3 cm), medium (3–6 cm), or large (> 6 cm) and assigned a score of 1, 2, or 3, respectively. AVM size represents an important determinant of safety of resection for multiple reasons. Larger malformations are more likely to abut critical anatomic structures at the nidus margins. As a result, resection of larger lesions places a greater volume of functional tissue at risk. The size of the malformation also reflects the arterial supply and number of arterial feeding pedicles. Increasing AVM diameter places the nidus into an expanding number of vascular territories, thereby increasing the quantity of feeding pedicles and parent vessels supplying the AVM. The surgical approaches required to safely resect larger AVMs must account for blood supply from multiple territories and provide safe avenues by which to access those vessels.[1] Finally, as with most surgical procedures, larger lesions require a longer amount of time to remove. Patients with larger malformations are subjected to the risks of prolonged anesthesia, increased blood loss, and prolonged brain retraction.

Based on angiography, venous drainage is segregated into two distinct categories, superficial and deep drainage. Lesions possessing only superficial venous drainage are scored a zero. Superficial venous drainage is defined by venous outflow directed through the cortical venous system. AVMs exhibiting any element of deep venous drainage are assigned a 1. Venous drainage corresponds with accessibility of the lesion, as deep venous drainage places arterialized veins in a medial and potentially difficult location to access. These veins are often the subependymal veins of the ventricles and may be difficult to control, adding to blood loss, length of surgery, and volume of tissue resected.

Eloquence is assigned to structures and regions of the brain with known quantifiable function that, if injured, will result in a disabling neurologic deficit (▶ Fig. 12.1; Spetzler–Martin eloquent areas). AVMs confined to noneloquent regions are scored a zero, while AVMs involving at least one eloquent area are scored a 1. AVM nidus usually displaces surrounding tissue from its anatomic location; thus, eloquence is defined by the normal location of the affected anatomy. Obviously, dissection within or adjacent to eloquent tissue places the patient at a greater risk of postoperative impairment and increases the risk of resection. Computed tomography (CT) and magnetic resonance imaging (MRI) are useful in determining the anatomic relationships of the nidus.

The grade of an individual AVM is calculated from the sum of the three scores, which can range from grade I to grade V. Grade I

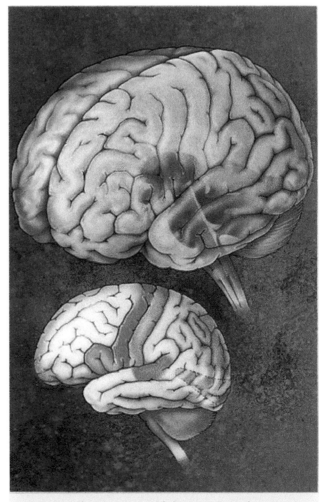

Fig. 12.1 Spetzler–Martin areas of eloquence. Deep eloquent areas are depicted in the upper image and include the hypothalamus, thalamus, brainstem, and cerebellar peduncles. Cortical eloquent areas are depicted in the lower image and include the primary motor area, primary sensory area, language areas, and primary visual area. (Adapted from Spetzler and Martin.[1])

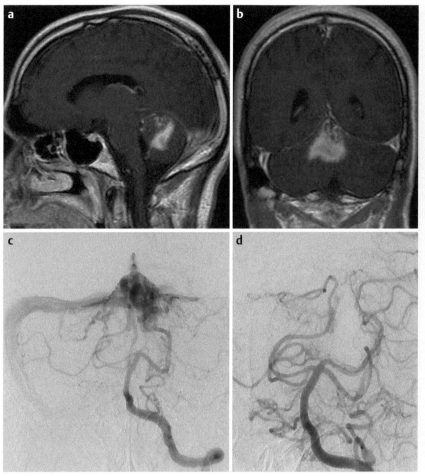

Fig. 12.2 Spetzler–Martin Grade II (S2V0E0) AVM. A 46-year-old man presented with a severe headache, nausea, and truncal ataxia. Sagittal **(a)** and coronal **(b)** MRI with gadolinium demonstrating a 3.2 × 2 × 2 cm AVM of the vermis and left tentorial surface of the cerebellum. **(c)** Preoperative left vertebral artery injection in the anteroposterior (AP) plane shows a hypertrophic left superior cerebellar artery feeding pedicle and superficial drainage to the tentorial sinuses. A supracerebellar-infratentorial approach was used to resect the AVM. **(d)** A postoperative left vertebral artery injection in the AP plane demonstrating complete resection of the AVM. The patient was discharged to rehab with persistent ataxia.

lesions are small, located in noneloquent regions, and display superficial drainage, and are therefore associated with limited morbidity and mortality with resection. Grade V lesions are large, involve eloquent anatomy, and display a component of deep venous drainage, rendering resection challenging, and are associated with significant operative risk. A total of 12 combinations of the grading criteria are possible. To test the validity of the system, the grading scale was applied to 100 AVMs resected by Spetzler and correlated with surgical complications. Complications were subdivided into minor deficits, major deficits, and mortality. There were no mortalities within the cohort. Grade I and II lesions were resected without major deficits. The percentage of major deficits progressively increased with each successive grade. Minor deficits were not observed in grade I AVM resections, and the incidence increased to 5 and 12% for grade II and III lesions, respectively. Grade IV and V lesions had the highest incidence of minor deficits. Examples of Spetzler–Martin grade II AVMs are seen in ▶ Fig. 12.2 and ▶ Fig. 12.3.

Further Classification of Spetzler–Martin Grade III AVMs

Due to its reliance on only three AVM characteristics, the Spetzler–Martin grading system is limited in the classification of intermediate grade lesions. This ambiguity is particularly true in regard to the scoring of grade III lesions, which are composed

of four distinct subtypes.[1] The initial Spetzler–Martin paper demonstrated an incidence of 16% for minor and major neurologic deficits.[1] In a follow-up study, Hamilton and Spetzler reported a 2.8% permanent morbidity for grade III AVM resection.[2] Heros et al found the incidence of surgical complications to be 11.4% for resection of grade III lesions.[3] De Oliveira et al initially proposed a reclassification of grade III AVMs into two additional subgroups, IIIA ("large") and IIIB ("small and eloquent"), thereby reducing the number of Spetzler–Martin grade III subtypes from four to two.[4] A total of 95.5% of patients with grade IIIA AVMs experienced good outcomes with embolization and resection, as opposed to only 70% of grade IIIB patients. A total of 27.8% of IIIB patients demonstrated a poor outcome and 2.1% died, which resulted in the authors recommending radiosurgery for this group.

Lawton and colleagues demonstrated the influence of size on outcomes following the resection of grade III AVMs.[5] Grade III lesions were subdivided into small (< 3 cm), medium/deep (3–6 cm), and medium/eloquent (3–6 cm) groups. Large AVMs (> 6 cm) were not encountered, leading the authors to conclude that these lesions are nonexistent or exceedingly rare despite the fact that the Spetzler–Martin system allows for their grading. This finding is likely due to the fact that AVMs with a diameter greater than 6 cm almost always abut or involve eloquent brain or possess at least one deep draining vein, thereby rendering them a grade IV lesion. A total of 97.1% of patients with

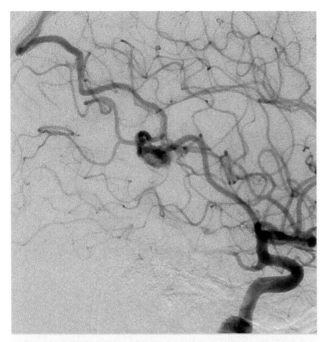

Fig. 12.3 Spetzler–Martin grade II (S1V0E1) AVM. A 42-year-old man presented to the clinic with a history of a remotely ruptured AVM located in the posterior left superior temporal gyrus. He reports a significant mixed aphasia resulted from the previous hemorrhage; however, he made significant improvement and is currently high functioning. Lateral projection of a left internal carotid injection demonstrates a compact 1.6 × 1.4 × 0.7 cm nidus fed by the angular branch of the middle cerebral artery. Superficial drainage via a single vein is directed to the superior sagittal sinus. The patient opted for radiosurgical intervention.

Table 12.2 Modification of the Spetzler–Martin grading scale

Grade	Size	Score	
		Venous drainage	Eloquence
I	1	0	0
II	1	0	1
II	1	1	0
II	2	0	0
III–	1	1	1
III	2	1	0
III +	2	0	1
III*	3	0	0
IV	2	1	1
IV	3	1	0
IV	3	0	1
V	3	1	1

*Note: Grade III AVMs are exceedingly rare, almost nonexistent.

The modifications to the original Spetzler–Martin grading system were made to further surgical risk stratification of the heterogeneous population of grade III AVMs. As with the original calculation, the grade is the sum of the size (S), venous drainage pattern (V), and eloquence (E) scores. Grade III– AVMs (S1V1E1) have a surgical risk close to that of a low-grade AVM; meanwhile, grade III + AVMs (S2V0E1) have a surgical risk close to that of a high-grade AVM.

Source: Lawton.[5]

small grade III AVMs remained unchanged or improved neurologically. In total, 92.9% of patients with medium/deep grade III lesions experienced no change or improvement in their condition. Patients in the medium/eloquent group fared worse, with only 85.2% remaining unchanged or improved. Within this cohort, 14.8% of patients suffered a decline in condition or died following surgery, representing two-thirds of the neurological morbidity and death in the study. Surgical risk of small AVM resection was 2.9%, while it was 7.1 and 14.8% for medium/deep and medium/eloquent lesions, respectively. The incidence of morbidity and mortality of small grade III lesions is low and rivals that of Spetzler–Martin grade II lesions. This finding is in contrast to the reported higher incidence of complications in the de Oliveira series, where smaller AVMs in eloquent anatomy were subject to poorer outcomes.[4] Conversely, in the Lawton series, resection of medium/eloquent AVMs is subject to considerably higher rates of morbidity and death that are comparable to grade IV AVMs.[5] Medium/deep lesions were associated with a surgical risk similar to the entire class of grade III AVMs.[1,5]

The authors proposed a modification to the Spetzler–Martin grading system to better define the risk of resection of the four grade III subtypes[5] (▶ Table 12.2). The four subtypes are relabeled with a "–" (lower surgical risk) or "+" (higher surgical risk). III– AVMs correspond to the small AVMs amenable to resection. III + AVMs represent the medium/eloquent group and are associated with the prohibitive risks seen with grade IV and V lesions. Grade III AVMs are medium/deep AVMs and occupy a

zone of intermediate risk, which the authors concede remain a decision-making dilemma. These lesions must be addressed on an individual basis, and treatment must be based on a combination of patient wishes, surgeon experience, and the clinical picture as a whole.[5] III* lesions are the > 6 cm AVMs that were not encountered in the study.

Lawton–Young AVM Grading System

Lawton and colleagues also proposed a grading scale to supplement the Spetzler–Martin score and add clarity to clinical decision making.[6] The Lawton–Young supplementary grading system considers three variables significantly correlated with surgical risk, diffuseness, patient age, and hemorrhagic versus nonhemorrhagic presentation. The scoring of the three categories is summated to arrive at a cumulative score ranging from 1 to 5 (▶ Table 12.3). Diffuseness is associated with elevated surgical risk due to the imprecise surgical boundaries that result when the nidus is not compact and easily defined. These vague margins increase the risk of nidal bleeding and transgression of eloquent structures. Age is considered to account for pediatric (< 20 years old) patients who tend to fare better following AVM resection due to limited systemic disease and a greater potential for neurologic recovery. Patients older than 40 years were assumed to have a greater incidence of systemic disease, thereby limiting their ability to tolerate surgery and recover from neurologic injury. Finally, the authors included hemorrhagic and nonhemorrhagic presentations, adding a point for nonhemorrhagic presentations. Hemorrhagic presentation was associated with a lower surgical risk due to hematoma-related fixed neurologic deficits that cannot be worsened by resection.[7] Additionally, the presence

Table 12.3 Lawton–Young supplementary grading system

Variable	Point score, full model		Spetzler–Martin grading scale		Supplemental grading scale	
	Definition	Weighting*	Definition	Points	Definition	Points
AVM size	Diameter (cm)	X1	<3 cm	1		
			3–6 cm	2		
			>6 cm	3		
Deep venous drainage	No	0	No	0		
	Yes	3	Yes	1		
Eloquence	No	0	No	0		
	Yes	2	Yes	1		
Age	Decades	X1			<20 years	1
					20–40 years	2
					>40 years	3
Unruptured presentation	No	0			No	0
	Yes	4			Yes	1
Diffuse	No	0			No	0
	Yes	2			Yes	1
Perforating artery supply	No	0				
	Yes	0				
Grade		Total (1–10)		Total (1–5)		Total (1–5)

*Weighting x1 for continuous variables = actual value x1.
Note: The Lawton–Young supplementary grading system on the right side of the table considers three additional variables (patient age, hemorrhagic presentation, and diffuseness) as predictors of neurological outcomes after microsurgical AVM resection. Deep perforating artery supply was initially shown to be associated with increased surgical risk, but this elevated risk was not supported in developing the supplementary grading system. The combined score on the left side of the table yielded the highest predictive accuracy of neurological outcomes after microsurgical AVM resection.

Source: Lawton et al.[6]

of a hematoma may create or enhance dissection planes or obliterate a portion of the arterial supply.

The predictive accuracy of this supplementary system was tested against the Spetzler–Martin scale and a 10-point scale that is composed of a sum of the two scores (the supplemented Spetzler–Martin grade).[6] The supplemented Spetzler–Martin grade was found to be the most predictive of surgical risk, while the original Spetzler–Martin score was the least predictive. The supplementary Lawton–Young score was significantly more accurate than the Spetzler–Martin score. The authors conclude that the supplementary score can be used to support the findings of the Spetzler–Martin score or provide an additional means by which to assess risk when there is a difference between the two scales.

12.3.2 AVM Classification and Endovascular Therapy

Spetzler–Martin Grading and Embolization

Advancements in endovascular intervention have greatly impacted current strategies for the management of AVMs. The advent of liquid embolic agents, particularly Onyx, flow-directed and detachable-tip microcatheters, and balloon-assisted techniques have expanded the armamentarium available to treating physicians. Embolization is currently used prior to surgical resection to reduce flow through the nidus, obliterate difficult to access deep feeders, and reduce intraoperative blood loss. Endovascular intervention is also used in conjunction with radiosurgical management, for palliation of symptoms and curative obliteration.[8,9,10,11,12,13]

Multiple authors have applied the Spetzler–Martin scale or its components to the endovascular management of AVMs with variable results. Hartmann et al reported no significant relationship between the Spetzler–Martin grade or its individual components and the incidence of postembolization complications.[14] Gobin et al found increasing embolization complication rates with increasing Spetzler–Martin grade in patients undergoing embolization and radiosurgery.[10] Viñuela et al demonstrated the incidence of embolization-associated complications to increase with each subsequent Spetzler–Martin grade.[15] Haw et al reported a significant association between the incidence of complications and the location of the nidus in eloquent tissue.[16] Kim et al applied the Spetzler–Martin grading to a series of patients treated with embolization performed as a curative procedure or as part of a multidisciplinary treatment regimen.[17] The relationship between the incidence of complications and grade was not significant, but did demonstrate a clear trend of increasing complications with increasing lesion grade.

The Buffalo Score

Endovascular embolization of AVMs subjects patients to many of the same risks as open surgical resection; however, the means by which these complications occur are drastically different. Ischemic complications arise from occlusion of normal arteries following embolism into an en passage vessel, reflux from a feeding pedicle, or thromboembolism from prolonged catheterization. Penetration of embolic material into the venous outflow prior to complete nidus obliteration results in outflow restriction and potentially subsequent rupture. Superselective catheterization of arterial feeders risks perforation and intracranial hemorrhage. To account for these unique complications, Dumont et al proposed a grading system, the Buffalo score, to assess the risk of endovascular intervention for a particular lesion.[18]

The grading system relies on three characteristics: the number of feeding pedicles, the diameter of the feeding pedicles, and the eloquence of the surrounding brain.[18] Based on angiography, the number of feeding pedicles is classified as one to two, three to four, or five or more. Embolization of each pedicle is an individual intervention; thus, an increasing number of pedicles is equated with an increasing possibility of iatrogenic injury.[17,18] The diameters of the feeding pedicles are measured within 1 cm of the nidus on angiography and classified into two groups, large (mostly, diameter > 1 mm) or small (mostly, diameter < 1 mm). Smaller pedicles are a more challenging target for superselection and are more prone to wire perforation and subsequent hemorrhage. Additionally, liquid embolic agents may have a greater tendency to reflux into normal parent vessels when injected into smaller diameter pedicles. The eloquence of tissue adjacent to the nidus represents the third risk factor.[1] Risk of neurologic deficit due to embolization is greater when embolizate is injected into eloquent regions. The cumulative grade for an individual lesion is calculated by combining the scores for each of the three variables (▶ Table 12.4).

AVMs at lowest risk of a complication following embolization are grade I lesions with a single arterial feeder that is greater than 1 mm in diameter and located in a noneloquent region. Grade V AVMs are associated with the highest risk of embolization and are located in eloquent tissue and possess five or more pedicles, the majority of which are < 1 mm. The grading system was applied to 50 consecutive patients who underwent AVM embolization, and the complication rates were as follows: grades 1 and 2, 0%; grade 3, 14%; grade 4, 50%; and grade 5, 75%. Interestingly, the incidence of endovascular complications also reflected the Spetzler–Martin grading; however, the correlation between the Buffalo score and the incidence of endovascular complications was stronger. ▶ Fig. 12.4 depicts a left mesial temporal lobe AVM which was treated with Onyx embolization and subsequent radiosurgery.

12.3.3 Radiosurgical Classification of AVMs

Radiosurgery has assumed a larger role in the management of small and medium-sized AVMs. Successful radiosurgical intervention is defined by complete obliteration of the AVM without the development of new or worsening neurologic deficits.[19] Complete nidus obliteration ranges between 65 and 90% and usually occurs after a latency period of 1 to 3 years, during which the risk of hemorrhage is sustained.[20,21,22,23,24,25,26,27] Nidus involution may also be associated with significant edema and radiation changes to eloquent anatomy, resulting in disabling neurologic deficits. The Spetzler–Martin grading system does not account for the AVM characteristics that influence outcome following radiosurgery.[24,28]

Pollock and Flickinger proposed a grading scale for the radiosurgical management of AVMs with Gamma Knife therapy.[19] Based on an analysis of patients undergoing stereotactic radiosurgery for AVMs at two institutions, the authors concluded that three factors are most predictive of obliteration and neurologic deficit rates: patient age, AVM volume, and location of the nidus. The statistical methods used to calculate the score are beyond the scope of this chapter, but the three variables are incorporated into an equation that assigns a total score for the AVM (▶ Table 12.5). When tested against the patient cohort, the calculated AVM score showed a significant correlation with clinical outcomes, while the Spetzler–Martin score did not correlate. All patients with a score of ≤ 1 had excellent clinical outcomes (AVM obliteration and no new/worsening neurologic deficit), while only 39% of patients with a score of ≥ 2 achieved an excellent outcome. The validity of the AVM radiosurgery score has been tested in additional studies. Andrade-Souza and colleagues reviewed 136 AVMs treated with radiosurgery over an 11-year period.[29] Patient AVMs with a score of < 1 were associated with a 91.7% incidence of excellent outcomes. Radiosurgery resulted in excellent outcomes in only 33.3% of AVMs scoring > 2. De Oliveira et al found a significant correlation between the modified Spetzler–Martin grade and excellent outcomes, although the correlation between the radiosurgery score and outcomes was statistically stronger.[4,29] Andrade-Souza et al tested the accuracy of the radiosurgery score in basal ganglia, internal capsule, and thalamic AVMs.[30] Radiosurgery of AVMs

Table 12.4 Buffalo score

Graded feature	Points assigned
Number of arterial pedicles	
1 or 2	1
3 or 4	2
5 or more	3
Diameter of arterial pedicles	
Most > 1 mm	0
Most ≤ 1 mm	1
Nidus location	
Noneloquent	0
Eloquent	1

Note: When calculating the Buffalo score, the AVM grade is the sum of the points assigned for the number of pedicles, diameter of the arterial pedicles, and the nidus location.

Source: Dumont et al.[18]

Table 12.5 AVM radiosurgery grading scale

Characteristic	Coefficient
AVM volume (cm³)	0.1
Patient age (years)	0.02
AVM location[a]	0.3
Frontal or temporal = 0	
Parietal, occipital, intraventricular, corpus callosum, or cerebellar = 1	
Basal ganglia, thalamic, or brainstem = 2	

Note: AVM score = (0.1)(AVM volume) + (0.02)(patient age) + (0.3)(AVM location).

[a]When AVM involved multiple sites, fractional values are used according to the number of sites (0.5 for two sites, 0.33 for three sites).

Source: Pollock and Flickinger.[19]

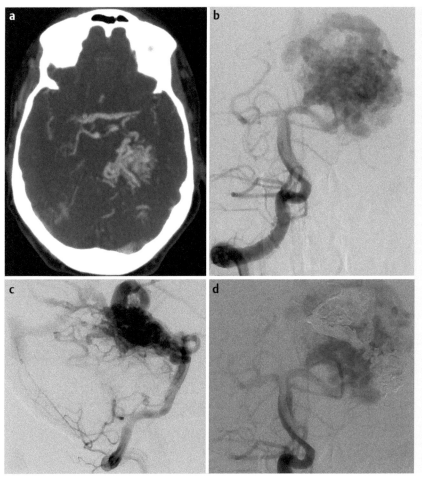

Fig. 12.4 Spetzler–Martin grade IV (S2V1E1) AVM. A 63-year-old woman presented following the acute onset of a severe headache. CTA **(a)** demonstrated a 4 × 3.2 × 2.6 left mesial temporal AVM. The AP **(b)** and lateral **(c)** projections of a right vertebral artery injection shows the distal left posterior cerebral artery (PCA) blood supply to the nidus. Multiple small feeders from the left anterior choroidal artery were also observed. Drainage is primarily to the serpiginous and dilated left basal vein of Rosenthal. The patient underwent the first of multiple planned Onyx embolizations **(d)** prior to radiosurgical treatment of the residual nidus.

with a score < 1.5 resulted in a 75% obliteration rate and a 10% rate of complications. Treatment of AVMs with a score > 1.5 had a 50% obliteration rate and a 27.3% incidence of complications. The overall incidence of excellent outcome was 70% for scores < 1.5 and 40.9% for those > 1.5, which represented a trend toward correlation. The AVM radiosurgery score has been shown to be equally reliable for linear accelerator–based radiosurgery and has since been simplified by classifying nidus location into a two-tiered system (basal ganglia/thalamus/brainstem vs. other).[29,30,31,32,33]

12.4 Classification of Dural Arteriovenous Fistulas

12.4.1 Background

Djindjian performed extensive work with superselective catheterization of the branches of the external carotid artery.[34] The findings contributed significantly to the understanding of vascular and neoplastic pathology of the skull base and dura. In 1977, dAVFs were classified on the pattern of venous drainage for the first time as a result of these studies.[35] Type I fistulas exhibited immediate venous drainage into a sinus or meningeal vein. Type II fistulas drained into a venous sinus, which then refluxed into a secondary sinus or cortical veins. Type III fistulas demonstrated venous drainage directly into a cortical vein

without an intervening sinus. Type IV fistulas drained into cortical veins, of which at least one possessed a giant venous pouch.[35] In relation to the clinical presentation, type I fistulas generally followed a benign course, and aggressive symptomatology increased with subsequent types. This scheme is an important milestone in the evolution of the understanding of intracranial dAVFs, yet the simplicity of the grading fails in a number of key areas addressed by the subsequent Cognard system.

12.4.2 Borden Classification System

The Borden Classification System of dAVFs was published in 1995 in an attempt to build upon the Djindjian system.[36] The authors incorporate spinal fistulas into the scheme and classify the various fistulas into three clinically relevant types that pertain to treatment. The pattern of venous drainage remains the defining characteristic in determining fistula type. Retrograde drainage of the fistula into the superficial cortical veins is termed "subarachnoid venous drainage." The authors introduce the term dural "arteriovenous fistulous malformation (AVFM)" to be inclusive of lesions that are composed of multiple fistulous connections. The Borden classification system also describes two subtypes, subtype a and subtype b, that are applied as a modifier to all three primary types. Subtype a fistulas are also known as simple fistulas and are defined by a single fistulous connection between a lone meningeal artery and a draining vein or sinus. Subtype b fistulas are multiple fistulas (complex fistulas) composed of multiple fistulous connections fed by multiple dural arterial pedicles.

Under this classification scheme, type I dural AVFMs are still those with venous drainage directly into a dural venous sinus or meningeal vein. These malformations may contain single or multiple fistulous connections between a meningeal artery and dural venous sinus or meningeal vein. The key components are a lack of subarachnoid venous drainage and maintenance of venous outflow in the normal anterograde direction. The clinical course of these lesions is relatively benign, and symptomatic presentations are commonly associated with pulsatile tinnitus and cranial nerve deficits.[37,38,39] Carotid-cavernous fistulas (CCFs) and spinal dAVFs are also included in this type. Type II dural AVFMs drain into a venous sinus that then exhibits reflux into cortical veins. There may be one or more fistulous connections that drain directly into the sinus. The arterialized blood within the sinus is then forced to travel from the sinus into the cortical veins in a retrograde direction. Patients present with symptoms referable to intracranial hypertension or hemorrhage. Spinal fistulas that drain into the epidural venous plexus and perimedullary veins are grouped with these lesions. The spinal epidural venous plexus is considered analogous to the cranial intradural sinuses and the perimedullary veins are comparable to the cortical veins.[40,41]

Like the Djindjian systems, the Borden type III dural AVFMs drain directly into cortical veins without an intervening dural venous sinus and, once again, can consist of a single or multiple fistulous connections. The cortical veins, which normally deliver blood in an anterograde direction to the sinus, do not flow into the sinus at all. Instead, venous blood flow into the veins travels in a retrograde direction. The authors described a number of scenarios in which this type of fistula may exist. The first is in the presence of a patent sinus. In these instances, the arterialized vein does not communicate with the dural sinus at the point of the fistula. This occurs if the meningeal artery communicates directly with the cortical vein. A scenario may also exist where a patent segment of sinus is trapped on either side by completely occlusive thrombus. Arterial blood from a meningeal artery that develops a fistulous connection with the patent segment would only have associated cortical veins by which to drain in a retrograde fashion.[36] A third possibility to explain the venous drainage of a type III AVFM would be a fistulous connection between a meningeal feeder and a venous structure naturally isolated from the dural sinuses, such as a venous lake.

The clinical course of these lesions is primarily malignant and patients frequently present with intracranial hemorrhage or symptoms of intracranial hypertension. Infratentorial type III dural AVFMs drain into the spinal perimedullary veins, resulting in spinal venous congestion and myelopathy.[42,43,44,45] Conversely, spinal dural AVFMs that drain intracranially via the perimedullary veins also represent type III lesions.[46,47]

12.4.3 The Cognard Classification System

The Cognard classification system was first published in 1995 and represented a review of a series of 205 consecutive patients with dural AVFs at a single institution.[48] The authors recorded the clinical presentation of the patients and the angiographic features of the fistulas. Patients were divided into two groups

Table 12.6 Aggressive versus nonaggressive neurological manifestations of cerebral dural AVFs

Aggressive	Nonaggressive
Intracranial hypertension (headache, nausea/vomiting, visual deficit/loss, papilledema)	Isolated headache
Intracranial hemorrhage	Bruit
Focal neurological deficit	Ocular symptoms unrelated to intracranial hypertension
Seizures	Vertigo[a]
Altered mental status	
Ascending myelopathy	
Vertigo[a]	

Note: In the development of the Cognard classification of dural AVFs, the team divided patients into two groups based on the presence or absence of aggressive neurological manifestations. Angiography was then used to characterize 5 distinct types based on the pattern of venous drainage and the presence or absence of venous ectasia. Analysis revealed that the aggressive behavior of dural AVFs was associated with the presence of cortical venous drainage.

[a]Cognard and colleagues defined vertigo as aggressive when pronounced and nonaggressive when isolated and minimal.

Source: Cognard et al.[48]

based on the presence or absence of aggressive neurologic symptoms. Aggressive and nonaggressive neurologic symptoms are defined in ► Table 12.6. Classification into five distinct types was based on the pattern of venous drainage and the presence or absence of venous ectasia. Retrograde drainage of the fistula into the veins of the cortical surface was termed "cortical venous drainage."

Type I fistulas exhibit anterograde drainage into a dural venous sinus. In the original study, 84 patients were diagnosed with type I venous drainage. Of these patients, 83 had nonaggressive neurologic symptoms, 47 of which were followed up for a mean of 40 months. The one patient with aggressive neurologic symptoms was an iatrogenic postoperative dAVF that developed after cerebellar hemangioblastoma resection. The high-flow fistula exhibited type I venous drainage into a dominant transverse sinus. However, the lack of a significant contralateral transverse sinus resulted in venous hypertension in the single draining sinus.

Type II fistulas represent a class of fistulas that can be further subdivided based on their angiographic appearance into one of three subtypes. These fistulas demonstrate anterograde venous drainage into a dural venous sinus; however, incomplete drainage results in reflux. Anterograde venous drainage into the sinus may arise secondary to multiple scenarios. Extremely high-flow fistulas may overwhelm the ability of a widely patent dural sinus to provide sufficient venous outflow, thereby resulting in reflux. Additionally, lower flow lesions may still display reflux in the presence of venous outflow obstruction or stenosis. Type IIa fistulas exhibit retrograde flow into a secondary sinus, while type IIb lesions are found to have retrograde venous drainage through cortical veins. Of the 27 fistulas demonstrating type IIa drainage, 67% presented with nonaggressive neurologic symptoms. Of those patients with aggressive neurologic manifestations, the vast majority were secondary to increased intracranial pressure. Findings included headaches, visual disturbances, papilledema, and tonsillar herniation; however, none of these fistulas presented with hemorrhage. Only 10 patients with type IIb venous drainage were identified, 3 of which manifested with aggressive symptoms (2 hemorrhages and 1 case of intracranial hypertension). Type IIa + b fistulas are those that demonstrate retrograde venous drainage into secondary dural sinuses and cortical veins. Cognard classified 18 fistulas with this drainage pattern, 12 of which presented with an aggressive clinical course. One patient presented with hemorrhage.

Type III fistulas drain directly into cortical veins. Of the 25 dural AVFs exhibiting this pattern of venous drainage, 19 (7%) resulted in aggressive neurologic symptoms. Of these 19 patients, 10 (40%) presented with intracranial hemorrhage. Thus, the incidence of hemorrhage in patients with type III drainage was higher than that of patients with either type IIb or IIa + b (11%). This distinction is an important one, as direct reflux into a cortical vein poses a significantly higher risk of hemorrhage when compared to indirect reflux into a cortical vein from an intervening sinus.

Type IV fistulas drain directly into cortical veins, of which at least one must demonstrate venous ectasia. The venous ectasia must measure greater than 5 mm in diameter and three times the diameter of the draining vein from which it arises. Out of 29 total patients with a type IV fistula, 28 (97%) presented with aggressive neurologic symptoms. A total of 19 (66%) suffered an intracranial hemorrhage. Type V fistulas drain through the perimedullary veins. A total of 12 patients presented with type V fistulas, all of whom suffered from aggressive neurologic symptomatology. Six patients developed progressive myelopathy, whereas five presented following a subarachnoid hemorrhage. One patient was symptomatic from a focal neurologic deficit.

The authors were able to identify additional clinically significant data that made considerable contributions to the current understanding of these lesions. The anatomic location of the fistula demonstrated a significant correlation with the presence or absence of aggressive neurologic symptoms. No patients with fistulas draining to the cavernous sinus presented with aggressive symptoms. Aggressive symptoms were present in fistulas involving the transverse sinus (27%), the torcula (100%), superior sagittal sinus (65%), tentorium (92%), and anterior skull base (88%). Importantly, all of the fistulas involving the anterior skull base and tentorium demonstrated cortical venous drainage, accounting for their relatively aggressive natural history. Ninety-five percent of all of the fistulas studied were fed solely by meningeal branches, while 5% received pedicles from meningeal and cortical arterial feeders. The presence or absence of a cortical arterial supply did not influence the neurologic symptomatology. Males (56.5%) were significantly more likely to experience aggressive symptomatology than females (29%). This finding was largely due to differences between anatomic location and venous drainage patterns between the two sexes. A total of 85% of dAVFs draining to the cavernous sinus and 58% of those draining to the transverse sinuses (the two locations with the lowest incidence of aggressive symptomatology) were found in women. Furthermore, women exhibited type I venous drainage in 50% of all cases, whereas only 29% of men with dAVFs demonstrated this pattern of drainage. A total of 57.5% of male fistulas resulted in cortical venous drainage (type IIb–V), whereas only 36% of women suffered from cortical reflux. Possible underlying etiologies of fistula formation were found in

26% of patients. Recent cranial trauma, cerebral thrombophlebitis, and neurologic surgery were the most frequently identified preceding events. Ear and nasal sinus infections within a week prior to presentation were also noted. No significant correlation between the presence of a possible etiology and the aggressiveness of symptom onset could be found.

12.4.4 Clinical Utility of Borden and Cognard Classifications

Davies et al reported on a series of 102 dAVFs in 98 patients encountered over an 11-year period at a single institution.[49] Two neuroradiologists classified all lesions by the Borden and Cognard classifications. The value of the Borden system in predicting the behavior of dural AVFs was examined. The Cognard system was evaluated for reproducibility and for any additional clinical utility gained by the more detailed categorization. Aggressive clinical presentation was defined by death, intracranial hemorrhage, or nonhemorrhagic neurological deficit (excluding cranial neuropathy associated with CCFs). The authors found a highly significant correlation between the Cognard and Borden types and presentation with intracranial hemorrhage or nonhemorrhagic neurological deficit. While the Borden classification benefits from its simplicity and ease with which the clinical course can be predicted, the Cognard classification provides a more detailed description of the angioarchitecture.

12.4.5 Lesion Location and Risk of Hemorrhage

The anatomic location of dAVFs has garnered interest as a potential variable affecting the risk of rupture.[48,50] Aminoff originally separated dAVFs into an anteroinferior group and posterosuperior group, which followed a more aggressive clinical course.[51] Davies et al reported aggressive clinical courses for 79% of tentorial fistulas, 75% of anterior cranial fossa fistulas, and 50% of superior sagittal sinus fistulas.[49] Awad et al found an aggressive neurological course to be most often associated with lesions involving the tentorial incisura.[50] Cognard et al demonstrated a significant relationship between anatomic location and the aggressiveness of symptomatology.[48] An aggressive clinical course was associated with lesions involving the torcula (100%), tentorium (92%), and anterior skull base (88%).[48] Patients with cavernous sinus fistulas did not develop aggressive symptoms, while fistulas of the transverse sinus followed an aggressive clinical course in 27% of cases. Lesion classification based on anatomic location can be misleading when attempting to predict the clinical course. Aggressive lesions have been observed in all possible anatomic locations.[49,50] The predilection for dAVFs of certain locations to behave more aggressively than others is likely due to the regional venous anatomy. Lesions of the anterior cranial fossa and tentorium are limited in venous outflow pathways, particularly in their access to dural venous sinuses. As a result, more often than not, venous drainage is "forced" to reflux into the cortical venous system.[49,52] This phenomenon is clearly depicted in the Cognard series, where all fistulas of the tentorium and anterior cranial fossa demonstrated cortical venous drainage (type III, IV, or V).[48] Conversely, 28% of the transverse sinus and 12% of the cavernous sinus fistulas displayed cortical venous drainage.

12.5 Classification of DAVFs of Specific Anatomic Locations

12.5.1 Carotid-Cavernous Fistula Classification

The previously discussed classification schemes of dAVFs include CCFs and provide sufficient criteria by which to classify these lesions. However, due to their unique location and relationship to the venous drainage of the orbit, CCFs may present with unique symptoms. Furthermore, the potential for these fistulas to receive arterial supply from the internal carotid artery, as well as the external carotid artery, identifies these lesions as a distinct and often complex clinical entity. Barrow et al published the most comprehensive and clinically useful classification system for CCFs in 1985 based on findings in 14 patients.[53] The Barrow classification system represents the most widely used system in practice and classifies CCFs based on the angioarchitecture of the lesion. The system accounts for all of the additional variables by which these lesions can be subdivided: spontaneous versus traumatic, high-flow versus low-flow, and angiographically direct versus indirect.

Type A fistulas represent a direct fistulous connection between a defect in the wall of the cavernous segment of the internal carotid artery and the cavernous sinus. The defect may be caused by the rupture of a cavernous carotid aneurysm (spontaneous) or, more commonly, by a traumatic tear in the arterial wall secondary to a blunt or penetrating head injury. These fistulas are the only high-flow and high-pressure lesions in the classification due to the direct connection between artery and sinus. All other fistulas are low flow secondary to their indirect fistulous connections with internal and external branches. Type B CCFs are indirect fistulas between the internal carotid artery meningeal branches and the cavernous sinus. Type C CCFs are the result of fistulous connections between the meningeal branches of the external carotid artery and the cavernous sinus. Type D fistulas exist between branches of the internal and external carotid arteries and the cavernous sinus.

Type A fistulas rarely undergo spontaneous resolution secondary to the high-flow and high-pressure nature of the fistulous connection. When left untreated, a majority of patients will develop progressive visual loss and aggressive neurologic symptoms. Low-flow CCFs often resolve spontaneously, with an incidence of 10 to 60% in the literature.[54,55,56,57,58] Thirty-six percent of low-flow fistulas in the Barrow publication resolved spontaneously.[53] Thus, in the absence of significant neurologic symptoms and visual deterioration, these lesions can initially be managed conservatively. Concerning angiographic features, such as cortical venous reflux, represent an indication for treatment because of the increased likelihood of intracranial hemorrhage.

12.5.2 Hypoglossal Canal dAVFs

Hypoglossal canal dAVFs (HCDAVFs) involve the anterior condylar venous confluence (ACC) and/or the anterior condylar vein (ACV) and are commonly fed by the neuromeningeal branch of the ascending pharyngeal artery.[59] These lesions account for approximately 3.6 to 4.2% of dAVFs, and exhibit complex patterns of venous drainage.[60,61] The communication of the ACC and ACV with the venous drainage of the orbit, posterior fossa sinuses, and vertebral venous plexuses results in the wide range of symptoms associated with these lesions. Spittau and colleagues provided the most clinically useful classification based on the pattern of venous drainage.[59] Type I fistulas demonstrate dominant venous drainage to the internal jugular vein and/or the vertebral venous plexus with or without reflux to the sigmoid, transverse, inferior petrosal, or cavernous sinuses. Type II lesions have dominant retrograde drainage to the cavernous sinus and/or orbital veins with or without anterograde drainage to the internal jugular vein and/or the vertebral venous plexus or cortical venous reflux. Type III fistulas exhibit dominant/exclusive drainage to cerebellar pial or perimedullary veins (cortical venous drainage).[59] A total of 75% of all HCDAVFs presented with pulse-synchronous tinnitus and was frequently the only symptom at presentation at type I lesions. A total of 30.8% of fistulas presented with orbital symptoms referable to reflux into the cavernous sinus. Hypoglossal nerve palsy only occurred with type I fistulas. Only 5% of HCDAVFs presented with intracranial hemorrhage, all of which were type III lesions. Cervical myelopathy was most commonly found in type III fistulas.

12.6 Conclusion

The number and complexity of the classification systems used to describe intracranial AVMs and dAVFs is a testament to the difficulty with which these lesions are managed. Variability in the anatomic location of occurrence, individual lesion angioarchitecture, and presenting symptomatology make accurate classification of lesions a vital step in preparing a treatment plan. The classification systems discussed here simplify these lesions by selecting the key features that are most likely to influence a particular mode of intervention.

References

[1] Speizler RF, Martin NA. A proposed grading system for arteriovenous malformations. 1986. J Neurosurg. 2008; 108(1):186–193

[2] Hamilton MG, Spetzler RF. The prospective application of a grading system for arteriovenous malformations. Neurosurgery. 1994; 34(1):2–6, discussion 6–7

[3] Heros RC, Korosue K, Diebold PM. Surgical excision of cerebral arteriovenous malformations: late results. Neurosurgery. 1990; 26(4):570–577, discussion 577–578

[4] de Oliveira E, Tedeschi H, Raso J. Comprehensive management of arteriovenous malformations. Neurol Res. 1998; 20(8):673–683

[5] Lawton MT, Project UBAMS, UCSF Brain Arteriovenous Malformation Study Project. Spetzler-Martin Grade III arteriovenous malformations: surgical results and a modification of the grading scale. Neurosurgery. 2003; 52(4): 740–748, discussion 748–749

[6] Lawton MT, Kim H, McCulloch CE, Mikhak B, Young WL. A supplementary grading scale for selecting patients with brain arteriovenous malformations for surgery. Neurosurgery. 2010; 66(4):702–713, discussion 713

[7] Lawton MT, Du R, Tran MN, et al. Effect of presenting hemorrhage on outcome after microsurgical resection of brain arteriovenous malformations. Neurosurgery. 2005; 56(3):485–493, discussion 485–493

[8] Dawson RC , III, Tarr RW, Hecht ST, et al. Treatment of arteriovenous malformations of the brain with combined embolization and stereotactic radiosurgery: results after 1 and 2 years. AJNR Am J Neuroradiol. 1990; 11(5):857–864

[9] Mathis JA, Barr JD, Horton JA, et al. The efficacy of particulate embolization combined with stereotactic radiosurgery for treatment of large arteriovenous malformations of the brain. AJNR Am J Neuroradiol. 1995; 16(2):299–306

[10] Gobin YP, Laurent A, Merienne L, et al. Treatment of brain arteriovenous malformations by embolization and radiosurgery. J Neurosurg. 1996; 85(1): 19–28

[11] Debrun GM, Aletich V, Ausman JI, Charbel F, Dujovny M. Embolization of the nidus of brain arteriovenous malformations with n-butyl cyanoacrylate. Neurosurgery. 1997; 40(1):112–120, discussion 120–121

[12] Han PP, Ponce FA, Spetzler RF. Intention-to-treat analysis of Spetzler-Martin grades IV and V arteriovenous malformations: natural history and treatment paradigm. J Neurosurg. 2003; 98(1):3–7

[13] van Beijnum J, van der Worp HB, Buis DR, et al. Treatment of brain arteriovenous malformations: a systematic review and meta-analysis. JAMA. 2011; 306(18):2011–2019

[14] Hartmann A, Pile-Spellman J, Stapf C, et al. Risk of endovascular treatment of brain arteriovenous malformations. Stroke. 2002; 33(7):1816–1820

[15] Viñuela F, Dion JE, Duckwiler G, et al. Combined endovascular embolization and surgery in the management of cerebral arteriovenous malformations: experience with 101 cases. J Neurosurg. 1991; 75(6):856–864

[16] Haw CS, terBrugge K, Willinsky R, Tomlinson G. Complications of embolization of arteriovenous malformations of the brain. J Neurosurg. 2006; 104(2): 226–232

[17] Kim LJ, Albuquerque FC, Spetzler RF, McDougall CG. Postembolization neurological deficits in cerebral arteriovenous malformations: stratification by arteriovenous malformation grade. Neurosurgery. 2006; 59(1):53–59, discussion 53–59

[18] Dumont TM, Kan P, Snyder KV, Hopkins LN, Siddiqui AH, Levy EI. A proposed grading system for endovascular treatment of cerebral arteriovenous malformations: Buffalo score. Surg Neurol Int. 2015; 6:3

[19] Pollock BE, Flickinger JC. A proposed radiosurgery-based grading system for arteriovenous malformations. J Neurosurg. 2002; 96(1):79–85

[20] Colombo F, Pozza F, Chierego G, Casentini L, De Luca G, Francescon P. Linear accelerator radiosurgery of cerebral arteriovenous malformations: an update. Neurosurgery. 1994; 34(1):14–20, discussion 20–21

[21] Friedman WA, Bova FJ, Mendenhall WM. Linear accelerator radiosurgery for arteriovenous malformations: the relationship of size to outcome. J Neurosurg. 1995; 82(2):180–189

[22] Lunsford LD, Kondziolka D, Flickinger JC, et al. Stereotactic radiosurgery for arteriovenous malformations of the brain. J Neurosurg. 1991; 75(4):512–524

[23] Miyawaki L, Dowd C, Wara W, et al. Five year results of LINAC radiosurgery for arteriovenous malformations: outcome for large AVMS. Int J Radiat Oncol Biol Phys. 1999; 44(5):1089–1106

[24] Pollock BE, Flickinger JC, Lunsford LD, Maitz A, Kondziolka D. Factors associated with successful arteriovenous malformation radiosurgery. Neurosurgery. 1998; 42(6):1239–1244, discussion 1244–1247

[25] Schlienger M, Atlan D, Lefkopoulos D, et al. Linac radiosurgery for cerebral arteriovenous malformations: results in 169 patients. Int J Radiat Oncol Biol Phys. 2000; 46(5):1135–1142

[26] Steiner L, Lindquist C, Adler JR, Torner JC, Alves W, Steiner M. Clinical outcome of radiosurgery for cerebral arteriovenous malformations. J Neurosurg. 1992; 77(1):1–8

[27] Yamamoto Y, Coffey RJ, Nichols DA, Shaw EG. Interim report on the radiosurgical treatment of cerebral arteriovenous malformations. The influence of size, dose, time, and technical factors on obliteration rate. J Neurosurg. 1995; 83(5):832–837

[28] Meder JF, Oppenheim C, Blustajn J, et al. Cerebral arteriovenous malformations: the value of radiologic parameters in predicting response to radiosurgery. AJNR Am J Neuroradiol. 1997; 18(8):1473–1483

[29] Andrade-Souza YM, Zadeh G, Ramani M, Scora D, Tsao MN, Schwartz ML. Testing the radiosurgery-based arteriovenous malformation score and the modified Spetzler-Martin grading system to predict radiosurgical outcome. J Neurosurg. 2005; 103(4):642–648

[30] Andrade-Souza YM, Zadeh G, Scora D, Tsao MN, Schwartz ML. Radiosurgery for basal ganglia, internal capsule, and thalamus arteriovenous malformation: clinical outcome. Neurosurgery. 2005; 56(1):56–63, discussion 63–64

[31] Zabel-du Bois A, Milker-Zabel S, Huber P, Schlegel W, Debus J. Stereotactic linac-based radiosurgery in the treatment of cerebral arteriovenous malformations located deep, involving corpus callosum, motor cortex, or brainstem. Int J Radiat Oncol Biol Phys. 2006; 64(4):1044–1048

[32] Zabel-du Bois A, Milker-Zabel S, Huber P, Schlegel W, Debus J. Pediatric cerebral arteriovenous malformations: the role of stereotactic linac-based radiosurgery. Int J Radiat Oncol Biol Phys. 2006; 65(4):1206–1211

[33] Pollock BE, Flickinger JC. Modification of the radiosurgery-based arteriovenous malformation grading system. Neurosurgery. 2008; 63(2):239–243, discussion 243

[34] Djindjian R. Super-selective arteriography of branches of the external carotid artery. Surg Neurol. 1976; 5(3):133–142

[35] Djindjian R, Merland, JJ. Superselective arteriography of the external carotid artery. New York, NY: Springer-Verlag; 1977:606–628

[36] Borden JA, Wu JK, Shucart WA. A proposed classification for spinal and cranial dural arteriovenous fistulous malformations and implications for treatment. J Neurosurg. 1995; 82(2):166–179

[37] Lalwani AK, Dowd CF, Halbach VV. Grading venous restrictive disease in patients with dural arteriovenous fistulas of the transverse/sigmoid sinus. J Neurosurg. 1993; 79(1):11–15

[38] Viñuela F, Fox AJ, Debrun GM, Peerless SJ, Drake CG. Spontaneous carotid-cavernous fistulas: clinical, radiological, and therapeutic considerations. Experience with 20 cases. J Neurosurg. 1984; 60(5):976–984

[39] Viñuela F, Fox AJ, Pelz DM, Drake CG. Unusual clinical manifestations of dural arteriovenous malformations. J Neurosurg. 1986; 64(4):554–558

[40] Cahan LD, Higashida RT, Halbach VV, Hieshima GB. Variants of radiculomeningeal vascular malformations of the spine. J Neurosurg. 1987; 66(3):333–337

[41] Pia, HW, Djindjian, R. Spinal Angiomas. Advances in Diagnosis and Therapy. 1st ed. Berlin: Springer-Verlag; 1978

[42] Gobin YP, Rogopoulos A, Aymard A, et al. Endovascular treatment of intracranial dural arteriovenous fistulas with spinal perimedullary venous drainage. J Neurosurg. 1992; 77(5):718–723

[43] Partington MD, Rüfenacht DA, Marsh WR, Piepgras DG. Cranial and sacral dural arteriovenous fistulas as a cause of myelopathy. J Neurosurg. 1992; 76(4): 615–622

[44] Pierot L, Chiras J, Meder JF, Rose M, Rivierez M, Marsault C. Dural arteriovenous fistulas of the posterior fossa draining into subarachnoid veins. AJNR Am J Neuroradiol. 1992; 13(1):315–323

[45] Wrobel CJ, Oldfield EH, Di Chiro G, Tarlov EC, Baker RA, Doppman JL. Myelopathy due to intracranial dural arteriovenous fistulas draining intrathecally into spinal medullary veins. Report of three cases. J Neurosurg. 1988; 69(6): 934–939

[46] Di Chiro G, Doppman JL. Endocranial drainage of spinal cord veins. Radiology. 1970; 95(3):555–560

[47] Djindjian R, Hurth M, Thurel C. Cervico-cranial phlebography of angiomas of the spinal cord. Neuroradiology. 1970; 1(1):42–46

[48] Cognard C, Gobin YP, Pierot L, et al. Cerebral dural arteriovenous fistulas: clinical and angiographic correlation with a revised classification of venous drainage. Radiology. 1995; 194(3):671–680

[49] Davies MA, TerBrugge K, Willinsky R, Coyne T, Saleh J, Wallace MC. The validity of classification for the clinical presentation of intracranial dural arteriovenous fistulas. J Neurosurg. 1996; 85(5):830–837

[50] Awad IA, Little JR, Akarawi WP, Ahl J. Intracranial dural arteriovenous malformations: factors predisposing to an aggressive neurological course. J Neurosurg. 1990; 72(6):839–850

[51] Aminoff MJ. Vascular anomalies in the intracranial dura mater. Brain. 1973; 96(3):601–612

[52] Malik GM, Pearce JE, Ausman JI, Mehta B. Dural arteriovenous malformations and intracranial hemorrhage. Neurosurgery. 1984; 15(3):332–339

[53] Barrow DL, Spector RH, Braun IF, Landman JA, Tindall SC, Tindall GT. Classification and treatment of spontaneous carotid-cavernous sinus fistulas. J Neurosurg. 1985; 62(2):248–256

[54] Bitoh S, Hasegawa H, Fujiwara M, Nakata M, Sakaki S. Spontaneous carotid-cavernous fistulas. Neurol Med Chir (Tokyo). 1981; 21(7):757–764

[55] Shields CB, Tutt HP. Spontaneous obliteration of carotid-cavernous fistulas. South Med J. 1981; 74(5):617–620

[56] Peeters FL, Kröger R. Dural and direct cavernous sinus fistulas. AJR Am J Roentgenol. 1979; 132(4):599–606

[57] Slusher MM, Lennington BR, Weaver RG, Davis CH , Jr. Ophthalmic findings in dural arteriovenous shunts. Ophthalmology. 1979; 86(5):720–731

[58] Voigt K, Sauer M, Dichgans J. Spontaneous occlusion of a bilateral caroticocavernous fistula studied by serial angiography. Neuroradiology. 1971; 2(4): 207–211

[59] Spittau B, Millán DS, El-Sherifi S, et al. Dural arteriovenous fistulas of the hypoglossal canal: systematic review on imaging anatomy, clinical findings, and endovascular management. J Neurosurg. 2015; 122(4):883–903

[60] Choi JW, Kim BM, Kim DJ, et al. Hypoglossal canal dural arteriovenous fistula: incidence and the relationship between symptoms and drainage pattern. J Neurosurg. 2013; 119(4):955–960

[61] Manabe S, Satoh K, Matsubara S, Satomi J, Hanaoka M, Nagahiro S. Characteristics, diagnosis and treatment of hypoglossal canal dural arteriovenous fistula: report of nine cases. Neuroradiology. 2008; 50(8):715–721

13 Step-by-Step Microsurgical Resection of Arteriovenous Malformations

Benjamin K. Hendricks and Aaron Cohen-Gadol

Abstract

Cerebral arteriovenous malformations (AVMs) represent a highly morbid and formidable neurosurgical challenge. Cerebral AVMs are managed with a unimodal or multimodal strategy, including microsurgical resection, stereotactic radiosurgery, and/or endovascular embolization. Microsurgical resection of these lesions is the most definitive strategy for occlusion but requires immense surgical prowess and endurance. The general principles for AVM microsurgical resection begin with an intimate understanding of the three-dimensional angioarchitecture involved. This serves as a basis for preoperative surgical planning and determination of appropriate endovascular preoperative interventions. The next fundamental step involves a surgical approach with a wide operative field providing optimal working angles for the nidal disconnection, and unanticipated maneuvers are potentially necessary if complications are encountered. Feeding arteries must then be sequentially dissected, occluded, and disconnected from the nidus. Identifying and disconnecting the arterial feeding vessels involves perinidal circumdissection with immense importance reliant on preserving the dominant draining veins. Following circumdissection and occlusion of the feeding arteries, the dominant draining veins are disconnected to complete the nidal resection. These lesions provide an immense surgical challenge hindering intraoperative efficiency. Therefore, the surgeon must have knowledge of time-saving and decision-making maneuvers to provide an efficient strategy for the resection. This chapter highlights the details and nuances of these fundamental steps for successful AVM microsurgical management, which are applicable to all cerebral AVMs.

Keywords: microsurgical, dissection, angioarchitecture, nidus, circumdissection, efficiency, fundamental, craniotomy

Key Points

- Understand the unique three-dimensional anatomic distribution of the arteriovenous malformation prior to attempting excision.
- Plan a generous exposure utilizing wide arachnoid dissection and gravity retraction to facilitate optimal working angles for the more tedious steps of excision.
- Feeding arteries must be located and appropriately sacrificed using microclips, bipolar cautery, or both.
- The exposure of the arteriovenous malformation nidus should proceed in a circumferential manner until the apex is visible, augmented by intraoperative navigation to ensure correct pial incision and transparenchymal trajectory.
- The surgeon must protect the dominant draining vein until the feeding arteries are sacrificed; if the vein is injured prior to sacrifice of the feeding arteries, the surgeon must control the venous bleeding without occluding the vein and focus on eliminating the feeding arteries.
- Timely removal of the arteriovenous malformation is the best method to control the bleeding.

13.1 Introduction

Arteriovenous malformations (AVMs) are an aberrant dysplastic connection between arteries and veins without intervening capillaries, which form a nidus and facilitate high-flow arteriovenous shunting. AVMs are an important cause of morbidity and mortality among neurosurgical patients and most commonly present with hemorrhage and less frequently with refractory seizures, chronic headaches, or focal neurologic deficits.[1] The average annual risk for AVM rupture is 2.2% per year and increases to 4.5% per year for rerupture.[2] The risk is increased with identification of an intranidal aneurysm(s) and for deep parenchymal AVMs.[2] With the increased utilization of magnetic resonance imaging (MRI) evaluation of the brain for unrelated reasons, AVMs are increasingly identified incidentally. Therefore, neurosurgeons must be aware of the indications for therapy and selection of an appropriate mode of treatment.

Management options for cerebral AVMs include microsurgical excision, angiographic embolization, and stereotactic radiosurgery, or a combination approach.[3,4,5,6,7] Goals for successful intervention for AVMs include prevention of (re)hemorrhage, hinder progression of mass effect–induced preintervention neurologic deficits, and/or provide seizure control. Large and/or complex lesions are often best managed with observation,[8,9] but large malformations can be made more amendable to radiotherapy or microsurgical excision by the use of preoperative embolization. The Spetzler–Martin grading scale has been adopted to guide recommendations for surgical management of AVMs, based on predicting prognosis from nidus size, eloquence of adjacent parenchyma, and the venous drainage pattern.[10] The grading system can be utilized to optimize the recommendation for microsurgical management based on characteristics of the AVM predictive of morbidity.[10,11]

In decisions regarding the use of radiosurgery, the Pollock–Flickinger score can be utilized to predict patient outcomes.[12] Endovascular embolization as a stand-alone technique for AVM obliteration is rarely utilized and generally reserved for small single pedicle AVMs, although with the advance of endovascular instrumentation and use of Onyx embolization medium, the stand-alone use of this modality is being studied for more complex lesions to determine its future applicability.[13,14,15] Embolization is more commonly utilized to devascularize feeders that will be difficult to surgically access, followed by definitive microsurgical excision.

13.2 Materials and Methods

This step-by-step approach to the microsurgical management of AVMs is based on literature review of foundational books discussing the principles of AVM operative management, primary clinical research articles describing the recent trends in management practices, and personal surgical experience.

13.3 Results

Successful AVM excision requires meticulous perioperative planning and diagnostic evaluation. A complete history and neurologic exam should be performed, followed by a thorough radiographic evaluation including computed tomography (CT), MRI, and catheter angiogram evaluation (▶ Fig. 13.1). Out of these modalities, the catheter angiogram provides the most valuable information regarding nidus hemodynamics and angioarchitecture. The patient's unique AVM should be scored based on the scoring scales discussed in the introduction to appropriately recommend the optimal modality for therapy. The remaining discussion within this section will guide the reader through the technical principles for microsurgical AVM excision.

Routine preoperative arterial pedicle embolization for augmentation of feeder devascularization can be performed based on surgeon preference. We believe aggressive overembolization of cortical pedicles, which are commonly targeted endovascularly, may result in an increase in the flow within parenchymal white matter perforators (▶ Fig. 13.2). This anomaly is likely explained on the principle that a cerebral AVM will endure and facilitate continued arteriovenous shunting, because of the AVM serving as the path of least resistance for any sources of hemodynamic flow. The enhanced flow through deep parenchymal feeders poses a greater intraoperative risk for hemorrhage during disconnection and these feeders are commonly inaccessible for embolization. Therefore, selective embolization of those feeders that are relatively inaccessible early in microsurgical dissection is reasonable. A preoperative discussion between the microsurgeon and interventionalist is warranted before embolization is undertaken.

13.3.1 Patient Positioning

Patient positioning begins with attention toward head position, which should involve consideration of cranial venous return and the anticipated operative corridor. The patient's head should be kept above the level of the heart, with the neck in slight extension, and avoiding severe unilateral rotation at the neck. These measures prevent intracranial venous hypertension, which is particularly important to avoid in the setting of AVM surgery. When planning patient positioning concerning the operative trajectory, the need for optimal working angles, maximizing exposure of feeding arteries, and minimizing risk to the major draining veins should be considered. The high risk for intraoperative bleeding and unique technical challenges associated with AVM surgery necessitate a generous operative corridor that provides numerous and flexible working angles to efficiently manage subcortical bleeding.

The major pitfalls encountered with patient positioning include failure to maximize gravity retraction and forgoing the use of free surfaces while attempting to access the lesion. The failure to maximize gravity retraction on the brain results in the need for use of aggressive fixed retraction, which increases cortical injury risk and, potentially, morbidity.

13.3.2 Craniotomy

Following appropriate patient positioning, the craniotomy can be planned with the assistance of neuronavigation based on MRI or preferably CT angiogram (CTA) data. The goal is to achieve a wide craniotomy with exposure of the AVM nidus, feeding arteries, draining veins, and a small region of normal parenchyma surrounding the AVM (▶ Fig. 13.3). Craniotomies

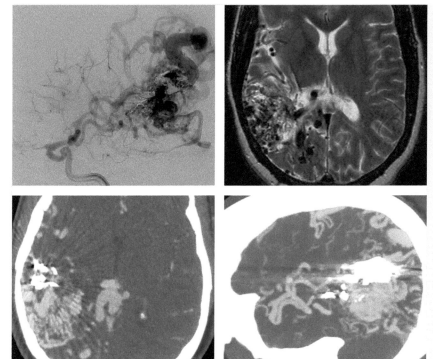

Fig. 13.1 Illustrative case demonstrating a large right-sided temporoparietal convexity AVM. Left upper is a lateral internal carotid artery (ICA) arteriogram demonstrating the primary feeding arteries coursing along the anterior pole of the nidus and derive from middle cerebral artery (MCA) branches. The primary draining vein is observed superoposteriorly along the nidus. The superior and posterior margins of the nidus are obscured by the presence of embolic material. Right upper is an MR image providing proximity information of the nidus relative to the adjacent ventricle and eloquent cortex, and discloses the presence of parenchymal feeders in at the ventricular trigone. Lower left and right are CTA images providing enhanced vascular anatomy relative to the surrounding parenchyma and cranium.

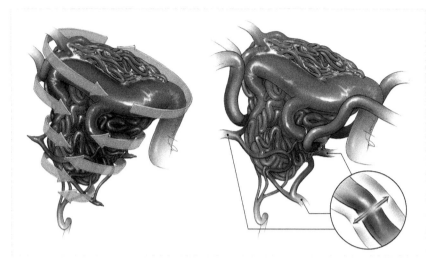

Fig. 13.2 Surgeon preference dictates use of preoperative arterial pedicle embolization. By endovascularly obliterating the major cortical pedicles, increased flow within parenchymal perforators is encouraged due to being the path of least resistance for hemodynamic flow. This enhanced flow increases the risk of hemorrhage from these vessels, which already pose a significant surgical challenge.

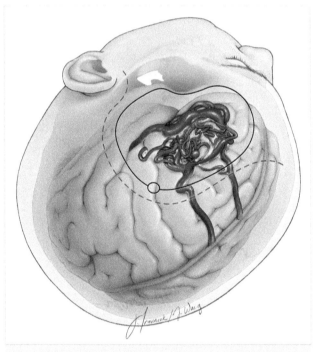

Fig. 13.3 Optimal head positioning, incision, and craniotomy are illustrated for a left frontal AVM. This craniotomy has been performed in a liberal manner to permit a generous durotomy and exposure of normal perinidal parenchyma. The craniotomy outline also demonstrates the utility of a wide craniotomy in avoiding inadvertent nidus transgression during drilling. Injury to a primary draining vein during this stage of the operation can be disastrous due to the difficulty in controlling the bleeding without completely occluding the vein.

and opening of cerebrospinal fluid (CSF) cisterns. If this is impractical, such as in the case of an interhemispheric craniotomy, a lumbar drain can be used to gradually drain CSF during the craniotomy, providing relaxation during parenchymal manipulation.

It is paramount to avoid penetrating the dura while drilling to create the craniotomy; therefore, a greater number of burr holes as well as making short passes with the craniotome decreases the risk for injury to the underlying engorged draining veins. The avoidance of this complication can be challenging because the draining veins within the dural leaves can often be large enough to erode the inner table of the calvarium. This complication can also be avoided by use of lumbar CSF drainage to facilitate thorough dissection of the decompressed dura away from the inner calvarial table before the footplate is employed.

13.3.3 General Steps and Nuances of Technique in AVM Resection

The universal mandatory steps for microsurgical excision of every AVM should be adhered to for each lesion. Violating any of these principles or their specific order increases the risk for adverse outcomes or complications.

Step 1: Three-Dimensional Understanding of the Malformation

Careful analysis of each sequence of the MRI, CTA, and preoperative angiogram should be undertaken, and planning of a well-thought-out strategy for approach undertaken. MRI is particularly helpful to map the functional cortices and their anatomical relationship to the nidus and the hematoma if the patient has suffered from a hemorrhage preoperatively. Distinction between feeding vessel aneurysms and nidal aneurysms should be made at this step in the operation. CTA should be used for intraoperative navigation due to its ability to provide a high-resolution depiction of the vascular anatomy in relation to adjacent parenchymal landmarks. The main draining veins and embolization material are useful as superficial landmarks to transpose the preoperative angiogram onto the operative field, which can be quite challenging with complex AVMs.

for AVMs should be made generously and not adherent to principles of minimally invasive surgery. The large craniotomy will permit optimal management of unforeseen bleeding, at which time it would not be feasible to enlarge the craniotomy timely for improved exposure.

To permit ideal manipulation of the nidus and parenchyma, the craniotomy can also be planned to provide early exposure

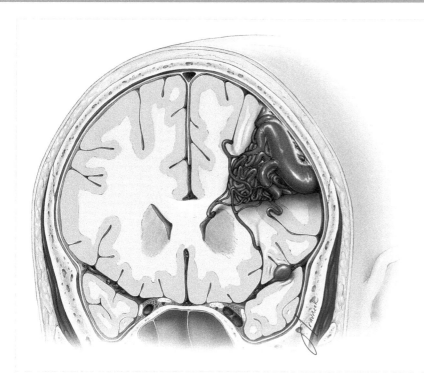

Fig. 13.4 Common depth of nidus angioarchitecture for a superficial convexity AVM is illustrated. The role the perinidal sulci have in hiding the feeding arteries is illustrated. This nidus also demonstrates how the primary draining vein can intermingle with the other cerebrovascular components of the aneurysm in the deeper segments near the apex necessitating a meticulous descent during dissection to avoid injuring this critical structure. Deep parenchymal arterial feeders are illustrated and highlight the challenge encountered by these structures due to their anatomical complexity and potential for significant hemorrhage.

It is imperative to thoroughly understand and "memorize" the location, morphology, and serpentigenous routes demonstrated by the angioarchitecture. Feeding arteries can be identified by the surface landmarks, large draining veins, and embolic material. The location of the main marginal feeding arteries should serve as the target for the initial dissection and disconnection. These large feeding arteries can nest themselves within the sulci surrounding the AVM, requiring meticulous subarachnoid dissection to expose the vessels. Preoperative identification of these vessels enhances the efficiency of the disconnection (▶ Fig. 13.4). Large deep white matter feeders should also be identified using CTA prior to nidus dissection to appropriately plan for adequate hemostatic maneuvers. These vessels lack the durability of the tunica media demonstrated in the superficial feeding vessels of the AVM, enhancing their friability and risk for hemorrhage when manipulated intraoperatively.[8]

If the AVM has ruptured preoperatively, the border of the AVM that was breached is targeted first to decompress the hematoma cavity and relax the brain. The border of the AVM that faces eloquent cortex should be targeted last, following disconnection of the majority of the AVM, so as to permit minimal manipulation of the adjacent parenchyma. These key areas of the AVM should be mentally outlined and a sequential disconnection plan devised prior to beginning the procedure.

Step 2: Creation of a Generous Exposure and Preparation for Disconnection

The principles discussed in the introduction regarding patient positioning should be followed to permit flexible working angles. Gravity retraction can be achieved through proper patient positioning to optimize the exposure of the AVM. This goal must be anticipated when initially positioning the patient for surgery so as to avoid manipulating the patient's head once the operation has begun.

The craniotomy principles discussed in the introduction should also be followed to provide a generous exposure of each arterial feeder and all the draining veins. Do *not* plan the size of the craniotomy according to the size of the angiographic nidus of the AVM alone but rather plan the size of the craniotomy to maximize the perinidal exposure. The dura should be opened widely with the goal of exposing normal parenchyma surrounding all sides of the AVM. In the setting of a previous hemorrhage, the process of turning the dural flap must be performed meticulously due to the heightened risk of adherent scarring between dura and an underlying pial vessel within the AVM. It is imperative to avoid early tearing of major draining veins because of the risk for occluding the veins when attempting to achieve hemostasis early in the dissection.

The surgeon must anticipate challenging dissection planes where deep white matter perforators can generate torrential bleeding that is difficult to control. In these locations, it is advisable to provide adequate space and ergonomic working angles to handle the tough moments during disconnection of the deep white matter feeders.

Step 3: Managing the Feeding Arteries

Following the creation of a wide dural exposure, the fissures and sulci adjacent to the AVM should be opened to identify the feeding arteries. Exposure of the feeding vessels often requires meticulous subarachnoid dissection, particularly overlying the AVM, because of the presence of thickened arachnoid bands. For this tedious task, jewelers' forceps can be used to grasp the margins of the arachnoid bands and tear/remove the thickened arachnoid layers to unveil the feeding arteries (▶ Fig. 13.5). It is imperative that during this step the draining veins are protected and not transgressed because managing hemorrhage from these vessels early in the dissection is difficult.

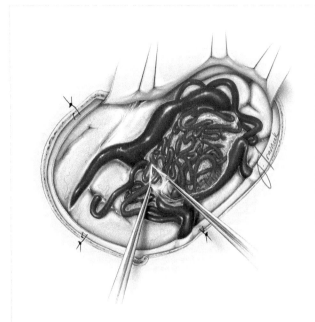

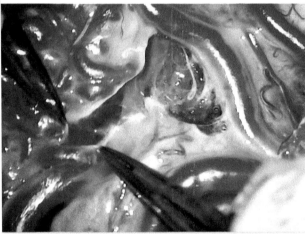

Fig. 13.5 The arachnoid dissection required to expose the feeding vessels is a test of the surgeon's endurance and patience. Dense arachnoid adhesions commonly overly the AVM and necessitate a meticulous technique of disconnection to avoid tearing the underlying vasculature. Use of jewelers' forceps is illustrated. The distinction between feeding arteries and draining veins at this stage should be attempted based on coloration but can be challenging due to the significant amount of arteriovenous shunting.

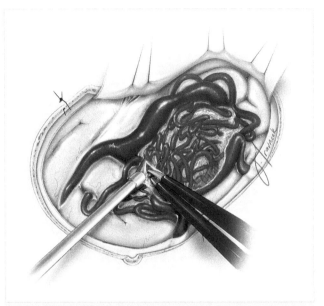

Fig. 13.6 Bipolar cautery is an effective method to achieve coagulation of the small- and medium-sized pial and cortical feeding arteries. The more robust tunica media of these vessels permits more rapid disconnection of these feeding arteries compared to the tenuous disconnection of deep parenchymal perforators. Despite the comparative ease of disconnecting the pial and cortical feeding arteries with bipolar coagulation, the surgeon must remain vigilant to protect en passage vessels along the cortical surface.

If early recognition of the contribution of a vein or an artery is imperative for assigning the steps of disconnection, a temporary occlusion trial of the feeding artery or draining vein can be performed. This technique is referred to as the temporary occlusion test, and is performed by gently squeezing the vessel using a pair of forceps or a temporary aneurysm clip. If the temporary occlusion results in engorgement of the AVM, the occluded vessel is predicted to be an important draining vein and should be kept intact until the end of AVM disconnection. If temporary occlusion of the vessel in question results in an increased bluish hue of the AVM, then the vessel is predicted to be an arterial feeder, although this generally is only observed when all arterial feeders have been occluded/disconnected.

Alternatively, intraoperative fluorescence angiography (FLOW800, Zeiss Meditech, Oberkochen, Germany) can also be effective in demonstrating the timing and velocity of vascular flow, which can help in distinguishing if the vessel contributes to the AVM and if it is a feeding artery versus a draining vein. There can be segments of the angioarchitecture that complicate differentiation between being arterial versus being venous because of the high-flow arterialization of the shunting veins. Differentiation of the vessels becomes more apparent in the end stages of AVM disconnection because of decreased shunting through arterialized veins resulting in return of the blue hue of the vessel, revealing its identity.

Localizing deep feeding arterial vessels for subcortical AVMs can be more challenging because of the lack of direct visualization. A draining vein at the surface may herald the path to a deep lesion without any surface presentation. Other subcortical AVMs may require localization using subtler surface cues such as superficial cortical arterialized veins or mildly dilated arterial feeders. These vessels can be traced down into the sulcus and ultimately to the AVM nidus.

The initial disconnection of the AVM should include small and medium cortical and pial feeding arteries which are amendable to coagulation. These thicker walled vessels do not possess the risk for uncontrollable hemorrhage that is demonstrated by subcortical deep white matter perforators. Therefore, the thicker walled cortical vessels should be efficiently disconnected from the nidus (▸ Fig. 13.6). Particularly large feeding arteries should be disconnected by first applying microclips to occlude the vessel lumen and then generously applying bipolar coagulation to proximal and distal segments of the vessel relative to the clip. Then, the vessel can be sharply sacrificed. While

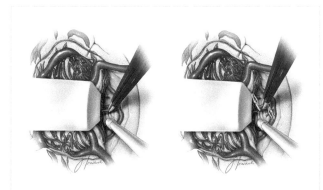

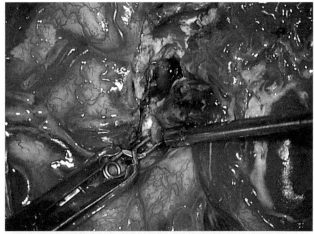

Fig. 13.7 Larger cortical and pial feeding arteries may be more appropriately disconnected with application of microclips followed by proximal and distal bipolar coagulation, and finally sharp disconnection. For these larger caliber arteries, bipolar coagulation alone may not be sufficient to occlude the lumen and facilitate coagulation.

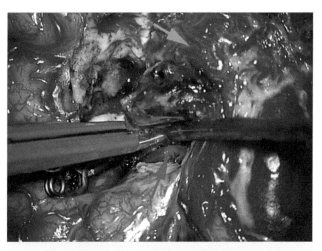

Fig. 13.8 Identification of en passage vessels (*black arrow*) can be challenging and requires vigilance by the surgeon. The characteristic appearance of normal cortical cerebrovasculature should be demonstrated by the en passage vessels, which can be differentiated from the serpentigenous and dilated appearance of the feeding arteries (*green arrow*).

performing the disconnection along the cortical and pial surfaces, the surgeon should be vigilant for the presence of en passage vessels (▶ Fig. 13.7). Differentiation of these vessels is often evident through the difference in configuration. The feeding arteries are often serpentigenous and distended, whereas en passage arteries appear as normal superficial cortical vessels (▶ Fig. 13.8). The en passage vessels should be preserved to avoid postoperative ischemic neurologic deficits.

The disconnection of small-caliber deep white matter parenchymal perforators that feed the AVM should be approached with an entirely different strategy. These vessels have a thin tunica media resulting in a limited presence of smooth muscle and elastic lamina.[8] This results in a less robust contraction of the lumen when exposed to a bipolar coagulation current.[8] Therefore, despite application of a seemingly sufficient coagulation current, these vessels may continue to bleed vigorously and recoil into the parenchyma, potentially resulting in occult intracerebral hemorrhage. The best strategy for disconnection of the deep parenchymal feeders involves removal of a small volume of white matter immediately surrounding the perforator to expose a more proximal segment of the vessel with relatively normal walls. Then, the surgeon can coagulate or clip-ligate the more native characterized vessel (▶ Fig. 13.9). One significant pitfall for perforator disconnection is in the setting of an underexposed

perforator that hemorrhages and the surgeon decides to pack the bleeding site with hemostatic material. The packing will provide the surgeon with a false sense of security regarding the acquisition of hemostasis and permits remote intracerebral hemorrhage with secondary cerebral herniation.

The angioarchitecture can dramatically change in the setting of preoperative radiosurgery, such that delicate parenchymal perforators transform into readily coagulable vessels. The parenchyma exposed to radiation will demonstrate gliosis, which can serve as a guide to localizing the thickened perforator vessels. This can permit a more efficient disconnection of parenchymal perforators.

Step 4: Strategic Circumdissection

Each AVM possesses its own unique angioarchitecture and marginal configuration. However, there are five key strategic steps for microdissection:
1. Subarachnoid/pial dissection.
2. Parenchymal dissection.
3. Ependymal dissection.
4. Inspection to ensure complete nidus disconnection.
5. Primary draining vein sacrifice permitting AVM removal.

Following initial cortical feeder disconnection, the dissection should proceed in a circumferential manner centered on the nidus progressing deeply until the nidus apex is exposed, which is generally near the periventricular ependyma (▶ Fig. 13.10). The surgeon should attempt to incorporate the native sulci and fissures into the initial circumdissection to minimize cortical gyrus transgression. During the descent to reach the apex of the nidus, the surgeon should always ensure the preservation of a wide surgical field. If hemorrhage is encountered in a suboptimally exposed surgical field during deep circumdissection, achieving hemostasis can be very challenging. The use of intraoperative CTA-based neuronavigation can assist in correct placement of the superficial pial incisions and ensure a correct

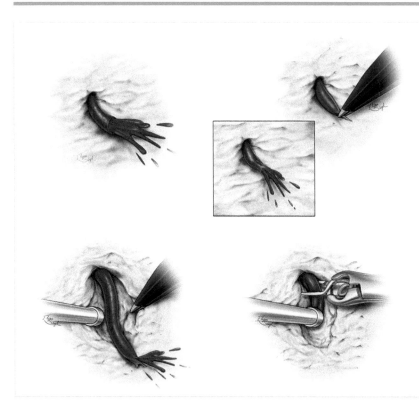

Fig. 13.9 Illustration of the challenge of coagulating a parenchymal perforator artery. Compared to the superficial cortical feeding arteries, these vessels demonstrate a smaller caliber and a less robust tunica media within the vascular wall. This histological difference results in less vasoconstriction in response to a bipolar current and subsequently these vessels can demonstrate persistent hemorrhage and retraction within the parenchyma. The left lower image illustrates the appropriate technique for coagulation of the parenchymal perforators, which first involves removal of a small volume of parenchyma adjacent to the vessel. The proximal segment of the vessel demonstrates a more native histology and therefore is more amendable to coagulation techniques, either bipolar coagulation or clip ligation.

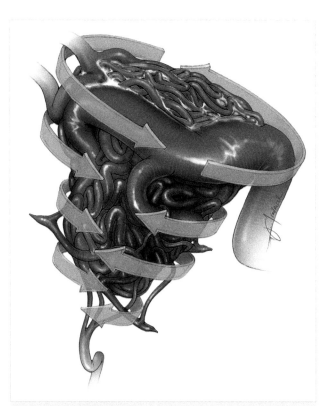

Fig. 13.10 The dissection of the nidus should proceed in a pattern of circumdissection beginning at the pial surface and terminating at the apex or periventricularly. The fissures and sulci within the superficial surface of the brain should be used to minimize parenchymal transgression and facilitate dissection planes.

trajectory of the deep parenchymal dissection particularly where the nidus margins are not readily apparent. The nidus should be localized and the dissection plane should be maintained outside its margins. Any transgression of the nidus should be strictly avoided during the descent to the apex.

Any coagulation of the nidus before its complete disconnection should be avoided because of the risk for hemorrhage. If a breach in the nidus wall is encountered as a result of transgressing the parenchyma too near the nidus lobules during deep circumdissection, the surgeon can place a small piece of thrombin-soaked cotton over the defect in the nidus. Gentle application of pressure on the cotton should tamponade the breach. Aggressive coagulation of the nidus in the setting of a breach should be avoided because of the resulting alteration in luminal hemodynamics that precipitates nidus rupture and secondary cerebral edema. The draining veins that wrap around the deeper sections of the nidus should also be protected.

Step 5: Protecting the Dominant Draining Vein(s)

Disconnecting the main draining vein(s) should be the last step of the operation, prior to removal of the nidus. These veins should be protected until all feeding arteries are disconnected from the nidus, at which point the veins become darker. This change should be observed by the surgeon prior to disconnecting the vein. If the surgeon is not sure of the change in color of the draining vein, a temporary clip test can be performed on the draining vein, observing for any enlargement of the nidus, which would signify the presence of residual feeding arteries (▶ Fig. 13.11). In the setting of residual arterial feeders, the

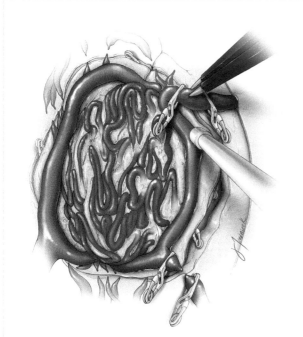

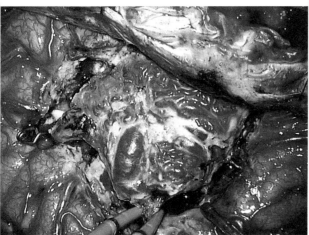

Fig. 13.11 The temporary occlusion test is a necessary step the surgeon must use prior to disconnecting any primary or secondary veins. If following occlusion of the vessel of interest the AVM appears to enlarge, the surgeon must pursue additional arterial feeder disconnection prior to transecting the vein.

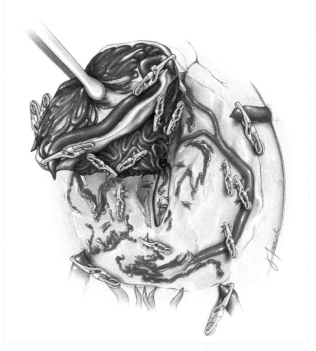

Fig. 13.12 Following test occlusion the primary draining veins are microclipped, bipolar coagulated, and sharply transected. In an attempt to avoid recurrence the excision bed should be examined for any remaining segments of the nidus and to achieve sufficient hemostasis. An en passage vessel along the right margin of the bed was preserved and can be visualized.

A major pitfall in AVM surgery is the management of inadvertent transgression of a main draining vein prior to isolating and disconnecting large feeding arteries. In this setting, the vein should not be occluded despite the risk for hemorrhage, because by occluding the vein there will be an acute rise in intranidal pressure that can precipitate AVM rupture and immediate cerebral edema.[16] The best strategy is to allow the vein to bleed while efficiently localizing and disconnecting the feeding arteries. In such a setting, a "commando" operation is necessary requiring the surgeon to remain calm, decisive, and in control.

Step 6: Efficient Excision of the AVM

The final steps of dissection for large AVMs should be expected to involve bleeding from the resection bed and the nidus. During these steps, it is important that the surgeon remain in control and focus on efficiently removing the AVM. At this stage of the operation, a timely excision is the best method to control hemorrhage. Following temporary clip test occlusion of the main draining vein and the lack of enlargement of the nidus, the remaining veins can be microclipped, bipolar coagulated, and transected (▶ Fig. 13.12). There are several pitfalls encountered during the final steps of excising the AVM.

The apex of AVMs commonly extends to ventricular ependyma and incorporates ependymal and choroid plexus vessels, even in the setting of negative periventricular angiographic findings. Therefore, to prevent recurrence of AVMs that demonstrate periventricular components, the circumdissection can be

vessels are often located in close proximity to the draining vein. If additional exposure is necessary when searching for residual arterial feeders, the primary draining vein can be mobilized to expose underlying arterial feeders or for nidus manipulation.

Within the angioarchitecture of an AVM, there are primary veins and secondary veins. These veins should be angiographically distinguished preoperatively based on the caliber of the vein and velocity of flow, such that the primary vein has the greatest diameter and capacitates the largest flow. If the distinction between the primary and secondary veins has been made accurately and a majority of the feeding arteries were disconnected during circumdissection, the secondary veins can be sacrificed prior to complete AVM disconnection. This optional step often permits enhanced mobility of the nidus, which may be necessary to access occult feeding arteries.

carried to the level of the ventricle. At this depth, the nidus can be disconnected from the ependymal and choroid plexus vessels. When attempting disconnection of choroidal arteries or ependymal vessels, bipolar electrocautery is generally sufficient because of a robust tunica media. However, disconnection this deep in the parenchyma can pose challenges regarding sufficient exposure of the vessel. In these settings, microclips can be applied to disconnect the vessel prior to its coagulation. The surgeon must be vigilant for retraction of the choroidal or ependymal feeding artery during attempted coagulation, because, if these vessels are not sufficiently coagulated, occult intraventricular hemorrhage and herniation syndromes can result. Therefore, unexpected brain herniation at this step of the operation should alert the operator to examine the ventricle to evacuate the blood and deal meticulously with the bleeding ependymal feeding vessels. This step is particularly important for pediatric patients, which may have ependymal or plexal contribution to the nidus and have an increased the risk for recurrence.[17,18]

While pursuing disconnection of a "vein" near the apex of the nidus, the surgeon may inadvertently truncate a deep segment of the AVM nidus. This can precipitate major complications including nidus rupture.[16] Thorough inspection of the ventricular wall can avoid these errors and the delayed/future risk of hemorrhage or AVM recurrence.

One commonly encountered pitfall during the latter steps of AVM excision is the presence of major feeding arteries adjacent to a primary draining vein. In an attempt to preserve the integrity of the draining vein, the feeding vessel may remain unnoticed and prevent the fundamental sign of blue discoloration of the vein. The surgeon will likely encounter this problem if the entire AVM appears disconnected except the primary draining vein, but the vein still appears red. In this setting, the surgeon should attempt to localize and disconnect an occult feeding artery in close proximity of the vein.

Following nidus excision, complete obliteration of arteriovenous shunting within the cerebrovasculature should be verified with intraoperative angiography. Residual regions of hyperperfusion directed outwardly from the nidus excision bed can be representative of minor arteriovenous shunting. These subtle shunts do not demand aggressive disconnection. Instead, the surgeon should observe these with regular follow-up imaging, particularly in pediatric patients, who are prone to recurrence and demand surveillance follow-up.[17,18]

Following angiographic confirmation of AVM removal, complete hemostasis is secured. The patient's mean arterial pressure should be raised up to 15 to 20 mm Hg above the baseline level and maintained for 10 to 15 minutes. Any bleeding is suspicious for residual AVM nidus and indicates a high risk of postoperative hematoma development. The only method to achieve hemostasis is to remove the residual AVM.

While pursuing homeostasis after AVM excision, coagulation of friable white matter should be minimized. Use of coagulation in the bed of excision will often result in enhanced bleeding. Instead, the surgeon should utilize multiple rounds of irrigation and meticulously observe for hemostasis. This can be a challenging step but patience is an essential component to achieving hemostasis along the nidus bed.

Illustrative examples of the sequential progression through the fundamental steps of AVM excision are shown in ▶ Fig. 13.13 and ▶ Fig. 13.14.

13.4 Discussion

The fundamental steps of AVM microsurgical excision discussed in this chapter provide a general standard approach applicable for all cerebral AVMs. This approach was devised from a culmination of techniques described by master surgeons[8,9,19,20] and personal expertise.[17] This approach incorporates advances in radiographic technology to understand the three-dimensional aspects of the nidus and the roadmap of the parenchymal perforators, prior to manipulation.

The major change AVM microsurgery will face in the future involves the contentious findings demonstrated by the randomized trial of unruptured brain AVMs (ARUBA) study.[21] Although uncertainty remains regarding the utility of the study in the face of its short follow-up data, the results of this study are likely to impact patient selection and evidence-based recommendations made by neurosurgeons relating to the appropriate management for AVMs. The results of multicentered randomized trials, such as ARUBA, will have a large impact on the future of microsurgical AVM management.[21] There will always be a role for microsurgical resection in specific lesions, particularly those with a history of rupture. The increased incorporation of less invasive treatment modalities, such as stereotactic radiosurgery and endovascular embolization, will also impact the prevalence of microsurgically appropriate cases.

13.5 Conclusion

AVM microsurgery remains the most definitive management strategy for occlusion of an AVM.[22] The microsurgical steps discussed in this chapter provide a foundation for surgical management of these lesions. The application of these principles to each AVM a surgeon encounters ensures a fundamental approach upon which the surgeon can apply novel techniques for lesions in differing location. A complete microsurgical AVM excision trials the surgeon's technical prowess, perseverance, and efficiency. The hallmarks of a matured AVM surgeon are evident through an intimate understanding of the three-dimensional anatomy of the AVM intraoperatively, the ability to make operative decisions without hesitation while maintaining elegance in technique, and, in situations with significant hemorrhage, the ability to remain mentally controlled and serve as the source of leadership during disaster.

Despite the frequency of complications and morbidity incurred during AVM microsurgery, the outcomes of these procedures can be optimized by appropriate patient selection, meticulous adherence to the principles of AVM excision, and the willingness of the surgeon to learn from his or her previous experiences treating these complicated lesions.

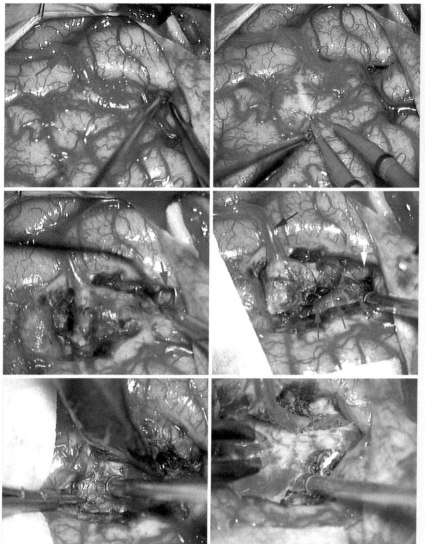

Fig. 13.13 This illustration serves to demonstrate the fundamental steps in AVM resection. This subcortical AVM was not readily apparent on the cortical surface and only demonstrated a single large vessel to herald its presence (upper left image). The subarachnoid and pial dissection was performed (upper right image). Further dissection revealed an en passage artery (*red arrow*, middle left image). Deeper parenchymal dissection exposed the nidus margin (middle right image). The identity of the cortically visualized vessel (*blue arrow*) remains unknown and is therefore not disconnected. An embolized vessel was identified (lower left image). Following complete AVM excision, the initial cortically visible vessel was identified as an en passage artery that was successfully protected (lower right image).

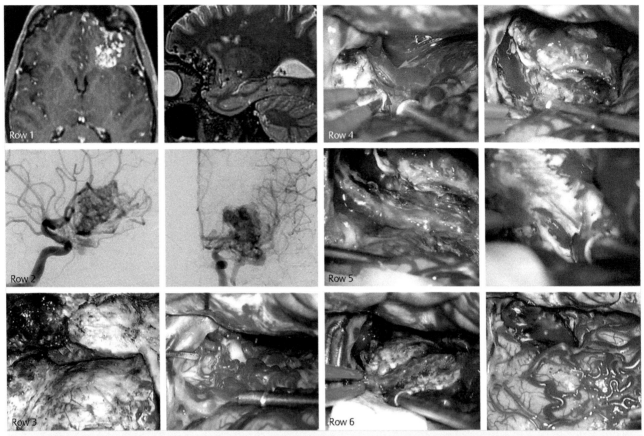

Fig. 13.14 Complete radiographic analysis of the AVM was undertaken (Rows 1 and 2). A generous osteotomy above the orbital roof facilitated an optimal operative trajectory (Row 3). Arachnoid and pial dissection was undertaken permitting the disconnection of MCA derived AVM feeding arteries. The nidus was skeletonized and revealed a prominent feeding artery (*red arrow*) adjacent to a primary draining vein (*purple arrow*) (Row 4). The primary draining vein was liberated from its surrounding tissue to permit mobilization and deeper access to the nidus. The deep parenchymal feeding arteries are identified and appropriately disconnected (Row 5). A temporary occlusion test of the primary draining vein is performed and does not demonstrate any enlargement of the nidus, indicative of complete AVM disconnection. The AVM was excised and the remaining cortical veins turn blue, indicating the lack of arteriovenous shunting (Row 6).

Reference

[1] Laakso A, Hernesniemi J. Arteriovenous malformations: epidemiology and clinical presentation. Neurosurg Clin N Am. 2012; 23(1):1–6

[2] Gross BA, Du R. Natural history of cerebral arteriovenous malformations: a meta-analysis. J Neurosurg. 2013; 118(2):437–443

[3] Pabaney AH, Reinard KA, Massie LW, et al. Management of perisylvian arteriovenous malformations: a retrospective institutional case series and review of the literature. Neurosurg Focus. 2014; 37(3):E13

[4] Natarajan SK, Ghodke B, Britz GW, Born DE, Sekhar LN. Multimodality treatment of brain arteriovenous malformations with microsurgery after embolization with onyx: single-center experience and technical nuances. Neurosurgery. 2008; 62(6):1213–1225, discussion 1225–1226

[5] See AP, Raza S, Tamargo RJ, Lim M. Stereotactic radiosurgery of cranial arteriovenous malformations and dural arteriovenous fistulas. Neurosurg Clin N Am. 2012; 23(1):133–146

[6] Colby GP, Coon AL, Huang J, Tamargo RJ. Historical perspective of treatments of cranial arteriovenous malformations and dural arteriovenous fistulas. Neurosurg Clin N Am. 2012; 23(1):15–25

[7] Spetzler RF, Ponce FA. A 3-tier classification of cerebral arteriovenous malformations. Clinical article. J Neurosurg. 2011; 114(3):842–849

[8] Lawton MT, Probst KX. Seven AVMs Tenets and Techniques for Resection. 1st ed. New York, NY: Thieme; 2014

[9] Spetzler RF, Kondziolka DS, Higashida RT, Kalani MYS. Comprehensive Management of Arteriovenous Malformations of the Brain and Spine. Cambridge: Cambridge University Press; 2015

[10] Spetzler RF, Martin NA. A proposed grading system for arteriovenous malformations. J Neurosurg. 1986; 65(4):476–483

[11] Theofanis T, Chalouhi N, Dalyai R, et al. Microsurgery for cerebral arteriovenous malformations: postoperative outcomes and predictors of complications in 264 cases. Neurosurg Focus. 2014; 37(3):E10

[12] Pollock BE, Flickinger JC. A proposed radiosurgery-based grading system for arteriovenous malformations. J Neurosurg. 2002; 96(1):79–85

[13] Lopes DK, Moftakhar R, Straus D, Munich SA, Chaus F, Kaszuba MC. Arteriovenous malformation embocure score: AVMES. J Neurointerv Surg. 2016; 8 (7):685–691

[14] Yu SC, Chan MS, Lam JM, Tam PH, Poon WS. Complete obliteration of intracranial arteriovenous malformation with endovascular cyanoacrylate embolization: initial success and rate of permanent cure. AJNR Am J Neuroradiol. 2004; 25(7):1139–1143

[15] van Rooij WJ, Jacobs S, Sluzewski M, van der Pol B, Beute GN, Sprengers ME. Curative embolization of brain arteriovenous malformations with onyx: patient selection, embolization technique, and results. AJNR Am J Neuroradiol. 2012; 33(7):1299–1304

[16] Torné R, Rodríguez-Hernández A, Lawton MT. Intraoperative arteriovenous malformation rupture: causes, management techniques, outcomes, and the effect of neurosurgeon experience. Neurosurg Focus. 2014; 37(3):E12

[17] Conger A, Kulwin C, Lawton MT, Cohen-Gadol AA. Endovascular and microsurgical treatment of cerebral arteriovenous malformations: Current recommendations. Surg Neurol Int. 2015; 6:39

[18] Gross BA, Storey A, Orbach DB, Scott RM, Smith ER. Microsurgical treatment of arteriovenous malformations in pediatric patients: the Boston Children's Hospital experience. J Neurosurg Pediatr. 2015; 15(1):71–77

[19] Yasargil MG. Microneurosurgery, Volume IIIB: AVM of the Brain, Clinical Considerations, General and Special Operative Techniques, Surgical Results. 1st ed. New York, NY: Thieme Medical Publishers, Inc.; 1988

[20] Yasargil MG. Microneurosurgery, Volume IIIA: AVM of the Brain, History, Embryology, Pathological Considerations, Hemodynamics, Diagnostic Studies, Microsurgical Anatomy. 1st ed. New York, NY: Thieme Medical Publishers, Inc.; 1987

[21] Mohr JP, Parides MK, Stapf C, et al. International ARUBA investigators. Medical management with or without interventional therapy for unruptured brain arteriovenous malformations (ARUBA): a multicentre, non-blinded, randomised trial. Lancet. 2014; 383(9917):614–621

[22] Pradilla G, Coon AL, Huang J, Tamargo RJ. Surgical treatment of cranial arteriovenous malformations and dural arteriovenous fistulas. Neurosurg Clin N Am. 2012; 23(1):105–122

14 Surgical Approaches and Nuances for Lobar Arteriovenous Malformations

Cameron G. McDougall, Jonathan White, and H. Hunt Batjer

Abstract

Frontal, temporal, parietal, and occipital arteriovenous malformations (AVMs) make up a significant proportion of cerebral AVMs. Many of these AVMs are favorably located in nonelo-quent areas of the brain with good cortical presentation. Because of this, if done well, it is possible to surgically remove these AVMs with a treatment risk that is lower than their untreated natural history. The first key to delivering good outcomes is proper patient selection. A detailed history, a careful review of the imaging, and an honest appraisal of the surgeon's ability are paramount. A decision then needs to be made about preoperative embolization. The risk of embolization must be balanced against the potential benefits of decreased blood loss, shorter operative times, and the clarity embolization brings to the angioarchitecture of the AVM. Once in the operating room, the patient must be positioned carefully to allow for full exposure of the AVM. When the microscope is finally brought into use, the pial surface must be broken circumferentially around the presenting surface of the AVM and then deepened evenly around the lesion. Careful hemostasis should be achieved as each margin is dissected to avoid having bleeding from multiple parts of the AVM at once. Once resection is thought to be complete, postoperative angiography is needed to make sure all early venous drainage has been eliminated. Patient care does not end when the procedure is over. A successful outcome is also dependent on attentive care in the intensive care unit during the first few days postresection.

Keywords: cerebral arteriovenous malformation, surgical technique, complication avoidance, microsurgery, endovascular embolization

Key Points

- With proper patient selection and good microsurgical dissection, a significant number of lobar arteriovenous malformations can be treated with a risk much lower than their untreated natural history.
- Excellent preoperative evaluation including a thorough neurological examination, detailed anatomic and functional imaging, and judicious use of preoperative embolization are important in achieving the best possible outcomes.
- Proper patient positioning, selection of the appropriate surgical approach, and meticulous intraoperative dissection will maximize technical success.
- Patient care does not end with the skin closure. Aggressive and attentive postoperative ICU care and diligent outpatient follow-up are needed.

14.1 Introduction

Frontal, temporal, parietal, and occipital arteriovenous malformations (AVMs) make up a significant proportion of cerebral AVMs. Many of these AVMs are favorably located in nonelo-quent areas of the brain with good cortical presentation. Because of this, if done well, it is possible to surgically remove these AVMs with a treatment risk that is lower than their untreated natural history. In this chapter, we will discuss nuances of patient selection, positioning, exposure, and microsurgical technique. Management of the patients before, during, and after surgery will also be reviewed.

14.2 Patient Selection

This represents the cornerstone of all AVM management and its importance cannot be overstated. There is significant controversy surrounding the optimal management of AVMs. The ARUBA study (a randomized study of unruptured brain AVMs) concluded that unruptured AVMs should not be treated and found an annual event (death or new stroke) rate of 2.2% in those managed medically and a 30.7% event rate in patients undergoing treatment.[1] This study has been criticized because a significant number of patients who were screened were never randomized. Furthermore, many authors would consider the event rate in the treatment arm of ARUBA to be on the extreme end of the spectrum.[2] If nothing else, this study suggests that if unruptured AVMs are to be treated then it must be done with a very low risk of complications.

The key to achieving this goal is in careful patient selection (in particular for the unruptured population). It can be helpful to categorize the process into three parts: (1) patient factors such as patient age, comorbidities, expectations, and concerns (e.g., hemorrhage anxiety); (2) presentation details such as pervious hemorrhage, associated seizure disorder, and current neurological deficits can influence the decision-making process; (3) AVM features, such as anatomical location and the presence of high-risk features (e.g., nidal/flow-related aneurysms), and the configuration of the AVM itself such as nidal compactness necessitate careful consideration.

A helpful scale for patient management is the Spetzler–Martin supplementary grading scale (▶ Table 14.1). It assigns the patient a score based on several factors found to be significant predictors of outcome following surgical treatment. Increasing scores are associated with an increased likelihood of a poor outcome. Scores > 6 were associated with a 55% chance of an adverse surgical outcome or death.[3] However, scales such as this serve only as a guide, and the decision to treat any patient with any modality must be made on an individualized basis and measured against the projected natural history of that specific AVM.

Table 14.1 The Spetzler–Martin supplementary grading system

Category	Points
Size	
<3 cm	1
3–6 cm	2
>6 cm	3
Venous drainage	
Superficial	0
Deep	1
Eloquence	
No	0
Yes	1
Age	
0–20 years	1
21–40 years	2
>40 years	3
Nidus	
Compact	0
Diffuse	1
Hemorrhage	
Yes	0
No	1

Patients who are younger and healthy with cortical AVMs that have good superficial representation in relatively noneloquent areas of the brain favor resection. Older, sicker, patients with deeply located AVMs or AVMs in eloquent locations favor observation or radiosurgery.

14.3 Patient Positioning

14.3.1 General Considerations

Proper position is crucial in all of cranial neurosurgery but is especially true of AVMs. The cases can be long, there is potential for significant blood loss, and, unlike a tumor, it can be extremely difficult to take out an AVM if the entire lesion is not well visualized under the craniotomy flap. When choosing a patient position, several factors must be taken into account. First, it is best if the lesion is in the center of the brain exposed by the bone flap. Next, the position must facilitate access to the proximal feeding vessels and allow visualization of the draining veins. The veins, which in general cannot be sacrificed until the majority or all of the arterial input has been taken, can tether the mass of the nidus. This limitation must be taken into account when positioning. Finally, the patient must be positioned in such a way that the surgeon is reasonably comfortable during the procedure. Long surgeries with the surgeon in some contorted position make for a long, painful day and lead to rushing and careless mistakes.

14.3.2 Frontal Lobe AVMs

Obviously, patient positioning will be dictated by AVM location. In the superficial frontal lobe, especially in the superior, middle, and inferior frontal gyrus, arterial supply is from anterior cerebral arteries and the distal middle cerebral arteries. The decision about positioning is usually straightforward with the head turned in such a way that lesion is in the most superior part of the exposure. Lesions on the orbital surface generally warrant a lateral exposure if they are far from the midline, allowing for a lateral subfrontal view. Orbital surface lesions with a more medial presentation are usually best accessed from the anterior subfrontal view, making a head neutral with significant extension the position of choice.

Lesions of the frontal lobe presenting to the interhemispheric fissure present several reasonable choices for positioning. One is a head neutral position with an interhemispheric approach and gentle retraction of the frontal lobe ipsilateral to the lesion from medial to lateral. This works well, particularly if the lesion is relatively superficial in the interhemispheric fissure. Another clever approach to a lesion presenting to the interhemispheric fissure is to place the patient lateral with the lesion side down. In this position, gravity naturally pulls the lesion-side brain down, giving a more natural medial-to-lateral retraction of the brain. Another benefit of this position is that excess bleeding tends to run out of the interhemispheric fissure, thus avoiding pooling of blood in the surgeon's line of sight.

14.3.3 Temporal Lobe AVMs

Like frontal lobe AVMs, temporal lobe AVMs are fed by distal middle cerebral artery (MCA) branches. Depending on how anterior and medially they present, they also have feeding from the anterior temporal artery and the anterior choroidal artery. Lesions that are more posterior can also recruit posterior cerebral artery feeding. It is important to keep this vasculature in mind when deciding what position to use.

AVMs of the anterior temporal lobe, whether presenting medially or laterally, can be exposed through a pterional exposure or one of its numerous modifications. A true lateral position or supine with the head rotated the appropriate amount usually works well for this approach. Lesions of the posterior temporal lobe that present to the lateral cortex require a more posterior exposure

14.3.4 Parietal Lobe AVMs

AVMs of the parietal lobe often extend anteriorly into the posterior temporal lobe or posteriorly into the occipital lobe. The details of this cortical presentation drive the patient position. Lesions with more anterior extension can be positioned supine with the head turned. For progressively more posterior lesions, it may be more comfortable to have the patient either in a semi-sitting position or prone. There is a "no man's land" between the posterior parietal lobe and the anterior occipital lobe that can sometimes make it difficult to decide which exposure is best.

14.3.5 Occipital Lobe AVMs

Like their frontal and temporal lobe counterparts, AVMs of the occipital lobe can present medially or posteriorly to the cortical surface, or they may present to the interhemispheric fissure. Lateral and posterior presenting AVMs may be positioned laterally, supine with the head turned, sitting, semi-sitting, or prone.

Each of these positions has its relative benefits and shortcoming. Sitting and semi-sitting have the advantage of allowing pooled blood to run off during surgery, facilitating visualization and maximizing the effectiveness of the bipolar. The disadvantage is the added time it takes to position properly and the added risk of hypotension and air embolism. The prone position is a good compromise depending on the AVM's presentation to the surface. The surgeon then has the choice of operating at the patient's head with the brain essentially upside down or working over the patient's tucked arm looking superiorly.

14.4 Exposure

14.4.1 General Considerations

Maximizing the AVM exposure and creating a safe working corridor is an important detail which is often overlooked. In general, it is best for the entire AVM to be visualized after exposure, including the draining vein if it presents to the surface. Working under the bone edge, especially if there is any problem in controlling intraoperative bleeding, can lead to serious problems. Exposure should also take into account the arterial feeders to the AVM. When possible, it is reassuring to have proximal control of the feeding vessel away from the AVM in the event of difficulty in controlling bleeding while working around the nidus. When possible, it is preferable to expose an adequate margin of normal brain around the AVM. This normal brain on the AVM's edge is vulnerable to injury, either by feeding vessels retracting into it during the AVM resection or from hemorrhage from normal perfusion pressure breakthrough bleeding. In many AVMs, it is not clear where the precise margin is during resection and so erring on the side of some extra exposure is wise.

After the skin and muscle have been reflected, the bone flap is elevated. The skin exposure and elevation of the bone flap can be bloody if there is external carotid or muscular collateral feeding of the AVM. The transosseous venous channels can be a source of important bleeding while turning the craniotomy as they can be arterialized.

Once the bone flap is removed, the dura is opened. This step should be never underestimated and should be preferentially done under the microscope. Great care must be taken not to injure the draining vein while opening the dura. The dura opening should be wide to take maximum advantage of the bony opening. It is easy to lose the benefits of a generous craniotomy by minimizing the extent of dura opening. The dura can be stellated into as many parts as necessary to maximize the opening. Not infrequently, especially near the venous sinuses, a large arterialized vein will enter the dura and then travel within the dura to reach the sinus. Cutting the dura on both sides of the vein and then leaving a small portion of dura over the vein allows exposure of the AVM without disruption of the venous drainage. At the end of the case, if the vein is arterialized, the vein along with the portion of dura left to protect it can be sacrificed. Whenever possible, nonarterialized veins should be preserved.

14.4.2 Frontal Lobe AVMs

Exposure of frontal lobe AVMs is dependent on location. Lesions of the convexity can be treated using a pterional-type exposure or one of its variants. More posterior lesions are exposed via a horseshoe-shaped flap with the lesion in the center. Lesions that present to the interhemispheric fissure can be exposed via a bicoronal incision. This exposure requires several subtle considerations. First, care must be used in placing the cranial fixation device such as the Mayfield head holder. Either the pins can get in the way of the exposure or they can be placed too far from the equator of the head allowing the head to slip. Even if the head holder shifts subtly during the case, the resulting movement can make the skin closure difficult. Occasionally, someone may have to crawl under the blood drapes to remove the fixed head holder and switch to a horseshoe-type holder in order to complete the closure.

When dissection within the interhemispheric fissure is needed, the sagittal sinus must be exposed. There are many options for this but the safest alternative is to place multiple burr holes on either side of the sinus, strip the dura of the sinus away from the bone flap, and then carefully complete the cutting of the bone immediately over the sinus. Fortunately, the dura of the sinus is very thick; unfortunately, the sinus can be arterialized and the normally easily controlled transosseous venous bleeding can be arterialized and difficult to control.

14.4.3 Temporal Lobe AVMs

AVMs of the temporal lobe can present to the lateral temporal cortex or the medial temporal surface facing the midbrain or tentorium. They may also face inferiorly the floor of the middle cranial fossa. Lesions of the anterior, superior, and middle temporal gyrus can be exposed via a standard pterional approach. If the lesion is also in the inferior temporal gyrus, it is useful to do an interfacial dissection of the temporal fascia. This allows exposure to the floor of the middle cranial fossa. This extended exposure is mandatory for middle cranial fossa presenting lesions in which a subtemporal look is necessary.

AVMs that present to the medial temporal lobe can be approached through a pterional exposure or one of its variants. If the lesion is anterior, such as in the uncus, the lesion may be immediately visualized with minimal frontal or temporal lobe retraction. If the lesion is more posterior, in and around the sylvian fissure, it may be necessary to split the fissure for optimal exposure. Many of the AVMs in this region may be fed by arterial input from small feeding vessels arising "en passage" from a large MCA that then continues on to supply normal brain. In this case it is crucial to preserve the MCA. During the exposure therefore, it is necessary to make the exposure sufficiently large to identify the distal vessel.

Lesions in the posterior temporal lobe can generally be exposed with a horseshoe flap, hopefully centered over the AVM. Deep lesions of the temporal lobe are more complex and are beyond the scope of this chapter.

14.4.4 Occipital and Parietal AVMs

AVMs of the occipital and parietal lobes are usually exposed either through a linear incision, if they are relatively small, or via a horseshoe flap with the lesion in the center, for more sizeable AVMs. AVMs presenting to the occipital interhemispheric fissure carry many of the same caveats discussed for interhemispheric frontal AVMs. The bone flap must be elevated from the arterialized sinus with care. The safest way to accomplish this is with multiple burr holes on both sides of the sinus. Similarly, although less often than frontally, important arterialized or nonarterialized veins may travel through the dura on their way to the sinus. The dura must therefore be opened carefully.

The occipital lobe, especially in the region of the interhemispheric fissure, should be considered eloquent because of the visual pathways and the visual cortex. Care must be taken not only to avoid injury to the surrounding brain during resection, but also in utilizing retraction. Prolonged retraction of the occipital lobe from medial to lateral to work in the interhemispheric fissure frequently results in a visual field deficit, which may not always be reversible. Placing the patient in the lateral position with the lesion-side down is one way to try to minimize retraction injury.

14.5 Navigation

There are multiple surgical adjuncts that when used correctly can assist with surgical resection of AVMs. Neuronavigation is an essential tool for safe surgical treatment of deep-seated AVMs. Lobar AVMs, in general, tend to have a cortical presentation that decreases the need for navigation, although navigation in such cases can be helpful in planning the safest and best approach to the lesion without adding risks. Navigation can help in planning a craniotomy that takes into account not only the location of the nidus but also the superficial draining veins and venous sinuses. Software is available that allows merging angiography (either digital subtraction angiography [DSA] or magnetic resonance angiography [MRA]) with the magnetic resonance imaging (MRI) used for registration, and this may aid easier identification of specific portions and components of the AVM during surgery.[4,5] Some microscopes allow their focal point to be used as a registration probe, which can be helpful in confirming that circumferential dissection of the AVM proceeds deeply toward the ependymal surfaces. Although useful, it must be kept in mind that as cerebrospinal fluid (CSF) is released and the brain shifts with resection, the accuracy of the navigation becomes less reliable.

Cranial features are unreliable, and probably the most important implication of the ARUBA study is that surgical treatment and its attendant risks must be minimized if surgery is to remain as a relevant treatment option. The popularization of stereotactic radiosurgery as a treatment option (and to a lesser extent, endovascular treatment) has forced neurosurgery to improve in order to remain relevant. Every effort should be made to control, minimize, and, when possible, eliminate perioperative risk. The downsides of navigation are small but the setup time can be significant (in particular, if some component of the system is not working properly). The registration platform can also become an obstacle if not correctly positioned during patient registration. Notwithstanding these limitations, strong consideration should be given to the use of neuronavigation in most craniotomies for AVM resection.

14.6 Embolization

The use of preoperative endovascular embolization has gone through several phases. It remains an important adjunct, but a balance must be struck between the risks associated with embolization and its potential benefits. The risks of embolization are not insignificant, and our own institutional data identified a 7.7% risk of adverse events associated with preoperative embolization of over 339 procedures (including a 2% risk of mortality).[6] More recently, embolization with Onyx has become more prevalent for AVM treatment and has largely replaced NBCA and PVA embolization techniques but does not appear to have changed the overall risks of embolization.[7]

Preoperative embolization must be carefully considered. Lower grade lobar AVMs with superficial feeding arteries may not require preoperative embolization and the risks can be forgone altogether. An individualized approach to this adjunct will help minimize the risks and ensure that only those who will truly benefit from embolization are treated. Preoperative embolization is not the same as preradiosurgical embolization or embolization used alone with an intent to cure or treat a high-risk feature.

The goals for embolization should be clear at the outset of the procedure. Embolization of specific arterial pedicles or AVM features should be discussed with the endovascular team before the procedure. This will ensure that the procedure focus only on those components of the AVM that will potentially complicate the surgical resection.

For lobar AVMs, this often means embolization of deep arterial feeders that will not be encountered until late in the dissection. Embolization can also be used to treat flow-related aneurysms that will not be easily accessible during the resection. Careful study of the Onyx cast after embolization can also help to orient the surgeon during the resection and facilitate microsurgical manipulation of the lesion.

For larger lesions, the embolization is best performed in stages in order to avoid sudden hemodynamic shifts that could predispose to normal perfusion pressure breakthrough. We generally prefer a 2-day interval, or longer, between embolization sessions in order to give the local cerebral circulation a chance to adjust to the increased flow. Staged embolization for larger AVMs will help to dissipate the hemodynamic risks associated with resection alone, thereby decreasing the overall risks of treatment.

Patient management following embolization requires diligent neurocritical care and should emphasize strict blood pressure control. Again, a calculated risk should only be undertaken when every opportunity to minimize the potential complications are seized upon. The judicious application of focused preoperative embolization can simplify AVM resection and decrease intraoperative blood loss. The risks of embolization should only be undertaken in order to decrease the surgical risks such that a balance resulting in the best possible patient outcome is achieved. For smaller lobar lesions, the lower risks of surgical resection should be balanced against the risks of embolization. Patients with larger lesions and those with more challenging surgical features will often benefit from preoperative embolization.

14.7 Monitoring and Mapping

Neurophysiologic monitoring in lobar AVM surgery is problematic. The most common monitoring tools used in other neurosurgical operations are somatosensory evoked potentials (SSEPs) and motor evoked potentials (MEPs). Lobar AVM surgery involving eloquent cortex necessitates exposure of that cortex, making SSEP and MEP monitoring impossible. Direct cortical stimulation using bipolar stimulation probes can be used to help precisely identify motor and sensory cortical regions but cannot deliver continuous feedback during the dissection.[8] Pyramidal white matter tracts can also be identified in a similar fashion with unipolar stimulation, but this mode of monitoring suffers from the same limitations. Awake cortical language mapping has also been described.[9] These techniques may be useful when working on AVMs encroaching on the motor and sensory gyri or their associated white matter pathways but have failed to gain wide acceptance for various reasons.

In general, monitoring adds a degree of complexity to an already challenging and often prolonged operation. Furthermore, unlike a low-grade glioma or an epileptogenic focus, the resection margin of an AVM is predefined and essentially cannot be modified. In regions of eloquence, this margin should be as tight to the lesion as humanly possible while never forgetting that inadvertent entry into the lesion can precipitate disaster. Lesions with a diffuse nidus involving eloquent cortex should not undergo resection without a thorough understanding on the part of both the patient and the surgeon that a postoperative deficit is likely.

Instead of direct cortical mapping, some authors prefer preoperative imaging techniques such as functional MRI (fMRI) and diffusion tensor imaging (DTI) to try and discern the relationships between functional regions of interest to the lesion.[10] These functional localization techniques may be helpful in terms of both determining the safety of surgical resection and planning the operative approach once surgery is selected. Some controversy exists surrounding the reliability of fMRI in AVMs as it relies on the detection of functional–metabolic coupling to detect active cortical regions during specific motor, language, or sensory tasks. The problem with this type of analysis in the perilesional region is that blood flow may not be normal in the tissue adjacent to an AVM and this may decrease ability of fMRI to detect the functional tissue of interest. A prospective, randomized trial evaluating the efficacy of fMRI in AVM surgery is currently under way.[11]

14.8 Intraoperative and Microsurgical Nuances

14.8.1 General Considerations

All the preparation thus far leads to the microsurgical stage of the resection. This section of the chapter will explore the equipment needed for a successful operation, the step-by-step anatomical aspects to the resection of the AVM, and a detailed description of the stages of the surgical resection.

14.8.2 Equipment

Each surgeon relies on specific tools with which he or she is most familiar and which are better suited for a specific task. For AVM surgery, the bipolar forceps is one of the most important tools. A bipolar with a suitable size blade is key. Blades that are too large make isolating small vessels difficult. Tips that are too small can be troublesome in delivering sufficient charge to the offending vessel. Given that the brain/AVM interface is frequently bloody, bipolar blades which stick to the tissue can be a problem. The simplest remedy for this potential issue is the use of an irrigating bipolar, or to have an assistant to irrigate as the main operator works around the AVM. More recently, a variety of "nonstick" bipolars have become available with varying degrees of efficacy. A second issue unique to AVM resection is the nature of the smaller vessels at the base of the AVM. These vessels are thin walled and lack a muscular layer, which makes them often resistant to coagulation. The use of small AVM clips can be helpful in addressing this issue.

A good operative microscope is also crucial to AVM resection. The microscope provides both magnification and illumination into the field. One limitation of the microscope is its depth of field. When working under high-power magnification, the depth of field of the microscope gets shorter. This means that only a smaller portion of the entire field is in focus at any one time. When working at the bottom of the resection bed, one needs to be mindful of the tissue that is not in perfect focus. A mouthpiece focus switch for the microscope, which allows the surgeon to adjust the focal point of the microscope without having to pass back any instruments, is very helpful in order to allow continuous focus by adjusting the focal length. A foot pedal or an autofocus is another option. Newer cameras and other imaging apparatuses are in development, which may greatly increase depth of field.

Another important consideration in the resection of an AVM is the use of retractors. Retraction may be necessary to view the presenting surface of the AVM, for example, with AVMs presenting to the interhemispheric fissure or the floor of the anterior or middle cranial fossa. Retraction may also be necessary during circumferential dissection of the nidus to gently retract the exposed portion of the nidus and allow the surgeon to expose deeper portions of the AVM. Multiple retractor systems are available, although none of them is completely without drawbacks. Anticipation of the directions of retraction that might be necessary will allow the surgeon the flexibility to retract smoothly, without having to constantly reposition the retractors.

The availability of high-quality, consistent suction is paramount. Devices that can regulate the magnitude of suction are available and allow for more subtle alterations in the power of the suction than can the surgeon's finger on a slotted sucker alone. Selection of the appropriate size sucker is also important. The smaller the sucker, the more easily manipulated through the vasculature at the base of the resection; however, a sucker of sufficient size is necessary to adequately clear the field of blood and debris. Suction tends to became clogged over time, especially in the face of significant bleeding. Having at least two, and ideally three, good suctions is prudent.

As with the microscope and suction, each surgeon prefers different number and types of microdissectors, microscissors, and other instruments to treat the AVM. Some surgeons use a different tool for every need, while others become facile with one or two pieces of equipment, which they use for all phases of the microdissection.

14.8.3 Intraoperative Anatomic Considerations

Under the microscope, the presenting surface of the AVM is analyzed and compared to the preoperative imaging. The direction and location of arterial feeders is reviewed and the final plan of which margin to approach first is made. The draining vein or veins as well as their anatomical pathways to the sinuses are inspected. If multiple veins are present, it may be possible to sacrifice one in the midportion of the dissection if the AVM is tethered in order to gain circumferential access to parts of the nidus. Indocyanine green fluorescein can be helpful at this point to confirm superficial feeders and draining veins. Finally, the initial pial incision is made. This is best done in a circumferential fashion to begin the process of devascularizing the AVM. Consideration should be given to the deeper extent of the AVM, which is often wider below the surface than at the surface. Wide opening of the arachnoidal planes of the sulci is important in order to uncover in a less traumatic fashion portions of the AVM buried underneath the cortical surface.

Once the pial cut is made, the resection continues deeper and deeper into the white matter. This cut should be close enough to the AVM to minimize disruption of adjacent brain tissue, but far away enough to avoid inadvertently entering the AVM. If the bleeding is brisk, the resection is probably in the AVM and the best course of action is to abandon that margin, obtain hemostasis, and begin again with a wider margin. As these margins are deepened, the various feeding vessels come into view. Vessels previously embolized with Onyx can be helpful intraoperative roadmaps to the extent of resection. Small feeding vessels entering the AVM nidus can be electrocoagulated and divided. Large ones can be clip-ligated on the proximal side and electrocoagulated on the AVM side prior to being divided.

The final deep margin of the AVM is the most difficult part. When possible, it is opportune to have a partner relieve you during some of the earlier, easier dissection, so that you can face the final battle rested. The bottom of the AVM frequently touches one of the ventricular surfaces. Numerous primitive vessels enter and exit the AVM from this ventricular surface. These vessels are difficult to control because they are deep, are bathed in a mixture of blood and CSF, and do not take a bipolar charge well. Be patient and avoid stirring up bleeding from multiple vessels. Small AVM clips when well placed are a blessing but too many, poorly placed, clips can obscure vision and short the bipolar charge.

If bleeding from a given margin becomes too brisk, it is best to pack it off and work a different part of the AVM for a while; later, consideration should be given to restart working on the bleeding margin at a greater distance from the nidus. If bleeding becomes life-threatening, it may be best to back out the microscope, switch to the largest suction, and rapidly resect a much wider margin in an effort to occlude the proximal vasculature. This may incur significant neurological deficit but help to avoid an intraoperative death. Fortunately, in the age of embolization, this is rarely necessary. Once the AVM is resected, it is wise to obtain additional hemostasis and sit and wait 15 to 20 minutes to observe the surrounding brain while the patient is at a slightly higher blood pressure to make sure the resection bed is stable.

14.9 Postoperative Care

In AVM surgery more than in other neurosurgical operations, the patient care episode is not over with the skin closure. On the contrary, particularly with AVM surgery, the skin closure can be just the beginning. It is wise to get an intraoperative angiogram at the end of the case in complex cases. This can be done intraoperatively prior to the closure if you are in a center fortunate enough to have this capability, but it can also be done by transporting the patient under anesthesia to the angiogram suite and performing the study. Even a small residual can put the patient at risk for early post-op hemorrhage.

In the ICU, blood pressure should be tightly controlled, sometimes even below baseline blood pressure, to minimize resection bed hemorrhage or bleeding into the surrounding brain. If the case is long, fluid balance, respiratory status, and coagulation disorders must all be addressed. A CT scan 12 hours or so after surgery can help identify, barring unexpected new neurological deficit, asymptomatic hemorrhage in the resection bed or surrounding brain. If postoperative hematoma requires a return to the operating room, one should be prepared to do AVM surgery, not just a hematoma evacuation. The brain surrounding the AVM, even with a negative arteriogram, can bleed as vigorously as during the initial AVM resection.

14.9.1 Results

The results of AVM surgery are variable and depend on many factors. Outcomes rely heavily on patient selection, and although the extrapolation of results from large single-center (and usually single-surgeon) series may not be valid, clear trends can still be observed. The original Spetzler–Martin grading scale was created to predict outcomes following surgical resection based on a retrospective series of 100 patients. Progressively higher grades demonstrated an increased risk of operative complications, while lower grade lesions had a very low risk.[12] This was later prospectively applied to 120 patients with similar findings, suggesting an increasing likelihood of a new postoperative neurological deficit with increasing scores.[13]

This system was further refined in the modified Spetzler–Martin grading system. In a series of 300 patients, no patients with scores of 1 or 3 were clinically worse or dead postoperatively. Five percent of patients with scores of 4 were clinically worse or dead following surgery. Patients with scores of 5 and 6 both had 19% chance of a poor outcome and those with a score of 7 had a 24% chance. Very few patients with scores > 7 underwent surgery.[3] When this scoring system was applied to a larger multicenter cohort of 1,009 patients with AVMs undergoing surgical resection in four different high-volume centers, the results were similar in the lower grade patients but increased for those with midgrade scores. Patients with a score of 4 had a 21% chance of a poor outcome, and those with grades 5 and 6 had a 54 and 56% chance of a poor outcome, respectively.[14]

The ARUBA study recommended against intervention for unruptured AVMs based on a 30.7% risk of stroke or death in the "intervention group." This heterogeneous group included all treatment modalities and surgery-specific outcomes from this study are unknown. Furthermore, there were very few surgical patients in the "intervention" group and a higher than expected number of patients undergoing embolization for cure. Whether this study has external validity remains controversial.

Because of their cortical involvement, seizures are common in lobar AVMs. Focusing solely on seizure outcomes in 103 patients with AVMs treated surgically, von der Brelie et al found that the seizure outcome was related to the severity of their preoperative seizure disorder. Overall, 76.7% of the patients with preoperative seizures were seizure-free postoperatively. However, those with drug-resistant epilepsy prior to surgery had only a 52% chance of seizure freedom.[15] The UCSF group evaluated 130 patients with preoperative epilepsy and found a much more favorable postsurgical epilepsy outcome, with 96% of patients becoming seizure-free or having only a single seizure postoperatively.[16]

14.10 Conclusion

With a 2.2% per year risk of rupture from the ARUBA data and numerous other studies suggesting patients with AVMs die early, it seems reasonable that patients with a long remaining lifespan, whose AVMs can be treated with a low morbidity, should be treated. Many of the AVMs discussed in this chapter fall into that category. Reasonably sized AVMs in noneloquent cortex that have good cortical presentation can have perioperative morbidity and mortality risks less than 5%.[12]

To achieve this low patient morbidity, significant experience and attention to detail are necessary. Patient selection is critical. Preoperative embolization to reduce intraoperative blood loss and to allow for a more gradual obliteration of the AVM can be helpful. Preoperative functional imaging and the use of navigation tools aid in a successful surgery. Proper positioning and a generous, well-placed bone flap are needed.

Intraoperatively, it is important to follow a well-rehearsed, stereotypical plan. The first step is identification of the feeding vessels and careful handling of the draining vein during the exposure. Next, the circumference of the presenting surface is mapped out and the pial surface is electrocoagulated and divided. A vigilant, circumferential dissection then takes place with care to avoid working too deep in one segment of the AVM. If the base of the resection cavity, usually at an ependymal surface, is made in the shape of a cone and not a pyramid, there will be room to ligate the remaining deep vasculature. Once this is complete, the draining vein or veins can be taken.

It is too early to claim victory when the intraoperative period is over. Postoperative angiography is needed to confirm complete resection. Close perioperative control of blood pressure and fluid balance as well as coagulation and electrolytes is required. Hemorrhage in the perinidal brain, whether symptomatic or not, must be managed aggressively. Finally, to truly achieve the best outcomes, the patients must be followed in the outpatient clinic until they have completed their recovery and a plan for delayed imaging is decided. Careful attention to detail can deliver AVM outcomes superior to their natural history.

References

[1] Mohr JP, Parides MK, Stapf C, et al. International ARUBA Investigators. Medical management with or without interventional therapy for unruptured brain arteriovenous malformations (ARUBA): a multicentre, non-blinded, randomised trial. Lancet. 2014; 383(9917):614–621

[2] Rutledge WC, Abla AA, Nelson J, Halbach VV, Kim H, Lawton MT. Treatment and outcomes of ARUBA-eligible patients with unruptured brain arteriovenous malformations at a single institution. Neurosurg Focus. 2014; 37(3):E8

[3] Lawton MT, Kim H, McCulloch CE, Mikhak B, Young WL. A supplementary grading scale for selecting patients with brain arteriovenous malformations for surgery. Neurosurgery. 2010; 66(4):702–713, discussion 713

[4] Bekelis K, Missios S, Desai A, Eskey C, Erkmen K. Magnetic resonance imaging/magnetic resonance angiography fusion technique for intraoperative navigation during microsurgical resection of cerebral arteriovenous malformations. Neurosurg Focus. 2012; 32(5):E7

[5] Gonzalez LF, Albuquerque FC, Boom S, Burling BS, Papadopoulos SM, Spetzler RF. Image-guided resection of embolized cerebral arteriovenous malformations based on catheter-based angiography. Neurosurgery. 2010; 67(2):471–475

[6] Taylor CL, Dutton K, Rappard G, et al. Complications of preoperative embolization of cerebral arteriovenous malformations. J Neurosurg. 2004; 100(5): 810–812

[7] Crowley RW, Ducruet AF, Kalani MY, Kim LJ, Albuquerque FC, McDougall CG. Neurological morbidity and mortality associated with the endovascular treatment of cerebral arteriovenous malformations before and during the Onyx era. J Neurosurg. 2015; 122(6):1492–1497

[8] Burchiel KJ, Clarke H, Ojemann GA, Dacey RG, Winn HR. Use of stimulation mapping and corticography in the excision of arteriovenous malformations in sensorimotor and language-related neocortex. Neurosurgery. 1989; 24(3): 322–327

[9] Gabarrós A, Young WL, McDermott MW, Lawton MT. Language and motor mapping during resection of brain arteriovenous malformations: indications, feasibility, and utility. Neurosurgery. 2011; 68(3):744–752

[10] Ellis MJ, Rutka JT, Kulkarni AV, Dirks PB, Widjaja E. Corticospinal tract mapping in children with ruptured arteriovenous malformations using functionally guided diffusion-tensor imaging. J Neurosurg Pediatr. 2012; 9(5):505–510

[11] Zhao B, Cao Y, Zhao Y, Wu J, Wang S. Functional MRI-guided microsurgery of intracranial arteriovenous malformations: study protocol for a randomised controlled trial. BMJ Open. 2014; 4(10):e006618

[12] Spetzler RF, Martin NA. A proposed grading system for arteriovenous malformations. J Neurosurg. 1986; 65(4):476–483

[13] Hamilton MG, Spetzler RF. The prospective application of a grading system for arteriovenous malformations. Neurosurgery. 1994; 34(1):2–6, discussion 6–7

[14] Kim H, Abla AA, Nelson J, et al. Validation of the supplemented Spetzler-Martin grading system for brain arteriovenous malformations in a multicenter cohort of 1009 surgical patients. Neurosurgery. 2015; 76(1):25–31, discussion 31–32, quiz 32–33

[15] von der Brelie C, Simon M, Esche J, Schramm J, Boström A. Seizure Outcomes in Patients With Surgically Treated Cerebral Arteriovenous Malformations. Neurosurgery. 2015; 77(5):762–768

[16] Englot DJ, Young WL, Han SJ, McCulloch CE, Chang EF, Lawton MT. Seizure predictors and control after microsurgical resection of supratentorial arteriovenous malformations in 440 patients. Neurosurgery. 2012; 71(3):572–580, discussion 580

15 Surgical Treatment of Cerebellar Arteriovenous Malformations

João Paulo Almeida, Vitor Yamaki, Mateus Reghin Neto, Feres Chaddad Neto, Albert Rhoton Jr., and Evandro de Oliveira

Abstract

Cerebellar arteriovenous malformations (AVMs) represent approximately 10% of all intracranial AVMs. Although less common, these lesions are associated with rates of hemorrhage, morbidity, and mortality higher than supratentorial AVMs. In this chapter, we evaluate the anatomical characteristics of the cerebellum and cerebellar AVMs and discuss the application of a new classification of cerebellar AVMs based on the microsurgical anatomy of this region. The smaller size of the cerebellum, the lack of perforating arteries and deep venous drainage system, and few eloquent areas when compared to the brain hemispheres are important characteristics to be considered for planning and treatment of cerebellar AVMs. Therefore, we propose an anatomical classification system for cerebellar AVMs based on size (< 2 cm: I; 2–4 cm: II; > 4 cm: III), location (superficial: A; deep: B; mixed: C), and extension to the dentate nucleus and superior cerebellar peduncles. The anatomical classification of cerebellar AVMs may be used for planning of microsurgical treatment of different types of AVMs in this region.

Keywords: arteriovenous, malformation, cerebellum, surgery, classification, anatomy

- Cerebellar arteriovenous malformations (AVMs) present specific natural history, clinical presentation, and anatomical characteristics.
- Hemorrhage of these lesions is associated with high rates of morbidity and mortality, which justifies the importance of their adequate treatment.
- Microsurgical resection is the gold standard treatment of cerebellar AVMs.
- Size, location, and involvement of the dentate nuclei play a major role in the surgical planning of cerebellar AVMs.

15.1 Introduction

Posterior fossa arteriovenous malformations (AVMs) account for 7 to 15% of all intracranial AVMs[1,2,3,4] and are mostly represented by cerebellar AVMs, a heterogeneous group that includes 75 to 81.2% of all the posterior fossa AVMs.[3,4] Even though cerebellar AVMs represent a minority of all intracranial AVMs, they carry a higher risk of rupture and are associated with considerable higher rates of morbidity and mortality.[2]

Cerebellar AVMs, unlike supratentorial malformations, present more frequently with hemorrhages.[2] Mortality rates of up to 66.7% have been associated with the rupture of posterior fossa AVMs.[5] Hernesniemi et al performed a retrospective analysis of 238 AVM patients with a mean follow-up period of 13.5 years.[6] According to this study, an infratentorial location is one of the most important risk factors for rupture. Univariate analysis demonstrates an annual rate of rupture of 11.6% in the first 5 years after admission, with a cumulative rupture rate of 45% in the first 5 years, as compared with an annual rate of 4.3% and a cumulative 5-year rate of 19% for supratentorial AVMs.

Microsurgical resection remains the gold standard treatment for cerebellar AVMs. Treatment selection must be performed according to the characteristics of each case, and the complete resection of the AVM must be the goal of treatment. Surgery is associated with excellent outcomes when performed by a dedicated vascular microneurosurgeon,[4,7,8,9] with reported rates of complete resection of 92 to 100% and morbidity and mortality of 9 to 17% and 4 to 8%, respectively.[4,5,7,8,9,10,11]

In this chapter, we aim to discuss the microsurgical anatomy of cerebellar AVMs and surgical techniques for resection of those lesions.

15.2 Methodology

The cerebellar anatomy review was based on analysis of studies from the Microsurgery Laboratory of the University of Florida, Gainesville, and the Microsurgery Laboratory of the Institute of Neurological Sciences–Hospital Beneficencia Portuguesa de Sao Paulo.

Based on the microsurgical anatomy of the cerebellum and posterior fossa, our philosophy for treatment of cerebellar AVMs is discussed through evaluation of selected cases treated by our team.

15.3 Results

15.3.1 Microsurgical Anatomy

The exquisite complexity of posterior fossa contents requires a thorough knowledge of microsurgical anatomy of this region. Such anatomic background guides the surgeon to the most appropriate approach.[7,12] Only then the surgeon is able to adequately evaluate the spatial location of the malformation (i.e., its relationships within the cerebellum and/or brainstem to the posterior fossa cranial nerves, arteries, and veins) based on the preoperative catheter digital subtraction angiography (DSA), magnetic resonance imaging (MRI) scans, and computed tomography (CT) scans.[13]

Anatomically, the cerebellum may be divided into three surfaces: tentorial, petrosal, and suboccipital.[14] Each of these is related with a cerebellar fissure, cerebellar artery, and specific draining veins. As described by Yasargil,[15] knowledge of this anatomy is crucial since arterial supply and venous drainage of AVMs usually follow the same vascular pattern of normal brain, which guides the surgeon during resection of the lesion.

The tentorial surface faces and conforms to the lower surface of the tentorium[14] (▶ Fig. 15.1). The anteromedial part of this surface, the apex, formed by the anterior vermis, is the highest

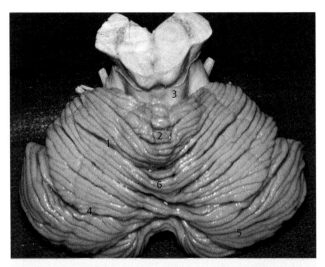

Fig. 15.1 Tentorial surface of the cerebellum. 1: primary fissure; 2: culmen; 3: cerebellomesencephalic fissure; 4: postclival fissure; 5: superior semilunar lobule; 6: declive. (Images from the personal collection of Dr. Evandro de Oliveira. Obtained at the Laboratory of Microneurosurgery, Dr. Albert Rhoton Jr, University of Florida, Gainesville.)

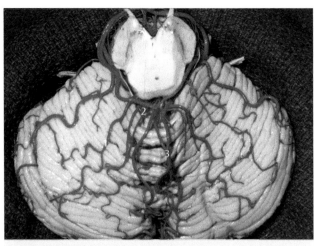

Fig. 15.2 Cerebellomesencephalic and cortical segments of the ACS. 1: hemispheric branches; 2: vermian branches; 3: precerebellar branches. (Images from the personal collection of Dr. Evandro de Oliveira. Obtained at the Laboratory of Microneurosurgery, Dr. Albert Rhoton Jr, University of Florida, Gainesville.)

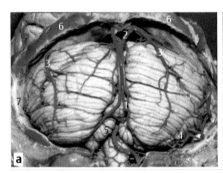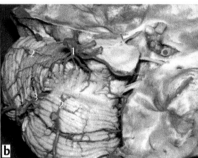

Fig. 15.3 (a,b) Venous drainage of the cerebellum. Superior hemispheric and vermian veins drain the tentorial surface of the cerebellum, while anterior hemispheric veins are the main responsible for the drainage of the petrosal surface and inferior vermian and hemispheric veins for the suboccipital surface. (Images from the personal collection of Dr. Evandro de Oliveira. Obtained at the Laboratory of Microneurosurgery, Dr. Albert Rhoton Jr, University of Florida, Gainesville.)

point on the cerebellum. This surface slopes downward from its anteromedial to its posterolateral edge. On the tentorial surface, the transition from the vermis to the hemispheres is smooth and not marked by the deep fissures on the suboccipital surface between the vermis and hemispheres. The cerebellomesencephalic or precentral cerebellar fissure is located between the posterior aspect of the midbrain and the tentorial surface, closely related with the upper roof of the IV ventricle. The superior cerebellar artery is mainly responsible for the arterial supply of this region[16] (▶ Fig. 15.2). The superior cerebellar artery (SCA) is the last branch of the basilar artery before its bifurcation into the posterior cerebral arteries. It arises in front of the midbrain, near the pontomesencephalic junction, below the oculomotor nerves; it runs toward the posterior surface of the brainstem, passing inferior to the trochlear (IV) nerve and superior to the trigeminal (V) nerve, encircling the midbrain. It then reaches the cerebellomesencephalic fissure, giving rise to the precerebellar arteries. After reaching this region, the SCA sends cortical branches to the tentorial surface of the cerebellar hemispheres and to the vermis. The venous drainage of the tentorial region is performed by the superior hemispheric and vermian veins, which drain toward the vein of Galen, torcula, and transverse sinuses (▶ Fig. 15.3).

The petrosal or anterior surface faces the posterior surface of the petrous bones, the brainstem, and the fourth ventricle[14] (▶ Fig. 15.4). The lateral or hemispheric part of the petrosal surface rests against the petrous bone and is retracted to expose the cerebellopontine angle (CPA). The median or vermian part of the petrosal surface has a deep longitudinal furrow, the anterior cerebellar incisura, which wraps around the posterior surface of the brainstem and fourth ventricle. The right and left halves of the petrosal surfaces are not connected from side to side by a continuous strip of vermis, as are the suboccipital and tentorial surfaces, because of the interposition of the fourth ventricle between the superior and inferior part of the vermis. The cerebellopontine fissure is formed by the folding of the cerebellar hemisphere around the lateral side of the pons and the middle cerebellar peduncle. It has a superior limb between the rostral half of the middle cerebellar peduncle and the superior part of the petrosal surface and an inferior limb between the caudal half of the middle cerebellar peduncle and the inferior part of the petrosal surface. The middle cerebellar peduncle fills the interval

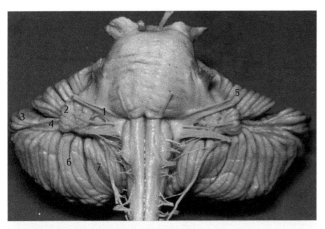

Fig. 15.4 Petrosal surface of the cerebellum. 1: facial and vestibulocochlear nerves; 2: flocculus; 3: superior semilunar lobule; 4: petrosal fissure; 5: quadrangular lobule; 6: inferior semilunar lobule; 7: biventral lobule. (Images from the personal collection of Dr. Evandro de Oliveira. Obtained at the Laboratory of Microneurosurgery, Dr. Albert Rhoton Jr, University of Florida, Gainesville.)

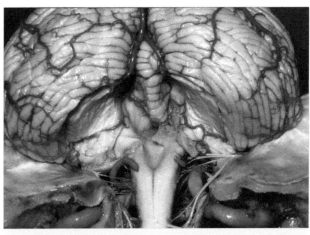

Fig. 15.6 Suboccipital surface of the cerebellum and its veins, after removal of the tonsils and biventral lobules. The inferior hemispheric and vermian veins are the main responsible for the drainage of this surface. (Images from the personal collection of Dr. Evandro de Oliveira. Obtained at the Laboratory of Microneurosurgery, Dr. Albert Rhoton Jr, University of Florida, Gainesville.)

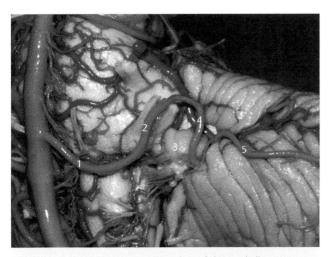

Fig. 15.5 Irrigation of the petrosal surface of the cerebellum. 1: anterior pontine segment of the AICA; 2: lateral pontine segment of the AICA; 3: flocculus; 4: floculopeduncular segment of the AICA; 5: cortical segment of the AICA; (Images from the personal collection of Dr. Evandro de Oliveira. Obtained at the Laboratory of Microneurosurgery, Dr. Albert Rhoton Jr, University of Florida, Gainesville.)

between the two limbs. The anterior inferior cerebellar artery (AICA) is the main arterial trunk related to the cerebellopontine fissure and petrosal surface of the cerebellum[16] (▶ Fig. 15.5). It originates anterior to the pons and runs in a posterolateral direction, in close association to the facial (VII) and vestibulocochlear (VIII) nerves in the CPA. After passing around the flocculus, it reaches the cerebellopontine fissure and then sends cortical branches to the petrosal surface of the cerebellum. The anterior hemispheric veins and the superior petrosal sinus are primarily responsible for the venous drainage of this region.

The suboccipital surface of the cerebellum, located between the sigmoid sinuses and below the transverse sinus, is the most complex of the three surfaces[14] (▶ Fig. 15.6). The suboccipital

surface presents a deep vertical cleft, the posterior cerebellar incisura. The vermis is folded into it and forms the cortical surface within this incisura. The lateral walls of the incisura are formed by the medial aspects of the cerebellar hemispheres. At the suboccipital surface, the vermis is located posterior to the fourth ventricle and above the foramen of Magendie. In this region, the superior portion of the vermis presents a pyramidal shape and it is, therefore, named pyramid. The inferior portion, the uvula, projects downward between the cerebellar tonsils, presenting a similar configuration to that observed at the oropharynx. The rostromedial borders of the tonsils are in close contact to the lateral borders of the uvula. The nodule, located deep to the uvula, is related to the inferior half of the fourth ventricle roof. The broadest portion of the vermis in the posterior cerebellar incisura is the pyramid–uvula junction. Inferiorly, the incisura is continuous with the vallecula cerebelli, a cleft between the tonsils that communicates with the foramen of Magendie. Located between the suboccipital surface of the cerebellum and the medulla, the cerebellomedullary fissure is one of the most complex fissures of the human brain. Its ventral wall is formed by the inferior medullary velum, posterior surface of the medulla, and tela choroidea. The posterior wall is composed by the uvula, tonsils, and biventral lobules. It extends superiorly to the level of the lateral recesses and communicates around the superior poles of the tonsils with the cisterna magna, through the foramen of Magendie with the fourth ventricle, and around the foramina of Luschka with the cerebellopontine fissures. The posterior inferior cerebellar artery (PICA) is the main vessel for arterial supply of the suboccipital region[16] (▶ Fig. 15.7). It originates from the distal portion of the intracranial vertebral artery, anterior to the medulla. It encircles the inferior portion of the brainstem, passing close to the hypoglossal (XII) nerve and, then, to the glossopharyngeal (IX), vagus (X) and spinal accessory (XI) nerve. It then usually forms a caudal and a cranial loop medially to the tonsil and finally reaches the cerebellomedullary fissure, close to the lower portion of the roof of the fourth ventricle. Once out of this fissure, PICA sends

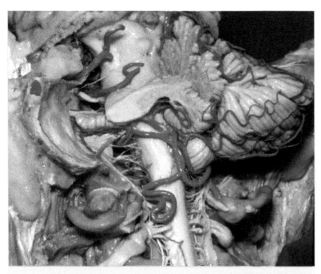

Fig. 15.7 Medial view of the right cerebellar hemisphere. The PICA originates from the distal portion of the intracranial vertebral artery. It encircles the inferior portion of the brainstem, passing close to the XII, IX, X, and XI nerves. It usually forms a caudal and a cranial loop medially to the tonsil toward the cerebellomedullary fissure. Once out of this fissure, PICA sends cortical branches to the suboccipital surface of the cerebellum. (Images from the personal collection of Dr. Evandro de Oliveira. Obtained at the Laboratory of Microneurosurgery, Dr. Albert Rhoton Jr, University of Florida, Gainesville.)

cortical branches to the inferior vermis, tonsils, and the suboccipital surface of the cerebellum.[12,15] The venous drainage of this region is based on the inferior hemispheric and vermian veins, which drain toward the transverse and/or tentorial sinuses and torcula.

15.3.2 Special Features of the Cerebellum and Cerebellar AVMs

Anatomical characteristics of the cerebellum, such as size, cerebellar regions, arterial supply, venous drainage, and eloquence, differentiate the cerebellar AVMs from their supratentorial counterparts.

Size

A previous study of our group evaluated the cerebellar dimensions based on the measurement of 40 cerebellar hemispheres. According to this study, the anteroposterior cerebellar axis represented the largest cerebellar axis (5.24 ± 0.30 cm, range: 4.48–5.8 cm). It was significantly larger than the craniocaudal axis ($p < 0.05$; 5.09 ± 0.28 cm, range: 4.7–5.79 cm) and tended to be larger than the horizontal axis (5.13 ± 0.26 cm, range: 4.63–5.59 cm), but significance was not reached in the latter comparison. None of the cerebellar hemispheres studied presented an axis ≥ 6 cm in diameter.

Cerebellar Regions

According to location, cerebellar AVMs may be classified in four different groups: tentorial, petrous, suboccipital, and vermian. Moreover, these lesions may be further classified according to their location in the cerebellar parenchyma, as follows: superficial, deep, and mixed. Superficial AVM are lesions restricted to the cortical surface of cerebellum; deep AVMs do not present extension into the cerebellar cortex, and mixed AVMs are defined as lesions with extension from the cortex to the deep cerebellar white matter (▶ Fig. 15.8, ▶ Fig. 15.9, ▶ Fig. 15.10).

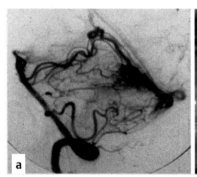
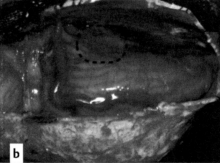

Fig. 15.8 Superficial tentorial AVM. **(a)** DSA demonstrates the superficial location of the nidus of this AVM at the tentorial cerebellar surface. Cortical branches of the SCA provide the arterial supply while the venous drainage is done by superior hemispheric veins. **(b)** Surgical exposure of the lesion after a suboccipital approach. The dashed line demonstrates the location of the AVM. (Images from the personal collection of Dr. Evandro de Oliveira.)

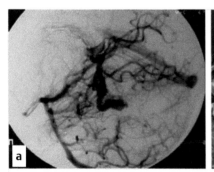
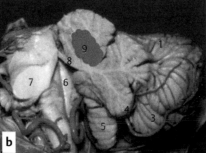

Fig. 15.9 Deep vermian AVM. **(a)** DSA shows a deep AVM nidus located in the deep cerebellar white matter of the vermis and in close relation with the roof of the IV ventricle, but that do not reach the cerebellar cortex. **(b)** Microsurgical dissection demonstrates the medial aspect of the right cerebellar hemisphere, sagittal view. 1: tentorial surface; 2: PICA—cortical hemispheric branches; 3: suboccipital surface; 4: PICA—cortical vermian branches; 5: tonsil; 6: floor of the IV ventricle; 7: middle cerebellar peduncle; 8: upper portion of the roof of the IV ventricle and fibers of the superior cerebellar peduncles; 9: deep vermian AVM. (Images from the personal collection of Dr. Evandro de Oliveira.)

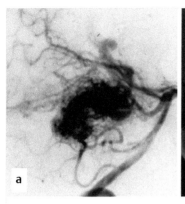
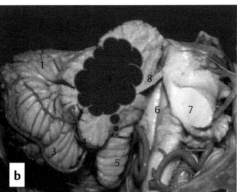

Fig. 15.10 Mixed vermian AVM. **(a)** DSA demonstrates a large lesion that extends from the cerebellum cortex to the deep cerebellar white matter and roof of the IV ventricle. In this case, arterial supply to the AVM was provided by SCA, AICA, and PICA. **(b)** Microsurgical dissection demonstrates the medial aspect of the right cerebellar hemisphere, sagittal view. 1: tentorial surface; 2: PICA–cortical hemispheric branches; 3: suboccipital surface; 4: PICA–cortical vermian branches; 5: tonsil; 6: floor of the IV ventricle; 7: middle cerebellar peduncle; 8: upper portion of the roof of the IV ventricle and fibers of the superior cerebellar peduncles; 9: deep vermian AVM. (Images from the personal collection of Dr. Evandro de Oliveira.)

Arterial Component

The SCA, AICA, and PICA, branches of the vertebral and basilar arteries, provide the cerebellar arterial supply. Didactically, the cerebellum irrigation may be divided as shown in ▶ Table 15.1; however, those vascular regions often overlap; for example, suboccipital AVMs are usually supplied by branches from SCA and PICA.

Compared to supratentorial AVMs, cerebellar AVMs are not supplied by perforating arteries. The presence of the central core, or insular block, justifies an important part of the anatomical differences between the supra- and infratentorial spaces. This eloquent region, located in the deep white matter of the brain hemispheres, distinct from the cortical portions of hemispheres, is supplied by perforating branches composed by lenticulostriate and thalamoperforating arteries. In the posterior fossa, however, perforators predominantly supply the brainstem. Thus, cerebellar AVMs are supplied by arterial feeders composed by superficial branches of the posterior fossa circulation.

Venous Drainage

In the supratentorial space, the presence of the central core justifies the importance of the deep venous system. The central core is the main region drained by the vein of Rosenthal and internal cerebral veins, the main veins of the deep venous

system. The absence of a large gray matter component deep in the cerebellum parenchyma is followed by the absence of a relevant deep venous system for cerebellar drainage. According to the Spetzler–Martin classification, only the superficial hemispheric veins draining to the straight or transverse sinuses are considered superficial draining veins. The application of this classification, as proposed, may lead to incorrect evaluation of the cerebellar AVM. In this scenario, superficially located veins, such as the superior vermian veins, may be considered part of the deep venous system due to drainage to the vein of the Galen complex; however, anatomically, those vessels are located superficial in cerebellum and should not be classified as deep veins. Thus, the venous drainage of the cerebellum is based only on a superficial draining system.

Eloquence

The deep cerebellar nuclei are eloquent areas in the cerebellum.[1] Among deep nuclei, the dentate nucleus is the most relevant functional structure, enrolled in planning, movement control, and cognitive functions.[12] It receives afferent connections from the olivocerebellar, reticulocerebellar, tectocerebellar, and spinocerebellar pathways, through middle and inferior cerebellar peduncles, while efferent connections include the cerebellorubral, dentatothalamic, and fastigioreticular pathways, which run through the superior cerebellar peduncles.[1] The dentate nucleus is located 5 mm lateral to the inferior part of the cerebellar vermis, posteroinferior to the middle cerebellar peduncle, and inferolateral to the inferior cerebellar peduncle. In the suboccipital region of cerebellum, the dentate nucleus can be reached through dissection of the biventral fissure followed by resection of the biventral lobules and tonsils.

15.3.3 Anatomical Classification

Although the Spetzler–Martin grading system[17] is extremely useful for the evaluation and prediction of outcomes of supratentorial AVMs, the special features of cerebellar AVMs justify the application of a specific system for these lesions. Considering the anatomic characteristics of the cerebellum, we classify cerebellar AVMs according to its location, depth in the

Table 15.1 Anatomy-based grading scale for cerebellar AVMs

Size	Score
<2 cm	I
2–4 cm	II
>4 cm	III
Deepness	
Superficial	A
Deep	B
Mixed	C
Eloquence	
Dentate nucleus	Yes*
	No

*See text for more information on the dentate nucleus.

cerebellar parenchyma, size, and involvement of dentate nucleus. With regard to location, we classified AVMs in four categories: tentorial, petrous, suboccipital, or vermian. Once the site of the lesion is defined, AVMs are classified following the criteria specified on ▶ Table 15.1. Lesions that present dentate nucleus involvement are represented by *. Clinical application of our grading scale is demonstrated in ▶ Fig. 15.11, ▶ Fig. 15.12, ▶ Fig. 15.13, ▶ Fig. 15.14.

15.4 Discussion

15.4.1 Philosophy of Treatment for Cerebellar AVMs

The surgical management of AVMs is still one of the most intricate problems in neurosurgery. Although direct surgical treatment remains the ultimate therapy for most cases, there have

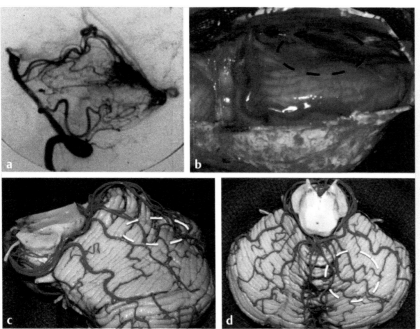

Fig. 15.11 Tentorial AVM (grade IA). **(a)** Cerebral angiography showing a cerebellar AVM in the tentorial region, small in size (<2 cm), superficial, without involvement of dentate nucleus (noneloquent). **(b)** Suboccipital craniotomy with exposure of the AVM. **(c,d)** Arterial supply of cerebellum; lateral **(c)** and superior **(d)** view. The AVM is supplied by the superior cerebellar artery and the venous drainage is done by superior hemispheric and vermians veins. (Images from the personal collection of Dr. Evandro de Oliveira.)

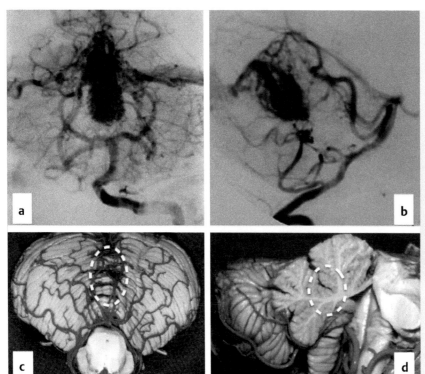

Fig. 15.12 Vermian cerebellar AVM (IIB). Vermian cerebellar AVM, size grade II, located deep in the cerebellar parenchyma **(b)**, without involvement of the dentate nucleus. **(a,b)** DSA showing the main feeders of the AVM, originated from the SCA and PICA. **(c)** Superior view of cerebellum demonstrating the territory of irrigation of the SCA. **(d)** Medial view of cerebellum demonstrating the course of the PICA and the area supplied by it. (Images from the personal collection of Dr. Evandro de Oliveira.)

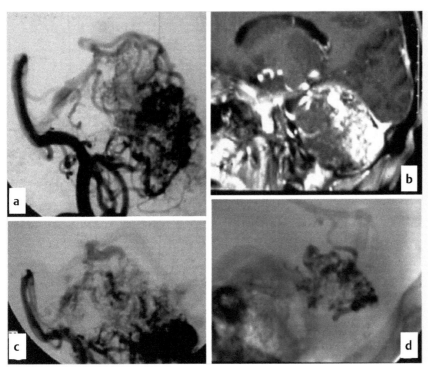

Fig. 15.13 Suboccipital cerebellar AVM (IIIC*).
(a) DSA showing the arterial supply of the AVM originated from the SCA, AICA, and PICA.
(b) Sagittal view of T1 contrast enhanced MRI scan showing the large suboccipital AVM **(c,d)**. Preoperative embolization and reduction of AVM nidus after endovascular treatment. (Images from the personal collection of Dr. Evandro de Oliveira.)

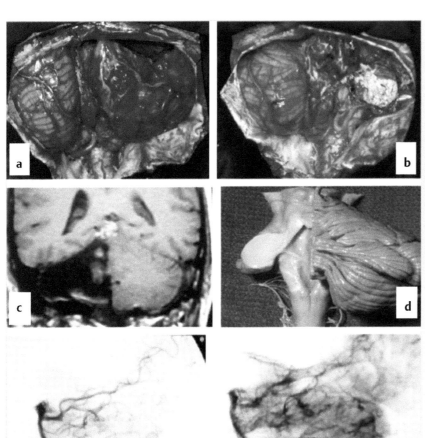

Fig. 15.14 Suboccipital cerebellar AVM (IIIC*)— surgical resection of the AVM presented in ▶ Fig. 15.13. **(a)** Surgical exposure of the AVM. **(b)** Operative view after AVM resection with preservation of the cerebellar peduncles. **(c)** Coronal T1-weighted contrast enhanced MRI scan showing total resection of the AVM. **(d)** Anatomical dissection demonstrating the resection of the cerebellar hemisphere with preservation of the cerebellar peduncles. **(e,f)** Postoperative DSA after total resection of AVM. (Images from the personal collection of Dr. Evandro de Oliveira.)

been a series of advances in neurological imaging, interventional neuroradiology, and radiosurgery that have contributed enormously to the management of these lesions. Together with the microsurgical technique, these advances and the developments in anesthesia and intraoperative monitoring have greatly improved the surgical results.

In order to better plan the operative strategy, the neurosurgeon who deals with AVMs should have a complete three-dimensional knowledge of the brain anatomy and a thorough understanding of the natural history of such lesions. Surgical indication should be based on the anatomical characteristics of the AVM in each patient. The surgeon should also compare his own surgical results with the long-term risks of leaving the AVM untreated.[7]

Although varying from case to case, some basic technical principles should be followed when planning the operation. The best strategy for each individual patient is discussed by a multidisciplinary team of specialists, led by the neurosurgeon who is the one to decide the role of each adjuvant therapy in the final treatment plan. As microsurgery requires that the surgeon be in the best of conditions, the idea of a team approach should also apply to the craniotomy. The main surgeon who will dissect and resect the AVM should not participate in the approach but rather come to surgery after all the bone work is done and the AVM is completely exposed.[7,12]

For the purpose of planning the surgical treatment of cerebellar AVMs, we utilize the grading system previously described, recently proposed by our group. Although simple, it guides the surgeon regarding the anatomical details that should be considered when planning the treatment of cerebellar AVMs. When there are no clinical contraindications, we recommend surgery to virtually all patients who present with those lesions. Exceptions include elderly patients with unruptured AVMs and patients that harbor cerebellar AVM with involvement of the dentate nuclei who do not accept the postoperative deficit associated with the surgical resection of those lesions. Small and medium size cerebellar AVMs (grade I and II) may be surgically approached without the need of preoperative embolization; however, we recommend endovascular treatment for all large (grade III) cerebellar AVMs prior to surgical resection. Radiosurgery, although effective in selected cases, has the disadvantage of leaving the patient unprotected from hemorrhagic events for a variable period of time. It may be useful for elderly patients with limited life expectancy or for neurologically intact patients who do not accept surgery and harbor a small AVM.

15.4.2 Surgery Technique for Resection of Cerebellar AVMs

It is our impression that posterior fossa AVMs that are not located in the brainstem are lesions for which surgical resection is significantly less difficult than those located in the supratentorial compartment.

These AVMs usually receive supply from branches of either the SCA, the PICA, and/or the AICA, which can frequently be easily accessed during surgery. All cortical and subcortical lesions related to the cerebellar hemispheres and to the vermis and located posteriorly to the flocculus usually do not involve the brainstem, and therefore can be resected with very low morbidity.

The surgical treatment of cerebellar AVMs follows similar principles to those applied to their supratentorial counterparts.[12] The craniotomy must be large enough to expose all the AVM as well as some extension of normal brain tissue around its borders. Small craniotomies play no role in the surgical treatment of AVMs. We recommend a suboccipital craniotomy with the patient in semi-sitting position for most cerebellar AVMs. As an exception, petrous AVMs benefit of a lateral extension of the suboccipital approach, with exposure of the transverse-sigmoid junction.

It is essential to follow the principles of good microsurgery: a clean operative field with minimal or no bleeding, opening of the cisterns and fissures, minimal retraction, and no damage to the normal vessels or to the brain tissue.

It is important to find and preserve the arachnoid plane. If the surgeon loses the arachnoid plane, there is a greater risk of entering the nidus before an adequate exposure of the lesion is achieved. Serious bleeding or damage to the normal brain may result of such action. The myth that AVM surgery produces profuse bleeding is wrong. With tenacity and careful and delicate work, bleeding can be controlled with bipolar cauterization, and clean operative fields can be obtained.

With the normal anatomy in mind, the surgeon must achieve proximal control of the vessels going to the AVM. Ideally, the surgeon must dissect all vessels around the AVM and only obliterate them very close to the lesion. This will avoid the obliteration of the so-called vessels *en passage*, which, although passing through the AVM, are in reality going to normal areas of the brain. Bipolar cauterization should be done only when the surgeon is sure that a specific vessel belongs to the AVM. The greatest difficulty lies in the coagulation of the deep feeders. These vessels are usually small, with a high flow, with fragile walls that are difficult to obliterate. After coagulation of most afferents, the arteriovenous shunt is interrupted and the AVM "dies." The last step is the resection of the lesion and cauterization of the draining veins.[12]

Although the perfect bipolar unit is yet to be developed, it is the most important surgical tool during the surgery of AVMs. Temporary mini-clips applied in small vessels prior to coagulation may be helpful. Very rarely, we use aneurysm clips or any other metallic clip to obliterate the vessels.

According to its location, cerebellar AVMs present different details that should be considered for surgical treatment.

Suboccipital

Suboccipital AVMs are mainly supplied by cortical branches of the SCA and venous drainage is performed by inferior hemispheric and vermian veins. Dentate nucleus may be involved in grades II/III B or C AVMs located in the inferior suboccipital region. Exposure of AVMs near the tonsils requires dissection of the cisterna magna, telovelar region, and lateral medullary cistern. Careful identification of PICA branches, inferiorly and medially to tonsils, and lower cranial nerves (IX, X, XI, XII) is important to avoid major neurovascular injuries.

Petrous

We recommend the lateral suboccipital craniotomy with the patient in a semi-sitting position for exposure of petrous AVMs.

Dissection of the cisterna magna and CPA for CSF drainage and cerebellum relaxation is recommended for improved exposure of the petrosal surface. Although this is a noneloquent cerebellar region, the VII and VIII cranial nerves, middle cerebellar peduncle, and pons surround the lesions located in this region. The arterial supply of petrosal AVMs is mostly provided by AICA branches. Relevant veins for petrous AVMs are the cerebellopontine and anterior hemispheric veins. Dissection of the posterior part of theses AVM may require resection of part of the cerebellar cortex.

Tentorial

AVM draining veins directed toward the transverse sinus must be preserved during initial dissection. Arterial irrigation mainly originates from cortical branches of SCA, which are found and coagulated at the beginning of surgery. Tangential nidus dissection aims to move the AVM toward the tentorium. After circumferential ligation of nidus feeders, hemispheric and superior vermian veins should be occluded and the AVM resected.

Vermian

Vermian branches of SCA and PICA usually provide the arterial supply for these lesions. The origin of SCA-derived feeders can be reached in the cerebellomesencephalic fissure, while the origin of PICA-derived feeders may observed at the telovelar region and at the suboccipital surface, where medial PICA branches may also provide feeders to the AVM. After identification and ligation of the arterial feeders, the nidus is circumferentially dissected, which may require resection of portion of the vermis, in order to maintain the dissection plane and avoid major bleeding from the nidus. Coagulation of the main drainage veins, usually composed by superior and inferior vermian veins, may then be performed and followed by complete resection of the AVM. Inferior vermian AVMs may be in close contact with the dentate nuclei. In those cases, whenever possible, careful delimitation of the nidus and delicate dissection of the lateral portions of the lesion may limit potential injuries to this structure.

15.5 Conclusion

Cerebellar AVMs are challenging lesions in neurosurgery. Management of these AVMs requires knowledge of their natural history, thorough clinical and radiological evaluation, and collaboration between neurosurgeons, endovascular surgeons, and radiosurgeons. Anatomical differences in size, arterial supply, venous drainage, and eloquent areas between the supratentorial space and the cerebellum justify the unique characteristics of cerebellar AVMs, which, in our view, favor surgical treatment of most of these lesions.

Finally, surgical treatment of cerebellar AVMs follows the basic principles of microneurosurgery, which requires a detailed anatomical knowledge of the brain structures and a refined microsurgical technique. We believe training in a microsurgical laboratory is essential for development of the surgical abilities required to adequately approach those lesions.

References

[1] Al-Shahi R, Warlow C. A systematic review of the frequency and prognosis of arteriovenous malformations of the brain in adults. Brain. 2001; 124(Pt 10): 1900–1926

[2] Arnaout OM, Gross BA, Eddleman CS, Bendok BR, Getch CC, Batjer HH. Posterior fossa arteriovenous malformations. Neurosurg Focus. 2009; 26 (5):E12

[3] Batjer H, Samson D. Arteriovenous malformations of the posterior fossa. Clinical presentation, diagnostic evaluation, and surgical treatment. J Neurosurg. 1986; 64(6):849–856

[4] Drake CG, Friedman AH, Peerless SJ. Posterior fossa arteriovenous malformations. J Neurosurg. 1986; 64(1):1–10

[5] Symon L, Tacconi L, Mendoza N, Nakaji P. Arteriovenous malformations of the posterior fossa: a report on 28 cases and review of the literature. Br J Neurosurg. 1995; 9(6):721–732

[6] Hernesniemi JA, Dashti R, Juvela S, Väärt K, Niemelä M, Laakso A. Natural history of brain arteriovenous malformations: a long-term follow-up study of risk of hemorrhage in 238 patients. Neurosurgery. 2008; 63(5):823–829, discussion 829–831

[7] de Oliveira E, Tedeschi H, Raso J. Multidisciplinary approach to arteriovenous malformations. Neurol Med Chir (Tokyo). 1998; 38 Suppl:177–185

[8] O'Shaughnessy BA, Getch CC, Bendok BR, Batjer HH. Microsurgical resection of infratentorial arteriovenous malformations. Neurosurg Focus. 2005; 19(2): E5

[9] Sinclair J, Kelly ME, Steinberg GK. Surgical management of posterior fossa arteriovenous malformations. Neurosurgery. 2006; 58(4) Suppl 2:ONS-189–ONS-201, discussion ONS-201

[10] Kelly ME, Guzman R, Sinclair J, et al. Multimodality treatment of posterior fossa arteriovenous malformations. J Neurosurg. 2008; 108(6):1152–1161

[11] Rodríguez-Hernández A, Kim H, Pourmohamad T, Young WL, Lawton MT, University of California, San Francisco Arteriovenous Malformation Study Project. Cerebellar arteriovenous malformations: anatomic subtypes, surgical results, and increased predictive accuracy of the supplementary grading system. Neurosurgery. 2012; 71(6):1111–1124

[12] de Oliveira E, Tedeschi H, Raso J. Comprehensive management of arteriovenous malformations. Neurol Res. 1998; 20(8):673–683

[13] Almeida JP, Medina R, Tamargo RJ. Management of posterior fossa arteriovenous malformations. Surg Neurol Int. 2015; 6:31

[14] Rhoton AL, Jr. Cerebellum and fourth ventricle. Neurosurgery. 2000; 47(3) Suppl:S7–S27

[15] Yasargil MG. Microneurosurgery. Stuttgart: Thieme Stratton; 1984

[16] Rhoton AL, Jr. The cerebellar arteries. Neurosurgery. 2000; 47(3) Suppl:S29–S68

[17] Spetzler RF, Martin NA. A proposed grading system for arteriovenous malformations. J Neurosurg. 1986; 65(4):476–483

16 Surgical Treatment of Intracranial Dural Arteriovenous Fistulas

Federico Cagnazzo, Thomas J. Sorenson, and Giuseppe Lanzino

Abstract

Intracranial dural arteriovenous fistulas (DAVFs) are pathological vascular connections between dural arteries and dural venous sinuses, dural veins, or meningeal veins, with the shunt usually located within the dural leaflets. The venous drainage pattern is the most important predictor of clinical behavior and possibility of treatment. Nowadays, most of intracranial DAVFs can be satisfactorily treated with an endovascular approach, and surgery has become a second line of treatment. However, surgical approach is a valid therapeutic strategy in symptomatic patients who need immediate cure, or when embolization is not feasible or safe due to the risk of collateral arterial branches embolization or inability to achieve a microcatheter position close enough to the shunt to achieve effective treatment. Accordingly, certain anatomical locations may still require surgical treatment, such as anterior ethmoidal, craniocervical junction, and tentorial DAVFs. Surgical disconnection of the draining vein is an effective strategy that allows occlusion of the fistula or promotes its conversion into a less aggressive lesion. Finally, surgery can be indicated after failed initial endovascular occlusion, or in a combined strategy with endovascular treatment.

Keywords: intracranial dural arteriovenous fistulas, surgical treatment, endovascular treatment, venous drainage

Key Points

- Intracranial dural arteriovenous fistulas (DAVFs) are rare vascular lesions, though potentially the cause of intracranial hemorrhage or neurological symptoms related to venous congestion.
- With the evolution of endovascular techniques, embolization represents a safe and effective treatment modality for most of these lesions.
- Despite advances of endovascular techniques, surgery remains a valid therapeutic strategy in those patients who need immediate cure and are not amenable to safe and effective embolization.
- Because of local anatomical conditions and/or characteristics of the feeding arteries, anterior ethmoidal, craniocervical junction, and tentorial DAVFs are those anatomical location that may still require surgical disconnection even in the modern endovascular era.
- The pattern of venous drainage influences clinical behavior. Surgical disconnection of the draining vein(s) is a feasible strategy that allows the occlusion of the fistula or promotes its conversion into a more benign lesion.

16.1 Introduction and General Principles

Intracranial dural arteriovenous fistulas (DAVFs) are pathological vascular connections between dural arteries and dural venous sinuses, dural veins, or meningeal veins, with the shunt usually located within the dural leaflets. The venous drainage pattern is the most important predictor of clinical behavior, natural history, risk of hemorrhage, and possibility of treatment.[1] Borden et al and Cognard et al underlined the relation between the cortical venous reflux and the clinical aggressiveness.[2,3] Angioarchitecture and venous outflow, as well as the location of the DAVF, are also critical for the treatment management. Therapeutic strategies include conservative monitoring, endovascular embolization (transarterial or transvenous), surgical excision, and radiosurgery.[4]

With the improvement of endovascular techniques, especially the advent of Onyx, embolization of DAVFs has become the first choice, and most intracranial DAVFs can be satisfactorily treated with an endovascular approach. With this paradigm shift, surgical management has become the second line of treatment usually utilized and indicated only in a certain subset of situations. Surgery is still required for cases in need of immediate cure (because of hemorrhage or aggressive neurological symptoms) and embolization is not feasible or safe because of high risk of embolization into collateral branches or inability to achieve favorable catheter position close enough to the shunt to provide effective treatment. Surgical treatment may also be evaluated after a failed endovascular embolization attempt or in a combined strategy with endovascular treatment.

16.2 Materials and Methods

The current literature regarding the surgical treatment of intracranial DAVFs was explored. We reported the results of the published surgical series in which the surgical approach was used alone or combined with endovascular treatment. The aim of this chapter is to describe the current surgical management of the intracranial DAVFs, and report the anatomical locations and angioarchitecture characteristics for which surgery is indicated.

16.3 Results and Discussion

16.3.1 General Principles

The potential approaches of surgical treatment include (1) occlusion of the involved sinus, (2) disconnection of the proximal portion of the draining vein in those with exclusive cortical venous drainage, or (3) disconnection of the dangerous portion of the cortical vein, without complete occlusion of the shunt turning a fistula with "dangerous" angioarchitecture into one with more benign features.

In general, treatment is indicated for symptomatic and clinically aggressive DAVFs. Borden type I fistulas have a very low risk of hemorrhage or nonhemorrhagic neurologic deficits, and observation with surveillance and palliation of symptoms with particulate embolization are viable choices. Alternatively, many Borden type II–III DAVFs show aggressive clinical behaviors, and treatment is often required. In a classic meta-analysis of 377 intracranial DAVFs, Awad et al noted that cortical venous drainage is often associated with progressive neurological deficits, increased intracranial pressure, and higher risk of hemorrhage.[5]

In a seminal publication now of historical value, Sundt and Piepgras described resection of the involved dural sinus before the development of endovascular treatment and modern microsurgical approaches. These authors described the results of 27 patients surgically treated with ligation and complete excision of the transverse sinus at the point of connection with the sigmoid sinus. The results were excellent in 22 patients and good in 1 patient. However, two patients died and two suffered poor outcome.[6] With refinement of endovascular techniques, the vast majority of DAVFs with involvement of a major dural sinus and retrograde cortical venous drainage are treated with endovascular techniques and surgery is rarely necessary. When surgery is necessary for an isolated arterialized sinus, skeletonization of the sinus with disconnection of arterialized veins and packing of the sinus with hemostatic agent without excision is the preferred surgical technique (▶ Fig. 16.1 and ▶ Fig. 16.2).

In those patients with DAVFs without sinus involvement and exclusive leptomeningeal drainage, simple disconnection of the proximal portion of the draining vein is a simple and effective technique (▶ Fig. 16.3). Collice et al described two types of DAVF: "sinus fistula," which occurs when the lumen of the sinus participates in the shunt, and "nonsinus fistula," which occurs when the shunt is confined into the wall of the sinus without communication to the inside of the parent sinus.[7] The authors introduced the concept of "disconnecting" the venous drainage in the nonsinus fistula DAVFs. Twenty cases of DAVFs with

"pure leptomeningeal drainage" were treated (9 with direct surgery, 11 with preoperative arterial embolization). Complete radioanatomical cure was obtained in 95% of cases with a low morbidity and mortality rate.

The similar treatment was reported by Thompson et al in four patients with DAVFs and leptomeningeal venous drainage. The authors treated two petrotentorial, one middle fossa, and one posterior fossa DAVF by interrupting the draining vein in the passage between dura and subarachnoid space. Improvement of neurological condition and complete occlusion were obtained in all four patients.[8] Although simple and very effective, surgical disconnection of the draining vein has become a less common procedure given that many of these DAVFs can be effectively treated with liquid embolic agents.

In DAVFs with involvement of a main sinus and retrograde leptomeningeal drainage, the treatment strategy can be to simply exclude the retrograde leptomeningeal drainage without complete occlusion of the DAVF if complete occlusion of the fistula cannot be safely obtained. This strategy converts the DAVF into a more benign type of vascular lesion. Davies et al of the University of Toronto Brain Vascular Malformation Study Group assessed a large series of 102 patients with aggressive cranial DAVFs. In cases of combined dural sinus drainage and cortical venous reflux, the authors performed a selective disconnection of the drainage vein, which leaves the fistula in the wall of the dural sinus untouched. Selective disconnection was performed in 23 DAVFs and the neurological and angiographic outcome was comparable to those with obliterated DAVFs.[9]

16.4 Surgical Treatment by Location

16.4.1 Anterior Cranial Fossa (Ethmoidal Fistulas)

Anterior cranial fossa DAVFs have been reported with much lower frequency than with other locations and represent fewer than 10% of all DAVFs.[10] Ethmoidal DAVFs can cause headache,

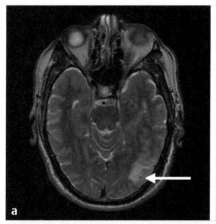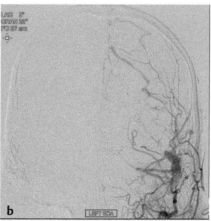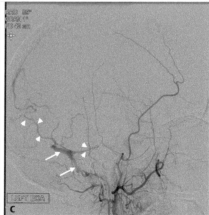

Fig. 16.1 A 63-year-old man presented with progressive visual symptoms. **(a)** MRI demonstrates evidence of T2 signal changes in the left parietal occipital area (*white arrow*). The remaining of the MRI suggests evidence of abnormal vascularity of the region, so catheter angiography was performed. Left external ICA injection anteroposterior (AP) **(b)** and lateral **(c)** views show a fistula of the isolated transverse sigmoid sinus junction (*arrows*) with retrograde cortical venous drainage through multiple veins (*arrowheads*).

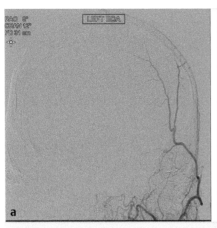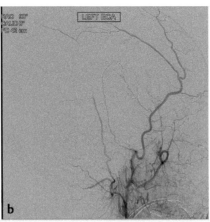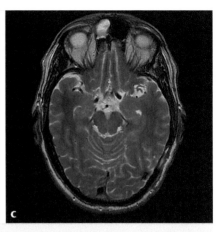

Fig. 16.2 Same patient as ▶ Fig. 16.1. Through a left parietal occipital craniotomy, the isolated left transverse sigmoid junction was exposed and the isolated sinus was packed with hemostatic agent and obliterated. Postoperative angiography, left external carotid artery injection, AP view **(a)** and lateral view **(b)** show complete occlusion of the fistula. Follow-up axial T2 MRI **(c)** shows resolution of the T2 changes at follow-up.

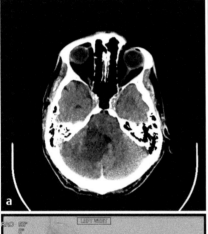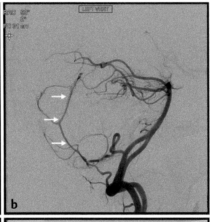

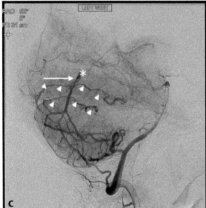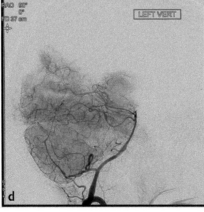

Fig. 16.3 In patients with exclusive leptomeningeal drainage, simple ligation of the proximal portion of the arterialized vein as it emerges from the dura results in complete obliteration and resolution of the fistula. This 54-year-old man presented with several-week history of intractable nausea, headache, and cognitive decline. CT of the head demonstrated edema of the right cerebellar hemisphere with compression of the fourth ventricle **(a)**. CT with contrast (not shown) suggested abnormally dilated vessels in the posterior fossa, and this prompted a catheter angiography. **(b)** Right vertebral artery injection, lateral view shows a dilated posterior meningeal artery *(arrows)* supplying a dural fistula localized under the posterior third of the tentorium. **(c)** In the late arterial phase, there is an early filling vein *(white arrows)* emanating from the undersurface of the tentorium *(asterisk)* with retrograde cortical venous drainage *(arrowheads)*. Because of inability to achieve distal microcatheter navigation of the feeding artery, the patient was treated with surgical disconnection by placing a surgical clip at the point of emergence of the arterialized vein from the tentorium. Follow-up catheter angiography **(d)** confirms complete angiographic obliteration of the fistula.

visual symptoms, seizures, or epistaxis. They can also occasionally hemorrhage and cause more aggressive symptoms.[11,12]

The principal blood supply to these DAVFs is derived from the ophthalmic artery (▶ Fig. 16.4 and ▶ Fig. 16.5) but the external carotid artery can also give arterial feeders. The pial veins of the anterior frontal lobe usually drain the ethmoidal DAVF into the superior sagittal sinus. More rarely, they can drain posteriorly toward the cavernous or sphenoparietal sinuses.[10,13] The

higher hemorrhage risk could be related to the increased pressures in fragile pial veins that drain into the superior sagittal sinus. Varices or pseudoaneurysms can also increase the risk of rupture.

Currently, endovascular techniques represent the best treatment option for most intracranial DAVFs. However, endovascular embolization of ethmoidal fistulas presents many limitations. The selective catheterization of the ophthalmic and

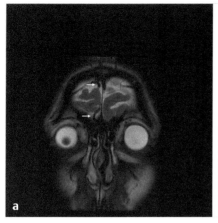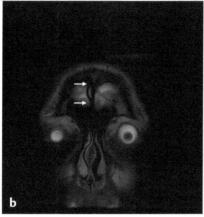

Fig. 16.4 This 45-year-old woman underwent MRI for investigation of new onset of headache. Coronal T2 MRI **(a,b)** suggests presence of abnormally dilated vessel in anterior frontal region (*white arrows*).

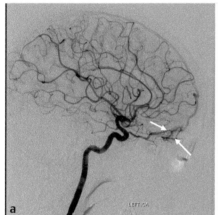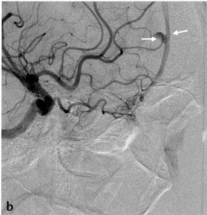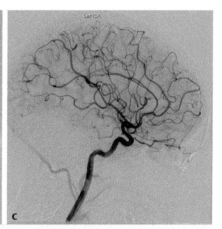

Fig. 16.5 (a) Lateral selective right internal carotid artery injection shows an AV fistula (*white arrows*) in the region in the anterior cranial fossa fed by branches of the ophthalmic artery. **(b)** Magnified oblique view demonstrates the nidal component of the fistula and the draining cortical vein corresponding to the dilated vessel identified on the MRI. There is a venous varix (*white arrows*) indicating partial venous outflow obstruction. The patient underwent a right frontal craniotomy and occlusion of the proximal draining vein as it emerged from the dura of the anterior cranial fossa. **(c)** Postoperative catheter angiography confirms complete exclusion of the fistula.

ethmoidal arteries is often technically challenging due to the small diameter and tortuous course. There is also considerable risk of reflux of the embolic agents into the ophthalmic artery (especially the central retinal artery) or into the supraclinoid internal carotid artery (ICA).[11,14]

For these reasons, surgery can be a safe and effective treatment in this location. The surgical access can be unilateral or, in the case of bilateral fistulas, bilateral.[15] The key point of the surgical treatment is the disconnection of the proximal portion of the draining vein, which usually emerges from the dura of the cranial base in close proximity to the cribriform plate (▶ Fig. 16.5). Disconnection can be achieved with clip ligation or coagulation and sectioning of the proximal vein. While approaching the site of fistula, frontal lobe manipulation and retraction must be minimized to avoid avulsing the draining vein. Focal venous dilatations are frequent in this location and are usually a site of hemorrhage or intraoperative rupture. Occlusion of the venous connection between the dural and the pial vessels allows their resolution, and there is no need to remove or coagulate these venous dilatations.[10] Intraoperative angiography and recently introduced indocyanine green videoangiography can be useful to document the complete obliteration of the DAVF.[15,16] In evaluating the preoperative angiography, close

attention must be directed to the study of the venous drainage, since, in some cases, ethmoidal DAVFs can be bilateral and each hemisphere has separate venous drainage.

Several series reported a high rate of success of the surgical treatment with relatively low incidence of complications. Lawton et al reported the results of a relatively large series of 16 surgically treated patients, describing complete occlusion of lesions in all patients and a 93% likelihood of good clinical outcome.[11] In a series of 16 ethmoidal DAVFs treated with modern techniques, Cannizzaro et al reported using surgical treatment for 54% of patients with excellent clinical results.[17]

Overall, surgery is a safe and effective option for anterior fossa DAVFs and it is often the best therapeutic modality for this specific fistula location even in the modern endovascular era. Moreover, the surgical approach is performed in noneloquent areas of the brain, and in case of hemorrhage, surgery also allows the possibility to remove any associated hematomas.

16.4.2 Cavernous Sinus Region

While direct carotid cavernous fistulas (CCFs) are a direct communication between the ICA and a vein in the region of the cavernous sinus usually related to trauma or rupture of a cavernous ICA aneurysm, so-called "indirect" CCFs are nothing but a variation of DAVFs draining through one of the parasellar veins.[18] Similar to DAVFs in other locations, DVAFs of the cavernous sinus region are usually treated with endovascular techniques or radiosurgery. Surgery is necessary only in exceptional cases.[19]

The cavernous sinus is an intracranial compartment that is not easily accessible by microsurgery, and surgical treatment can be evaluated only in selected conditions. Different surgical treatments have been described: suturing, clipping, trapping the fistula, packing the cavernous sinus, or ligating the ICA.[20] Overall success rates using surgical intervention in the treatment of CCFs have been reported at between 31 and 79%.[21,22,23]

In recent series, surgery is used when the endovascular access is not feasible or after the failure of embolization. Tu et al reported results from a series of 19 patients previously treated with endovascular embolization.[24] Surgical intervention was used after the incomplete result of an endovascular approach. The obliteration was obtained in 94% of cases. Similar results were reported by Day and Fukushima after nine patients underwent direct surgical intervention following endovascular failure for a type D CCFs. The obliteration rate was 100%, but all patients experienced a transient diplopia and trigeminal neuralgia, and two patients had a temporary and permanent hemiparesis.[23]

With the evolution of endovascular treatments, the role of surgery becomes limited only for selected cases of CCF. In special situations, when the cavernous sinus cannot be reached transvenously, surgery could be used to provide the access through the petrosal vein, or the superior ophthalmic vein for a retrograde catheterization to allow the embolization of the fistula.[25,26]

16.4.3 Tentorial DAVFs

Tentorial DAVFs are often characterized by an aggressive clinical behavior because of the consistent presence of retrograde leptomeningeal venous outflow.[27] Many studies reported hemorrhage rates of between 58 and 74%, and progressive neurological symptoms in 79% to 92% of cases although more recent series have observed an increasing percentage of patients with minimally symptomatic or even incidental lesions.[5,28,2930] When symptomatic, prompt and radical treatment is indicated.

Until a few years ago, tentorial DAVFs represented one of the most common indications for direct surgery for DAVFs. However, with recent advances in liquid embolic agents, most of these fistulas can be effectively and safely be treated with Onyx or similar agents.[31] Surgery is necessary only in those cases after failed endovascular therapy or when endovascular therapy is hazardous or not feasible (▶ Fig. 16.3).

Lawton et al reported a large surgical series of 31 tentorial DAVFs divided into six types. The authors performed a specific operative treatment based on the specific type, and all DAVFs were embolized preoperatively from a transarterial access. A specific approach was used for each type of DAVF, and the strategy was to interrupt the draining vein. Complete obliteration was obtained in 94% cases with low complication rate.[32]

Other authors have reiterated the efficacy of venous drainage disconnection in the surgical treatment of tentorial DAVFs. Tomak et al reported another large series of 22 patients with tentorial Borden type III DAVF treated between 1988 and 2000.

Seven patients (32%) underwent selective surgical disconnection of their venous drainage with complete resolution of the fistula.[27]

Tentorial DAVFs can be cured with selective disconnection of the venous drainage without extensive nidal resection, which is usually associated with higher blood loss and higher procedural complications. This strategy can cure or convert a malignant fistula into a more benign version. Additionally, presurgical transarterial embolization to the venous side (especially with Onyx) or transvenous embolization can be used in a multimodality strategy to promote a safe and complete eradication of the fistula.

16.4.4 Transverse-Sigmoid Sinus DAVFs

The transverse-sigmoid sinus is the most common location for DAVFs. Awad et al reported 62.9% DAVFs occurred in the transvers-sinus sinus in a systematic analysis of 377 DAVFs.[5] Their clinical presentation in about 50% of cases is a pulse synchronous bruit, or headache. More aggressive symptoms, such as intracranial hypertension, hemorrhage, or ascending myelopathy are less frequent and occur in about 27% of patients.[3] Treatment is usually indicated in more aggressive lesions with cortical venous drainage or nonhemorrhagic neurological deficits. This treatment is usually performed with an endovascular transarterial or transvenous approach that carries a higher possibility of complete occlusion of the fistula. In our institution, transverse/sigmoid sinus DAVFs without aggressive neurological symptoms are effectively and safely treated with a combination of radiosurgery followed by particle embolization.[33,34]

The surgical resection of the involved sinus was described by Sundt and Piepgras, but this radical approach is merely of historical interest and unnecessary given it is associated with complications.[6] In cases of incomplete occlusion after endovascular treatment, surgery can be performed with the intent of occluding the sinus (▶ Fig. 16.1 and ▶ Fig. 16.2) and/or disconnect arterialized veins. In a large surgical series reported by Kakarla et al, the authors identified two types of transverse-sigmoid sinus fistula, each with a different surgical treatment. In nine patients, the entire sinus was involved, skeletonized, and obliterated with coils. In the remaining 11 patients, it was possible to identify a single leptomeningeal venous drainage, which was obliterated. Good outcome was obtained in 95%. Only three patients had a residual DAVF that was treated with postoperative embolization.[35]

16.4.5 Convexity-Superior Sagittal Sinus DAVFs

DAVFs involving the superior sagittal sinus (SSS) are rare compared to other locations, and account for about 8% of intracranial DAVFs.[3] This kind of fistula most often involves the midportion of the sagittal sinus. The point of the fistula can be also located in the dural layers of the convexity. These fistulas have often bilateral arterial feeders from the middle meningeal artery or other branches derived from the external carotid artery. Superior sagittal sinus fistulas often exhibit a retrograde venous drainage into the parasagittal cortical veins. With modern advanced imaging, it has become clear that many of these fistulas utilize a venous "pocket" that often runs parallel to the main sinus.

When necessary, microsurgery can involve different strategies: skeletonization of the sinus, disconnection of all arterialized vein, or a combination with endovascular treatment.

In a series reported by Van Dijk et al, four patients had a convexity DAVF with direct cortical venous reflux (nonsinus type), and five patients had an SSS fistula (two sinus type and three nonsinus type). The simple coagulation and occlusion of the drainage vein was performed with a good angiographic results and outcome.[36]

16.4.6 Craniocervical Junction DAVFs

DAVFs at the craniocervical junction are uncommon. The clinical presentation commonly includes acute subarachnoid hemorrhage and myelopathy. Subarachnoid hemorrhage is more common in DAVFs of the craniocervical junction draining cranially toward the brainstem, whereas myelopathy is more common in these DAVFs with caudal drainage toward the spinal cord. Less frequent symptoms include brainstem dysfunction, radiculopathy, cranial nerve palsy, and occipital neuralgia.[37,38,39]

The arterial supply often derives from the meningeal branches of the vertebral artery or from the occipital artery and ascending pharyngeal artery. The DAVF drainage can involve different venous systems, and the pattern of venous outflow can cause different clinical presentations. The perimedullary veins are usually involved, and they drain arterialized blood through the pial coronal venous plexus into the spinal cord via the radial veins. This causes venous congestion and myelopathy. Sometimes, the drainage may occur superiorly into the intracranial venous system. Increasing intravenous pressure and fast venous outflow can promote varix formation, resulting in subarachnoid hemorrhage.[40]

Radiological and clinical diagnoses can be challenging because a craniocervical DAVF is a rare vascular anomaly often characterized by a complex, deep-seated vascular anatomy. Among intracranial DAVFs, craniocervical junction DAVFs are best suited to surgery as the main therapeutic option since endovascular techniques present some limitations. Specifically, arterial feeders are usually small and tortuous, and often they arise directly from the vertebral artery, so endovascular navigation is a challenge and the risk of embolic complications is higher. Additionally, venous access is not easy and is often not feasible because of the small diameter of the draining vessels. Once the fistula is localized, surgery consists of simple disconnection of the draining vein as it emerges from the dura.

Zhao et al performed a systematic review of the literature and reported that 34 of 56 patients (61%) with craniocervical DAVFs were treated with surgical ligation of the feeding artery or interruption of the draining vein. In 31 patients (55%), surgery was the first treatment, while surgery was performed as secondary treatment after incomplete occlusion of endovascular treatment in three cases. Radiological follow-up showed complete occlusion of the fistula in all patients.[40]

16.5 Conclusion

Endovascular embolization is the preferred treatment for most intracranial DAVFs, though surgery is indicated for specific situations. These cases may include ethmoidal, tentorial, and craniocervical junction fistulas, complex arterial and venous angioarchitecture, failed initial endovascular occlusion, or impossible catheterization of feeding arteries or draining veins.

References

[1] Liu JK, Dogan A, Ellegala DB, et al. The role of surgery for high-grade intracranial dural arteriovenous fistulas: importance of obliteration of venous outflow. J Neurosurg. 2009; 110(5):913–920

[2] Borden JA, Wu JK, Shucart WA. A proposed classification for spinal and cranial dural arteriovenous fistulous malformations and implications for treatment. J Neurosurg. 1995; 82(2):166–179

[3] Cognard C, Casasco A, Toevi M, Houdart E, Chiras J, Merland JJ. Dural arteriovenous fistulas as a cause of intracranial hypertension due to impairment of cranial venous outflow. J Neurol Neurosurg Psychiatry. 1998; 65(3):308–316

[4] Natarajan SK, Ghodke B, Kim LJ, Hallam DK, Britz GW, Sekhar LN. Multimodality treatment of intracranial dural arteriovenous fistulas in the Onyx era: a single center experience. World Neurosurg. 2010; 73(4):365–379

[5] Awad IA, Little JR, Akarawi WP, Ahl J. Intracranial dural arteriovenous malformations: factors predisposing to an aggressive neurological course. J Neurosurg. 1990; 72(6):839–850

[6] Sundt TM , Jr, Piepgras DG. The surgical approach to arteriovenous malformations of the lateral and sigmoid dural sinuses. J Neurosurg. 1983; 59(1):32–39

[7] Collice M, D'Aliberti G, Arena O, Solaini C, Fontana RA, Talamonti G. Surgical treatment of intracranial dural arteriovenous fistulae: role of venous drainage. Neurosurgery. 2000; 47(1):56–66, discussion 66–67

[8] Thompson BG, Doppman JL, Oldfield EH. Treatment of cranial dural arteriovenous fistulae by interruption of leptomeningeal venous drainage. J Neurosurg. 1994; 80(4):617–623

[9] Davies MA, Ter Brugge K, Willinsky R, Wallace MC. The natural history and management of intracranial dural arteriovenous fistulae. Part 2: aggressive lesions. Interv Neuroradiol. 1997; 3(4):303–311

[10] Im SH, Oh CW, Han DH. Surgical management of an unruptured dural arteriovenous fistula of the anterior cranial fossa: natural history for 7 years. Surg Neurol. 2004; 62(1):72–75, discussion 75

[11] Lawton MT, Chun J, Wilson CB, Halbach VV. Ethmoidal dural arteriovenous fistulae: an assessment of surgical and endovascular management. Neurosurgery. 1999; 45(4):805–810, discussion 810–811

[12] Halbach VV, Higashida RT, Hieshima GB, Wilson CB, Barnwell SL, Dowd CF. Dural arteriovenous fistulas supplied by ethmoidal arteries. Neurosurgery. 1990; 26(5):816–823

[13] Gliemroth J, Nowak G, Arnold H. Dural arteriovenous malformation in the anterior cranial fossa. Clin Neurol Neurosurg. 1999; 101(1):37–43

[14] Lefkowitz M, Giannotta SL, Hieshima G, et al. Embolization of neurosurgical lesions involving the ophthalmic artery. Neurosurgery. 1998; 43(6):1298–1303

[15] Schuette AJ, Cawley CM, Barrow DL. Indocyanine green videoangiography in the management of dural arteriovenous fistulae. Neurosurgery. 2010; 67(3):658–662, discussion 662

[16] Youssef PP, Schuette AJ, Cawley CM, Barrow DL. Advances in surgical approaches to dural fistulas. Neurosurgery. 2014; 74 Suppl 1:S32–S41

[17] Cannizzaro D, Peschillo S, Cenzato M, et al. Endovascular and surgical approaches of ethmoidal dural fistulas: a multicenter experience and a literature review. Neurosurg Rev. 2016. DOI: 10.1007/s10143-016-0764-1

[18] Lanfzino G, Meyer FB. Carotid-cavernous fistulas. In: Winn HR, ed. Youmans Neurological Surgery. 6th ed. Philadelphia, PA: Elsevier/Saunders; 2011:3991–3999

[19] Wachter D, Hans F, Psychogios MN, Knauth M, Rohde V. Microsurgery can cure most intracranial dural arteriovenous fistulae of the sinus and non-sinus type. Neurosurg Rev. 2011; 34(3):337–345, discussion 345

[20] Ellis JA, Goldstein H, Connolly ES , Jr, Meyers PM. Carotid-cavernous fistulas. Neurosurg Focus. 2012; 32(5):E9

[21] Ringer AJ, Salud L, Tomsick TA. Carotid cavernous fistulas: anatomy, classification, and treatment. Neurosurg Clin N Am. 2005; 16(2):279–295, viii

[22] Gemmete JJ, Chaudhary N, Pandey A, Ansari S. Treatment of carotid cavernous fistulas. Curr Treat Options Neurol. 2010; 12(1):43–53

[23] Day JD, Fukushima T. Direct microsurgery of dural arteriovenous malformation type carotid-cavernous sinus fistulas: indications, technique, and results. Neurosurgery. 1997; 41(5):1119–1124, discussion 1124–1126

[24] Tu YK, Liu HM, Hu SC. Direct surgery of carotid cavernous fistulae and dural arteriovenous malformations of the cavernous sinus. Neurosurgery. 1997; 41 (4):798–805, discussion 805–806

[25] Hara T, Hamada J, Kai Y, Ushio Y. Surgical transvenous embolization of a carotid-cavernous dural fistula with cortical drainage via a petrosal vein: two technical case reports. Neurosurgery. 2002; 50(6):1380–1383, discussion 1383–1384

[26] Yu SC, Cheng HK, Wong GK, Chan CM, Cheung JY, Poon WS. Transvenous embolization of dural carotid-cavernous fistulae with transfacial catheterization through the superior ophthalmic vein. Neurosurgery. 2007; 60(6):1032–1037, discussion 1037–1038

[27] Tomak PR, Cloft HJ, Kaga A, Cawley CM, Dion J, Barrow DL. Evolution of the management of tentorial dural arteriovenous malformations. Neurosurgery. 2003; 52(4):750–760, discussion 760–762

[28] Picard L, Bracard S, Islak C, et al. Dural fistulae of the tentorium cerebelli. Radioanatomical, clinical and therapeutic considerations. J Neuroradiol. 1990; 17(3):161–181

[29] Davies MA, TerBrugge K, Willinsky R, Coyne T, Saleh J, Wallace MC. The validity of classification for the clinical presentation of intracranial dural arteriovenous fistulas. J Neurosurg. 1996; 85(5):830–837

[30] Cannizzaro D, Brinjikji W, Rammos S, Murad MH, Lanzino G. Changing Clinical and Therapeutic Trends in Tentorial Dural Arteriovenous Fistulas: A Systematic Review. AJNR Am J Neuroradiol. 2015; 36(10): 1905–1911

[31] Puffer RC, Daniels DJ, Kallmes DF, Cloft HJ, Lanzino G. Curative Onyx embolization of tentorial dural arteriovenous fistulas. Neurosurg Focus. 2012; 32(5):E4

[32] Lawton MT, Sanchez-Mejia RO, Pham D, Tan J, Halbach VV. Tentorial dural arteriovenous fistulae: operative strategies and microsurgical results for six types. Neurosurgery. 2008; 62(3) Suppl 1:110–124, discussion 124–125

[33] Loumiotis I, Lanzino G, Daniels D, Sheehan J, Link M. Radiosurgery for intracranial dural arteriovenous fistulas (DAVFs): a review. Neurosurg Rev. 2011; 34(3):305–315, discussion 315

[34] Link MJ, Coffey RJ, Nichols DA, Gorman DA. The role of radiosurgery and particulate embolization in the treatment of dural arteriovenous fistulas. J Neurosurg. 1996; 84(5):804–809

[35] Kakarla UK, Deshmukh VR, Zabramski JM, Albuquerque FC, McDougall CG, Spetzler RF. Surgical treatment of high-risk intracranial dural arteriovenous fistulae: clinical outcomes and avoidance of complications. Neurosurgery. 2007; 61(3):447–457, discussion 457–459

[36] van Dijk JM, TerBrugge KG, Willinsky RA, Wallace MC. Selective disconnection of cortical venous reflux as treatment for cranial dural arteriovenous fistulas. J Neurosurg. 2004; 101(1):31–35

[37] Zhou LF, Chen L, Song DL, Gu YX, Leng B. Tentorial dural arteriovenous fistulas. Surg Neurol. 2007; 67(5):472–481, discussion 481–482

[38] Llácer JL, Suay G, Piquer J, Vazquez V. Dural arteriovenous fistula at the foramen magnum: Report of a case and clinical-anatomical review. Neurocirugia (Astur). 2016; 27(4):199–203

[39] Niwa J, Matsumura S, Maeda Y, Ohoyama H. Transcondylar approach for dural arteriovenous fistulas of the cervicomedullary junction. Surg Neurol. 1997; 48(6):627–631

[40] Zhao J, Xu F, Ren J, Manjila S, Bambakidis NC. Dural arteriovenous fistulas at the craniocervical junction: a systematic review. J Neurointerv Surg. 2016; 8 (6):648–653

17 Surgery of Basal Ganglia, Thalamic, and Brainstem Arteriovenous Malformations

Venkatesh S. Madhugiri, Mario Teo, and Gary K. Steinberg

Abstract

Arteriovenous malformations (AVMs) of the basal ganglia, thalamus, and brainstem are among the most challenging lesions neurosurgeons are called upon to treat. These deep-seated AVMs account for 2 to 12% of all intracranial AVMs, have a higher risk of hemorrhage than more superficial lesions, and frequently require complex multimodal management paradigms. Endovascular embolization is usually a prelude to surgery. Residual lesion after endovascular therapy and/or surgery can be managed by radiosurgery. The optimal surgical approach is based on the location of the lesion and its proximity to an ependymal or cortical surface. For AVMs of the basal ganglia and thalamus, six main surgical approaches are used individually or in combination: (1) frontal interhemispheric transcallosal, (2) parietal interhemispheric transcallosal, (3) occipital transtentorial infrasplenial, (4) supracerebellar infratentorial, (5) transsylvian, and (6) transcortical. For brainstem AVMs, the approaches are based on six described anatomic locations of the lesions using the safe entry zone, and we often favor the "occlusion in situ" technique. Pial brainstem AVMs can be safely excised or surgically obliterated, whereas parenchymal brainstem AVMs are best managed by nonsurgical means. Furthermore, several intraoperative adjuncts are useful for the safe resection of these deep-seated lesions, including neuronavigation, mild hypothermia, strict control of the mean arterial pressure (also postoperatively), electrophysiological monitoring, and ICG or digital subtraction angiography..

Keywords: AVM, brainstem, basal ganglia, thalamic, endovascular embolization, hemorrhage, microsurgery, radiosurgery

Key Points

- Deep-seated arteriovenous malformations (AVMs) usually have a higher risk of hemorrhage than more superficial lesions.
- No single treatment modality can usually achieve a complete cure. Endovascular embolization is frequently a prelude to surgery or radiosurgery. Residual AVM after endovascular therapy and/or surgery can be managed by radiosurgery.
- Several preoperative and intraoperative adjuncts such as neuronavigation, controlled mild hypothermia, strict control over the mean arterial pressure during and after surgery, electrophysiology, ICG and intraoperative angiography are required for the safe resection of these lesions.
- Surgical approach is tailored to the location of the lesion and its proximity to an ependymal or pial surface.
- Pial brainstem AVMs can be safely excised, whereas parenchymal brainstem AVMs are best managed by nonsurgical means.

17.1 Introduction

Arteriovenous malformations (AVMs) of the basal ganglia, thalamus, and brainstem are among the most challenging lesions that neurosurgeons are called upon to treat. These relatively rare lesions usually require complex multimodal management paradigms.[1] AVMs involving the basal ganglia and thalamus comprise about 2 to 12% of all AVMs, whereas brainstem lesions are rarer still and probably account for 2 to 6% of all intracranial AVMs.[2,3] The mortality rate for a first hemorrhage from all AVMs has been reported to be about 10%, and about 13 and 20% for subsequent rebleeds.[4] The annual risk of hemorrhage is 2 to 3% per year, except in the first year after a bleed when the chance of rebleed is approximately 6%. There is some evidence to suggest that deep and centrally located lesions, such as those in the basal ganglia, thalamus, and brainstem, have a more aggressive course than AVMs in more superficial locations in the brain.[1] In one large series, 71.9% of these patients presented with hemorrhage, with an annual rebleed rate of 11.4% during a 6.6-year follow-up.[5] Our Stanford series of 96 basal ganglia and thalamic AVM patients (69% presenting with hemorrhage) demonstrated a rebleed rate of 9.6%/year after diagnosis, but before any treatment. This is a worrisome issue, given that a bleed in these areas can be devastating—hemorrhage in patients with deep AVMs can not only lead to profound motor and sensory deficits but also to cognitive and memory disorders.[6] Only about a fifth (21.9%) of patients who are diagnosed with an AVM in the basal ganglia or thalamus are likely to be neurologically intact at the time of their original presentation, irrespective of whether they presented with a bleed or not.[7] Brainstem AVMs have an equally high risk of bleeding—up to 88.5% of patients presented with hemorrhage in some series. Brainstem hemorrhage can have devastating consequences, including immediate death or deep coma in up to 40% of patients.[8,9] Hemorrhage from these lesions could easily extend into the ventricles and obstruct the cerebrospinal fluid (CSF) pathways. Management of the lesion itself would then be complicated with the addition of hydrocephalus. Indeed, the presence of hydrocephalus in patients who present with a ruptured AVM could portend a poorer prognosis.[10]

There are several issues to be considered while managing these lesions. The first would be to recognize patterns of clinical presentation in those patients who do not present with hemorrhage so that early diagnosis and treatment of unruptured lesions can be achieved. Various series have reported rates of presentation with hemorrhage of 70 to 88%.[1,7] Other clinical symptoms and signs include headache in 27.1%, neurological deficits including hemiparesis in 61.5%, visual field defects in 12.5%, dysphasia in 14.6%, and seizures in 13.5%.[7] The second issue would be to formulate effective multimodal management strategies. Not only do these patients present with more severe deficits, but surgery outcomes are not as good as for AVMs in other locations.[11] The availability of endovascular (embolization) therapy (EVT) and radiosurgery has made it possible to cure some of these lesions. However, no single technique can usually achieve a cure when applied in isolation.[1] In up to 16% of patients in our series of deep AVMs, all three modalities of treatment were invoked.[2] In the Stanford AVM series, only 4 of 124 patients (3.2%) with basal ganglia/thalamic AVMs were completely cured without surgery—1 with EVT and 3 with a combination of EVT and radiosurgery.[2]

EVT is usually performed as a prelude to surgery to reduce the vascularity of the lesion. Endovascular embolization prior to surgical excision is not always feasible because many of these lesions derive their blood supply from deep perforating arteries, including the lenticulostriate arteries, insular perforators, thalamoperforators, and anterior and posterior choroidal arteries. The long, short, and circumflex brainstem perforators that would ultimately supply intraparenchymal brainstem AVMs are difficult to embolize as well. In one large series, only 41% of these lesions could be effectively embolized prior to surgery.[12] Other series have reported complete obliteration rates of 14.5 to 20% with EVT alone.[13,14]

Radiosurgery is a viable option for basal ganglia and thalamic AVMs, especially for those lesions that have not bled. A cure can be effected after a single session of radiosurgery in as many as 61.9% of patients. In one series, the annual risk of hemorrhage after radiosurgery was 9.5% in the first year, 4.7% in the second year, and 0% thereafter.[15] Radiosurgery does not confer complete protection from hemorrhage until the AVM is completely obliterated. In a large radiosurgery series, 88% of patients presented with hemorrhage. After radiosurgery, 14.3% experienced bleeds during follow-up, with a mortality of 50%. This is an important factor to consider when recommending radiosurgery for these lesions. Radiosurgery is a good option for brainstem lesions as well, and the efficacy seems undiminished because of the location of these lesions in the posterior fossa.[16]

Although these basal ganglia, thalamic, and brainstem lesions are deep seated and difficult to access, there are definite indications for microsurgery. One indication is to evacuate large hematomas that could cause herniation. AVMs that are not completely obliterated after multiple sessions of radiosurgery or embolization are another potential indication for surgery. Lesions that abut a ventricular wall could potentially be accessed more easily than those that are completely intraparenchymal. This chapter discusses the surgical strategies to tackle these lesions.

17.2 Patient Selection

As already discussed, hemorrhage rates for patients with basal ganglionic and thalamic AVMs could be significantly higher than those with lesions in other locations. In a review of untreated patients with more than 500 patient-years of follow-up (who were ultimately referred to Stanford for evaluation), the pretreatment annual rupture rate was 9.6% per year. Periventricular AVM location and deep venous drainage have been identified as independent risk factors for hemorrhage in large natural history studies, including one from Finland.[17] A history of previous hemorrhages correlates with bleed recurrence in the AVMs of the thalamus and basal ganglia.[7,17,18] Hemorrhage from a basal ganglia or thalamic AVM also carries a risk of serious morbidity, with up to 85% of post-bleed patients developing

hemiparesis or hemiplegia. The higher risk of hemorrhage and greater morbidity from hemorrhage should be factored into the decision as to whether to treat basal ganglia and thalamic AVMs. Given the high rates of hemorrhage and the devastating consequences thereof, observation may not be a reasonable option.

Brainstem AVMs also have annual hemorrhage rates as high as 15 to 17.5%, which makes observation and follow-up difficult to justify as a management strategy.[19,20] Hemorrhage from brainstem AVMs is associated with a poor prognosis, with death in as many as one-third of treated and two-thirds of untreated patients.[21,22] The Lawton-Young AVM grading system incorporates patient age (< 20, 20–40 years, or > 40 years), hemorrhagic presentation (ruptured vs. unruptured), and compactness of the nidus (compact vs. diffuse) in addition to the variables in the Spetzler-Martin grading system.[23] This scale could be used as a part of the decision-making process as it scores patients with prior hemorrhage higher—these are also the patients who would require immediate management rather than observation.

Poor candidates for surgery would be patients with severe comorbidities, elderly patients, and patients with devastating neurological deficits. Patients with lesions located within the posterior limb of the internal capsule should receive treatment with non-microsurgical techniques because of the high risk of permanent deficits. In patients with asymptomatic AVMs, the risk of surgical morbidity should be carefully weighed against the natural history of the lesion and patient-specific factors. Patients presenting with hemorrhage are known to have a worse natural history and poorer outcomes after rehemorrhage; thus, carefully tailored low morbidity treatments with a goal of AVM obliteration can decrease future hemorrhage risk and the associated morbidity.

17.3 Imaging and Embolization

Preoperative high-quality magnetic resonance imaging (MRI) and digital subtraction angiography (DSA) are essential to understanding an AVM's angioarchitecture and cerebral location. The presence of associated aneurysms, high flow shunts, and venous varices should be noted. In some cases, preoperative MR tractography can be useful to localize the traversing tracts and understand their disposition relative to the nidus, aid in surgical approach selection, and enhance intraoperative neuronavigation. We highly recommend that a navigation protocol MRI with an MR angiogram be performed the day prior to surgery to guide the approach to and resection of deep AVMs. CISS-3D or FIESTA sequences could also be of use in tracing the feeding vessels and draining veins. Thalamic and basal ganglionic AVMs are generally fed by the medial and lateral lenticulostriate arteries, recurrent arteries of Heubner, thalamogeniculate arteries, thalamoperforating arteries, and anterior and posterior choroidal arteries. Almost all AVMs in the basal ganglia and thalamus have deep venous drainage. In patients with AVMs amenable to embolization, we recommend staged embolizations spaced at least 1 week apart. We never attempt to embolize more than 30% of the AVM at any session because more aggressive embolization can cause swelling and hemorrhage. It should be borne in mind that embolization, even as a prelude to surgery, is not entirely without risk. In a series of supratentorial AVMs treated with partial or complete embolization, 6.9% of patients developed permanent neurologic deficits after embolization. The risk factors for postprocedure deterioration were identified as location in eloquent areas and exclusive deep venous drainage.[24]

17.4 Anesthetic Technique and Electrophysiology

Surgery is usually performed with the patient under general anesthesia. Several surgeons have reported performing AVM excision with the patient awake. This technique appears to be especially useful to map cortical and subcortical speech areas using intraoperative stimulation.[25,26] The safety that is afforded with the patient awake should be balanced against the tight anesthesia and hemodynamic control that are usually required for AVM excision. The patient's mean arterial pressure (MAP) should be controlled between 70 and 80 mm Hg throughout induction of anesthesia and surgical exposure. MAP should be reduced further to between 60 and 70 mm Hg during resection of the AVM through emergence from anesthesia. We also recommend mild hypothermia with a target core temperature of 33 to 34 °C achieved via a cooling blanket and/or cold saline infusion via femoral venous catheters. Experimental evidence and some clinical studies have shown mild hypothermia to be protective against cerebral ischemic insults.[27] Electrophysiological monitoring and mapping are important tools in the resection of AVMs. The use of continuous bilateral upper and lower somatosensory-evoked potentials (SSEPs) and motor-evoked potentials (MEPs) along with cortical and subcortical mapping can be invaluable in decreasing the risks associated with the surgical and endovascular management of these lesions. We routinely use electrophysiologic monitoring for all patients undergoing microsurgical excision of deep AVMs.

17.5 Surgical Techniques

Adequate exposure is critical to resecting deep vascular malformations. Virtual reality-based software may be especially useful in the preoperative planning of the stepwise surgical strategy.[28,29] It is critical to identify the arterial feeders, which form the initial points of attack, early on in the procedure. Their position should be predicted from the preoperative DSA and MRI, and neuronavigation should be used in localizing them intraoperatively. They should then be divided close to the nidus while preserving the draining veins. Several millimeters of a feeding artery should be exposed prior to coagulation or using microclips—this is because of the tendency of these feeders to retract into the brain parenchyma once they are cut. The veins are usually arterialized and should not be mistaken for feeding arteries, given inadvertent sacrifice of draining veins early on in the procedure can lead to AVM swelling and rupture. Intraoperative indocyanine green (ICG) angiography and the use of the Charbel Transonic flowmeter, which indicates direction of flow, may be useful in distinguishing arteries from arterialized veins.[29] Microsurgical resection is performed under high-power magnification with very fine irrigating bipolar coagulation forceps or the Spetzler-Malis nonstick bipolar, using low coagulation

power to limit the spread of current to surrounding brain tissue.[30] The nidus is then dissected from the surrounding brain as the surgeon looks for gliotic and hemosiderin-stained brain as a plane. The plane of dissection should remain as close to the periphery of the nidus as possible to minimize the risk of injuring normal brain. However, occasionally "dirty coagulation" may need to be performed of the deep, small, difficult vessels inside apparently normal brain around the AVM.[31] One group recommends the neuroendoscope as a useful tool to develop the plane of dissection, especially in those AVMs that abut the ventricular surface.[32] The final step is to divide the draining veins. Intraoperative angiography is often helpful to confirm the excision of the nidus while operating on these complex lesions.[33] In one series, 22.22% of patients had a residual nidus on intraoperative angiography that required further excision.[34] Several series also report the use of ICG angiography to confirm excision, but we do not consider this as valuable as catheter angiography because the dye does not visualize deeper aspects of the AVM.[29]

Careful hemostasis should be achieved and confirmed by gently raising the MAP to normal levels as well as by using the Valsalva maneuver before the dura is closed. The surgical bed should be lined with Surgicel (Ethicon, Inc., Somerville, NJ) to induce hemostasis of small vessels. If the ventricle was entered, a ventricular catheter is often placed prophylactically. The dura is then closed primarily or with the aid of a dural substitute. We use 4–0 braided nylon suture for dural closure. The bone is replaced with titanium plates and screws, the galea is closed with 2–0 absorbable sutures, and staples are placed in the skin.

17.5.1 Surgery for Basal Ganglionic and Thalamic AVMs

There are six main surgical approaches used individually or in combination for AVMs of the basal ganglia and thalamus, depending on lesion location: (1) frontal interhemispheric transcallosal, (2) parietal interhemispheric transcallosal, (3) occipital transtentorial infrasplenial, (4) supracerebellar infratentorial, (5) transsylvian, and (6) transcortical (frontal or parietal). The point of closest presentation of the lesion to a ventricular or pial surface influences the surgical trajectory as does the proximity of a hematoma cavity to these surfaces. We may use a ventriculostomy or lumbar drain for brain relaxation before positioning. However, this is not necessary if an intraventricular approach is utilized, given that CSF can be drained directly with the opening of the ventricle. Additional steps to induce brain relaxation include hyperventilation, diuresis, or both. The groin should also be prepared for possible intraoperative angiography.

Interhemispheric Transcallosal Approach— Frontal and Parietal

AVMs that present to a ventricular surface are best exposed via a transcallosal route (▶ Fig. 17.1). Lesions of the medial aspect of the caudate are best approached via an anterior transcallosal approach and those of the posterior medial thalamus and pulvinar via a posterior transcallosal approach. For the frontal approach, the patient is positioned supine with the head slightly elevated above the heart and flexed 20 to 30 degrees.

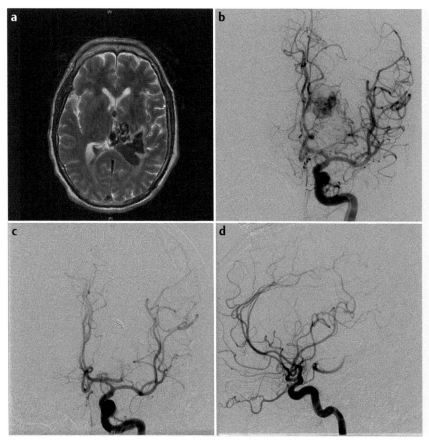

Fig. 17.1 A Spetzler-Martin grade III thalamic arteriovenous malformation (AVM) treated by multimodal management. The patient presented with a massive intraventricular hemorrhage. He underwent embolization of some of the posterior cerebral artery feeders followed by partial surgical resection of the nidus and CyberKnife to the residual lesion. **(a)** Axial T2-weighted image showing an AVM in the left thalamus with hemorrhage extending into the lateral ventricles. **(b)** Anteroposterior view of an angiography showing the nidus, supplied predominantly by the left posterior cerebral artery and draining into the vein of Galen. **(c,d)** Posttreatment angiography. The anteroposterior **(c)** and lateral **(d)** views show no residual nidus.

Alternatively, an ipsilateral side-down, lateral position could be used so that the frontal lobe falls away from the falx under the influence of gravity. A paramedian trapdoor incision is made on the side of the AVM. We usually place two-thirds of the flap anterior and one-third of the flap posterior to the coronal suture. For the parietal approach, the patient is placed in a park-bench position and the anterior margin of the craniotomy is posterior to the postcentral gyrus. The bone flap should be planned after reviewing the coronal and sagittal MRI sequences so as to locate the positions of the draining veins into the sagittal sinus. The bone flap is made large enough in the anterior-posterior direction to allow preservation of these cortical draining veins. The bone flap is usually taken across the midline, exposing the superior sagittal sinus. The dura is incised based on the sinus and tacked up, giving a wider access to the interhemispheric fissure. When large cortical draining veins prevent exposure from one side, a dural incision and approach may be performed from the contralateral side. Although it is thought that the division of one cortical draining vein may not lead to a significant problem, this is not necessarily true. The size and drainage territory of the sacrificed vein, the development of the Sylvian system, and collateral drainage all determine if venous infarction would occur or not.[35]

Once entry to the interhemispheric fissure is effected, retractors are used to visualize the corpus callosum, and the operating microscope is brought into the field. Care must be taken to avoid overly aggressive retraction of the medial frontal lobe because lower limb weakness and/or venous infarction can result from this maneuver. The callosomarginal and pericallosal arteries are identified and the pericallosal arteries should be separated in the midline. A callosotomy is then performed and the lateral ventricle is entered. Image guidance is employed to help determine the site of callosotomy and the site of corticectomy based on the location of the AVM in the caudate or thalamus. If the AVM is not on the surface of the thalamus, an approach into the thalamus through the pulvinar (posterior part of the thalamus) can be performed. The AVM is then resected using the microsurgical principals described in the beginning of this section.

Transsylvian Approach

AVMs located in the putamen and extending to the insular cortex could be excised via the transsylvian approach. A classical frontotemporal craniotomy is performed, exposing the sylvian fissure. Neuronavigation is used to determine the point closest to the AVM from the superficial sylvian fissure and the fissure is opened. The most critical part of this approach would be to differentiate AVM feeders from en passage branches of the middle cerebral artery. Typically, the branches of the middle cerebral artery would need to be skeletonized for one to appreciate the anatomy and avoid coagulating a normal traversing branch.

Transcortical (Frontal or Parietal)

Lesions located in the lateral basal ganglia or thalamus, not extending to the insular cortex or ependymal surface, can be excised via a transcortical approach (► Fig. 17.2, ► Fig. 17.3).

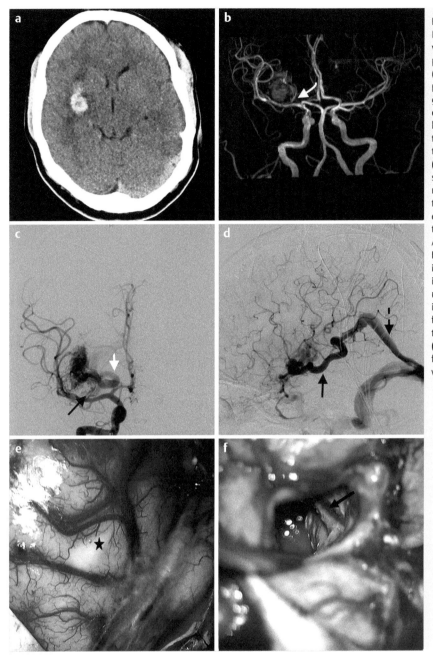

Fig. 17.2 Basal ganglionic Spetzler-Martin grade III arteriovenous malformation (AVM), operated via a right pterional approach. The patient presented with sudden loss of consciousness. **(a)** Axial CT image at presentation. This patient presented with a hemorrhage in the right basal ganglia. He underwent an MRI as part of his evaluation. **(b)** MR angiography shows an AVM located just superior to the right M1 segment of the middle cerebral artery. The *white arrow* points to an enlarged lenticulostriate feeder. **(c)** Anteroposterior projection of a digitally subtracted angiography showed a nidus measuring 2 × 1.5 cm, supplied by feeders from the lenticulostriate perforators (*black arrow*). An early draining vein is seen on the medial aspect of the nidus (*white arrow*). **(d)** Lateral view of the AVM. The venous drainage into the basal vein of Rosenthal (*arrow*) and thence to the straight sinus is seen (*broken arrow*). **(e,f)** Intraoperative images. A conventional pterional craniotomy was made. **(e)** The site of corticectomy was on the inferior frontal gyrus, just abutting the sylvian fissure (*black star*). The hematoma and feeders to the nidus could be accessed via this approach. **(f)** The hematoma has been evacuated and the first of the lenticulostriate feeders is visible in the walls of the hematoma cavity (*arrow*).

Image guidance is critical to define the nearest cortical entry zone to reach the AVM (► Fig. 17.2e). The presence of a hematoma that reaches the cortical surface is invaluable in this approach. Navigation that incorporates real-time ultrasound can be more valuable than conventional navigation while using this approach.[29] Microsurgical techniques are standard as described earlier. Sometimes a combination of treatment modalities and surgical approaches is required. Staged treatments are reasonable options to limit morbidity (► Fig. 17.3, ► Video 17.1).

Occipital Transtentorial Infrasplenial

This valuable approach is useful for lesions located in the pulvinar, tectal plate of the midbrain, as well as in the superior vermis and cerebellum.[36,37,38] The patient is positioned in a lateral or three-quarter prone position to allow the occipital lobe to fall away from the falx by gravity, minimizing the need for retraction. The craniotomy should ideally expose the superior sagittal sinus and the dura is opened with its base toward the sinus. Usually, there are no bridging veins in this location and the occipital lobe can be retracted readily. The tentorium can be divided lateral to the straight sinus, from the free edge of the incisura back to the transverse sinus if need be, providing access to the ambient and quadrigeminal cisterns.

Infratentorial Supracerebellar

AVMs in the pulvinar, posterior midbrain, and tectal plate regions can be accessed via an infratentorial supracerebellar approach.[39] The patient is positioned in the modified prone Concorde position with the surgeon operating from below. Mild retraction of

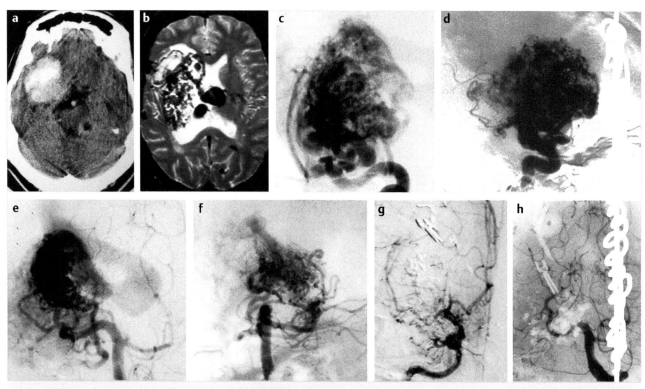

Fig. 17.3 A 28-year-old man presented initially with a bleed from a giant grade V right frontoparietal arteriovenous malformation (AVM) involving the thalamus and basal ganglia. Despite treatment with proton beam radiosurgery, he suffered three subsequent bleeds resulting in left upper extremity weakness. (a) Axial CT showing his fourth hemorrhage. (b) Axial MR showing the AVM. Nine years after radiosurgery, there was no change in the angiographic appearance of the AVM noted on right carotid anteroposterior (AP) (c) and lateral (d) or vertebrobasilar AP (e) and lateral (f) views. He underwent four sessions of embolization followed by three sessions of microsurgical resection with cure of the AVM. Final postoperative carotid AP (g) and vertebrobasilar AP (h) views. He experienced no new neurologic deficits except for a quadrantanopsia.

the superior vermis and/or cerebellar hemispheres is often necessary. Alternatively, one can use the sitting or semi-sitting position with the head above the heart and chin tucked down

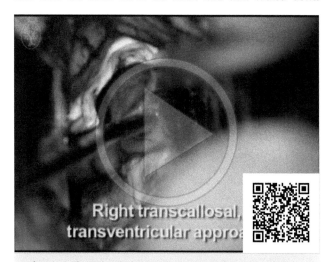

Video 17.1 This video demonstrates resection of a giant grade V frontoparietal arteriovenous malformation (AVM) with intraventricular extension after radiosurgery and embolization treatment. This is the same lesion as in ▶ Fig. 17.3. The patient underwent four sessions of embolization followed by three separate sessions of microsurgical resection via the transcallosal transventricular, frontal transcortical, and parietal transcortical routes, with cure of the AVM. https://www.thieme.de/de/q.htm?p=opn/tp/293510101/9781626237308_c017_v001&t=video

slightly; however, this position carries a risk of air embolism. A midline skin incision from the inion to C2 is performed, and the neck muscles are dissected in the midline. The suboccipital bone is exposed down to the foramen magnum, and the arch of C1 is identified. The confluence of sinuses (torcular Herophili) is localized using image guidance. A suboccipital craniotomy that extends a centimeter superior to the transverse sinuses is performed. This allows retraction of the tentorium and therefore opening of the supracerebellar space. The dura is opened in a **V** shape and tacked up, pulling the transverse sinuses cranially. The cerebellar hemispheres usually fall away from the tentorium once the arachnoid is opened and the CSF is drained. Superior vermian and cerebellar veins are usually encountered along the midline, draining into the straight sinus, and laterally above the cerebellar hemispheres, draining into the venous lakes of the tentorium. The midline veins are slightly stretched, coagulated near the cerebellar surface, and cut, allowing access to the quadrigeminal cistern and pineal region. The internal cerebral veins, the basal veins of Rosenthal, and the cerebellomesencephalic veins join to form the vein of Galen. These veins need to be gently separated to gain access to the pulvinar. The disadvantage of the supracerebellar infratentorial over the occipital transtentorial approach is the need to separate the venous complex. Although the latter approach has the advantage of exposure above the vein of Galen, it allows access only to the midline and ipsilateral half of the cerebellomesencephalic fissure. Image guidance is used to define the shortest distance to the AVM. Aforementioned microsurgical techniques are used to resect the AVM.

17.5.2 Surgery for Brainstem AVMs

Brainstem AVMs pose a formidable challenge to the neurosurgeon. They are located in the area of the human body with the highest concentration of critical structures. The mere act of entry into the brainstem could leave a patient with permanent deficits and thus, surgical experience with these lesions has been limited.[40,41,42,43,44,45] Brainstem AVMs can be divided into two types—those that are located within the substance of the brainstem itself and superficial pial lesions. Microsurgical excision is not usually the best option for lesions located within the brainstem—radiosurgery is often the treatment modality of choice. Several safe entry zones to access the interior of the brainstem have been described; nevertheless, excision of an AVM located within the substance of the brainstem may lead to unacceptable morbidity.[46,47,48] A technique of in situ occlusion has been described for superficial pial AVMs, as the process of circumferential dissection of the feeders and the nidus (which may be partly buried in or adherent to the brainstem) could lead to postsurgical deficits.[3,49,50] Therefore, the arterial feeders are identified but not dissected off the pia; they are then coagulated and cut, using ICG angiography liberally to ensure that the veins are being spared. Once all the arterial feeders have been cut, the draining veins are coagulated and either clipped or cut sequentially. Thus, the nidus is isolated both from the arterial and the venous sides. No attempt is made to remove the nidus; it is left in situ.

Pial AVMs of the brainstem have been divided into six groups based on their anatomic location[3]: (1) anterior midbrain lesions located between the cerebral peduncles and related to the III nerve, (2) posterior midbrain lesions located on the tectal plate, (3) anterior pontine lesions located between the basilar sulcus medially and trigeminal (CN V) root laterally and between the pontomesencephalic sulcus superiorly and pontomedullary sulcus inferiorly, (4) lateral pontine lesions located between the CN V root medially and the cerebellopontine fissure laterally, (5) anterior medullary lesions located between the anterolateral sulci and anterior to hypoglossal nerve (CN XII) rootlets, and (6) lateral medullary lesions located lateral to the preolivary sulcus and posterior to hypoglossal nerve rootlets, in the location of the P2 segment of the posterior inferior cerebellar artery.[3] AVMs located in the rhomboid fossa are rare but would be approached via a midline suboccipital approach. The surgical approach to these lesions depends on the location and the source of feeding arteries. Anterior midbrain AVMs can be approached via a transsylvian exposure as already described, with the addition of an orbitozygomatic osteotomy if required. Posterior midbrain AVMs can be approached via the supracerebellar, infratentorial, or occipital transtentorial routes (vide supra). Anterior pontine AVMs are usually unilateral and, thus, both anterior and lateral pontine AVMs can be approached via a retrosigmoid approach.[3] Midbrain or pontomesencephalic AVMs are exposed via a subtemporal or subtemporal transpetrosal approach if they present to the lateral or anterior surfaces of these structures[30] (▶ Fig. 17.4). Anterior and lateral medullary AVMs are resected via a far lateral approach.

Retrosigmoid Approach for Brainstem AVMs

The retrosigmoid approach is useful for pontine AVMs that are located anteriorly or laterally. For this standard approach,

patients are positioned either lateral or supine with the head turned after placing a pad beneath the ipsilateral shoulder or in a park-bench position.[51] The goal of positioning is to make the mastoid the uppermost point in the surgical field and to align the petrous bone vertically toward the floor. Alternatively, a semi-sitting position could also be employed.[52] Monitoring of all relevant cranial nerves is performed—for pontine AVMs, we monitor nerves V, VII, and VIII. Superior or inferior extension of the nidus itself or the feeders would mandate monitoring additional nerves. SSEPs and MEPs are routinely monitored from all four limbs. The skin incision is usually in the form of a lazy S and extends from above the transverse sinus laterally, curves to the midline near the foramen magnum, and extends inferiorly in the midline into the upper neck. Once the muscles have been detached from their attachment to the occipital bone, a retrosigmoid craniotomy that exposes the edge of the transverse and sigmoid sinuses is performed. The dura is opened in a "**K**" shape, based on the sinuses. CSF is released from the lateral cerebellomedullary cistern so as to relax the cerebellum and place a retractor on the hemisphere. Further surgery proceeds as described earlier. Navigation based on a preoperative MR angiography sequence would help identify the arterial feeders and proceed with the coagulation in situ technique.

Far Lateral Approach for Medullary Pial AVMs

The patient is placed in a modified park-bench position with the lower part of the body almost neutral in a supine position. A horseshoe skin incision is made extending from just behind (medial to) the mastoid groove to the midline (▶ Fig. 17.5, ▶ Fig. 17.6; ▶ Video 17.2). Alternatively, a lazy **S**-shaped skin incision could be used, beginning in the retroauricular area, descending vertically through the midpoint between the inion and mastoid, and curving in its lower part to the midline of the neck.[53] The muscles of the neck are detached from the occipital bone and reflected in a single layer to expose the occipital bone from the mastoid to midline and from the transverse sinus superiorly to C1 inferiorly. The ipsilateral half of the posterior arch of C1 is exposed by subperiosteal dissection. The vertebral artery needs to be dissected free from the arch of C1. A C1 hemilaminotomy is then performed, followed by a small retromastoid craniotomy that exposes the sigmoid sinus. The lateral edge of the foramen magnum rim is drilled away and drilling continues laterally into the condylar fossa and the medial third of the condyle. The dura is incised medial to the dural entry of the vertebral artery in a **C** shape (▶ Fig. 17.6). This exposure renders any retraction of the cerebellum, brainstem, or the spinal cord unnecessary[54] (▶ Video 17.2).

17.6 Postoperative Management and Outcome

All patients should be managed for 24 to 48 hours in an intensive care unit. Tight control of blood pressure is probably the most critical component of postoperative care. We set the MAP goals at 65 to 75 mm Hg if good hemostasis was obtained at the end of the case and at 60 to 65 mm Hg if hemostasis was difficult or there was any brain swelling. On the second postoperative day, we relax the MAP goals to between 75 and 90 mm Hg.

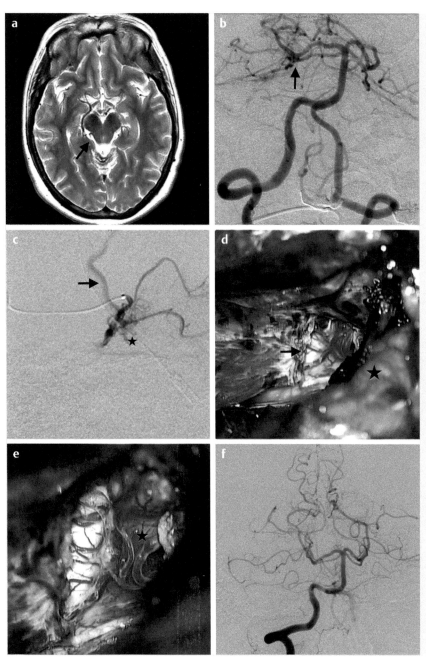

Fig. 17.4 Brainstem (midbrain) Spetzler-Martin grade III arteriovenous malformation (AVM). This patient presented with a hemorrhage. **(a)** Axial T2-weighted MRI image showing hemosiderin staining in the superior vermis and abnormal vessels on the posterolateral pial surface of the midbrain on the left side (*arrow*).
(b) Angiography, anteroposterior (AP) view showing the nidus (*arrow*) filled by the right superior cerebellar artery. **(c)** Superselective catheterization of the distal right superior cerebellar artery showing the nidus (*star*) and vein draining into the straight sinus (*arrow*).
(d) Intraoperative view. A subtemporal approach showing the temporal lobe retracted (*star*) and the tentorium coagulated and cut (*arrow*), while carefully preserving the IV nerve. **(e)** Zoomed in surgical view showing the pial AVM (*star*).
(f) Postoperative angiography, AP view, showing no residual nidus.

Subsequently, the patient is allowed to run normotensive pressures and is transferred to the floor if the postoperative course is uneventful by the third day. There are two theories as to why postoperative brain swelling and hemorrhage occur in patients who have had an AVM excision. The classic normal perfusion pressure breakthrough theory presupposes that CO_2 reactivity and autoregulation are abolished.[55] Thus, brain vessels remain maximally dilated to maintain adequate blood flow to normal brain tissue. After AVM resection, increased amounts of blood are redirected to these chronically dilated low-resistance vessels. Lack of usual autoregulatory control means that the proximal vessels are unable to increase resistance to the new perfusion pressure to protect the capillaries. These events cause edema or hemorrhage. The occlusive hyperemia theory, on the other hand, postulates that stagnation of arterial flow in former AVM feeders leads to edema and hemorrhage. In addition, obstruction of the veins that drain brain areas adjacent to the excised nidus leads to further engorgement, hyperemia, and further arterial stagnation.[56] Several strategies have been described to prevent this dreaded complication, including hyperventilation, hyperoxia, and use of nitric oxide.[57] We advocate maintaining low to normal blood pressure in the postoperative period in patients undergoing brain AVM resection, whether or not embolization was used preoperatively.

Postoperative anticonvulsants are indicated for patients who have seizures preoperatively. Unless the case was done in a hybrid angiography-operative suite, we also routinely perform a follow-up cerebral angiogram during the postoperative stay.

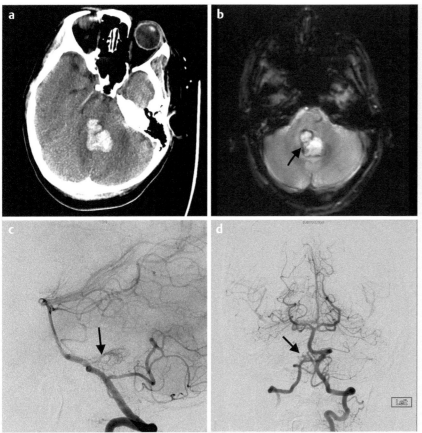

Fig. 17.5 Preoperative images of a brainstem (pontine) arteriovenous malformation (AVM). **(a)** Axial CT image shows a large bleed in the dorsolateral pons, extending into the middle cerebellar peduncle. **(b)** An axial T2 MR image, showing flow voids around the brainstem (*arrow*). **(c)** Lateral and **(d)** anteroposterior views of a left vertebral injection angiography, showing the nidus (*arrow*) near the right pontomedullary junction, supplied by a branch of the V4 segment of the right vertebral artery.

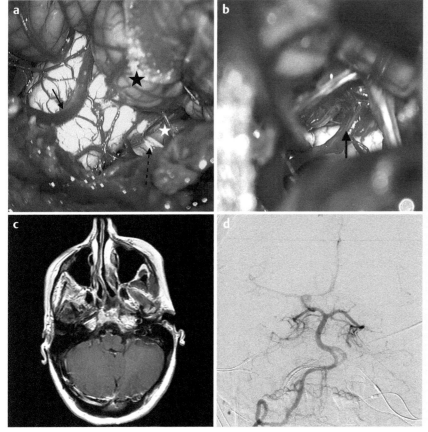

Fig. 17.6 Intraoperative and postsurgical images of the arteriovenous malformation (AVM) described in ▶ Fig. 17.5. This patient was operated on via a far lateral approach. **(a)** Initial view after dural opening and retracting the cerebellum (*black star*). The right PICA (*arrow*), vertebral artery (*white star*), and some lower cranial nerve rootlets are seen (*broken arrow*). **(b)** Magnified view of the pial AVM and the feeding arterial pedicle (*arrow*). **(c)** Postoperative gadolinium contrast-enhanced axial T1-weighted MR image showing postresection changes and no abnormal vessels. **(d)** Postsurgical angiography, AP view, showing no residual nidus.

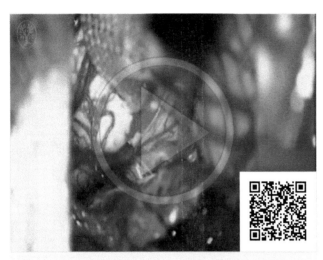

Video 17.2 Resection of a dorsolateral pontine arteriovenous malformation (AVM) via a far lateral approach. This surgical video demonstrates partial resection and coagulation of the AVM described in ► Fig. 17.5 and ► Fig. 17.6. The patient is positioned prone and a suboccipital craniotomy is performed. The occipital condyle is drilled to gain access to the lateral surface of the brainstem. The tonsil and cerebellar hemisphere are retracted and surgery proceeds. A part of the nidus was excised and some vessels adherent to the pial surface of the brainstem were coagulated in situ. ► Fig. 17.6d demonstrates complete obliteration of the nidus. https://www.thieme.de/de/q.htm?p=opn/tp/293510101/9781626237308_c017_v002&t=video

Several factors have been found to correlate with improved/unchanged functional status (vs. worsened functional status) at the time of last follow-up. These include treatment modality used (surgery had the best outcome, followed by SRS and worst outcome with embolization alone), pretreatment modified Rankin scale (mRS), and Spetzler-Martin score.[58] In our series of 122 patients with basal ganglionic and thalamic AVMs treated by multimodal approaches, 32% had excellent outcomes (mRS = 0 or 1), 49% had good outcomes (mRS = 2 or 3), and 6.6% had poor outcomes (mRS = 4 or 5). Thus, 81% had a good or excellent outcome after treatment. The mortality rate in this series was 8.2%; of these nine patients, four rebled and died during nonsurgical therapy. Other series have reported excellent to good outcomes in 93.4% of patients with basal ganglionic or thalamic AVMs treated with microsurgery. Motor function improved or remained unchanged in 80% of surgically treated patients.[5] Thus, microsurgery in conjunction with EVT and radiosurgery can eradicate a large proportion of these lesions with acceptable morbidity.

References

[1] Lawton MT, Hamilton MG, Spetzler RF. Multimodality treatment of deep arteriovenous malformations: thalamus, basal ganglia, and brain stem. Neurosurgery. 1995; 37(1):29–35, discussion 35–36

[2] Paulsen RD, Steinberg GK, Norbash AM, Marcellus ML, Marks MP. Embolization of basal ganglia and thalamic arteriovenous malformations. Neurosurgery. 1999; 44(5):991–996, discussion 996–997

[3] Han SJ, Englot DJ, Kim H, Lawton MT. Brainstem arteriovenous malformations: anatomical subtypes, assessment of "occlusion in situ" technique, and microsurgical results. J Neurosurg. 2015; 122(1):107–117

[4] Wilkins RH. Natural history of intracranial vascular malformations: a review. Neurosurgery. 1985; 16(3):421–430

[5] Sasaki T, Kurita H, Saito I, et al. Arteriovenous malformations in the basal ganglia and thalamus: management and results in 101 cases. J Neurosurg. 1998; 88(2):285–292

[6] Mahalick DM, Ruff RM, Heary RF, U HS. Preoperative versus postoperative neuropsychological sequelae of arteriovenous malformations. Neurosurgery. 1993; 33(4):563–570, discussion 570–571

[7] Fleetwood IG, Marcellus ML, Levy RP, Marks MP, Steinberg GK. Deep arteriovenous malformations of the basal ganglia and thalamus: natural history. J Neurosurg. 2003; 98(4):747–750

[8] Han SJ, Englot DJ, Kim H, Lawton MT. Brainstem arteriovenous malformations: anatomical subtypes, assessment of "occlusion in situ" technique, and microsurgical results. J Neurosurg. 2015; 122(1):107–117

[9] Torné R, Rodríguez-Hernández A, Arikan F, et al. Posterior fossa arteriovenous malformations: significance of higher incidence of bleeding and hydrocephalus. Clin Neurol Neurosurg. 2015; 134:37–43

[10] Aboukaïs R, Marinho P, Baroncini M, et al. Ruptured cerebral arteriovenous malformations: outcomes analysis after microsurgery. Clin Neurol Neurosurg. 2015; 138:137–142

[11] Shi YQ, Chen XC. Surgical treatment of arteriovenous malformations of the striatothalamocapsular region. J Neurosurg. 1987; 66(3):352–356

[12] Potts MB, Young WL, Lawton MT, UCSF Brain AVM Study Project. Deep arteriovenous malformations in the basal ganglia, thalamus, and insula: microsurgical management, techniques, and results. Neurosurgery. 2013; 73(3):417–429

[13] Hurst RW, Berenstein A, Kupersmith MJ, Madrid M, Flamm ES. Deep central arteriovenous malformations of the brain: the role of endovascular treatment. J Neurosurg. 1995; 82(2):190–195

[14] Richling B, Bavinzski G. Arterio-venous malformations of the basal ganglia. Surgical versus endovascular treatment. Acta Neurochir Suppl (Wien). 1991; 53:50–59

[15] Andrade-Souza YM, Zadeh G, Scora D, Tsao MN, Schwartz ML. Radiosurgery for basal ganglia, internal capsule, and thalamus arteriovenous malformation: clinical outcome. Neurosurgery. 2005; 56(1):56–63, discussion 63–64

[16] Ding D, Starke RM, Yen C-P, Sheehan JP. Radiosurgery for cerebellar arteriovenous malformations: does infratentorial location affect outcome? World Neurosurg. 2014; 82(1–2):e209–e217

[17] Hernesniemi JA, Dashti R, Juvela S, Väärt K, Niemelä M, Laakso A. Natural history of brain arteriovenous malformations: a long-term follow-up study of risk of hemorrhage in 238 patients. Neurosurgery. 2008; 63(5):823–829, discussion 829–831

[18] Gross BA, Du R. Natural history of cerebral arteriovenous malformations: a meta-analysis. J Neurosurg. 2013; 118(2):437–443

[19] Koga T, Shin M, Terahara A, Saito N. Outcomes of radiosurgery for brainstem arteriovenous malformations. Neurosurgery. 2011; 69(1):45–51, discussion 51–52

[20] Nozaki K, Hashimoto N, Kikuta K, Takagi Y, Kikuchi H. Surgical applications to arteriovenous malformations involving the brainstem. Neurosurgery. 2006; 58(4) Suppl 2:ONS-270–ONS-278, discussion ONS-278–ONS-279

[21] Drake CG, Friedman AH, Peerless SJ. Posterior fossa arteriovenous malformations. J Neurosurg. 1986; 64(1):1–10

[22] Fults D, Kelly DL, Jr. Natural history of arteriovenous malformations of the brain: a clinical study. Neurosurgery. 1984; 15(5):658–662

[23] Lawton MT, Kim H, McCulloch CE, Mikhak B, Young WL. A supplementary grading scale for selecting patients with brain arteriovenous malformations for surgery. Neurosurgery. 2010; 66(4):702–713, discussion 713

[24] Pan J, He H, Feng L, Viñuela F, Wu Z, Zhan R. Angioarchitectural characteristics associated with complications of embolization in supratentorial brain arteriovenous malformation. AJNR Am J Neuroradiol. 2014; 35(2):354–359

[25] Gamble AJ, Schaffer SG, Nardi DJ, Chalif DJ, Katz J, Dehdashti AR. Awake craniotomy in arteriovenous malformation surgery: the usefulness of cortical and subcortical mapping of language function in selected patients. World Neurosurg. 2015; 84(5):1394–1401

[26] Abdulrauf SI. Awake craniotomies for aneurysms, arteriovenous malformations, skull base tumors, high flow bypass, and brain stem lesions. J Craniovertebr Junction Spine. 2015; 6(1):8–9

[27] Iwama T, Hashimoto N, Todaka T, Sasako Y, Inamori S, Kuro M. Resection of a large, high-flow arteriovenous malformation during hypotension and hypothermia induced by a percutaneous cardiopulmonary support system. Case report. J Neurosurg. 1997; 87(3):440–444

[28] Ng I, Hwang PY, Kumar D, Lee CK, Kockro RA, Sitoh YY. Surgical planning for microsurgical excision of cerebral arterio-venous malformations using virtual reality technology. Acta Neurochir (Wien). 2009; 151(5):453–463, discussion 463

[29] Wang H, Ye ZP, Huang ZC, Luo L, Chen C, Guo Y. Intraoperative ultrasonography combined with indocyanine green video-angiography in patients with cerebral arteriovenous malformations. J Neuroimaging. 2015; 25(6):916–921

[30] Steinberg GK, Chang SD, Gewirtz RJ, Lopez JR. Microsurgical resection of brainstem, thalamic, and basal ganglia angiographically occult vascular malformations. Neurosurgery. 2000; 46(2):260–270, discussion 270–271

[31] Hernesniemi J, Romani R, Lehecka M, et al. Present state of microneurosurgery of cerebral arteriovenous malformations. Acta Neurochir Suppl (Wien). 2010; 107:71–76

[32] Yamada S, Iacono RP, Mandybur GT, et al. Endoscopic procedures for resection of arteriovenous malformations. Surg Neurol. 1999; 51(6):641–649

[33] Hashimoto H, Iida J, Hironaka Y, Sakaki T. Surgical management of cerebral arteriovenous malformations with intraoperative digital subtraction angiography. J Clin Neurosci. 2000; 7 Suppl 1:33–35

[34] Ellis MJ, Kulkarni AV, Drake JM, Rutka JT, Armstrong D, Dirks PB. Intraoperative angiography during microsurgical removal of arteriovenous malformations in children. J Neurosurg Pediatr. 2010; 6(5):435–443

[35] Park J, Hamm IS. Anterior interhemispheric approach for distal anterior cerebral artery aneurysm surgery: preoperative analysis of the venous anatomy can help to avoid venous infarction. Acta Neurochir (Wien). 2004; 146(9):973–977, discussion 977

[36] Sato T, Sasaki T, Matsumoto M, et al. Thalamic arteriovenous malformation with an unusual draining system–case report. Neurol Med Chir (Tokyo). 2004; 44(6):298–301

[37] Santi L, Tomita T. The occipital transtentorial approach for cerebellar arteriovenous malformation in a child. Childs Nerv Syst. 2000; 16(3):129–133

[38] Salcman M, Nudelman RW, Bellis EH. Arteriovenous malformations of the superior cerebellar artery: excision via an occipital transtentorial approach. Neurosurgery. 1985; 17(5):749–756

[39] Sanai N, Mirzadeh Z, Lawton MT. Supracerebellar-supratrochlear and infratentorial-infratrochlear approaches: gravity-dependent variations of the lateral approach over the cerebellum. Neurosurgery. 2010; 66(6) Suppl Operative:264–274, discussion 274

[40] Arnaout OM, Gross BA, Eddleman CS, Bendok BR, Getch CC, Batjer HH. Posterior fossa arteriovenous malformations. Neurosurg Focus. 2009; 26(5):E12

[41] Batjer H, Samson D. Arteriovenous malformations of the posterior fossa. Clinical presentation, diagnostic evaluation, and surgical treatment. J Neurosurg. 1986; 64(6):849–856

[42] Chyatte D. Vascular malformations of the brain stem. J Neurosurg. 1989; 70(6):847–852

[43] Hosoda K, Fujita S, Kawaguchi T, Yamada H. A transcondylar approach to the arteriovenous malformation at the ventral cervicomedullary junction: report of three cases. Neurosurgery. 1994; 34(4):748–752, discussion –752–753

[44] Solomon RA, Stein BM. Management of arteriovenous malformations of the brain stem. J Neurosurg. 1986; 64(6):857–864

[45] Sugiura K, Baba M. Total removal of an arteriovenous malformation embedded in the brain stem. Surg Neurol. 1990; 34(5):327–330

[46] Yagmurlu K, Rhoton AL , Jr, Tanriover N, Bennett JA. Three-dimensional microsurgical anatomy and the safe entry zones of the brainstem. Neurosurgery. 2014; 10 Suppl 4:602–619, discussion 619–620

[47] Recalde RJ, Figueiredo EG, de Oliveira E. Microsurgical anatomy of the safe entry zones on the anterolateral brainstem related to surgical approaches to cavernous malformations. Neurosurgery. 2008; 62(3) Suppl 1:9–15, discussion 15–17

[48] Kyoshima K, Kobayashi S, Gibo H, Kuroyanagi T. A study of safe entry zones via the floor of the fourth ventricle for brain-stem lesions. Report of three cases. J Neurosurg. 1993; 78(6):987–993

[49] Steiger HJ, Hänggi D. Retrograde venonidal microsurgical obliteration of brain stem AVM: a clinical feasibility study. Acta Neurochir (Wien). 2009; 151(12):1617–1622

[50] Velat GJ, Chang SW, Abla AA, Albuquerque FC, McDougall CG, Spetzler RF. Microsurgical management of glomus spinal arteriovenous malformations: pial resection technique: clinical article. J Neurosurg Spine. 2012; 16(6):523–531

[51] Tatagiba MS, Roser F, Hirt B, Ebner FH. The retrosigmoid endoscopic approach for cerebellopontine-angle tumors and microvascular decompression. World Neurosurg. 2014; 82(6) Suppl:S171–S176

[52] Samii M, Metwali H, Samii A, Gerganov V. Retrosigmoid intradural inframeatal approach: indications and technique. Neurosurgery. 2013; 73(1) Suppl Operative:ons53–ons59, discussion ons60

[53] Moscovici S, Umansky F, Spektor S. "Lazy" far-lateral approach to the anterior foramen magnum and lower clivus. Neurosurg Focus. 2015; 38(4):E14

[54] Ito M, Yamamoto T, Mishina H, Sonokawa T, Sato K. Arteriovenous malformation of the medulla oblongata supplied by the anterior spinal artery in a child: treatment by microsurgical obliteration of the feeding artery. Pediatr Neurosurg. 2000; 33(6):293–297

[55] Spetzler RF, Wilson CB, Weinstein P, Mehdorn M, Townsend J, Telles D. Normal perfusion pressure breakthrough theory. Clin Neurosurg. 1978; 25:651–672

[56] al-Rodhan NR, Sundt TM , Jr, Piepgras DG, Nichols DA, Rüfenacht D, Stevens LN. Occlusive hyperemia: a theory for the hemodynamic complications following resection of intracerebral arteriovenous malformations. J Neurosurg. 1993; 78(2):167–175

[57] Rangel-Castilla L, Spetzler RF, Nakaji P. Normal perfusion pressure breakthrough theory: a reappraisal after 35 years. Neurosurg Rev. 2015; 38(3):399–404, discussion 404–405

[58] Potts MB, Jahangiri A, Jen M, et al. UCSF Brain AVM Study Project. Deep arteriovenous malformations in the basal ganglia, thalamus, and insula: multimodality management, patient selection, and results. World Neurosurg. 2014; 82(3–4):386–394

18 Hemorrhage from Arteriovenous Malformations and Its Management

Ross Puffer and Giuseppe Lanzino

Abstract

Arteriovenous malformations (AVMs) are responsible for up to 4% of primary intracerebral hemorrhages, and in population-based studies, the incidence of hemorrhage at presentation is 50–65%. The current AVM literature was searched to determine rates of hemorrhage and outcome after rupture. Recommendations for the medical management of intracranial hemorrhage have been taken from the most recent American Heart Association/American Stroke Association guidelines, as well as notable trials that were performed to determine adequate blood pressure guidelines after primary intracerebral hemorrhage, such as ADAPT and INTERACT. We found that treatment guidelines follow those of primary intracerebral hemorrhage. Systolic blood pressure < 140 mmHg, treatment of raised ICP and normoglycemia, but despite best medical management, patients can experience complications including include seizures, vasospasm (rare), and deep venous thrombosis. Ultimately, AVM associated hemorrhages have better functional outcomes when compared to primary intracerebral hemorrhages.

Keywords: arteriovenous malformation, complications, hemorrhage, management

Key Points

- Between 50 and 65% of arteriovenous malformations (AVMs) present with hemorrhage.
- The timeframe of progression and involvement of multiple vascular territories may lead the clinician to consider AVM as a source of a hemorrhage.
- Treatment guidelines follow those of primary intracerebral hemorrhage: Systolic blood pressure < 140 mm Hg, treatment of raised intracranial pressure and normoglycemia.
- Complications after AVM rupture include seizures, vasospasm (rare), and deep venous thrombosis.
- AVM-associated hemorrhages have better functional outcomes when compared to primary intracerebral hemorrhages.

18.1 Introduction

Arteriovenous malformations (AVMs) are responsible for up to 4% of primary intracerebral hemorrhages, and in population-based studies, the incidence of hemorrhage at presentation is 50 to 65%.[1,2,3] Hemorrhage from AVM ruptures often occurs within the brain parenchyma, but up to 34% of patients can present with intraventricular hemorrhage (IVH) either isolated or associated with hemorrhage in other compartments, and 24% may have some elements of subarachnoid hemorrhage (SAH) as well.[2,3,4] In many cases (93%), the intracranial

hemorrhage occurs due to rupture of the AVM nidus; however, the hemorrhage can also be related to AVM-associated arterial aneurysms (approximately 7% of cases).[3] Patients with AVMs may experience a microhemorrhage which is clinically silent but evident on imaging.[5] Functional outcome after AVM rupture is better than in patients with primary intracerebral hemorrhage. In a recent study, patients who suffered ICH from an AVM had significantly better National Institute of Health Stroke Scale (NIHSS) score at 30-day follow-up than patients with spontaneous (non-AVM related) ICH (mean NIHSS of 3.9 ± 6.2 vs. 13.6 ± 9.5, respectively).[6] Often, AVM patients are younger, have lower blood pressure at admission, and higher GCS than patients with spontaneous ICH.[7] Despite these better reported outcomes when compared to spontaneous ICH, the fatality rate after AVM rupture has been found to be 11% at 1 month, increasing to 13% at 2 years. At 1 year postrupture, 40% of patients are dead or dependent (modified Rankin scale [mRS] ≥ 3).[7]

With advances in noninvasive imaging techniques, it has become apparent that several patients with the so-called unruptured AVMs have indeed radiological evidence of prior bleeding as indicated by T2 and FLAIR changes in the parenchyma around the AVM and in some cases frank cyst formation, most likely the result of previous subclinical bleeding. This is corroborated by direct and histopathological analysis after AVM excision.[5] These patients are considered to have suffered from a subclinical hemorrhage with no or very mild symptoms at the time of rupture. The true significance of these findings in relation to the natural history of these AVMs is unknown. However, this observation underscores that not all unruptured AVMs are the same, given that some patients may have suffered a prior hemorrhagic episode without noticeable clinical effects.[5]

18.2 Materials and Methods

The current AVM literature was searched to determine rates of hemorrhage and outcome after rupture. Recommendations for the medical management of intracranial hemorrhage have been taken from the most recent American Heart Association/American Stroke Association guidelines, as well as notable trials that were performed to determine adequate blood pressure guidelines after primary intracerebral hemorrhage, such as ADAPT and INTERACT.[8,9,10]

18.3 Results and Discussion

18.3.1 Initial Management of a Ruptured Arteriovenous Malformation

As discussed previously, AVMs may present with hemorrhage in 50 to 65% of cases, and the symptoms present at onset depend on the location and severity of the hemorrhage.[2,3] Small localized bleeds or simple SAH may manifest with headache with various characteristics in relation to the degree of blood extravasation and location. Hemorrhages near the cortical surface may lead to clinical seizures (in up to 33% of patients), and indeed an initial seizure as clinical presentation of an AVM warrants careful evaluation because seizures can be a symptom of hemorrhage even in the absence of headache. Deeper lesions and lesions adjacent to eloquent areas may present with motor, sensory, language, or visual symptoms.[11] AVM-associated hemorrhages can involve multiple vascular territories, and this may be a clue leading the clinician to an AVM as the cause rather than primary intracerebral hemorrhage. These symptoms may progress over minutes to hours from accumulation of blood products, local brain compression, and elevated intracranial pressure (ICP). The temporal relationship of symptom progression is often distinct from that of aneurysmal SAH, given its progression over minutes to hours rather than sudden, acute onset of maximum intensity in cases of aneurysmal SAH. Large parenchymal bleeds and/or intraventricular extension can be associated with rather rapid decline of the level of consciousness and progression to coma.

Initial management largely follows the same guidelines as primary intracerebral hemorrhage, with cardiorespiratory support and transfer to specialized medical attention as mainstays of initial management. After initial stabilization, neuroimaging should be obtained to determine the location, size, and possible source of intracranial hemorrhage. This should be completed using CT as the first screening image modality (class I, level A evidence).[9]

CT angiography can be obtained if an AVM is considered a possible source of the hemorrhage because of location, clinical factors, and patient age. This modality allows for rapid identification of an AVM in patients who may need urgent decompressive surgery and may also demonstrate associated aneurysms. Despite advances in modern CT angiography techniques, catheter-based angiography remains the gold standard. Nonetheless, vascular imaging should be considered if an AVM is thought to be the source (class IIa, level B).[9] If the patient does not require emergent, decompressive surgery, a catheter-based angiography should be performed within 24 hours if possible. This allows for the identification of any associated aneurysms, as well as the possible source of the intracranial hemorrhage (▶ Fig. 18.1).[12]

After the initial evaluation is complete, these patients should be managed in the intensive care unit (ICU) setting, preferably with staff accustomed to caring for critically ill neurology/neurosurgery patients. Patients with primary intracerebral hemorrhage have been found to have a lower overall mortality when cared for by dedicated neurological intensive care nurses and staff members (class I, level B).[9,13]

18.3.2 Medical Management

There are multiple management considerations for patients in the ICU setting after suffering a hemorrhage from an AVM. Blood pressure management guidelines are taken from

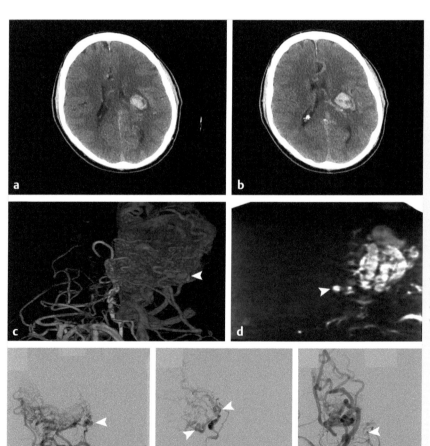

Fig. 18.1 Selective occlusion of rupture point in ruptured arteriovenous malformations (AVMs). This 63-year-old man had a known AVM diagnosed in 2007 after a seizure. No treatment was recommended because of the unruptured status and the risks of treatment. Nine years later, he presented with sudden headache and left-sided weakness. Head CT shows a deep hemorrhage (a,b). (c) Catheter angiography, left vertebral artery injection, shows a diffuse AVM with perinidal aneurysms (*arrowhead*). (d) Three-dimensional angiography shows the mass of the AVM and the perinidal aneurysms (*arrowhead*). (e) Dynamic CT shows that the perinidal aneurysms are in direct continuity with the hemorrhage and at the epicenter of it. Thus, these aneurysms are most likely the source of the hemorrhage. (f) Superselective catheterization of the feeding pedicle provides better definition of the perinidal dysplastic aneurysms (*arrowheads*). (g) The pedicle harboring the aneurysms was occluded with detachable coils (*arrowhead*) to decrease the risk of rehemorrhage.

available studies designed to generate guidelines for primary intracranial hemorrhage management. Studies have demonstrated that systolic blood pressures sustained about 140 mm Hg may be associated with hematoma expansion and worsened outcome.[14] While historically there was concern that rapid lowering of systolic blood pressure would lead to decreased perihematoma blood flow in edematous brain, recent multicenter trials, including ADAPT and INTERACT, have demonstrated that rapid blood pressure lowering does not significantly decrease perihematoma blood flow, is safe, and may lead to better functional outcomes.[8,10] Even though these studies were performed on patients who experienced primary intracerebral hemorrhage not associated with an AVM, it is recommended that in the setting of AVM-associated hemorrhage, systolic blood pressure should be maintained below 140 mm Hg to avoid hematoma expansion.

AVM-associated hemorrhage can lead to raised ICP, if the hematoma is large enough or if there is hydrocephalus in the presence of IVH. In cases with a contained hematoma and minimal IVH, ICP monitoring is likely not required. However, if evidence of hydrocephalus is present on imaging, or the clinical exam cannot be reliably followed (GCS < 8), ICP monitoring can be considered, either via external ventricular drainage or ICP monitor placement. The authors would recommend external ventricular drainage in any case with evidence of hydrocephalus, as this allows for both monitoring and treatment of any raised ICP. When an ICP monitor is utilized, cerebral perfusion pressure should be maintained between 50 and 70 mm Hg (class IIb, level C).[9] Before considering any invasive monitoring or placement of an EVD, AVM location and pattern of drainage should be identified as to avoid mechanical manipulations in an area involved by the AVM.

Blood glucose should be monitored in the ICU setting, and prior studies have demonstrated that hyperglycemia can lead to poor outcome in ICH patients.[15,16,17] Some authors have advocated tight blood glucose monitoring and control utilizing intravenous insulin infusions to maintain blood glucose between 80 and 110. However, recent evidence suggests that aggressive regulation of blood glucose to these levels may be harmful in that it may lead to more hypoglycemic episodes, which have also been linked to poor outcomes.[18,19,20,21] Current recommendations suggest that blood glucose should be monitored in the ICU setting and normoglycemia is recommended (class I, level C).[9]

18.3.3 Complications

Rebleeding can occur after AVM-associated hemorrhage. In the authors' experience, there is a subset of AVM patients who are at risk of rebleeding, often with severe or even devastating complications. These patients tend to have evidence of outflow obstruction with venous stasis and frank venous varices on vascular imaging. In other cases, it is likely that the AVM draining pathways may have undergone varying degrees of thrombosis that may have precipitated the initial rupture and the remaining draining vein may be under unusual stress potentially increasing the risk of early rebleeding. Hematoma compression of venous outflow tracts can lead to further hemodynamic changes within the AVM itself, possibly leading to further bleeding episodes. In some cases, the presence of a pseudoaneurysm, usually along the path of a small perforating vessel

feeding the AVM, can be the origin of the bleeding (▶ Fig. 18.1). Such cases must be monitored closely with repeat imaging, given these pseudoaneurysms can undergo progression (with further growth and rerupture) or even regression (with spontaneous thrombosis). Patients with AVM-associated arterial aneurysms should be treated like any other patient with aneurysmal SAH if there is clinical and radiological evidence linking the bleed to the aneurysm as a potential source. However, early rebleeding from an AVM is relatively uncommon outside of these special situations. Delayed cerebral vasospasm is rarely demonstrated in AVM-associated hemorrhages, with a recent study demonstrating the incidence of asymptomatic vasospasm on catheter-based angiography of 6.3%.[22] This is significantly less than the incidence of asymptomatic vasospasm after aneurysmal SAH, which has been reported to be as high as 70%.[23,24,25] It has been thought that differences in the hemodynamics of blood extravasation as well as a potential decreased concentration of oxygenated hemoglobin in blood from ruptured venous varices within the AVM may be the cause of lower rates of cerebral vasospasm, although no dedicated studies have been performed to further determine the underlying reason behind the decreased incidence of delayed vasospasm.

Seizures may occur after AVM-associated hemorrhage, and current recommendations state that clinical seizures, when present, should be treated with antiepileptic medications (class I, level A).[9] In patients with altered mental status, and especially in cases where the neurologic exam cannot fully be explained by the hematoma, EEG can be used to diagnose possible underlying seizure activity (class IIa, level B).[9] Furthermore, patients who demonstrate seizure activity on EEG should be treated with antiepileptic medications (class I, level C). Antiepileptic medications should not be used in patients who have not demonstrated either clinical or electrographic seizure activity, given that studies on the use of antiepileptic medications in ICH, specifically phenytoin, in patients without a documented seizure have demonstrated worse outcomes in those receiving phenytoin prophylaxis at 90 days post-bleed.[26,27] Thus, there is a recommendation against the use of prophylactic antiepileptics in patients with AVM-associated hemorrhages (class III, level B).[9] Prophylactic antiepileptic medications can be considered in patients who undergo surgery for cortical-based AVMs.

In many cases, patients suffering from an AVM-associated hemorrhage are bedbound for a period of their recovery. There is a high risk of deep venous thromboembolism in these patients, and recommendations state that pneumatic compression devices should be utilized (class I, level B).[2] There is no current consensus as to the timing for safe initiation of prophylactic heparin anticoagulation. Two trials have been performed in the primary intracerebral hemorrhage population, demonstrating no increased risk of rebleeding and no difference in incidence of deep venous thrombosis on post-bleed day 4 compared to post-bleed day 10 in patients started on low-dose subcutaneous heparin.[28,29] The current recommendations state that imaging demonstrating stability in the hematoma and no evidence of further bleeding should be performed prior to the initiation of any heparin anticoagulation. When this has been completed, prophylactic use of low-dose subcutaneous low-molecular-weight heparin or unfractionated heparin can be considered for prophylaxis against deep venous thrombosis (class IIb, level B).[9]

18.3.4 Timing of Surgery after AVM Hemorrhage

While the overall risk of rebleeding in all comers is low, there are specific architectural features of an AVM that may portend a higher risk of re-hemorrhage, such as single venous outflow with or without stasis and ectasia as well as the presence of associated aneurysms.[2,30,31,32,33,34] In patients who require emergent decompression and evacuation of a hematoma, it is advisable to only attempt full AVM resection with small, well-defined, superficial AVMs. In patients with large and more complex AVMs, we recommend simple clot evacuation as the initial procedure, followed by neurologic recovery and stabilization, at which point definitive intervention can be performed.[35] The extra time allows the residual hematoma to liquefy, the associated perihematoma edema to resolve leading to improved surgical planes, and visualization. It is important to determine the venous outflow after AVM hemorrhage to determine whether or not the patient is at risk for hyperacute rebleeding due to outflow tract thrombosis. Often times, AVM hemorrhage can be related to sudden thrombosis of the venous outflow or changes in the intrinsic hemodynamics of the AVM due to compression or thrombosis. In these patients, early surgical or endovascular intervention may be warranted to decrease the risk of a hyperacute rebleed that may be devastating. In patients being taken for surgery, a conventional angiography the day prior to surgery is advised to identify any changes to the microcirculation immediately before surgery.

18.3.5 Special Considerations— Pregnancy

AVM rupture during pregnancy and ultimate intervention can be difficult. Special care needs to be taken with any management decisions to ultimately protect the life of the mother while avoiding any danger to the fetus if at all possible. Modifications to the medical management and anesthetic management need to be considered during any possible intervention to avoid any detrimental effects on the fetus. If definitive treatment of the AVM is not considered emergent, surgery or intervention may be delayed until after delivery; however, the obstetrician should be notified because significant alterations in blood pressure during delivery may put the AVM at risk of hemorrhage. If intervention is required, AVM resection can be considered for small, superficial, ruptured AVMs. Mannitol and induced hypotension should be avoided during surgery due to the risk of fetal hypoxia and severe electrolyte abnormalities. Care should be taken to avoid significant blood loss during any attempted AVM resection in these circumstances.

18.4 Conclusion

AVM-associated intracerebral hemorrhage is distinct from aneurysmal SAH and even primary intracerebral hemorrhage. It can be the presenting finding in more than 50% of AVMs, and there are several aspects of a hemorrhage that can lead the clinician to the underlying diagnosis of AVM. Management specific to AVM-associated hemorrhage has not been well studied, so current guidelines follow those for managing primary intracerebral hemorrhage in the ICU setting. Despite the similarities in management, AVM-associated hemorrhage has been shown to have better functional outcomes at follow-up when compared to primary intracerebral hemorrhage.

References

[1] Al-Shahi R, Warlow C. A systematic review of the frequency and prognosis of arteriovenous malformations of the brain in adults. Brain. 2001; 124(Pt 10): 1900–1926

[2] Brown RD , Jr, Wiebers DO, Torner JC, O'Fallon WM. Frequency of intracranial hemorrhage as a presenting symptom and subtype analysis: a population-based study of intracranial vascular malformations in Olmsted Country, Minnesota. J Neurosurg. 1996; 85(1):29–32

[3] Cordonnier C, Al-Shahi Salman R, Bhattacharya JJ, et al. SIVMS Collaborators. Differences between intracranial vascular malformation types in the characteristics of their presenting haemorrhages: prospective, population-based study. J Neurol Neurosurg Psychiatry. 2008; 79(1):47–51

[4] Al-Shahi R, Bhattacharya JJ, Currie DG, et al. Scottish Intracranial Vascular Malformation Study Collaborators. Scottish Intracranial Vascular Malformation Study (SIVMS): evaluation of methods, ICD-10 coding, and potential sources of bias in a prospective, population-based cohort. Stroke. 2003; 34 (5):1156–1162

[5] Abla AA, Nelson J, Kim H, Hess CP, Tihan T, Lawton MT. Silent arteriovenous malformation hemorrhage and the recognition of "unruptured" arteriovenous malformation patients who benefit from surgical intervention. Neurosurgery. 2015; 76(5):592–600, discussion 600

[6] Choi JH, Mast H, Sciacca RR, et al. Clinical outcome after first and recurrent hemorrhage in patients with untreated brain arteriovenous malformation. Stroke. 2006; 37(5):1243–1247

[7] van Beijnum J, Lovelock CE, Cordonnier C, Rothwell PM, Klijn CJ, Al-Shahi Salman R, SIVMS Steering Committee and the Oxford Vascular Study. Outcome after spontaneous and arteriovenous malformation-related intracerebral haemorrhage: population-based studies. Brain. 2009; 132(Pt 2):537–543

[8] Butcher KS, Jeerakathil T, Hill M, et al. ICH ADAPT Investigators. The intracerebral hemorrhage acutely decreasing arterial pressure trial. Stroke. 2013; 44(3):620–626

[9] Morgenstern LB, Hemphill JC , III, Anderson C, et al. American Heart Association Stroke Council and Council on Cardiovascular Nursing. Guidelines for the management of spontaneous intracerebral hemorrhage: a guideline for healthcare professionals from the American Heart Association/American Stroke Association. Stroke. 2010; 41(9):2108–2129

[10] Anderson CS, Huang Y, Arima H, et al. INTERACT Investigators. Effects of early intensive blood pressure-lowering treatment on the growth of hematoma and perihematomal edema in acute intracerebral hemorrhage: the Intensive Blood Pressure Reduction in Acute Cerebral Haemorrhage Trial (INTERACT). Stroke. 2010; 41(2):307–312

[11] Hoffer ASJ, Bambakidis NC, et al, eds. Spontaneous Intracerebral Hemorrhage. 3rd ed. Philadelphia, PA: Elsevier; 2012

[12] Zacharia BE, Vaughan KA, Jacoby A, Hickman ZL, Bodmer D, Connolly ES, Jr. Management of ruptured brain arteriovenous malformations. Curr Atheroscler Rep. 2012; 14(4):335–342

[13] Diringer MN, Edwards DF. Admission to a neurologic/neurosurgical intensive care unit is associated with reduced mortality rate after intracerebral hemorrhage. Crit Care Med. 2001; 29(3):635–640

[14] Willmot M, Leonardi-Bee J, Bath PM. High blood pressure in acute stroke and subsequent outcome: a systematic review. Hypertension. 2004; 43 (1):18–24

[15] Fogelholm R, Murros K, Rissanen A, Avikainen S. Long term survival after primary intracerebral haemorrhage: a retrospective population based study. J Neurol Neurosurg Psychiatry. 2005; 76(11):1534–1538

[16] Kimura K, Iguchi Y, Inoue T, et al. Hyperglycemia independently increases the risk of early death in acute spontaneous intracerebral hemorrhage. J Neurol Sci. 2007; 255(1–2):90–94

[17] Passero S, Ciacci G, Ulivelli M. The influence of diabetes and hyperglycemia on clinical course after intracerebral hemorrhage. Neurology. 2003; 61(10): 1351–1356

[18] Finfer S, Chittock DR, Su SY, et al. NICE-SUGAR Study Investigators. Intensive versus conventional glucose control in critically ill patients. N Engl J Med. 2009; 360(13):1283–1297

[19] Oddo M, Schmidt JM, Carrera E, et al. Impact of tight glycemic control on cerebral glucose metabolism after severe brain injury: a microdialysis study. Crit Care Med. 2008; 36(12):3233–3238

[20] van den Berghe G, Wouters P, Weekers F, et al. Intensive insulin therapy in critically ill patients. N Engl J Med. 2001; 345(19):1359–1367

[21] Vespa PM. Intensive glycemic control in traumatic brain injury: what is the ideal glucose range? Crit Care. 2008; 12(5):175

[22] Gross BA, Du R. Vasospasm after arteriovenous malformation rupture. World Neurosurg. 2012; 78(3–4):300–305

[23] Charpentier C, Audibert G, Guillemin F, et al. Multivariate analysis of predictors of cerebral vasospasm occurrence after aneurysmal subarachnoid hemorrhage. Stroke. 1999; 30(7):1402–1408

[24] Ecker A, Riemenschneider PA. Arteriographic demonstration of spasm of the intracranial arteries, with special reference to saccular arterial aneurysms. J Neurosurg. 1951; 8(6):660–667

[25] Murayama Y, Malisch T, Guglielmi G, et al. Incidence of cerebral vasospasm after endovascular treatment of acutely ruptured aneurysms: report on 69 cases. J Neurosurg. 1997; 87(6):830–835

[26] Messé SR, Sansing LH, Cucchiara BL, Herman ST, Lyden PD, Kasner SE, CHANT investigators. Prophylactic antiepileptic drug use is associated with poor outcome following ICH. Neurocrit Care. 2009; 11(1):38–44

[27] Naidech AM, Garg RK, Liebling S, et al. Anticonvulsant use and outcomes after intracerebral hemorrhage. Stroke. 2009; 40(12):3810–3815

[28] Boeer A, Voth E, Henze T, Prange HW. Early heparin therapy in patients with spontaneous intracerebral haemorrhage. J Neurol Neurosurg Psychiatry. 1991; 54(5):466–467

[29] Dickmann U, Voth E, Schicha H, Henze T, Prange H, Emrich D. Heparin therapy, deep-vein thrombosis and pulmonary embolism after intracerebral hemorrhage. Klin Wochenschr. 1988; 66(23):1182–1183

[30] ApSimon HT, Reef H, Phadke RV, Popovic EA. A population-based study of brain arteriovenous malformation: long-term treatment outcomes. Stroke. 2002; 33(12):2794–2800

[31] Hillman J. Population-based analysis of arteriovenous malformation treatment. J Neurosurg. 2001; 95(4):633–637

[32] Mast H, Young WL, Koennecke HC, et al. Risk of spontaneous haemorrhage after diagnosis of cerebral arteriovenous malformation. Lancet. 1997; 350 (9084):1065–1068

[33] Stapf C, Labovitz DL, Sciacca RR, Mast H, Mohr JP, Sacco RL. Incidence of adult brain arteriovenous malformation hemorrhage in a prospective population-based stroke survey. Cerebrovasc Dis. 2002; 13(1):43–46

[34] Stapf C, Mast H, Sciacca RR, et al. New York Islands AVM Study Collaborators. The New York Islands AVM Study: design, study progress, and initial results. Stroke. 2003; 34(5):e29–e33

[35] Heros RC. Arteriovenous malformation-associated intracerebral hemorrhage. World Neurosurg. 2012; 78(6):586–587

19 Fundamentals of Endovascular Treatment for Arteriovenous Malformations and Arteriovenous Fistulas

Badih Daou, Pascal Jabbour, Stavropoula I. Tjoumakaris, and Robert H. Rosenwasser

Abstract

Endovascular management of cerebral arteriovenous malformations (AVMs) and arteriovenous fistulas (AVFs) has evolved tremendously over the past few decades and has become one of the primary treatment modalities to manage these lesions. Endovascular embolization of AVFs can be accomplished through a transarterial or transvenous approach depending on the location and complexity of the AVF and its vascular characteristics. The potential roles of embolization in AVF management include complete elimination of the AVF, palliation of disabling neurological symptoms, or a decrease in the flow through the AVF before other surgical or radiosurgical interventions are performed. Endovascular management of AVMs can be used for presurgical embolization of large AVMs, embolization of AVMs before radiosurgical intervention and for treating residual lesions that persist after radiosurgery, palliative embolization in patients with progressive or refractory neurological deficits, and finally as a primary treatment for curative embolization of small AVMs and AVMs that are not candidates for other surgical or radiosurgical approaches. N-butyl cyanoacrylate (NBCA) and Onyx liquid embolic agent are the most widely used agents for the embolization of AVFs and AVMs. Management of AVMs and AVFs requires a multidisciplinary team with expertise in the different treatment strategies available. Endovascular therapy has become a highly utilized, safe, and effective tool in the management of cerebral AVMs and AVFs either alone as a curative intervention or as an adjunct to other interventions.

Keywords: arteriovenous fistula, arteriovenous malformation, embolization, endovascular treatment, NBCA, Onyx

19.1 Introduction

The management of cerebrovascular malformations including arteriovenous malformations (AVMs) and arteriovenous fistulas (AVFs) has evolved tremendously over the past few decades. With the development of catheter and guidewire technology and novel embolic materials, endovascular management of these malformations has gained significant popularity and has become common practice. Intracranial AVMs are vessel abnormalities that constitute a connection between the arterial and venous systems with a lack of an intervening capillary bed.[1] The intervening network of vessels between the distal aspects of the arterial feeders and the proximal aspects of the draining veins is called the *nidus* and is the primary target of embolization.[2] In contrast, AVFs are direct fistulous connections between cerebral arteries and veins in the absence of an intervening nidus.[3] They can be stratified based on arterial supply into dural AVF and pial AVF. Dural arteriovenous fistulas (DAVFs) are arteriovenous shunts from a dural arterial supply to a dural venous channel, typically supplied by pachymeningeal arteries and located near a major venous sinus.[4] Pial arteriovenous fistulas (PAVFs) are rare vascular abnormalities that account for only 1.6% of all intracranial vascular malformations.[5] They are composed of one or more pial and cortical arterial feeders with a single venous channel and they are not located within the leaflets of the dura.[6] Intracranial AVMs and AVFs are relatively uncommon lesions, but the occurrence of these lesions can result in severe neurological symptoms, including seizures, headaches, focal neurological deficits, neuro-ophthalmologic symptoms, and more importantly intracerebral hemorrhage and death.[3,7,8,9,10] There are several treatment modalities available to manage AVMs and AVFs and these include expectant management, surgical, radiosurgical, and endovascular techniques, or a combination of these approaches. The appropriate treatment strategy depends on a multitude of factors and should be tailored according to patient characteristics (age, comorbidities, and clinical presentation) and characteristics related to the malformation including the location, classification, natural history of the lesion, and angiographic features. The objective of this chapter is to review and highlight the role of endovascular treatment in the management of AVMs and AVFs.

19.2 Materials and Methods

The materials included in this chapter represent an analysis of published articles, including published institutional results along with the authors' experience in the endovascular management of cerebral AVMs and AVFs.

Key Points

- There has been a tremendous evolution in the endovascular management of arteriovenous malformations (AVMs) and arteriovenous fistulas (AVFs) over the past few decades and represents a safe and effective primary treatment option for many lesions.
- Potential roles for embolization of AVFs include complete elimination, palliation of symptoms, or as an adjunct prior to surgery or radiosurgery.
- Endovascular embolization of AVMs may be performed as a preoperative adjunct prior to resection or radiosurgery, to treat residual lesions after prior intervention, and as palliative treatment to reduce neurological symptoms (such as from steal) and less commonly to achieve complete nidus obliteration in select lesions.
- Management of AVMs and AVFs is best accomplished in the setting of a multidisciplinary team.

19.3 Results

19.3.1 Arteriovenous Fistulas

Endovascular management has become the primary treatment modality of AVFs. Endovascular embolization of the fistula can be accomplished through a transarterial or transvenous route. Both approaches are usually performed through transfemoral access by catheterization of the femoral artery or femoral vein, respectively. The choice between the two access routes and the aim of the endovascular intervention depend on the location and complexity of the AVF, its vascular characteristics, and the potential complications inherent to each technique. The potential roles of embolization include complete elimination of the AVF, palliation of disabling neurological symptoms, or a decrease in the flow through the AVF before other surgical or radiosurgical interventions are undertaken.

There are several embolic materials that have been used for endovascular management of AVFs, including particles, liquid silicone, ethyl alcohol, polyvinyl alcohol, platinum microcoils, and cyanoacrylates. Liquid embolic agents are the most commonly used materials to manage AVFs, including N-butyl cyanoacrylate (NBCA; Trufill; Codman, Raynham, MA) (▶ Fig. 19.1) and Onyx liquid embolic agent (eV3 Neurovascular; Covidien, Irvine, CA) which is an ethylene vinyl alcohol polymer dissolved in dimethyl sulfoxide (DMSO).

19.3.2 Arteriovenous Malformations

Similarly, embolic materials used in the management of intracranial AVMs are divided into solid or liquid agents. Solid materials include polyvinyl alcohol particles, fibers, microballoons, and microcoils. Liquid agents include cyanoacrylate monomers such as NBCA and IBCA (*I*-butyl cyanoacrylate) as well as polymer solutions such as ethylene vinyl alcohol polymer. Other liquid agents include absolute ethanol which is not commonly used. The principal agents currently in use for treating brain AVMs are NBCA and Onyx.

The aim of the endovascular intervention differs based on the characteristics of the lesion. Endovascular management can be used for presurgical embolization of large or giant cortical AVMs (▶ Fig. 19.2), embolization of AVMs before radiosurgical intervention and for treating residual lesions that persist after radiosurgery, palliative embolization in patients with progressive or refractory neurological deficits, and in patients with large AVMs and AVMs that may be difficult to manage surgically or with radiosurgery, as well as finally as a primary treatment for curative embolization of small AVMs and AVMs that are not candidates for other surgical or radiosurgical approaches. Endovascular treatment can also be used to eliminate AVM-associated aneurysms, especially in acutely ruptured cases where the aneurysm is the source of hemorrhage.

19.4 Discussion

Most of the data available regarding endovascular treatment of AVMs and AVFs stem from level III, IV, and V evidences with level I and level II studies significantly lacking from the literature.

19.4.1 Endovascular Management of AVFs

Although endovascular management has become the mainstay of DAVF therapy, the best approach to manage each lesion should be individualized with involvement of a multidisciplinary team to evaluate each case. A meticulous evaluation of the patient's characteristics and clinical presentation and location, classification, and type of the lesion should be performed prior to treatment. The decision to manage AVFs through an endovascular approach should be based on an assessment of the risk of the intervention against the natural history of the lesion.

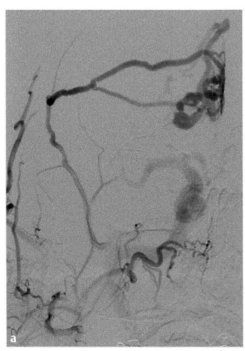
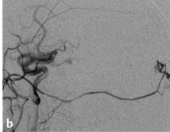
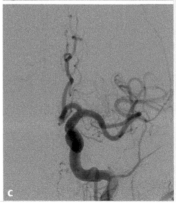

Fig. 19.1 (a) A 56-year-old male patient who presented with an occipital hemorrhage. Angiography with right external carotid artery injection showed a dural arteriovenous fistula fed by feeders from the middle meningeal artery, draining into the superior sagittal sinus with cortical venous drainage. **(b)** Left external carotid artery injection showing the middle meningeal feeders of the fistula. **(c)** Embolization with N-butyl cyanoacrylate was performed. Follow-up angiography showed complete occlusion of the fistula and associated cortical venous drainage after a single embolization session.

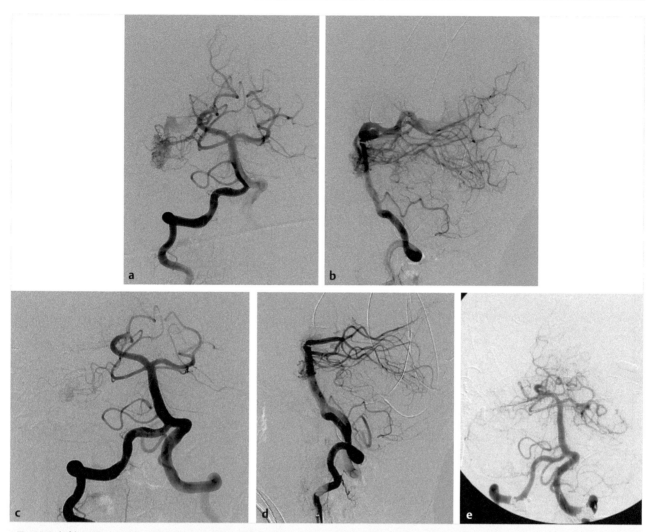

Fig. 19.2 (a,b) A 58-year-old male patient who was found to have an arteriovenous malformation (AVM) during evaluation for headaches. Angiography with right vertebral artery injection showed a right-sided temporal lobe Spetzler-Martin grade II AVM, fed by multiple feeders of the distal posterior cerebral artery on the right and posterior temporal arteries and draining deeply through two draining veins. **(c,d)** Preoperative embolization with Onyx was performed. Control angiography with selective right vertebral artery injection was performed showing 50% decrease in size of the AVM. **(e)** Surgical resection was performed. Control angiography showed 100% occlusion of the AVM.

Transvenous Access for AVF Management

Transvenous embolization aims at causing thrombosis of the venous side of the lesion and disconnection of leptomeningeal or cortical reflux with preservation of normal venous drainage.[4,11] Transvenous embolization often includes the obliteration of the adjacent dural venous sinus.[11] The transvenous approach has been primarily employed in the management of DAVFs, involving the cavernous, transverse, and sigmoid sinuses by allowing access to the affected venous sinus after which coils, balloons, or liquid embolic agents can be deployed.[12,13,14] However, the transvenous route may not be an option for many DAVFs, including tentorial incisura DAVFs and anterior cranial fossa lesions, which frequently behave aggressively.[6] Transvenous embolization of DAVFs involving the superior sagittal sinus is less optimal as well.[11,15] Patient selection for transvenous embolization depends on several important factors.[16] First, the segment of the sinus to be occluded must be in

proximity to the fistula and receive its entire venous drainage. Second, the diseased sinus should not be crucial to normal venous outflow and can be occluded. For this reason, cerebral venous drainage should be carefully assessed before transvenous embolization can be undertaken to determine the alternate pathways for cerebral venous drainage and avoid potential venous infarction or hemorrhage. Third, complete occlusion of the involved sinus segment is essential to avoid diversion of the flow into confluent cerebral veins and worsening of the cerebral venous drainage which may result in an acute venous infarct or hemorrhage.[16] Transvenous embolization is used in the management of large, complex DAVFs that have an accessible venous drainage. It is especially useful when the AVF has multiple arterial feeders. Occlusion of the venous side of DAVFs is usually well tolerated if the involved sinus is arterialized and does not serve as a site of drainage of normal circulation.[4] Usually, the pathologic segment is often associated with retrograde leptomeningeal venous drainage and these channels may be easier to obliterate using transvenous embolization. The main advantages of this approach are related to the ease of access to the fistulous site and the ability to obliterate the fistula in a single session.[11] Transvenous embolization is associated with a high efficacy and low complication rate.[17,18] The rates of complete angiographic obliteration of the AVF by the transvenous route have ranged mainly between 71 and 87.5%.[11,15,17,19] Complications associated with this approach include venous sinus thrombosis and infarction, vessel injury or rupture, disruption of the venous drainage, and altered hemodynamic patterns resulting in hemorrhage and worsening neurological deficits. Permanent complications have been reported in 4 to 7% of cases.[11,15,17,19]

Transarterial Access for AVF Management

The success of transarterial embolization in completely eliminating the DAVF depends on the number of accessible arterial feeders. This approach is most successful in achieving complete elimination of the lesion when the fistula has a small number of feeders, whereas DAVFs with a large number of feeders are rarely successfully treated with transarterial embolization alone. In DAVFs with multiple feeders, transarterial embolization may result in obliteration of the filling of the AVF after one injection, but the DAVF might still continue to draw feeders from other sources which may lead to development of new collaterals that may be more difficult to treat.[4,16] These partially treated DAVFs may later recur and result in hemorrhage. If, however, transarterial embolization results in occlusion of the common receptacle for all arterial feeders and disconnects any associated venous outflow, the embolization can be curative. Transarterial embolization can be used for the purpose of symptomatic palliation of disabling neurological symptoms through occlusion of arterial feeders without achieving complete obliteration of the fistula.[6] DAVFs that are followed expectantly or treated palliatively should be monitored closely with serial diagnostic imaging. Transarterial embolization can improve the safety and efficacy of other interventions as well by decreasing flow through the DAVF before other interventions are undertaken, such as surgical, radiosurgical, or transvenous management.[20,21] Transarterial embolization might offer advantages over transvenous access in certain cases.[16] Transvenous access to the fistula might be limited by venous sinus occlusion or high-grade stenosis in certain cases. Similarly, transvenous access to high-grade AVFs draining directly into remote small cerebral veins may result in significant complications. Complex fistulas may require management using a multi-staged approach, combining transarterial and transvenous techniques to eliminate cortical venous drainage and occlude the fistula. Kirsch et al reported in a study of 150 patients with DAVFs that immediate occlusion occurred in 30% of patients after transarterial embolization versus 81% with transvenous treatment alone. After combined transarterial/transvenous treatment, the angiographic cure rate was 54%.[14]

Alternative Access for AVF Management

In some cases, transfemoral access might not be possible because of unfavorable anatomy, tortuous vasculature, or femoral vascular pathology. Alternative transarterial access routes include the transradial approach, transcarotid access either percutaneously or through carotid cutdown, or direct puncture of a cavernous or ophthalmic fistula through the orbit.[22] Alternative transvenous routes include percutaneous cannulation of the facial vein, angular vein, superior ophthalmic vein, inferior ophthalmic vein, or direct transorbital puncture of the cavernous sinus.[22] A hybrid approach using surgical exposure of the superior ophthalmic vein or cavernous sinus followed by endovascular catheterization is also another option.[23]

Classification of AVFs and Endovascular Management

Angiography is essential for definitive diagnosis of AVFs and to provide a detailed evaluation of the arterial supply, anastomoses, and venous anatomy prior to embolization.[6] Treatment of DAVFs is guided by the classification of these lesions. One of the most well-recognized classification systems was reported by Djindjian and colleagues.[24,25] According to this system, type I DAVFs are characterized by normal anterograde drainage into a venous sinus or meningeal vein; type II lesions drain into a sinus, with reflux into adjacent sinuses or cortical veins, type III DAVFs drain directly into cortical veins with retrograde flow into the cerebral venous compartment, and type IV DAVFs have drainage directly into a venous pouch (venous lake or venous ectasia).

Cognard and colleagues developed another classification system based on a modified version of the Djindjian's classification.[26,27,28] They defined five types of DAVFs. Type I DAVFs were characterized by normal antegrade flow into the affected dural sinus. Type II lesions were associated with an abnormal direction of venous drainage within the affected dural sinus and were classified into three subtypes: type IIa, lesions with retrograde flow exclusively into a sinus or sinuses; type IIb, lesions with retrograde venous drainage into the cortical veins only; and type IIa + b, lesions with retrograde drainage into sinuses and cortical veins. Type III DAVFs had direct drainage into cortical veins without venous ectasia, whereas type IV DAVFs had direct drainage into cortical veins with venous ectasia greater than 5 mm in diameter and three times larger than the diameter of the draining vein. Type V DAVFs had drainage into spinal perimedullary veins. Type I DAVFs are considered benign, and do not usually require treatment. There is no evidence demonstrating significant benefits to prophylactic treatment of unruptured DAVFs that are not associated with leptomeningeal cortical venous drainage.[4] Expectant follow-up of these lesions using serial MRI and angiographic evaluation should be performed. Type IIa AVFs are best treated with transarterial embolization, whereas the best management strategy for type IIb and IIa + b lesions DAVFs is more challenging and these lesions usually require both transarterial and transvenous embolization to achieve complete cure.[6] For types III to V, the efficacy of endovascular management alone decreases and often complete occlusion of the fistula requires combined transarterial and occasionally transvenous embolization and surgical techniques to successfully eliminate the cortical venous drainage.[6]

Borden et al based their classification system on the venous anatomy and identified three categories.[29] Type I DAVFs drain directly into venous sinuses or pachymeningeal veins. Type II DAVFs drain into dural sinuses or pachymeningeal veins with retrograde drainage into subarachnoid veins. Type III DAVFs drain only into subarachnoid veins without any dural sinus or meningeal venous drainage. Borden type I DAVFs are mostly benign as well. Regardless of the classification system, the main factor indicating an aggressive clinical course appears to be the presence of leptomeningeal cortical venous drainage. Treatment of these lesions should be highly encouraged in asymptomatic patients and/or in patients with incidentally discovered lesions with leptomeningeal venous drainage.

Agents Used in Endovascular Treatment of AVFs

NBCA has been one of the main liquid embolic agents used for transarterial embolization of DAVFs with fairly good results.[30,31,32] Kim et al evaluated 121 DAVFs treated with transarterial glue embolization and reported angiographic cure in 29.8% of patients (immediate cure in 14% and progressive complete thrombosis of the residual shunt in 15.7%).[32] Surgical intervention or transvenous coil embolization was necessary for 45.2% of all cases. In a study that included 11 patients treated with transarterial injection of NBCA, 63.6% of patients were cured following the endovascular intervention.[32] Guedin et al reported a rate of complete closure of the AVF in 34 of 38 (89.5%) patients with Borden type II or III DAVFs and occlusion of cerebral venous drainage in all other patients who were treated with transarterial embolization using NBCA with no permanent morbidities or mortalities.[30]

The use of NBCA has some drawbacks. It is an adhesive agent that has a rapid rate of polymerization, which makes it somewhat difficult to use and may increase the risk of microcatheter retention or avulsion of the feeding artery upon removal of the microcatheter.[33] The injection must be performed fast and in a continuous fashion, which may decrease the precision of injection and result in suboptimal penetration into the target site. Both preparation and delivery of NBCA require an experienced user. Use of a wedged microcatheter technique with low-concentration glue may maximize glue penetration into the venous drainage route.[23]

Onyx offers several advantages over NBCA which allow for safer and more efficient treatment of DAVFs. Owing to its lava-like flow pattern and its nonadhesive nature, Onyx facilitates longer, slower, and more controlled injections with better penetration of the fistula.[23] Onyx can penetrate the depths of the AVF with high efficiency, which facilitates the embolization of a large portion of the lesion from a single pedicle injection decreasing the need for multiple embolization attempts.[23] In addition, Onyx injection can be discontinued for angiographic assessment of the embolization and evaluation of collaterals that may become evident during the course of embolization. Furthermore, Onyx is less adherent to the microcatheter than NBCA with possibly a lower risk of catheter retention and arterial rupture.[22] On the other hand, Onyx has some disadvantages in AVF management when compared to NBCA. An increase in fluoroscopy and procedure times and procedure costs has been reported with Onyx.[23,34] Cranial nerve injury, DMSO-induced angiotoxicity, and potential for distal embolization into the venous system and the pulmonary circulation are potential drawbacks as well.[23] Onyx comes in three different concentrations (6, 6.5, and 8%) with increasing viscosity. Although Onyx

comes in readymade vials containing EVOH, DMSO, and tantalum powder, it must be shaken for 20 minutes before injection to maximize its radiopacity.[35]

Various rates of successful treatment have been reported with the liquid embolic agent Onyx, with most results characterized by remarkably high cure rates with an important number of treatments being completed in one session.[28,36,37,38,39] Macdonald et al performed embolization of 52 DAVFs: transvenous embolization was successful in 11 of 15 patients, and transarterial embolization was successful in 27.3% in the non-Onyx group versus 72.7% in the Onyx group.[36] Abud et al reported their experience with transarterial Onyx embolization of 44 DAVFs and reported complete occlusion in all but nine patients, five of whom were successfully treated by transvenous embolization with coils and Onyx.[37] Furthermore, complete cure was achieved with a single procedure in 81% of patients. Stiefel et al reported angiographic cure in 72% of DAVFs (21/29 DAVFs) treated with Onyx embolization, mainly using a transarterial embolization with complications occurring in 9.7% with permanent morbidity in 2.4% of patients.[38] In a prospective study of 30 patients with DAVFs (10 grade II, 8 grade III, and 12 grade IV fistulas), Cognard et al reported that complete angiographic cure occurred in 24 of 30 patients (80%) with only two complications, including a temporary cranial nerve palsy and postprocedure hemorrhage.[28] Hu et al reported a complete angiographic cure rate of 79% in patients with DAVFs treated with transarterial embolization.[39] More specifically, when Onyx was used as the sole embolic agent, angiographic cure was observed in 87% of DAVFs.[39] Our published institutional results show that endovascular treatment was successful in achieving complete obliteration of the fistula in 28 of 39 patients (71%) after a mean number of 2.1 interventions, 21 patients by endovascular means alone, and 7 patients with combined endovascular and surgical approaches. The transarterial approach using Onyx embolization was the preferred treatment and most successful treatment (occlusion rate of 75%) with elimination of CVD in up to 85% of patients with Onyx embolization.[4] In general, cure rates between 63 and 100% have been reported with Onyx embolization of DAVFs.[22]

Onyx has also been used with transvenous access, especially in the management of carotid-cavernous fistulas (CCFs) with significant and rapid improvement in neuroophthalmologic symptoms (► Fig. 19.3). Elhammady et al performed transvenous embolization of eight CCFs and transarterial embolization of four CCFs and achieved complete obliteration of all lesions in a single session with resolution of symptoms in all patients by 2 months.[40] They observed three cranial nerve palsies.[40] Suzuki et al reported complete cure and resolution of symptoms in three cases with spontaneous CCFs treated with transvenous Onyx embolization.[41] Our institutional experience using Onyx embolization of CCFs through surgical cannulation of the superior ophthalmic vein showed complete obliteration in 8 out of 10 patients and a significant reduction in fistulous flow in the other 2 patients, which later progressed to near-complete occlusion on angiographic follow-up.[23] All patients experienced a complete clinical recovery and did not have any complications or recurrence. In another study by Zaidat et al, Onyx was successfully used in combination with coils or stents in five cases with complete occlusion.[42] Liquid embolic agents can be used alone or in combination with coils or balloons of the feeding

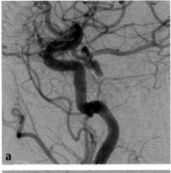

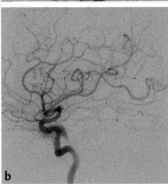

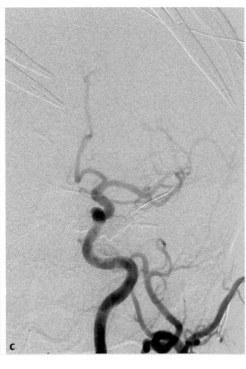

Fig. 19.3 (a) A 48-year-old female patient who presented with proptosis and chemosis. Right internal carotid artery catheterization showed a carotid-cavernous fistula (CCF) with small meningeal feeders. (b) Left internal carotid artery catheterization showed multiple meningeal feeders going into the cavernous sinus. (c) Surgical exposure for the left-sided superior ophthalmic vein was performed followed by catheterization of the superior ophthalmic vein and embolization with Onyx. Control angiography showed 100% occlusion of the CCF.

artery or venous outflow. Balloon-assisted and coil-assisted embolization can help in achieving a controlled delivery of the embolic agent into the fistula and can be useful in protecting the patency of arterial collaterals and critical venous pathways by limiting distal flow of the embolic agent.

19.4.2 Endovascular Management of AVMs

Endovascular therapy provides a minimally invasive approach for the management of AVMs with intraprocedural angiographic evaluation and the possibility of achieving immediate occlusion.

Presurgical Embolization of AVMs

Endovascular management can be used for presurgical embolization of large or giant cortical AVMs to reduce the blood flow within the nidus or to embolize deep, surgically inaccessible feeder arteries. Spetzler et al reported that complete excision was achieved in 18 of 20 patients who had presurgical embolization with no mortality and three nondisabling morbidities.[43] Viñuela et al studied 101 patients with cerebral AVMs and reported that patients who had presurgical embolization had an obliteration rate of 96% with low severe morbidity and mortality rates (1.98% each).[44] Weber et al performed preoperative embolization in 47 patients using Onyx and reported a mean nidus reduction of 84% after embolization.[45] Furthermore, 46 of 47 patients (98%) had complete obliteration of the AVM following surgery.[45] Jafar et al compared patients who had presurgical embolization to patients who received only surgical treatment and found that preoperative embolization of AVMs reduces operative time and intraoperative blood loss, makes surgical resection easier, and does not present with significantly more complications than surgery alone.[46] Pasqualin et al reported that patients treated with preoperative embolization had less postoperative neurological deficits, decreased intraoperative bleeding and fewer deaths, and had a lower incidence of postoperative epilepsy when compared with patients who underwent only surgical management.[47] Although surgical resection remains the standard for the definitive eradication of most brain AVMs, endovascular embolization has the potential to improve the safety and efficacy of the procedure.[48] In general, presurgical embolization decreases the nidus size of the AVM, occludes deep and surgically inaccessible arterial feeding vessels, occludes intranidal aneurysms and high-flow fistulas, decreases blood loss and length of the procedure, and facilitates surgical management.[2] Furthermore, preoperative embolization might be able to convert high Spetzler-Martin grade lesions to lower-grade lesions, thus turning potentially inoperable lesions into operable lesions.[48] Ideal targets are large Spetzler-Martin grade III or IV AVMs that can be embolized to microsurgically accessible targets.[43,46] Preoperative embolization has also been shown to be cost-effective when compared with surgery alone.[49]

Preradiosurgical Embolization of AVMs

Endovascular management can be used for embolization of AVMs before radiosurgical intervention to reduce the nidus size. Smaller lesions (< 3 cm in diameter) have a higher cure rate and a lower morbidity rate following radiosurgery.[48] Preradiosurgical embolization may also be used to occlude arterial feeders or intranidal aneurysms to reduce the risk of hemorrhage as well as target large high-flow AVMs which are less sensitive to radiosurgery.[2] Gobin et al performed endovascular embolization to reduce the size of the cerebral AVMs prior to radiosurgical treatment in 125 patients and reported that embolization resulted in complete occlusion in 11.2% of AVMs and reduced 76% of AVMs enough to allow radiosurgery.[50] Furthermore, after radiosurgery, 65% of the remaining AVMs were cured, increasing to 79% when the nidus was less than 2 cm in diameter.[50] However, the use of embolization prior to radiosurgery remains controversial due to contradictory results reported in the literature. In a review of 1,988 patients, embolization prior to radiosurgery was found to decrease the AVM obliteration rate (41% with previous embolization vs. 59% without previous embolization) but without increasing the rate of hemorrhage and permanent neurological deficits.[51] The risk-to-benefit ratio should be carefully assessed in each case. Embolization has also been shown to be safe and effective in treating residual lesions that persist after radiosurgery. Marks et al reported that a significant volume reduction (mean of 74%) was achieved in five of six patients who had endovascular treatment after radiosurgery.[52]

Palliative Embolization of AVMs

Endovascular treatment has been used for palliative embolization in patients with progressive or refractory neurological deficits secondary to high flow or venous hypertension and seizures, in patients with large AVMs and AVMs that may be difficult to manage surgically or with radiosurgery and to treat AVMs with high-risk features.[2,48] However, a study of 27 patients by Kwon et al that compared palliative embolization to medical treatment alone showed that embolization increases the rate of complications without a significant difference in the rate of clinical improvement.[53] Miyamoto et al observed in a study of 46 patients that palliative treatment of AVMs does not prevent bleeding and may even worsen the posttreatment course compared with the natural history of cerebral AVMs.[54] Partial AVM embolization is not recommended as a broad treatment strategy for AVMs[47]; however, it can be used as a temporary solution as a part of a treatment plan aimed at staged AVM obliteration as collaterals tend to develop rapidly.

Curative Embolization of AVMs

Even though endovascular embolization is usually performed as an adjuvant therapy for other interventions in the management of cerebral AVMs, curative embolization can be used as the primary treatment for some AVMs that are not candidates for other surgical or radiosurgical approaches. There are several factors that determine the efficacy of embolization for curative purposes. Smaller AVMs are more likely to be cured following embolization. Pierot et al found that AVMs less than 3 cm in maximal diameter were nearly five times more likely to be cured compared to AVMs ≥ 3 cm in diameter.[33] In addition, AVMs with a low number of arterial feeders are more likely to achieve complete cure following endovascular management. Superficial AVMs, AVMs in noneloquent locations, and those with an overall lower Spetzler-Martin grade are more likely to be cured as well.[55] Immediate angiographic cure rates have been reported to range from 5% to more than 94%.[55] Delayed recanalization seems to be a problem even for smaller AVMs.[2] To minimize recanalization, the operator should make sure that the embolic agent penetrates the AVM nidus rather than simply occlude its feeders.[56]

Complications and Safety of Endovascular Management of AVMs

Endovascular embolization of AVMs is not without its risks. Ischemic and hemorrhagic strokes resulting in transient or permanent neurological deficits are the main complications. Intracerebral hemorrhage can be the result of arterial dissection or perforation by the microwire or microcatheter, transition of a large amount of the embolic agent on the venous side of the AVM leading to immediate rupture, and rupture of an associated aneurysm and vascular injuries during retrieval of the catheter.[2,48] Ischemic stroke may result from arterial dissection related to microcatheter or guidewire manipulation, inadvertent occlusion of normal arterial branches by the embolic material, reflux of the embolic agent into normal cerebral vasculature, and showering of glue droplets during retrieval of the microcatheter.[2,35] Complications such as groin hematoma or dissection and other complications related to endovascular intervention such as contrast allergy, infection, and nephrotoxicity may occur as well.[35] Various rates of complications and morbidity have been reported with endovascular embolization of AVMs. This is mainly due to the different patient selection, agents used, and the reason for using embolization. Taylor et al reviewed 339 preoperative AVM embolization procedures performed in 201 patients using several embolic agents, including PVA particles (80.2%), NBCA (13.3%), detachable coils (9.3%), and Onyx (1.5%). Mortality was reported in 2% of patients, permanent neurological deficits in 9% of patients, temporary neurological deficits in 3.5% of patients, and vascular complications without neurological compromise in 9% of patients.[57] Haw et al performed 513 embolization procedures in 306 patients using NBCA for various reasons. They observed 62 overall hemorrhagic, ischemic, and technical complications with a permanent morbidity rate of 4.9% and a mortality rate of 2.6%.[58] Sahlein et al reported one of the lowest morbidity and mortality rates in the literature. They evaluated 130 patients with 131 brain AVMs treated with NBCA. The permanent morbidity and mortality rates were 0.8%.[59] This study also reported a higher rate of complete AVM cure (33%) as compared to other reports.[59] Starke et al studied 377 adjuvant embolization procedures with NBCA in 202 patients. New clinical deficits after embolization were observed in 14% of patients, with persistent neurologic deficits occurring in 2.5% of patients.[60] They performed an analysis of factors that may increase the risk of clinical deficits after endovascular intervention and reported that complex AVMs with treatment plan specifying more than one embolization procedure, AVMs with a diameter of less than 3 cm or more than 6 cm, and AVMs with a deep venous drainage and in eloquent location were more likely to result in new clinical deficits.[60] Pierot et al reported, in a prospective multicenter study of 117 patients using Onyx, an overall hemorrhagic complication rate of 8.5% with a morbidity rate of 5.1% and mortality rate of 4.3%.[33] Katsaridis et al reported, in a study of 101 patients who underwent a total of 219 embolization procedures using Onyx, a 5.9% rate of hemorrhagic complications and a 14.9% rate of neurologic deficits, 7.9% being permanent deficits and 7% being reversible deficits.[61] Mortality was observed in 3% of patients.[61] Panagiotopoulos et al retrospectively studied 82 patients with cerebral AVMs treated with Onyx: 119 embolization procedures were performed (1.45/patient). Permanent morbidity was

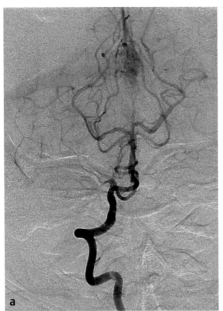
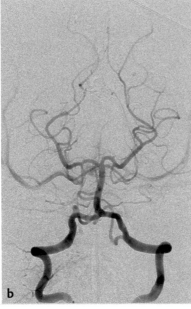

Fig. 19.4 (a) A 43-year-old female patient who presented with cerebellar hemorrhage. Left vertebral artery injection showed an arteriovenous malformation (AVM) of the superior cerebellar vermis fed by branches of the superior cerebellar artery primarily with venous outflow restriction in a superiorly draining vein emptying into the straight sinus. **(b)** Onyx embolization was performed. Complete obliteration of the AVM was achieved from a single treatment session.

reported in 3.8% of patients, whereas mortality was 2.4% (due to intracerebral hemorrhage). Furthermore, 12.2% of patients had nondisabling neurologic deficits, and 7.3% of patients had disabling neurologic deficits.[62]

Agents Used in Endovascular Treatment of AVMs

NBCA was approved by the U.S. Food and Drug Administration (FDA) in 2000 for the preoperative treatment of brain AVMs. Similarly, Onyx received FDA approval in 2005.

In AVMs embolized with NBCA, the rate of hemorrhagic complications has ranged from 0.9 to 13%, morbidity rate from 2 to 7.9%, and mortality rate from 0.5 to 7%.[11] Overall, the rate of hemorrhagic complications is between 4 and 12.2% with Onyx embolization, with most studies reporting rates between 6 and 9%.[11] The reported morbidity rates range from 3.5 to 15.5% and the mortality rates range from 0 to 3.2%. The rate of complete occlusion with Onyx embolization ranges from 8.3 to 53.9% with most recent studies reporting a rate around 50%, whereas the rate of complete occlusion with NBCA has been reported to be lower (between 5.6 and 33.3%).[11] Most of the comparisons between these two liquid embolic agents have been indirect. A trial by Loh et al that directly compared NBCA and Onyx in preoperative embolization concluded that the rate of adverse events was similar and the operative blood loss and resection time were comparable as well.[63] The efficacy of Onyx in achieving ≥ 50% reduction in AVM volume was nonsignificantly higher than NBCA (96 vs. 85.2%, respectively). However, Onyx is usually preferred for multiple reasons in cerebral AVM management: (1) Onyx has a nonadhesive nature which decreases the risk of adherence of the delivery catheter tip to the vessel wall and catheter retention within the AVM nidus; (2) it has less thrombogenicity and causes less inflammation than NBCA as no protein denaturation occurs; (3) Onyx allows for longer, slower, and more controlled injections with better penetration; and (4)

Onyx offers better handling during later surgical intervention (▶ Fig. 19.4).[11,63]

19.5 Conclusion

The therapeutic armamentarium to treat cerebrovascular malformations is continuously evolving which allows for highly individualized management strategies to be implemented based on the characteristics of each lesion. Management of AVMs and AVFs requires a multidisciplinary team with expertise in the different treatment strategies available. Endovascular management including transarterial and transvenous embolization, surgical treatment, and radiosurgery can be used alone or in combination as required for each individual case. Endovascular therapy has become a highly utilized tool in the management of cerebral AVMs and AVFs either alone as a curative intervention or as an adjunct to other interventions. Endovascular treatment of cerebrovascular malformations is safe and effective in the management of these complex lesions.

References

[1] Friedlander RM. Clinical practice. Arteriovenous malformations of the brain. N Engl J Med. 2007; 356(26):2704–2712

[2] Bruno CA , Jr, Meyers PM. Endovascular management of arteriovenous malformations of the brain. Interv Neurol. 2013; 1(3–4):109–123

[3] Gross BA, Du R. Diagnosis and treatment of vascular malformations of the brain. Curr Treat Options Neurol. 2014; 16(1):279

[4] Ghobrial GM, Marchan E, Nair AK, et al. Dural arteriovenous fistulas: a review of the literature and a presentation of a single institution's experience. World Neurosurg. 2013; 80(1–2):94–102

[5] Hoh BL, Putman CM, Budzik RF, Ogilvy CS. Surgical and endovascular flow disconnection of intracranial pial single-channel arteriovenous fistulae. Neurosurgery. 2001; 49(6):1351–1363, discussion 1363–1364

[6] Jabbour P, Tjoumakaris S, Chalouhi N, et al. Endovascular treatment of cerebral dural and pial arteriovenous fistulas. Neuroimaging Clin N Am. 2013; 23 (4):625–636

[7] Gross BA, Du R. Natural history of cerebral arteriovenous malformations: a meta-analysis. J Neurosurg. 2013; 118(2):437–443

[8] da Costa L, Wallace MC, Ter Brugge KG, O'Kelly C, Willinsky RA, Tymianski M. The natural history and predictive features of hemorrhage from brain arteriovenous malformations. Stroke. 2009; 40(1):100–105

[9] Hernesniemi JA, Dashti R, Juvela S, Väärt K, Niemelä M, Laakso A. Natural history of brain arteriovenous malformations: a long-term follow-up study of risk of hemorrhage in 238 patients. Neurosurgery. 2008; 63(5):823–829, discussion 829–831

[10] Gross BA, Du R. The natural history of cerebral dural arteriovenous fistulae. Neurosurgery. 2012; 71(3):594–602, discussion 602–603

[11] Gandhi D, Chen J, Pearl M, Huang J, Gemmete JJ, Kathuria S. Intracranial dural arteriovenous fistulas: classification, imaging findings, and treatment. AJNR Am J Neuroradiol. 2012; 33(6):1007–1013

[12] Halbach VV, Higashida RT, Hieshima GB, Mehringer CM, Hardin CW. Transvenous embolization of dural fistulas involving the transverse and sigmoid sinuses. AJNR Am J Neuroradiol. 1989; 10(2):385–392

[13] Halbach VV, Higashida RT, Hieshima GB, Hardin CW, Pribram H. Transvenous embolization of dural fistulas involving the cavernous sinus. AJNR Am J Neuroradiol. 1989; 10(2):377–383

[14] Kirsch M, Liebig T, Kühne D, Henkes H. Endovascular management of dural arteriovenous fistulas of the transverse and sigmoid sinus in 150 patients. Neuroradiology. 2009; 51(7):477–483

[15] Roy D, Raymond J. The role of transvenous embolization in the treatment of intracranial dural arteriovenous fistulas. Neurosurgery. 1997; 40(6):1133–1141, discussion 1141–1144

[16] Jabbour P, Tjoumakaris S, Chalouhi N, et al. Endovascular treatment of cerebral dural and pial arteriovenous fistulas. Neuroimaging Clin N Am. 2013; 23(4):625–636

[17] Yoshida K, Melake M, Oishi H, Yamamoto M, Arai H. Transvenous embolization of dural carotid cavernous fistulas: a series of 44 consecutive patients. AJNR Am J Neuroradiol. 2010; 31(4):651–655

[18] Klisch J, Huppertz HJ, Spetzger U, Hetzel A, Seeger W, Schumacher M. Transvenous treatment of carotid cavernous and dural arteriovenous fistulae: results for 31 patients and review of the literature. Neurosurgery. 2003; 53(4):836–856, discussion 856–857

[19] Urtasun F, Biondi A, Casaco A, et al. Cerebral dural arteriovenous fistulas: percutaneous transvenous embolization. Radiology. 1996; 199(1):209–217

[20] Friedman JA, Pollock BE, Nichols DA, Gorman DA, Foote RL, Stafford SL. Results of combined stereotactic radiosurgery and transarterial embolization for dural arteriovenous fistulas of the transverse and sigmoid sinuses. J Neurosurg. 2001; 94(6):886–891

[21] Goto K, Sidipratomo P, Ogata N, Inoue T, Matsuno H. Combining endovascular and neurosurgical treatments of high-risk dural arteriovenous fistulas in the lateral sinus and the confluence of the sinuses. J Neurosurg. 1999; 90(2):289–299

[22] Vanlandingham M, Fox B, Hoit D, Elijovich L, Arthur AS. Endovascular treatment of intracranial dural arteriovenous fistulas. Neurosurgery. 2014; 74 Suppl 1:S42–S49

[23] Chalouhi N, Dumont AS, Tjoumakaris S, et al. The superior ophthalmic vein approach for the treatment of carotid-cavernous fistulas: a novel technique using Onyx. Neurosurg Focus. 2012; 32(5):E13

[24] Davies MA, TerBrugge K, Willinsky R, Coyne T, Saleh J, Wallace MC. The validity of classification for the clinical presentation of intracranial dural arteriovenous fistulas. J Neurosurg. 1996; 85(5):830–837

[25] Djindjian R, Merland JJ, Theron J. Super-selective arteriography of the external carotid artery. New York, NY: Springer Verlag; 1977:606–628

[26] Cognard C, Casasco A, Toevi M, Houdart E, Chiras J, Merland JJ. Dural arteriovenous fistulas as a cause of intracranial hypertension due to impairment of cranial venous outflow. J Neurol Neurosurg Psychiatry. 1998; 65(3):308–316

[27] Cognard C, Gobin YP, Pierot L, et al. Cerebral dural arteriovenous fistulas: clinical and angiographic correlation with a revised classification of venous drainage. Radiology. 1995; 194(3):671–680

[28] Cognard C, Januel AC, Silva NA , Jr, Tall P. Endovascular treatment of intracranial dural arteriovenous fistulas with cortical venous drainage: new management using Onyx. AJNR Am J Neuroradiol. 2008; 29(2):235–241

[29] Borden JA, Wu JK, Shucart WA. A proposed classification for spinal and cranial dural arteriovenous fistulous malformations and implications for treatment. J Neurosurg. 1995; 82(2):166–179

[30] Guedin P, Gaillard S, Boulin A, et al. Therapeutic management of intracranial dural arteriovenous shunts with leptomeningeal venous drainage: report of 53 consecutive patients with emphasis on transarterial embolization with acrylic glue. J Neurosurg. 2010; 112(3):603–610

[31] Kim DJ, Willinsky RA, Krings T, Agid R, Terbrugge K. Intracranial dural arteriovenous shunts: transarterial glue embolization–experience in 115 consecutive patients. Radiology. 2011; 258(2):554–561

[32] Agid R, Terbrugge K, Rodesch G, Andersson T, Söderman M. Management strategies for anterior cranial fossa (ethmoidal) dural arteriovenous fistulas with an emphasis on endovascular treatment. J Neurosurg. 2009; 110(1):79–84

[33] Pierot L, Cognard C, Herbreteau D, et al. Endovascular treatment of brain arteriovenous malformations using a liquid embolic agent: results of a prospective, multicentre study (BRAVO). Eur Radiol. 2013; 23(10):2838–2845

[34] Velat GJ, Reavey-Cantwell JF, Sistrom C, et al. Comparison of N-butyl cyanoacrylate and onyx for the embolization of intracranial arteriovenous malformations: analysis of fluoroscopy and procedure times. Neurosurgery. 2008; 63(1) Suppl 1:ONS73–ONS78, discussion ONS78–ONS80

[35] Gailloud P. Endovascular treatment of cerebral arteriovenous malformations. Tech Vasc Interv Radiol. 2005; 8(3):118–128

[36] Macdonald JH, Millar JS, Barker CS. Endovascular treatment of cranial dural arteriovenous fistulae: a single-centre, 14-year experience and the impact of Onyx on local practise. Neuroradiology. 2010; 52(5):387–395

[37] Abud TG, Nguyen A, Saint-Maurice JP, et al. The use of Onyx in different types of intracranial dural arteriovenous fistula. AJNR Am J Neuroradiol. 2011; 32(11):2185–2191

[38] Stiefel MF, Albuquerque FC, Park MS, Dashti SR, McDougall CG. Endovascular treatment of intracranial dural arteriovenous fistulae using Onyx: a case series. Neurosurgery. 2009; 65(6) Suppl:132–139, discussion 139–140

[39] Hu YC, Newman CB, Dashti SR, Albuquerque FC, McDougall CG. Cranial dural arteriovenous fistula: transarterial Onyx embolization experience and technical nuances. J Neurointerv Surg. 2011; 3(1):5–13

[40] Elhammady MS, Wolfe SQ, Farhat H, Moftakhar R, Aziz-Sultan MA. Onyx embolization of carotid-cavernous fistulas. J Neurosurg. 2010; 112(3):589–594

[41] Suzuki S, Lee DW, Jahan R, Duckwiler GR, Viñuela F. Transvenous treatment of spontaneous dural carotid-cavernous fistulas using a combination of detachable coils and Onyx. AJNR Am J Neuroradiol. 2006; 27(6):1346–1349

[42] Zaidat OO, Lazzaro MA, Niu T, et al. Multimodal endovascular therapy of traumatic and spontaneous carotid cavernous fistula using coils, n-BCA, Onyx and stent graft. J Neurointerv Surg. 2011; 3(3):255–262

[43] Spetzler RF, Martin NA, Carter LP, Flom RA, Raudzens PA, Wilkinson E. Surgical management of large AVM's by staged embolization and operative excision. J Neurosurg. 1987; 67(1):17–28

[44] Viñuela F, Dion JE, Duckwiler G, et al. Combined endovascular embolization and surgery in the management of cerebral arteriovenous malformations: experience with 101 cases. J Neurosurg. 1991; 75(6):856–864

[45] Weber W, Kis B, Siekmann R, Jans P, Laumer R, Kühne D. Preoperative embolization of intracranial arteriovenous malformations with Onyx. Neurosurgery. 2007; 61(2):244–252, discussion 252–254

[46] Jafar JJ, Davis AJ, Berenstein A, Choi IS, Kupersmith MJ. The effect of embolization with N-butyl cyanoacrylate prior to surgical resection of cerebral arteriovenous malformations. J Neurosurg. 1993; 78(1):60–69

[47] Pasqualin A, Scienza R, Cioffi F, et al. Treatment of cerebral arteriovenous malformations with a combination of preoperative embolization and surgery. Neurosurgery. 1991; 29(3):358–368

[48] Ogilvy CS, Stieg PE, Awad I, et al. Stroke Council, American Stroke Association. Recommendations for the management of intracranial arteriovenous malformations: a statement for healthcare professionals from a special writing group of the Stroke Council, American Stroke Association. Circulation. 2001; 103(21):2644–2657

[49] Jordan JE, Marks MP, Lane B, Steinberg GK. Cost-effectiveness of endovascular therapy in the surgical management of cerebral arteriovenous malformations. AJNR Am J Neuroradiol. 1996; 17(2):247–254

[50] Gobin YP, Laurent A, Merienne L, et al. Treatment of brain arteriovenous malformations by embolization and radiosurgery. J Neurosurg. 1996; 85(1):19–28

[51] Xu F, Zhong J, Ray A, Manjila S, Bambakidis NC. Stereotactic radiosurgery with and without embolization for intracranial arteriovenous malformations: a systematic review and meta-analysis. Neurosurg Focus. 2014; 37(3):E16

[52] Marks MP, Lane B, Steinberg GK, et al. Endovascular treatment of cerebral arteriovenous malformations following radiosurgery. AJNR Am J Neuroradiol. 1993; 14(2):297–303, discussion 304–305

[53] Kwon OK, Han DH, Han MH, Chung YS. Palliatively treated cerebral arteriovenous malformations: follow-up results. J Clin Neurosci. 2000; 7 Suppl 1:69–72

[54] Miyamoto S, Hashimoto N, Nagata I, et al. Posttreatment sequelae of palliatively treated cerebral arteriovenous malformations. Neurosurgery. 2000; 46(3):589–594, discussion 594–595

[55] Potts MB, Zumofen DW, Raz E, Nelson PK, Riina HA. Curing arteriovenous malformations using embolization. Neurosurg Focus. 2014; 37(3):E19

[56] Viñuela F, Fox AJ, Pelz D, Debrun G. Angiographic follow-up of large cerebral AVMs incompletely embolized with isobutyl-2-cyanoacrylate. AJNR Am J Neuroradiol. 1986; 7(5):919–925

[57] Taylor CL, Dutton K, Rappard G, et al. Complications of preoperative embolization of cerebral arteriovenous malformations. J Neurosurg. 2004; 100(5):810–812

[58] Haw CS, terBrugge K, Willinsky R, Tomlinson G. Complications of embolization of arteriovenous malformations of the brain. J Neurosurg. 2006; 104(2):226–232

[59] Sahlein DH, Mora P, Becske T, Nelson PK. Nidal embolization of brain arteriovenous malformations: rates of cure, partial embolization, and clinical outcome. J Neurosurg. 2012; 117(1):65–77

[60] Starke RM, Komotar RJ, Otten ML, et al. Adjuvant embolization with N-butyl cyanoacrylate in the treatment of cerebral arteriovenous malformations: outcomes, complications, and predictors of neurologic deficits. Stroke. 2009; 40 (8):2783–2790

[61] Katsaridis V, Papagiannaki C, Aimar E. Curative embolization of cerebral arteriovenous malformations (AVMs) with Onyx in 101 patients. Neuroradiology. 2008; 50(7):589–597

[62] Panagiotopoulos V, Gizewski E, Asgari S, Regel J, Forsting M, Wanke I. Embolization of intracranial arteriovenous malformations with ethylene-vinyl alcohol copolymer (Onyx). AJNR Am J Neuroradiol. 2009; 30(1):99–106

[63] Loh Y, Duckwiler GR, Onyx Trial Investigators. A prospective, multicenter, randomized trial of the Onyx liquid embolic system and N-butyl cyanoacrylate embolization of cerebral arteriovenous malformations. Clinical article. J Neurosurg. 2010; 113(4):733–741

20 Endovascular Treatment of Arteriovenous Malformations of the Supratentorial Compartment

Stephan Munich and Demetrius K. Lopes

Abstract

Supratentorial arteriovenous malformations (AVMs) represent the majority of cerebral AVMs. However, they represent a heterogenous group of AVMs ranging from small, superficial lesions located in silent regions of the brain to deep, eloquently located lesions with complex angioarchitecture. Endovascular embolization has been increasingly utilized for the treatment of the full range of supratentorial AVMs. While traditionally endovascular techniques have been utilized preceding surgical resection or stereotactic radiosurgery, recently, they are more frequently being employed as a stand-alone treatment strategy. Angiographic cure is possible with endovascular techniques in many lesions and may avoid the complications associated with surgical resection and radiation. Curative endovascular embolization likely will become even more commonplace as the development of endovascular techniques continues to evolve.

Keywords: arteriovenous malformations, ARUBA, embolization, microsurgery, n-butyl cyanoacrylate, Onyx, stereotactic radiosurgery

- Endovascular embolization can be used effectively preceding surgical resection and stereotactic radiosurgery.
- Endovascular techniques can also serve as an effective stand-alone method to achieve angiographic cure of supratentorial arteriovenous malformations (AVMs).
- The development of new liquid embolic mediums and microcatheters has allowed for more controlled and effective endovascular embolization.
- With continued experience and development of endovascular technologies, the utilization of endovascular embolization to cure supratentorial AVMs is expected to expand.

20.1 Introduction

Arteriovenous malformations (AVMs) are abnormal connections of arterial and venous circulations, consisting of an intervening tangle of thin-walled vessels (nidus). They are rare vascular lesions, occurring in 15 to 18 per 100,000 adults in the general population with a detection rate of 1.21 per 100,000 person-years.[1,2,3] Hemorrhage is the most common presentation, with AVMs generally considered to carry an annual hemorrhage risk of 2 to 4%.[4] As with other intracranial lesions, the vast majority of AVMs occur in the supratentorial compartment. Therefore, consequent to their location, supratentorial AVMs may also present with seizure, headaches, or focal neurologic deficit. The ability to provide low-risk, effective, and durable treatment of these lesions is paramount. This is especially true following the recent publication of the Medical Management With or Without Interventional Therapy for Unruptured Brain Arteriovenous Malformations (ARUBA) trial, in which the necessity of treatment recently has been questioned.[5] In this chapter, we discuss the role of endovascular strategies in the contemporary management of supratentorial AVMs. We will also discuss technical aspects unique to endovascular techniques and their utilization for the treatment of supratentorial AVMs.

20.2 Preoperative Assessment and Workup

Following the initial clinical and radiographic evaluation, the most important first step in the management of the AVM is the determination of whether it should be treated. Generally accepted indications for treatment of AVMs include repeated, symptomatic hemorrhages, seizures (particularly when there is intolerance to anti-epileptic medications or those refractory to medical management), focal neurologic deficit, and patient preference.

The recent publication of a randomized trial of unruptured brain arteriovenous malformations (ARUBA) trial questioned the necessity of treatment of unruptured (and particularly, asymptomatic) AVMs. The authors found that their primary endpoint (i.e., the composite of death or symptomatic stroke) occurred in 10.1% of patients undergoing medical management and in 30.7% of those undergoing AVM treatment. While a detailed discussion of the multiple shortcomings of this study is beyond the scope of this chapter, perhaps its most obvious and influential limitation is the short length of follow-up (mean 33.3 months; SD 19.7 months).[6,7] With an annual hemorrhage risk of 2 to 4%, the potential threat of AVM rupture, therefore, is clearly affected by the patient's age and overall life expectancy, with young and healthy patients accumulating more risk over their lifetime (risk of hemorrhage = 1 − [annual risk of not bleeding] expected years of remaining life).[8] Therefore, despite the conclusions of the authors of the ARUBA study, the decision to not treat an AVM in a young and healthy patient should be undertaken with caution.

In addition to the aforementioned generalized hemorrhage risk, the application of various risk scores has been developed to aid in decision making. The Spetzler–Martin score is the most widely known and utilized.[9] Though it is frequently used to describe the radiographic appearance/location of AVMs, it was designed to characterize surgical difficulty and morbidity associated with surgical resection. Therefore, its application to lesions planned for endovascular or radiosurgical treatment must be done with caution and understanding that the continuum of associated morbidity described by this score may be skewed. On the light of this, we, as well as others, recently have proposed grading scales specific to the nuances of endovascular treatment (▶ Table 20.1).[10,11,12,13,14]

Table 20.1 Endovascular-specific arteriovenous malformation (AVM) grading scales

AVMES (Lopes et al[11])

AVM nidus size	1 (<3 cm)
	2 (3–6 cm)
	3 (>6 cm)
Number of arterial pedicles	1 (1–3)
	2 (4–6)
	3 (>6)
Number of draining veins	1 (1–3)
	2 (4–6)
	3 (>6)
Vascular eloquence	0 (noneloquent)
	1 (eloquent)

Buffalo score (Dumont et al[12])

Number of arterial pedicles	1 (1–2)
	2 (3–4)
	3 (>5)
Diameter of arterial pedicles	0 (most > 1 mm)
	1 (most ≤ 1 mm)
Nidus location	0 (noneloquent)
	1 (eloquent)

Bell et al[14]

Number of arterial pedicles	1 (<3)
	2 (3–5)
	3 (≥6)
Eloquence of adjacent areas	0 (noneloquent)
	1 (eloquent)
Presence of AVF component	0 (no AVF)
	1 (AVF)

Abbreviations: AVF, arteriovenous fistula; AVMES, arteriovenous malformation embocure score.

In our proposed AVM embocure score (AVMES), we found the number of arterial pedicles, the number of draining veins, the size of the AVM nidus, and the presence of "vascular eloquence" to be collectively relevant in the prediction of complete angiographic embolization and the expected risk of complication. The concept of vascular eloquence is unique to the AVMES. It is defined as arterial pedicle proximity to the internal carotid artery (ICA; an AVM was considered to possess vascular eloquence if its arterial pedicle was less than 20 mm from the ICA or first segment of cerebral arteries); it aims to describe a risk idiosyncratic to endovascular treatment strategies. Specifically, a proximal injury (e.g., reflux of Onyx occurring during embolization of an arterial pedicle arising from a short M1 parent vessel) would cause significant neurologic deficit, making these lesions significantly more risky to treat endovascularly.

In lesions with AVMES of 3, there was a 100% rate of angiographic obliteration and a 0% rate of major complication. Conversely, in lesions with AVMES of greater than 5, complete angiographic cure was obtained in only 20%, with major morbidity occurring in 30%. Application of this, as well as other "endovascular-specific" scores, is critical to the preoperative assessment and treatment planning of patients with AVMs. Though AVMES and other "endovascular-specific" scores assess the potential for success and morbidity associated with stand-alone endovascular therapy, they also serve as tools for the multidisciplinary assessment of these complex vascular lesions.

Endovascular therapy has become an integral part of the management of supratentorial AVMs. It offers a minimally invasive and effective treatment strategy. Though previously considered only in combination with surgical resection or stereotactic radiosurgery, increasingly it is being utilized as the sole treatment modality to obtain complete radiographic AVM obliteration.[15,16,17,18] In this chapter, we will discuss issues unique to the endovascular treatment of supratentorial AVMs, as well as the role of endovascular strategies both as a stand-alone and adjunctive modality. We will also discuss technical considerations encountered during endovascular treatment.

20.3 Intraoperative Considerations

20.3.1 Anesthesia

Endovascular embolization may be performed with the patient under general anesthesia or conscious sedation. Our preference is for general anesthesia since it eliminates any patient head movement, providing superior quality images without motion artifact. Procedural success does not rely on patient cooperation and this method may be particularly well suited for pediatric patients, patients with underlying cognitive and/or psychiatric disturbances, or others unable to remain still for the procedure, especially on prolonged embolization treatments (embocure cases). During the administration of general anesthesia, the neurologic exam is lost and recognition of intraoperative complication or intolerance of the procedure may be delayed. In order to address this concern, neurophysiologic monitoring such as electroencephalogram, motor-evoked potentials, and somatosensory-evoked potentials and in-depth knowledge of the vascular anatomy are of paramount importance when general anesthesia is utilized.

The primary benefit to AVM embolization under conscious sedation is preservation of the neurologic exam and possibility of performing provocative testing of the arterial pedicles. In this way, the patient can be examined serially throughout the procedure to ensure tolerance to the treatment. Microcatheterization and AVM embolization under conscious sedation require strict cooperation by the patient in order to permit high-quality imaging and avoidance of complications. Blood pressure control is particularly important in patients undergoing embolization under conscious sedation since anxiety and discomfort during various parts of the procedure may cause rises in blood pressure. Conscious sedation and provocative testing should be reserved for specific situations when an AVM arterial pedicle physiological testing is desired prior to embolization. Provocative testing has been shown to decrease treatment-related morbidity to less than 5%.[19] Its "real-time," intraoperative use is unique to endovascular treatment strategies and it can be utilized both in patients under general anesthesia with neuromonitoring and in patients under conscious sedation, but it is more ideal in those being treated under conscious sedation. Tawk et al described their experience with provocative testing in patients undergoing treatment of occipital lobe AVMs under conscious sedation.[20] Once the microcatheter was in its desired position within the arterial pedicle, a baseline neurologic exam was obtained. Amobarbital 75 mg was injected and the patient's neurologic exam was compared to the findings on baseline examination. If no new neurologic deficits developed, then the selected feeder was embolized. Although the authors describe their experience with the treatment of only AVMs of the occipital lobe, this technique is easily applicable to the treatment of AVMs in other locations.

Alternatively, Feliciano et al use propofol for their provocative testing under conscious sedation (off-label).[21] The authors performed neurologic examinations before and after the injection of propofol 7 mg through a microcatheter positioned in a given arterial pedicle. While the authors did not experience any adverse events related to this technique, it should be noted that cardiopulmonary dysfunction may occur.

When performing provocative testing on the patient being treated under general anesthesia, interpretation of the neurophysiologic monitoring is used instead of the neurologic exam. Coordination between the neurophysiologist, anesthesiologist and the treating physician is essential to safe and accurate interpretation of the provocative testing. The use of these tests allows the physician to assess the safety of embolization in a "pedicle by pedicle" fashion, assuring the safety of each injection of liquid embolic. However, this provocative testing should not be a substitute to understanding the vascular anatomy and AVM angioarchitecture.

20.3.2 Hemodynamic Monitoring

Hemodynamic monitoring is particularly important during the endovascular treatment of AVMs. Routinely, we maintain systolic blood pressure between 90 and 120 mm Hg during and for 24 hours after the procedure. Though anecdotal, we believe this to allow a more controlled embolization, perhaps decreasing the risk of unintentional, premature venous occlusion by the travel of liquid embolic through the AVM nidus to the draining vein(s).

Strict control of blood pressure is also essential to avoidance of normal perfusion pressure breakthrough and resultant hemorrhage. Maintenance of low to normal blood pressure for at least 24 hours postprocedure permits recovery of the autoregulatory capacity of the cerebral vasculature and minimizes the risk of hemorrhage.

20.3.3 Choice of Embolic Agent

Onyx

Though first described in the 1990s, Onyx (ev3 Inc, Plymouth, MN) was approved by the Food and Drug Association (FDA) for the treatment of AVMs in 2005.[22,23] It is an ethylene vinyl alcohol copolymer and, contrary to previous liquid embolic agents, is cohesive but not adhesive. This results in less adherence to microcatheters and vessel walls and, therefore, was intended to reduce the risk of complications associated with microcatheter removal. Because of its cohesive nature, rather than adhesive nature, a certain degree of reflux is permissible when using Onyx without necessarily compromising the removal of the microcatheter. A detailed description of Onyx was previously published by Ayad et al; a brief overview follows here.[24]

Onyx occlusion of a vessel lumen is initiated after the diffusion of dimethyl sulfoxide (DMSO) into the blood from the outer surface of the Onyx cast.[25] The precipitation of Onyx occurs from "outside-in"—it has been compared to the hardening of lava from a volcano.[24] Solidification occurs over several minutes to hours, permitting better anterograde penetration compared to n-butyl cyanoacrylate (n-BCA). Once solidified, Onyx feels rubbery, rather than hard and brittle, like n-BCA. This may make an Onyx-embolized AVM easier to dissect, thereby making resection more amenable.[26]

Onyx formulations used for AVM embolization are 18 and 34, which represent different viscosities. The different viscosities allow variable penetration of the nidus before polymerization occurs. While Onyx itself causes very little intravascular or perivascular inflammatory reactions, DMSO is capable of causing vasospasm and endothelial necrosis. For this reason, DMSO must be injected slowly.

Onyx and more recently Squid and Phil are liquid embolics of similar properties (e.g., nonadhesive) but different viscosities. This category of liquid embolic is our preferred method for embolization of supratentorial AVMs. They allow a better penetration of the nidus over a prolonged injection time compared to acrylates such as n-BCA.

n-Butyl Cyanoacrylate

n-BCA is a free-flowing liquid embolic that polymerizes via an anionic mechanism (i.e., upon contact with blood). n-BCA requires mixing with ethiodized oil by the treating physician to achieve the desired polymerization time. Higher concentrations of n-BCA result in a faster polymerization rate. Though it may be tedious in routine AVM treatment, the ability to control polymerization rate may serve useful when treating complex AVMs, particularly those with fistulous components.[13] According to in vitro testing described in the product information brochure, n-BCA polymerization times may range from immediately upon contact with plasma (0:1 ethiodized oil:n-BCA ratio) to 16 seconds (5:1 ethiodized oil:n-BCA ratio).

n-BCA is adhesive in nature. While this allows reliable vessel occlusion, it also adheres to the microcatheter. Therefore, reflux is ill tolerated when using n-BCA and proficiency with this technique is critical to safe and effective treatment. However, when utilized by experienced endovascular surgeons, the utilization of n-BCA has not been shown to be associated with any increase in morbidity or mortality.[27]

20.3.4 Choice of Microcatheter

Safe and effective endovascular embolization of supratentorial AVMs requires that the physician place the microcatheter at the pedicle serving only the AVM. Placement of the microcatheter too proximal in the intracranial circulation may result in unintended embolization of proximal, uninvolved vasculature resulting in ischemic neurologic consequences and not occluding the nidus of the AVM. Therefore, navigation through the cervical and cranial vasculature is essential to endovascular embolization.

The first advance in the development of microcatheters came in the form of flow-directed microcatheters (e.g., Magic, Balt, Montmorency, France). The basis for these catheters is the high-flow nature of AVMs compared to the surrounding, normal circulation. Because of this difference in flow, the soft, floppy tip of these microcatheters is preferentially directed into fistulous arterial pedicles.

Marathon and UltraFlow (ev3 Inc) were developed subsequently as over-the-wire microcatheters allowing for some steering of the microcatheter using 0.008- and 0.010-inch microguidewires. More recently, detachable tip microcatheters like Sonic (Balt, Montmorency, France) and Apollo (ev3 Inc) have also proven effective in the endovascular embolization of AVMs (▶ Fig. 20.1).[28,29,30] These detachable tip microcatheters allow for an atraumatic microcatheter removal as long as the liquid embolic agent does not reflux beyond (i.e., proximal to) the detachable tip marker. These newer generation microcatheters have been used with both Onyx and n-BCA.[28,29]

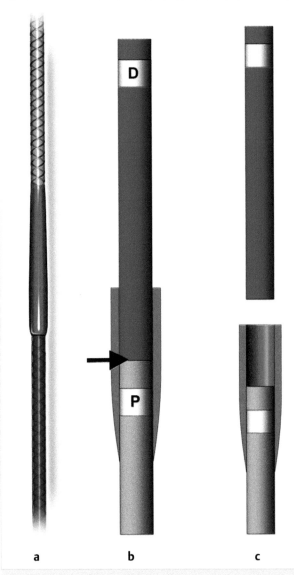

Fig. 20.1 Apollo detachable tip microcatheter—inner diameter 0.013 inch (**a**). The proximal (P) and distal (D) markers are seen (**b**). The separation point (*arrow*) occurs 1.25 mm distal to the proximal marker. The presence of the detachable tip (**c**) reduces the risk of catheter entrapment. (These images are provided courtesy of Medtronic Neurovascular, Irvine CA, USA.)

20.4 Stand-Alone Endovascular Embolization

The concept of curative endovascular embolization of cerebral AVMs is relatively new and remains controversial. Rates of endovascular cures had been reported to be 5 to 10%.[31,32,33,34] Many cite lack of very long-term follow-up and anecdotal experience(s) of recanalization as the basis for skepticism of the durability of stand-alone endovascular embolization. However, with the advent of new liquid embolics, increasing experience, and continued development of endovascular technology, AVMs may more frequently be recommended for curative embolization (▶ Fig. 20.2).

Yu et al described their experience using cyanoacrylate for AVM embolization with curative intent in 10 carefully selected patients.[35] Selection criteria included the following: AVM nidus no larger than 3 cm, no more than three arterial feeders, and relatively easy accessibility of the AVM nidus with the microcatheter. The authors experienced no procedure-related complications and achieved complete nidus occlusion in six patients. After a mean follow-up of 23 months (range 17–32 months), all AVMs remained occluded angiographically.

Similarly, Saatci et al described their use of Onyx for AVM embolization.[36] In their series of 350 patients, 178 experienced angiographic obliteration of the AVM by Onyx embolization alone. After a mean follow-up of 42 months (range: 12–96 months), all but two AVMs (99%) remained occluded. It should be noted that the majority of these patients (155 [87%]) had small AVMs (Spetzler–Martin grade I or II).

Continued experience with endovascular techniques/technology and the development of Onyx have led to a greater pursuit of curative endovascular embolization. Van Rooij et al reported their technique with curative embolization of supratentorial AVMs.[37] Twenty-four patients in whom curative embolization was considered had small- and medium-sized (mean size: 2.2 cm; range: 1–3 cm), superficially located AVMs, arterial feeders accessible with microcatheters and that allowed for Onyx reflux of 2 to 3 cm, a well-delineated nidus, and easily visible draining veins. Complete angiographic obliteration was achieved in a single treatment session in all patients. Angiography performed at 3 months demonstrated complete occlusion in all but 1 (96%) of the surviving patients.

Though detailed assessments of specific supratentorial locations are beyond the scope of this chapter, special attention should be given to so-called "deep AVMs" because these may be particularly well suited for stand-alone endovascular therapy given that surgical resection may be associated with significant morbidity. Mendes et al recently reported their experience with the endovascular management of deep AVMs.[38] They observed complete obliteration of these deep AVMs in 82% of the cases, with procedure-related complications occurring in 14%.

Not all supratentorial AVMs may be good candidates for curative endovascular embolization. In the aforementioned studies, lesions were carefully selected for intended endovascular cure. Common selection criteria among these studies include small AVMs with favorable angioarchitecture. Saatci found only 12.5% of Spetzler–Martin grade III–V lesions were able to be cured with endovascular embolization alone.[36] This sentiment was recently confirmed by Möhlenbruch et al who reported

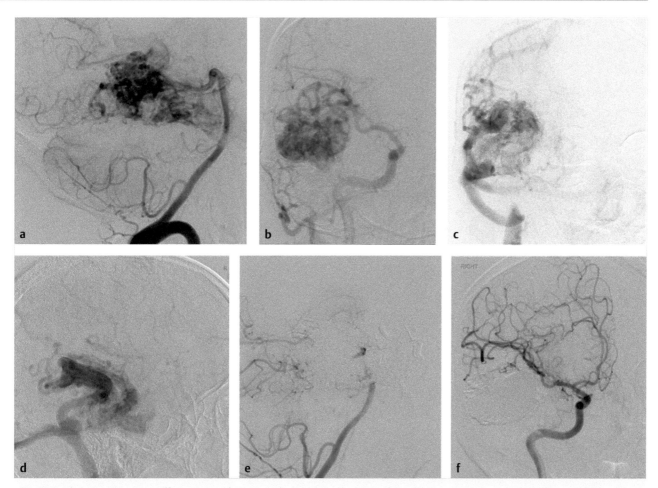

Fig. 20.2 A large arteriovenous malformation can be seen on the lateral vertebral artery (**a**) and anteroposterior common carotid artery (**b**) injections. The venous drainage is complex with multiple, tortuous draining veins (**c,d**). Complete occlusion was achieved using only endovascular embolization with Onyx (**e,f**).

complete occlusion of 100% ($n = 24$) of small- and medium-sized supratentorial AVMs (mean size: 2.2 cm; range: 1–3 cm) in one Onyx embolization session.[39] Jordan et al echoed this finding, reporting AVM diameter smaller than 3 cm to be a predictive factor for total occlusion, with an odds ratio of 50.9.[40] Larger AVMs may be limited in their ability to be cured with endovascular therapy alone due to finite penetration of the liquid embolic. As arterial feeders are occluded, they eliminate potential corridors to nidal penetration by embolic material. In this way, large AVMs may retain areas of active AVM nidus and have no endovascular corridor for microcatheterization or flow of liquid embolic.

Van Rooij et al also stress the importance of visualization of the proximal venous circulation emanating from the nidus; in this way, venous filling with Onyx can be easily recognized.[37] As previously mentioned, through the development of the authors' AVMES, we found the number of arterial pedicles, the number of draining veins, the size of the AVM nidus, and the presence of "vascular eloquence" to collectively affect the ability of the treating physician to achieve complete endovascular obliteration. Similar to the studies summarized here, we found a larger number of arterial pedicles and draining veins, a large AVM nidus, and proximal arterial feeders to make AVMs more difficult to cure with endovascular embolization alone.[11]

Patients with neurologic symptoms attributable to mass effect from surrounding edema may be less suitable for intended cure with endovascular treatment alone. The long-term effects of a retained mass of embolic material on these symptoms, cognition, and epilepsy remain unknown. Additionally, radiographic artifact from embolic material can limit interpretation of subsequent imaging and make patients with other intracranial lesions requiring serial follow-up imaging less suitable candidates for this approach.

As with any treatment technique, curative endovascular embolization has its flaws. However, recent experiences suggest that it is a safe and effective strategy for properly selected AVMs. The implementation of endovascular-specific assessment scales/scores, such as the AVMES,[11] may help clinicians identify those lesions suitable for stand-alone endovascular treatment. With growing endovascular experience and the continued development of endovascular technologies, the indications for curative endovascular embolization are expected to expand.

20.4.1 Transvenous Techniques

Traditionally, transarterial embolization is the preferred method of accessing supratentorial AVMs. However, in cases of difficult transarterial access, transvenous embolization may

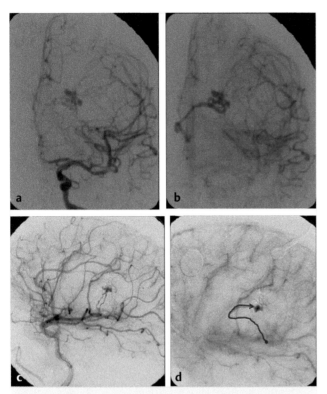

Fig. 20.3 AP view of digital subtraction angiography (a) showing a small, deep arteriovenous malformation with multiple small arterial feeders. This afferent angioarchitecture is prohibitive to complete embolization via transarterial techniques. The venous phase (b) demonstrates uncomplicated venous drainage with a single draining vein. Transarterial (c) and transvenous (d) approaches were used to achieve complete embolization.

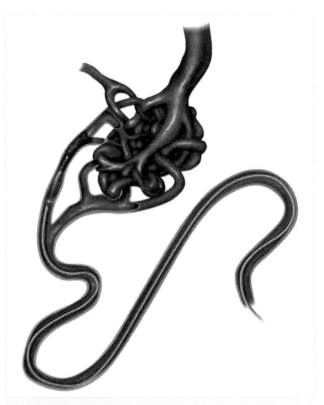

Fig. 20.4 Balloon-assisted embolization. The balloon catheter is docked in the desired position. The balloon is inflated and liquid embolic is injected. Inflation of the balloon helps prevent undesired reflux. (These images are provided courtesy of Microvention, Tustin, CA, USA.)

provide an effective alternative. The presence of small (often many) tortuous arterial feeders is particularly unfavorable for transarterial access.[41] The presence of a uncomplicated venous drainage (e.g., a single draining vein, few draining veins with simple transvenous access) is necessary for transvenous embolization. Transvenous techniques can be used alone, in cases with difficult arterial access, or in conjunction with transarterial techniques (▶ Fig. 20.3).

We typically achieve transvenous access through the femoral vein. A guide catheter is placed in the internal jugular. Given the tortuous venous anatomy, we prefer to use an intermediate catheter (distal access catheter [DAC], Concentric Medical, Mountain View, CA). Arterial access is often still required when transvenous embolization is pursued. A balloon can be inflated across the small arterial feeders to prevent embolization of the liquid embolic through the nidus and into the arterial circulation.

20.4.2 Balloon-Assisted Techniques

Balloon-assisted embolization relies on the use of a dual-lumen balloon (e.g., Scepter, Microvention, Tustin, CA; Ascent, Codman Neurovascular, Raynham, MA) that is compatible with the embolic to be used (▶ Fig. 20.4). Dual-lumen balloons consist of a central lumen through which liquid embolic is injected and a side lumen through which the balloon is inflated. The balloon catheter is navigated to its desired location in the arterial

pedicle where it is inflated by injecting contrast through the side lumen. The balloon is most stable in a curved segment. Selective injection can be performed through the central lumen to confirm the proper pedicle is selected and catheter location. Injection of liquid embolic then proceeds through the central lumen.

Constant and critical evaluation of the balloon is necessary in order to recognize any deflation or proximal migration. Balloon-assisted embolization may aid in preventing reflux into parent arteries. Additionally, the ability to arrest anterograde flow with balloon inflation within the arterial feeder may allow more controlled embolization. In this way, injection of liquid embolic is controlled more by the endovascular surgeon than by the patient's blood flow. Recent reports have demonstrated this technique to be safe and effective.[42,43,44,45]

20.4.3 Dual-Catheter Techniques

Traditional techniques for treating AVMs with multiple arterial feeders include staged embolization, in which liquid embolic is injected pedicle by pedicle. When multiple pedicles are present, there is significant arterial inflow that may result in difficulty in controlling the progression of liquid embolic during treatment, thereby causing premature venous occlusion. Recently, dual-catheter techniques have been described in which embolization proceeds simultaneously from multiple pedicles (▶ Fig. 20.5).[46,47]

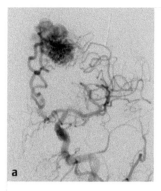
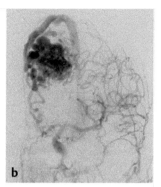
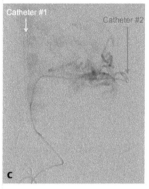
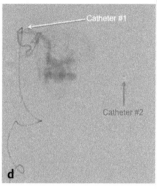
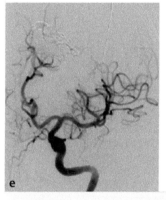
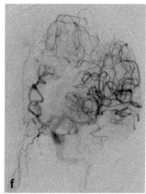

Fig. 20.5 Mid-arterial phase AP view of digital subtraction angiography (a) showing arteriovenous malformation (AVM) with afferent blood supply from both the anterior cerebral artery (ACA) and middle cerebral artery (MCA). Venous drainage is uncomplicated (b). The AVM was embolized using a dual-catheter technique, with one catheter in the ACA limb and a second catheter in the MCA limb. Selective injections through each microcatheter (c,d) demonstrate nidus targets for embolization. Follow-up angiogram (e,f) demonstrates complete occlusion of the AVM.

Typically, bilateral femoral artery access is achieved. A microcatheter is taken through each coaxial system and placed into the nidus via separate arterial pedicles. Simultaneous injection of liquid embolic is performed. By simultaneously blocking two afferent arterial limbs, the nidus may more selectively fill and the risk of premature venous occlusion may be decreased. Furthermore, since a greater portion of nidus is addressed, the number of required procedures to achieve complete occlusion may be decreased.

Recent reports have found this technique particularly useful in small AVMs with multiple arterial pedicles. In one small series, treatment of multifeeder AVMs with a dual-catheter

technique resulted in fewer hemorrhagic complications and lower procedure-related morbidity compared to single catheter techniques. Wider application and additional study of this technique is needed.

20.4.4 Pressure Cooker Technique

The pressure cooker technique was recently described by Chapot et al and is intended to create a plug to prevent liquid embolic reflux (▶ Fig. 20.6).[48] A detachable tip microcatheter is placed at the desired location within the AVM nidus. A second microcatheter is navigated alongside the first, with its tip positioned between the tip of the first catheter and the detachment zone marker. A plug is created by advancing coils and/or acrylic glue (e.g., *n*-BCA) through the second microcatheter.

Creation of the plug may serve several purposes. First, it prevents retrograde reflux into parent arteries. This may allow more proximal injection of embolic material and, therefore, more complete embolization. Secondly, by halting anterograde flow through the selected pedicle, it may allow for more controlled embolization of AVMs with fistulous components. Finally, by decreasing afferent flow to the AVM, the liquid embolic becomes more in the control of the endovascular surgeon and the risk of premature venous occlusion may be decreased.

20.5 Endovascular Embolization and Surgical Resection

Endovascular embolization entered the arena of AVM treatment as an adjunctive therapy whose primary function was to reduce the size of active AVM and augment the safety of surgical resection.[49,50] Occlusion of critical arterial feeders, particularly those that may be hidden by the AVM or other critical structures during operative resection, may improve morbidity of the surgical procedure.[51] Utilization of preoperative embolization to make large and/or inoperable AVMs amenable to surgical resection may be the most significant clinical impact of this multimodality strategy.

Perhaps one of the best examples of this benefit of preoperative endovascular embolization is one of the earliest. One year after publication of the renowned Spetzler–Martin scale, Spetzler et al described their experience of staged preoperative embolization of and grade V AVMs previously considered inoperable.[50] There was no mortality and only one disabling morbidity (5%). This represents an improvement in the same authors' outcomes of surgical resection of grade V AVMs in which they experienced a 12% rate of major morbidity.[9]

Nagashima et al compared surgical resection of cerebral AVMs before and since the dawn of the "embolization era," defined at the authors' institution as after 1992.[52] They observed surgery-related complications in 15% of patients treated in the pre-embolization era, while the complication rate was 3% in the embolization era. Similarly, unexpected residual AVM nidus occurred in 12% treated in the pre-embolization era, while this occurred in only 3% in the embolization era.

While Onyx embolization has become the liquid embolic medium of choice over the last decade, the choice of liquid embolic may not be critical to the benefits of preoperative embolization. Wong et al compared their experience using

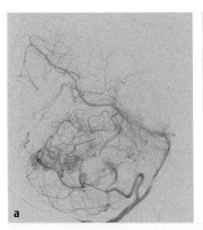 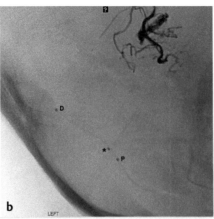 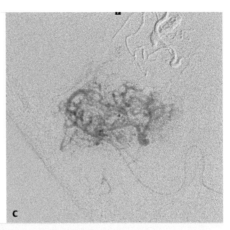

Fig. 20.6 Mid-arterial phase lateral view (**a**) of posterior fossa arteriovenous malformation (AVM; previous embolization performed at an outside facility is seen in the superior portion of the AVM). The lateral fluoroscopic image (**b**) demonstrates the position of the two microcatheters used in application of the pressure-cooker technique. The proximal (P) and distal (D) markers of the detachable tip microcatheter are seen. A second microcatheter is positioned within the detachable tip zone (marker indicated by *). From this catheter, an *n*-butyl cyanoacrylate plug was created. Onyx was then injected into the AVM through the first microcatheter (microinjection, **c**).

n-BCA for preoperative endovascular treatment to patients undergoing surgical resection without preoperative embolization.[53] They observed a statistically significant benefit of intraoperative blood loss and a trend toward shorter operative time in patients with Spetzler–Martin grade III and IV AVMs. No differences were observed in patients with Spetzler–Martin grade I or II lesions. Jafar et al reported no difference in intraoperative blood loss, operative time, or surgical complications in patients undergoing preoperative *n*-BCA embolization compared to those undergoing surgery without embolization.[54] However, they noted AVMs to be larger (3.9 vs. 2.3 cm) and have a higher Spetzler–Martin grade (3.2 vs. 2.5) in the group undergoing embolization. This led the authors to conclude "preoperative *n*-BCA embolization…makes lesions of larger size and higher grade the surgical equivalent of lesions of smaller size and lower grade."

Weber et al reported their experience in preoperative Onyx embolization of 47 AVMs (46 of which were supratentorially located). This strategy resulted in a mean nidus reduction of 84%. Preoperative Onyx embolization followed by surgical resection resulted in angiographic cure in 100% of patients with available follow-up (mean 13 months) with a 17% rate of disabling neurologic deficit. Similarly, Rodríguez-Boto et al described their initial experience in treating 13 complex supratentorial AVMs (Spetzler–Martin grade III–V) with preoperative Onyx embolization.[55] They report 100% cure in all patients with a 15.4% rate of disabling complications, both occurring after the surgical resection stage of treatment. These reports suggest that preoperative AVM embolization with Onyx provides a basis for safe microsurgical resection.

However, it is important to note that preoperative embolization carries the risks of both treatment modalities, namely those associated with endovascular embolization and surgical resection. Taylor et al examined the morbidity observed in 130 patients undergoing 324 endovascular embolization procedures prior to surgical resection.[56] Mortality was 1.2%, while permanent neurologic deficit occurred with 6.5% of procedures and temporary neurologic deficit was observed after 7% of procedures. These results demonstrate the safety associated with the endovascular component of a preoperative embolization treatment strategy. Additional analysis in this study revealed a trend toward poor outcome with increasing patient age and a trend away from poor outcome with more recent treatment date. These trends emphasize the learning curve associated with endovascular (and multimodality) AVM treatment.

The timing of surgical resection after preoperative embolization is an important consideration when utilizing this multimodal treatment strategy. On the one hand, allowing for recovery after the embolization may permit adjustment and normalization of the perinidal vasculature. However, on the other hand, incomplete embolization may subject the patient to a higher risk of hemorrhage, especially if there has been any compromise of the venous outflow. Kinouchi et al report early hemorrhage (3–13 days after embolization) occurring in 3 (8.1%) of the 37 patients that they treated with preoperative embolization, leading them to conclude that surgery should be undertaken as soon as possible following embolization.[57]

It should be noted that preoperative embolization is no substitute for surgical skill. Whereas many studies suggest that preoperative endovascular embolization may make high-grade lesions more amenable to resection without morbidity, the good outcomes observed in these studies may also be a function of the microsurgical skill(s) of the authors.[49,50,51,54] Even with preoperative embolization, Hartmann et al found increasing AVM size, deep venous drainage, and eloquent location to be predictors of treatment complication.[58] Therefore, even after preoperative embolization, delicate AVMs still require the attention and respect of the surgeon during resection.

20.6 Endovascular Embolization and Stereotactic Radiosurgery

The strategy of endovascular embolization prior to stereotactic radiosurgery serves a similar purpose as preoperative embolization, namely, it aims to change an AVM unsuitable for stereotactic radiosurgery alone to one that is amenable to radiosurgery. Specifically, by performing partial embolization of a large nidus, the residual AVM needing treatment is of a smaller size and more suitable for radiation treatment. Given that both endovascular embolization and stereotactic radiosurgery may be performed without general anesthesia, this strategy may be particularly well suited for patients with significant medical comorbidities, in whom the risks of general anesthesia and craniotomy may be intolerable.

Huo et al recently reported their large series of 162 patients undergoing Gamma knife radiosurgery following partial endovascular AVM embolization.[59] Preradiosurgical embolization resulted in a decrease in the median nidus volume from 14.3 to 9.01 cm^3. Embolization-related complications occurred in 14.8%. The mean duration between embolization and radiosurgery was 151 days. The overall AVM obliteration was reported as a worrisome 56.8%. However, further analysis revealed the rate of obliteration to be highly dependent on the amount of residual nidus after embolization (i.e., the amount of active AVM needing radiosurgical treatment). For residual AVM volume of less than 3 cm^3, the obliteration rate was 94.12%; for volumes of 3 to 10 cm^3, the obliteration rate was 61.29%; for volumes of greater than 10 cm^3, the obliteration rate was 33.33%. Indeed, multivariate analysis confirmed a decrease in AVM nidal volume to be the only factor independently associated with AVM obliteration. Using this treatment strategy, the authors observed a rate of only 3.1% of permanent clinical deterioration.

Similar results were observed by Kano et al in their case-control comparison of patients who underwent endovascular embolization prior to Gamma knife stereotactic radiosurgery compared to those who did not.[60] The authors found no statistically significant difference in the AVM obliteration between the two groups. However, similar to the report by Huo et al, they found the radiation AVM target volume (i.e., the amount of residual AVM after embolization) to have a statistically significant effect on the rate of obliteration—the obliteration rate at 5 years when target volume was greater than 8 cm^3 was 34%, whereas it was 67% when the target volume was less than 8 cm^3.

Concern regarding the utilization of this treatment strategy for the management of large AVMs previously was addressed by Blackburn et al when they reported their experience in treating 21 patients with large (nidus > 3 cm; mean: 4.2 cm) AVMs.[61] They found complete AVM obliteration in 81%. Endovascular complications resulted in minor permanent neurologic deficits in 14% and no major permanent deficits. Radiation-related complications occurred in 5% resulting in minor permanent neurologic deficits.

These reports highlight the importance of entering into the radiosurgery phase of this multimodal treatment strategy with a reasonable target volume of residual AVM. Thus, when radiosurgery is planned after endovascular embolization, reduction in nidus size must be pursued to its greatest extent. Failure to do so serves only to subject the patient to the risks of endovascular embolization, without providing the benefit.

There have been no studies specifically designed to assess the effects of different embolic material on the rate of AVM obliteration following post-embolization radiosurgery. However, though not statistically significant, Huo et al observed a lower obliteration rate in patients treated at least once with Onyx compared to those in whom Onyx was not used for embolization (53.1 vs. 62.5%, respectively).

Stereotactic radiosurgery is traditionally performed after endovascular embolization. Given the radiographic properties and potential distortion of various embolic materials, radiation dose planning is particularly important. Shtraus et al demonstrated that the difference between the attenuation of water and Onyx was 3%.[62] The authors caution that, without dose corrections accounting for this difference, high doses of radiation required for the treatment of AVMs may be delivered inaccurately. This difference in attenuation may be particularly important when the target volume is in eloquent areas.

Image distortion caused by embolic material also may be evident on the dose planning CT and/or MRI. One potential solution to planning image distortion created by embolic material, and our practice, is to perform cerebral angiography with the Gamma knife head frame on immediately prior to the treatment session. In this way, digital subtraction angiography images are utilized for treatment planning.

The treatment strategy of endovascular embolization followed by stereotactic radiosurgery utilizes two minimally invasive techniques and may be particularly fitting in deep or eloquently located AVMs. By decreasing the size of active AVM nidus, endovascular embolization may make large lesions that would otherwise be refractory to radiation treatment suitable for radiation. Critical to the success of this treatment strategy is sufficient nidus embolization (i.e., nidal volume reduction) such that the target lesion for radiation is satisfactorily small.

20.7 Conclusion

Given the novelty of endovascular techniques, long-term outcomes for endovascularly treated AVMs are just recently becoming available. If complete embolization cannot be achieved, additional therapy (i.e., surgical resection or radiation therapy) is obligatory, given that it has been demonstrated that partial embolization may be associated with post-treatment hemorrhage.

Endovascular embolization traditionally has been utilized as an adjunctive method with surgical resection (for surgically amenable lesions) or stereotactic radiosurgery (for deep, eloquent lesions). However, with increasing experience with endovascular techniques and the development of new microcatheters and liquid embolic mediums, it is more commonly being used as a stand-alone treatment with curative intent.

References

[1] Stapf C, Mohr JP, Pile-Spellman J, Solomon RA, Sacco RL, Connolly ES , Jr. Epidemiology and natural history of arteriovenous malformations. Neurosurg Focus. 2001; 11(5):e1

[2] Berman MF, Sciacca RR, Pile-Spellman J, et al. The epidemiology of brain arteriovenous malformations. Neurosurgery. 2000; 47(2):389–396, discussion 397

[3] van Beijnum J, van der Worp HB, Buis DR, et al. Treatment of brain arteriovenous malformations: a systematic review and meta-analysis. JAMA. 2011; 306(18):2011–2019

[4] Ondra SL, Troupp H, George ED, Schwab K. The natural history of symptomatic arteriovenous malformations of the brain: a 24-year follow-up assessment. J Neurosurg. 1990; 73(3):387–391

[5] Mohr JP, Parides MK, Stapf C, et al. international ARUBA investigators. Medical management with or without interventional therapy for unruptured brain

arteriovenous malformations (ARUBA): a multicentre, non-blinded, randomised trial. Lancet. 2014; 383(9917):614–621

[6] Russin J, Cohen-Gadol AA. Editorial: What did we learn from the ARUBA trial? Neurosurg Focus. 2014; 37(3):E9

[7] Russin J, Spetzler R. Commentary: the ARUBA trial. Neurosurgery. 2014; 75 (1):E96–E97

[8] Kondziolka D, McLaughlin MR, Kestle JR. Simple risk predictions for arteriovenous malformation hemorrhage. Neurosurgery. 1995; 37(5):851–855

[9] Spetzler RF, Martin NA. A proposed grading system for arteriovenous malformations. J Neurosurg. 1986; 65(4):476–483

[10] Munich SA, Lopes DK. Arteriovenous malformation embocure score (AVMES): reply. J Neurointerv Surg. 2015(Sep):3

[11] Lopes DK, Moftakhar R, Straus D, Munich SA, Chaus F, Kaszuba MC. Arteriovenous malformation embocure score: AVMES. J Neurointerv Surg. 2016; 8 (7):685–691

[12] Dumont TM, Kan P, Snyder KV, Hopkins LN, Siddiqui AH, Levy EI. A proposed grading system for endovascular treatment of cerebral arteriovenous malformations: Buffalo score. Surg Neurol Int. 2015; 6:3

[13] Bell DL, Leslie-Mazwi TM, Hirsch JA. Arteriovenous malformation embocure score (AVMES): response. J Neurointerv Surg. 2015(Sep):11

[14] Bell DL, Leslie-Mazwi TM, Yoo AJ, et al. Application of a Novel Brain Arteriovenous Malformation Endovascular Grading Scale for Transarterial Embolization. AJNR Am J Neuroradiol. 2015; 36(7):1303–1309

[15] Andreou A, Ioannidis I, Lalloo S, Nickolaos N, Byrne JV. Endovascular treatment of intracranial microarteriovenous malformations. J Neurosurg. 2008; 109(6):1091–1097

[16] Katsaridis V, Papagiannaki C, Aimar E. Curative embolization of cerebral arteriovenous malformations (AVMs) with Onyx in 101 patients. Neuroradiology. 2008; 50(7):589–597

[17] Panagiotopoulos V, Gizewski E, Asgari S, Regel J, Forsting M, Wanke I. Embolization of intracranial arteriovenous malformations with ethylene-vinyl alcohol copolymer (Onyx). AJNR Am J Neuroradiol. 2009; 30(1):99–106

[18] Reig AS, Rajaram R, Simon S, Mericle RA. Complete angiographic obliteration of intracranial AVMs with endovascular embolization: incomplete embolic nidal opacification is associated with AVM recurrence. J Neurointerv Surg. 2010; 2(3):202–207

[19] Sadato A, Taki W, Nakahara I, et al. Improved provocative test for the embolization of arteriovenous malformations–technical note. Neurol Med Chir (Tokyo). 1994; 34(3):187–190

[20] Tawk RG, Tummala RP, Memon MZ, Siddiqui AH, Hopkins LN, Levy EI. Utility of pharmacologic provocative neurological testing before embolization of occipital lobe arteriovenous malformations. World Neurosurg. 2011; 76(3–4): 276–281

[21] Feliciano CE, de León-Berra R, Hernández-Gaitán MS, Torres HM, Creagh O, Rodríguez-, Mercado R. Provocative test with propofol: experience in patients with cerebral arteriovenous malformations who underwent neuroendovascular procedures. AJNR Am J Neuroradiol. 2010; 31(3):470–475

[22] Terada T, Nakamura Y, Nakai K, et al. Embolization of arteriovenous malformations with peripheral aneurysms using ethylene vinyl alcohol copolymer. Report of three cases. J Neurosurg. 1991; 75(4):655–660

[23] Yamashita K, Taki W, Iwata H, et al. Characteristics of ethylene vinyl alcohol copolymer (EVAL) mixtures. AJNR Am J Neuroradiol. 1994; 15(6):1103–1105

[24] Ayad M, Eskioglu E, Mericle RA. Onyx: a unique neuroembolic agent. Expert Rev Med Devices. 2006; 3(6):705–715

[25] Szajner M, Roman T, Markowicz J, Szczerbo-Trojanowska M. Onyx(®) in endovascular treatment of cerebral arteriovenous malformations - a review. Pol J Radiol. 2013; 78(3):35–41

[26] Duffner F, Ritz R, Bornemann A, Freudenstein D, Wiendl H, Siekmann R. Combined therapy of cerebral arteriovenous malformations: histological differences between a non-adhesive liquid embolic agent and n-butyl 2-cyanoacrylate (NBCA). Clin Neuropathol. 2002; 21(1):13–17

[27] Crowley RW, Ducruet AF, Kalani MY, Kim LJ, Albuquerque FC, McDougall CG. Neurological morbidity and mortality associated with the endovascular treatment of cerebral arteriovenous malformations before and during the Onyx era. J Neurosurg. 2015; 122(6):1492–1497

[28] Altschul D, Paramasivam S, Ortega-Gutierrez S, Fifi JT, Berenstein A. Safety and efficacy using a detachable tip microcatheter in the embolization of pediatric arteriovenous malformations. Childs Nerv Syst. 2014; 30(6):1099–1107

[29] Paramasivam S, Altschul D, Ortega-Gutiarrez S, Fifi J, Berenstein A. N-butyl cyanoacrylate embolization using a detachable tip microcatheter: initial experience. J Neurointerv Surg. 2015; 7(6):458–461

[30] Maimon S, Strauss I, Frolov V, Margalit N, Ram Z. Brain arteriovenous malformation treatment using a combination of Onyx and a new detachable tip microcatheter, SONIC: short-term results. AJNR Am J Neuroradiol. 2010; 31(5): 947–954

[31] Deruty R, Pelissou-Guyotat I, Mottolese C, Bascoulergue Y, Amat D. The combined management of cerebral arteriovenous malformations. Experience with 100 cases and review of the literature. Acta Neurochir (Wien). 1993; 123(3–4):101–112

[32] Fournier D, TerBrugge KG, Willinsky R, Lasjaunias P, Montanera W. Endovascular treatment of intracerebral arteriovenous malformations: experience in 49 cases. J Neurosurg. 1991; 75(2):228–233

[33] Hurst RW, Berenstein A, Kupersmith MJ, Madrid M, Flamm ES. Deep central arteriovenous malformations of the brain: the role of endovascular treatment. J Neurosurg. 1995; 82(2):190–195

[34] Wilms G, Goffin J, Plets C, et al. Embolization of arteriovenous malformations of the brain: preliminary experience. J Belge Radiol. 1993; 76(5): 299–303

[35] Yu SC, Chan MS, Lam JM, Tam PH, Poon WS. Complete obliteration of intracranial arteriovenous malformation with endovascular cyanoacrylate embolization: initial success and rate of permanent cure. AJNR Am J Neuroradiol. 2004; 25(7):1139–1143

[36] Saatci I, Geyik S, Yavuz K, Cekirge HS. Endovascular treatment of brain arteriovenous malformations with prolonged intranidal Onyx injection technique: long-term results in 350 consecutive patients with completed endovascular treatment course. J Neurosurg. 2011; 115(1):78–88

[37] van Rooij WJ, Jacobs S, Sluzewski M, van der Pol B, Beute GN, Sprengers ME. Curative embolization of brain arteriovenous malformations with onyx: patient selection, embolization technique, and results. AJNR Am J Neuroradiol. 2012; 33(7):1299–1304

[38] Mendes GA, Silveira EP, Caire F, et al. Endovascular management of deep arteriovenous malformations: single institution experience in 22 consecutive patients. Neurosurgery. 2016; 78(1):34–41

[39] Möhlenbruch M, Bendszus M, Rohde S. Comment on: curative embolization of brain arteriovenous malformations with onyx: patient selection, embolization technique, and results. Clin Neuroradiol. 2012; 22(2):181–182

[40] Jordan JA, Llibre JC, Vazquez F, Rodríguez RM. Predictors of total obliteration in endovascular treatment of cerebral arteriovenous malformations. Neuroradiol J. 2014; 27(1):108–114

[41] Kessler I, Riva R, Ruggiero M, Manisor M, Al-Khawaldeh M, Mounayer C. Successful transvenous embolization of brain arteriovenous malformations using Onyx in five consecutive patients. Neurosurgery. 2011; 69(1):184–193, discussion 193

[42] Jagadeesan BD, Grigoryan M, Hassan AE, Grande AW, Tummala RP. Endovascular balloon-assisted embolization of intracranial and cervical arteriovenous malformations using dual-lumen coaxial balloon microcatheters and Onyx: initial experience. Neurosurgery. 2013; 73(2) Suppl Operative:ons238–ons243, discussion ons243

[43] Paramasivam S, Niimi Y, Fifi J, Berenstein A. Onyx embolization using dual-lumen balloon catheter: initial experience and technical note. J Neuroradiol. 2013; 40(4):294–302

[44] Spiotta AM, James RF, Lowe SR, et al. Balloon-augmented Onyx embolization of cerebral arteriovenous malformations using a dual-lumen balloon: a multicenter experience. J Neurointerv Surg. 2015; 7(10):721–727

[45] Spiotta AM, Miranpuri AS, Vargas J, et al. Balloon augmented Onyx embolization utilizing a dual lumen balloon catheter: utility in the treatment of a variety of head and neck lesions. J Neurointerv Surg. 2014; 6(7):547–555

[46] Abud DG, Riva R, Nakiri GS, Padovani F, Khawaldeh M, Mounayer C. Treatment of brain arteriovenous malformations by double arterial catheterization with simultaneous injection of Onyx: retrospective series of 17 patients. AJNR Am J Neuroradiol. 2011; 32(1):152–158

[47] Renieri L, Consoli A, Scarpini G, Grazzini G, Nappini S, Mangiafico S. Double arterial catheterization technique for embolization of brain arteriovenous malformations with onyx. Neurosurgery. 2013; 72(1):92–98, discussion 98

[48] Chapot R, Stracke P, Velasco A, et al. The pressure cooker technique for the treatment of brain AVMs. J Neuroradiol. 2014; 41(1):87–91

[49] Natarajan SK, Ghodke B, Britz GW, Born DE, Sekhar LN. Multimodality treatment of brain arteriovenous malformations with microsurgery after embolization with onyx: single-center experience and technical nuances. Neurosurgery. 2008; 62(6):1213–1225, discussion 1225–1226

[50] Spetzler RF, Martin NA, Carter LP, Flom RA, Raudzens PA, Wilkinson E. Surgical management of large AVM's by staged embolization and operative excision. J Neurosurg. 1987; 67(1):17–28

[51] Weber W, Kis B, Siekmann R, Jans P, Laumer R, Kühne D. Preoperative embolization of intracranial arteriovenous malformations with Onyx. Neurosurgery. 2007; 61(2):244–252, discussion 252–254

[52] Nagashima H, Hongo K, Kobayashi S, et al. Embolization of Arteriovenous Malformation. Efficacy and Safety of Preoperative Embolization Followed by Surgical Resection of AVM. Interv Neuroradiol. 2004; 10 Suppl 2:54–58

[53] Wong SH, Tan J, Yeo TT, Ong PL, Hui F. Surgical excision of intracranial arteriovenous malformations after preoperative embolisation with N-butylcyanoacrylate. Ann Acad Med Singapore. 1997; 26(4):475–480

[54] Jafar JJ, Davis AJ, Berenstein A, Choi IS, Kupersmith MJ. The effect of embolization with N-butyl cyanoacrylate prior to surgical resection of cerebral arteriovenous malformations. J Neurosurg. 1993; 78(1):60–69

[55] Rodríguez-Boto G, Gutiérrez-González R, Gil A, Serna C, López-Ibor L. Combined staged therapy of complex arteriovenous malformations: initial experience. Acta Neurol Scand. 2013; 127(4):260–267

[56] Taylor CL, Dutton K, Rappard G, et al. Complications of preoperative embolization of cerebral arteriovenous malformations. J Neurosurg. 2004; 100(5):810–812

[57] Kinouchi H, Mizoi K, Takahashi A, Ezura M, Yoshimoto T. Combined embolization and microsurgery for cerebral arteriovenous malformation. Neurol Med Chir (Tokyo). 2002; 42(9):372–378, discussion 379

[58] Hartmann A, Mast H, Mohr JP, et al. Determinants of staged endovascular and surgical treatment outcome of brain arteriovenous malformations. Stroke. 2005; 36(11):2431–2435

[59] Huo X, Jiang Y, Lv X, Yang H, Zhao Y, Li Y. Gamma Knife surgical treatment for partially embolized cerebral arteriovenous malformations. J Neurosurg. 2016; 124(3):767–776

[60] Kano H, Kondziolka D, Flickinger JC, et al. Stereotactic radiosurgery for arteriovenous malformations after embolization: a case-control study. J Neurosurg. 2012; 117(2):265–275

[61] Blackburn SL, Ashley WW , Jr, Rich KM, et al. Combined endovascular embolization and stereotactic radiosurgery in the treatment of large arteriovenous malformations. J Neurosurg. 2011; 114(6):1758–1767

[62] Shtraus N, Schifter D, Corn BW, et al. Radiosurgical treatment planning of AVM following embolization with Onyx: possible dosage error in treatment planning can be averted. J Neurooncol. 2010; 98(2):271–276

21 Endovascular Treatment of Arteriovenous Malformations of the Infratentorial Compartment

Celene B. Mulholland, M. Yashar S. Kalani, and Felipe C. Albuquerque

Abstract

Endovascular treatment of arteriovenous malformations of the infratentorial compartment is generally part of a multifaceted approach, given the rarity and the complexity of these lesions, which often present with hemorrhage. Although not often the definitive treatment, cerebral angiography is essential for characterizing the lesion and guiding further treatment.

Keywords: embolization, endovascular therapy, hemorrhage, infratentorial, microsurgical resection, posterior fossa, stereotactic radiosurgery

Keypoints

- Infratentorial arteriovenous malformations (AVMs) account for 7 to 15% of arteriovenous malformations.
- Patients with infratentorial AVMs are more likely to present with hemorrhage than patients with supratentorial AVMs.
- Endovascular management may be key to surgical resection.

21.1 Introduction

Infratentorial arteriovenous malformations (AVMs) account for only 7 to 15% of cerebral AVMs. However, their risk of rupture is substantially higher than that of supratentorial AVMs, and 80% of symptomatic patients with infratentorial AVMs present with hemorrhage.[1,2] Thus, the rate of hemorrhage is twice that of supratentorial AVMs.[3]

Management of patients with ruptured and unruptured AVMs of the infratentorial compartment requires a multidisciplinary approach. Endovascular embolization is generally used in addition to either microsurgical resection or stereotactic radiosurgery.

This chapter examines the role of endovascular management in the treatment of infratentorial AVMs. In it, we review endovascular treatment for both ruptured and unruptured AVMs.

21.2 Materials and Methods

A MEDLINE-based search of the neurosurgical literature was performed to identify all articles published between January 1980 and July 2016 that included the keywords "posterior fossa arteriovenous malformation," "infratentorial," and "endovascular." Retrieved articles were then reviewed to abstract the most up-to-date approaches to, and outcomes for, endovascular treatment of infratentorial AVMs.

Furthermore, we also drew upon our long-time institutional experience in treating numerous patients with infratentorial AVMs. Thus, the preoperative and postoperative angiograms and the intraoperative video that we have included reflect how AVMs are evaluated and treated within the clinical setting.

21.3 Results

A multitude of articles were identified and reviewed to extract relevant information about endovascular treatment. Articles that examined the role of endovascular treatment of posterior fossa AVMs were reviewed in depth. Articles that provided background epidemiologic data were also reviewed.

21.4 Discussion

Although posterior fossa AVMs compose only a small percentage of all AVMs, the propensity of patients with them to present with hemorrhage and neurologic decline highlights the importance of understanding the stages of their treatment. Endovascular embolization is generally considered an adjuvant to either microsurgical resection or stereotactic radiosurgery in the treatment of AVMs of the infratentorial compartment.[4] Digital subtraction angiography is the gold standard for characterizing these lesions, and it is of utmost importance preoperatively.

Infratentorial AVMs are classified according to the Spetzler-Martin grading scale, which takes into consideration the size of the AVM, its eloquent location, and its venous drainage (▶ Fig. 21.1). Additionally, it is important to identify their location in the cerebellar hemisphere, tonsils, pontocerebellar region, vermis, or brainstem. The location and grade of an AVM will often dictate the most appropriate treatment modality. For example, some authors report that they do not treat brainstem AVMs with microsurgery and instead either observe or treat them with radiosurgery with or without prior embolization.[5]

Treatment options for unruptured posterior fossa AVMs include observation, stereotactic radiosurgery, microsurgical resection, and endovascular embolization.[6] Location and grade influence the choice of treatment.[1,7]

In regard to ruptured AVMs of the infratentorial compartment, the treatment and timing of endovascular intervention depend on the location of the AVM, the status of the patient, and the other modalities that will be used in the management of the AVM. Given the high rates of hemorrhage of AVMs, it is not uncommon for patients to require emergent posterior fossa decompression or emergent evacuation of a cerebellar hematoma.[2] In this acute period, endovascular intervention may consist of embolization of a ruptured aneurysm.[2] A conventional angiogram should be obtained for all patients.

▶ Fig. 21.2 illustrates a cerebellar Spetzler-Martin grade II AVM in a patient who presented with cognitive changes but no evidence of hemorrhage. The patient underwent embolization of the AVM without complication. During embolization, two feeders off the superior cerebellar artery were embolized and one feeder off the anterior inferior cerebellar artery was embolized. Postoperative angiograms showed the Onyx cast and the resulting reduction in the size of the lesion (▶ Fig. 21.3). ▶ Fig. 21.4 and ▶ Fig. 21.5 illustrate a patient who presented with a cerebellar hemorrhage but did not require posterior

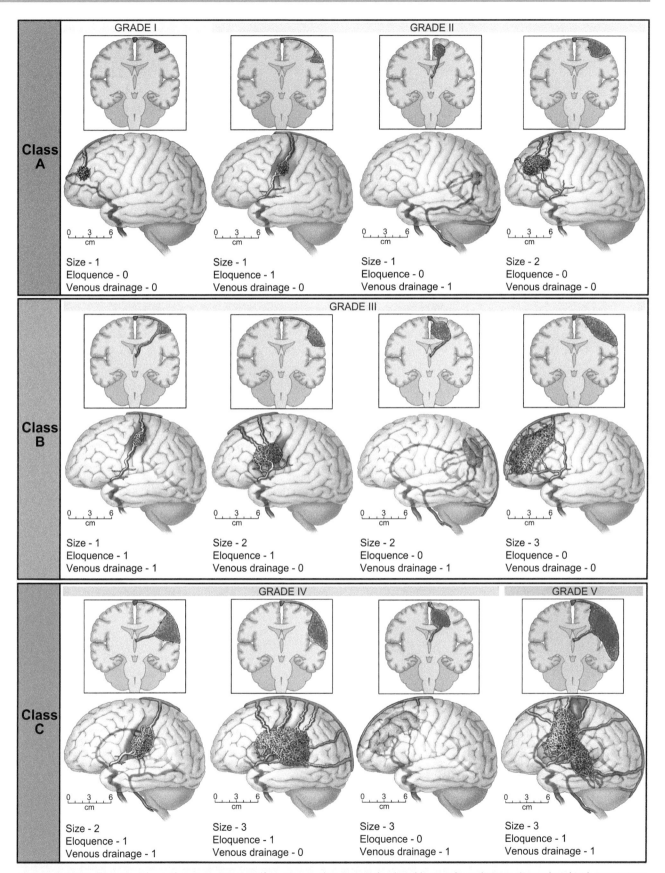

Fig. 21.1 Artist's illustration shows the arteriovenous malformation grading system developed by Spetzler and Martin. (Reproduced with permission from Spetzler RF, Ponce FA. A 3-tier classification of cerebral arteriovenous malformations. J Neurosurg 2011;114(March):842–849.)

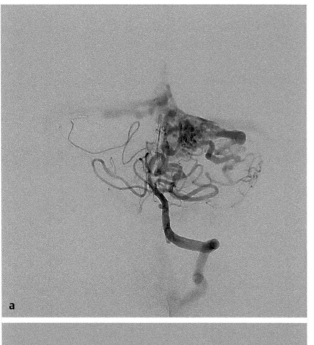

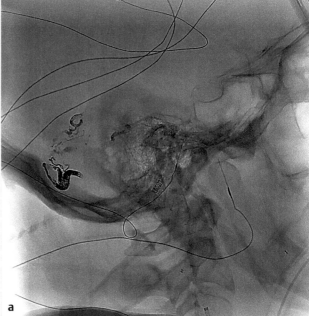

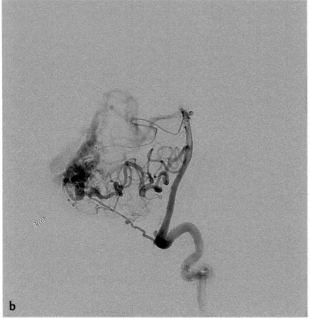

Fig. 21.2 Preoperative **(a)** anteroposterior and **(b)** lateral angiograms show a posterior fossa arteriovenous malformation that was deemed grade II on the Spetzler-Martin scale. (Used with permission from Barrow Neurological Institute, Phoenix, Arizona.)

Fig. 21.3 Postoperative **(a)** lateral angiogram demonstrating Onyx cast and **(b)** lateral angiogram demonstrating lesion size in the patient in ▶ Fig. 21.2 who had a Spetzler-Martin grade II arteriovenous malformation that was treated with embolization. (Used with permission from Barrow Neurological Institute, Phoenix, Arizona.)

fossa decompression. Angiography demonstrated a left cerebellopontine AVM in this patient, for whom embolization achieved angiographic cure. The AVM was embolized through the superior division of the left superior cerebellar artery and the left anterior and inferior cerebellar arteries.

For both ruptured and unruptured AVMs, the goal of endovascular embolization is to decrease the size of the lesion before microsurgical resection or stereotactic radiosurgery.[4,8] ▶ Video 21.1 shows how preoperative embolization to decrease the size of the lesion can prove to be successful. During treatment, superselective angiography to evaluate the nidus and any en passage vessels is of utmost importance. In a 2016 study by Lai et al,[8] 20 of 54 patients with posterior fossa AVMs were treated with embolization before undergoing radiosurgery or microsurgical resection. The mean devascularization rate was 46.9% in the 20 patients. Complications reported in various studies include intraprocedural or postprocedural hemorrhages and infarctions that are related to direct nidus injury or migration of embolic material and occlusion of draining veins.[1,4,7]

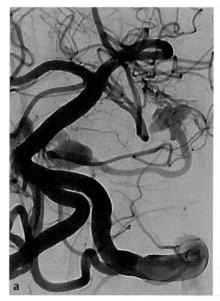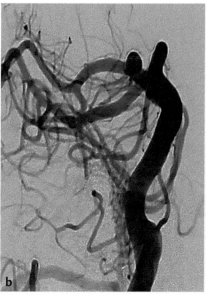

Fig. 21.4 (a) Anteroposterior and **(b)** lateral angiograms show a cerebellopontine arteriovenous fistula. (Used with permission from Barrow Neurological Institute, Phoenix, Arizona.)

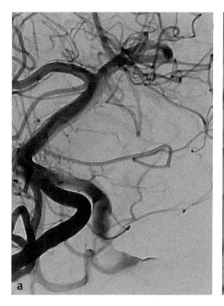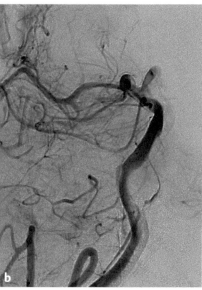

Fig. 21.5 Postoperative **(a)** anteroposterior and **(b)** lateral angiograms of the same patient in ▶ Fig. 21.4 show angiographic cure of the cerebellopontine arteriovenous malformation. (Used with permission from Barrow Neurological Institute, Phoenix, Arizona.)

As mentioned earlier, endovascular intervention is often used as part of a multimodality treatment approach to posterior fossa AVMs. However, in a 2016 study, Robert et al[1] examined endovascular embolization as a single-modality treatment. They treated 69 posterior fossa AVMs with endovascular management as the first-line therapy. Of those 69 patients, 9 patients subsequently underwent microsurgical resection and 6 underwent radiosurgery. Robert et al[1] reported an overall AVM obliteration rate of 72.5% ($n = 50$), whereas 5.8% ($n = 4$) underwent further treatment and 11.6% ($n = 8$) were incompletely treated.

Although it is well understood that posterior fossa AVMs have a higher risk of hemorrhage than their supratentorial counterparts, it is not well known if there are other characteristics, aside from the presence of an associated aneurysm, that increase the risk of hemorrhage. No studies have examined the long-term outcomes of patients with endovascular emboliza-

tion alone or of embolization of associated aneurysms alone. Unfortunately, a randomized control trial at this juncture is unlikely; thus, retrospective studies of larger databases may better elucidate the outcomes for this group of patients (▶ Video 21.1).

21.5 Conclusion

AVMs of the infratentorial compartment are rare lesions with a propensity to hemorrhage, resulting in possibly devastating neurologic complications. Endovascular embolization should be used as part of a multimodality treatment of posterior fossa AVMs that includes microsurgical resection or stereotactic radiosurgery. Endovascular embolization can also be used emergently to treat associated aneurysms when microsurgical clipping is not an option.

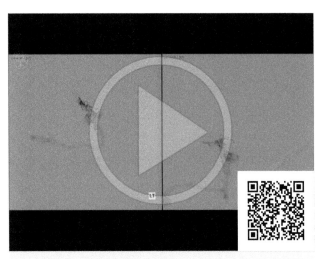

Video 21.1 Demonstration of complete occlusion of posterior fossa arteriovenous malformation. (Used with permission from Barrow Neurological Institute, Phoenix, Arizona.) https://www.thieme.de/de/q.htm?p=opn/tp/293510101/9781626237308_c021_v001&t=video

References

[1] Robert T, Blanc R, Ciccio G, et al. Endovascular treatment of posterior fossa arteriovenous malformations. J Clin Neurosci. 2016; 25:65–68

[2] Torné R, Rodríguez-Hernández A, Arikan F, et al. Posterior fossa arteriovenous malformations: Significance of higher incidence of bleeding and hydrocephalus. Clin Neurol Neurosurg. 2015; 134:37–43

[3] Khaw AV, Mohr JP, Sciacca RR, et al. Association of infratentorial brain arteriovenous malformations with hemorrhage at initial presentation. Stroke. 2004; 35(3):660–663

[4] Almeida JP, Medina R, Tamargo RJ. Management of posterior fossa arteriovenous malformations. Surg Neurol Int. 2015; 6:31

[5] Magro E, Chainey J, Chaalala C, Al Jehani H, Fournier JY, Bojanowski MW. Management of ruptured posterior fossa arteriovenous malformations. Clin Neurol Neurosurg. 2015; 128:78–83

[6] Arnaout OM, Gross BA, Eddleman CS, Bendok BR, Getch CC, Batjer HH. Posterior fossa arteriovenous malformations. Neurosurg Focus. 2009; 26(5):E12

[7] Kelly ME, Guzman R, Sinclair J, et al. Multimodality treatment of posterior fossa arteriovenous malformations. J Neurosurg. 2008; 108(6):1152–1161

[8] Lai LF, Chen JX, Zheng K, et al. Posterior fossa brain arteriovenous malformations: Clinical features and outcomes of endovascular embolization, adjuvant microsurgery and radiosurgery. Clin Neuroradiol. 2016. DOI: 10.1007/s00062-016-0514-3

22 Endovascular Treatment of Dural Arteriovenous Fistulas of the Brain

Edoardo Boccardi and Luca Valvassori

Abstract

The endovascular treatment of dural arteriovenous fistulas (DAVFs) of the brain has greatly improved with the advent of precipitating liquid embolics based on the solvent dimethyl sulfoxide (DMSO). The success of the procedure is directly related to the occlusion of the (first segment of the) draining vein; a thorough understanding of the anatomical details is therefore mandatory. The treatment techniques may differ depending on whether the draining vein is represented by a dural sinus or a pial vein, and different anatomical features will suggest an arterial or venous approach, knowing that catheterization of cerebral veins needs a somewhat different technical approach compared to arterial catheterization. The introduction and development of new materials (liquid embolics, detachable tip microcatheters, performing guidewires, large and long compliant balloons for sinus temporary occlusion) allow today a very high rate of cure with a limited procedural risk. Most frequently the relatively rare periprocedural complications are hemorrhagic, related to venous thrombosis or to the possible rupture of small pial feeders. Surgery remains an excellent therapeutic alternative especially in DAVFs draining in a pial vein.

Keywords: dural arteriovenous fistula, embolization, dimethyl sulfoxide, sinus occlusion, sinus coiling, venous catheterization

- For practical purposes and for better understanding the different treatment approaches, dural arteriovenous fistulas (DAVFs) are classified in two main groups: (1) the ones draining first in a sinus and (2) the ones draining directly in a pial vein.
- Brain vessels (arteries or veins) as everywhere else in the body constitute one single giant network, where everything is potentially connected with anything else.
- Catheterization of the veins is quite more challenging than catheterization of arteries. It requires a learning of the complexity of venous anatomy and a specific training.
- The pretreatment analysis of the DAVF is aimed at finding the exact point of fistula, that is the very first segment of the draining vein: "the foot of the vein," which will represent the target of the treatment.
- The advent of liquid embolic materials, based on the solvent dimethyl sulfoxide, has greatly improved the success rate of the endovascular approach to DAVFs.

22.1 Introduction

Over the years, a few hundred dural arteriovenous fistulas (DAVFs) have been diagnosed, treated, and followed by our multidisciplinary team consisting of neurologists, neurointensivists, neurosurgeons, and neuroradiologists at the authors' institution. The material for this chapter comes from direct experience of the authors, treating DAVFs of the brain in the neuroradiology department of the Niguarda Hospital in Milan for the last 30 years.

A few introductory considerations are required to understand our philosophy in the endovascular treatment (EVT) of DAVFs:

Over the past 40 years, several classifications have been proposed for DAVFs of the brain. Djindjian and Merland,[1] Borden et al,[2] Cognard et al,[3] and more recently Geibprasert et al[4] have all contributed with important works. However, we will not follow any specific classification because we feel that in the context of treatment each one has limitations. For the purpose of this chapter, we will divide intracranial DAVFs in two groups: DAVFs *located directly on a vein* and those *located on a sinus*. (▶ Fig. 22.1)

- In most DAVFs, the bulk of the arterial flow is coming from the meningeal arteries, but it is not unusual to find feeders coming from the pial brain network (▶ Fig. 22.2) both on sinuses and on pial veins. The more you look for the more you find. It is usually inconsequential, but it may become an important issue in a few cases. At times, the small shunts are located on the vein a little more distal than the dura emergence of the vein. We have seen cases where a surgical disconnection of the vein achieved complete elimination of the meningeal shunts, but a little pial shunt on the brain surface was maintained. Such pial feeders may have been responsible for delayed hemorrhages after treatment (sinus occlusion) of a DAVF, much like rupture of residual nidus of a brain arteriovenous malformation (AVM) after the occlusion of the draining vein (see below). It is important to analyze the presence of possible pial feeders in DAVFs.
- Finally, a lesson learned treating DAVFs and AVMs is that the brain and head arterial vessels constitute an immense network very much connected at all levels. It is not only the well-known communicating arteries or the more discrete leptomeningeal collaterals that are able to connect different arterial territories: these connections are almost everywhere and given time and flow demand any link is possible: superficial brain arteries with deep ones, meningeal arteries with brain vessels, and vice versa. Not only the bone, the diploe, but also the muscles and skin may take part in the process. These are not new vessels that form in response to angiogenetic stimuli, but rather dilatations of preexisting very small channels, which increase in size only because of flow demand.

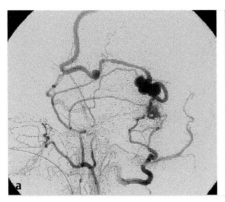
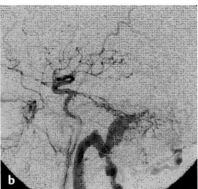

Fig. 22.1 (a) Dural arteriovenous fistula (DAVF) on a pial vein (Labbé vein): external carotid artery injection. The drainage is retrograde in veins reaching the superior sagittal sinus. (b) DAVF of the sigmoid sinus: common carotid artery injection. The drainage is orthograde toward the jugular vein.

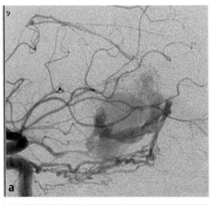
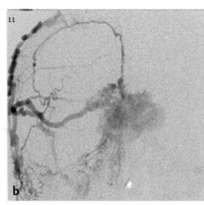
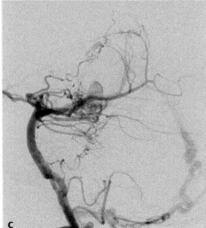
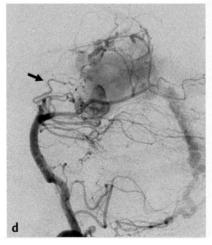

Fig. 22.2 (a) Dural arteriovenous fistula (DAVF) at the falcotentorial junction: right internal carotid artery injection. Feeders coming from tentorial branches of the meningohypophyseal trunk. (b) Right external carotid artery injection: feeders from the middle meningeal artery. (c) Feeders coming from the posterior meningeal artery. (d) Pial feeders from the transmesencephalic and retromesencephalic arteries (arrows).

The venous system has obviously the same properties, even though it is usually not quite easy to understand, or possibly the whole venous system is not well understood and these patterns may be there but not easy to recognize.

22.2 Endovascular Treatment of Intracranial DAVFs

As with all arteriovenous fistulas, EV cure is obtained only with occlusion of the proximal segment of the draining vein (the "foot" of the vein), where the arteriovenous shunts (A-V shunts) are actually located. This vein may be (1) a pial vein (running in the subarachnoid space on the surface of the cortex or otherwise) or (2) a sinus. There are profound clinical and methodological differences between the two forms. From an EV approach, there are also important technical issues that separate these two types. In general, it is better to avoid sacrifice of a sinus, except in selected cases, which will be discussed later. On the other hand, it is usually safe to occlude the foot of a pial vein (▶ Fig. 22.3).

22.2.1 Occlusion of the Pial Vein

Endovascularly the occlusion of the foot of the pial vein may be achieved in two ways: accessing it through the venous route or

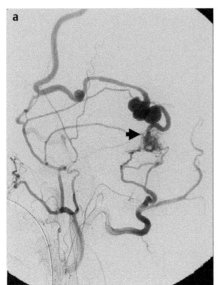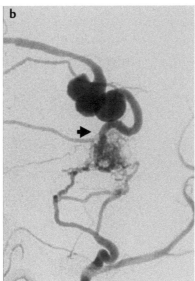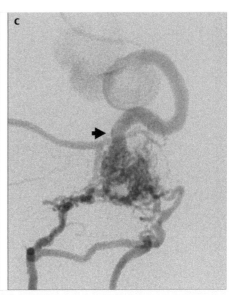

Fig. 22.3 (a-c) The "foot" of the vein (*arrows*) at progressive enlargements.

filling it through an arterial approach. The common use of the venous approach dates back to the early 1990s, when the detachable coils became available. It was preferred to the arterial approach because it offered high rates of cure, compared to the frequent complete or partial failures with intra-arterial injections of particles or glue.

The Venous Approach

It is always essential to have a complete and thorough study of the angiographic anatomy, but this is especially true in case one decides to reach the DAVF navigating the veins. First of all, the location and morphology of the foot of the vein, which is the procedure's target point, has to be well understood. Then one has to define the possible venous routes to reach it. It may be very hard to find an accessible route, because of the very complex venous network on the surface of the brain and because of the change in morphology of the draining veins, due to the increased amount and speed of arterialized flow. It is not infrequent to see tortuous dilated veins, with local varicosities, which may prevent any useful catheterization.

Catheter navigation in the venous tree has multiple technical differences with arterial navigation. First and most important is the *fragility* of the venous compared to the arterial structure. It is commonly held to be true that veins are easily occluded, dissected, or even ruptured when forceful pressures are utilized. While it is a risk that must always be kept in mind, it is remarkable how at times cortical veins may well tolerate very aggressive maneuvers.

Secondly one very important aspect of venous catheterization is that the *road map* is much less intelligible: that is, it is difficult to have all the veins completely and fully injected with contrast medium. If one injects from the arteries, most veins will be only faintly opacified and some will be all but invisible. If one injects from the vein, the vessels distal to the catheter (the ones to navigate forwardly) will not be seen: only those in the direction one is coming from will be shown. This is a major difference with arterial catheterization where the use of an angiographic "roadmap" is always very useful and well depicts

the way to go. It is therefore better to keep in mind that there are always many more veins than one has actually seen.

One third point is the variability of venous *branching*, where there are a lot more collaterals, connections, turnarounds, creating a multipotential network much more developed than on the arterial side. When navigating the veins, it is then easy to miss the main road and to catheterize secondary vessels (not known, not visible, not readily recognized), losing time and confidence.

Finally veins offer much less *support* to navigation of catheters and guide wires. Veins are more easily deformed and displaced, and therefore cannot counter the push of our devices. But more importantly their size is potentially much bigger than thought, that is, once inside a vein, one understands that the contrast injection has shown only a minimal part of the real caliber of the vessel. A vessel that looked a couple of millimeters in size may accept a wire loop three or four times that, or more. The precise position and direction of wires and catheters become therefore much more difficult.

All these negative features become evident when trying to catheterize a cortical vein backward from a sinus: the large size of the sinus offers no support, the outlet of the vein is often more complex than thought, and there are many unperceived venous branches in the proximity, both on the sinus wall and on the first segment of the vein. The problem has recently been partly solved by the introduction of longer intermediate catheters that provide the support veins do not give.

Once we have reached the correct position with a microcatheter—the correct position being the very initial part of the draining vein, the "foot"—we should be clear in our mind about the target of our treatment. The goal should be to fill and occlude the foot of the vein for a limited segment, not too long in order to avoid the occlusion of branching veins, possibly causing consequences on the normal drainage of the brain (► Fig. 22.4). Occluding a segment of 1 to 2 cm is usually more than enough.

Today we have ample choice of occluding devices or materials. The most popular are the detachable coils, normally used for aneurysms. They are very easy to use, reliable, well

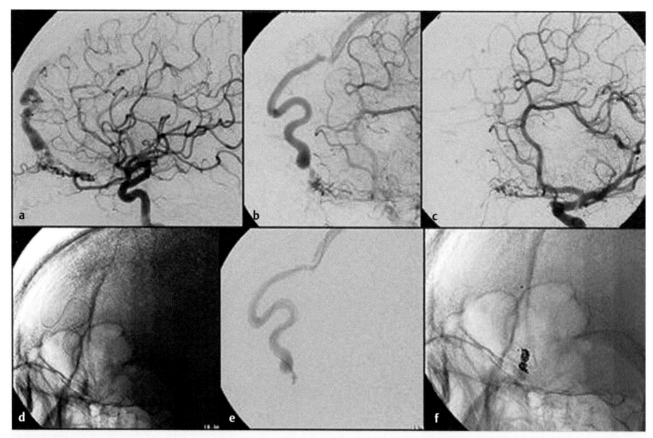

Fig. 22.4 **(a,b)** Lateral and oblique view: dural arteriovenous fistula of the crista galli. **(c)** Cure post-transvenous treatment with coils. **(d,e)** Microcatheter in the frontal vein. **(f)** Coils in the foot of the vein.

controllable, and well known. One should try to obtain a very dense tangle in a short segment of vein. There might be times though when the progressive coiling will displace the catheter more proximally, away from the correct location, with suboptimal results. In order to avoid that, one should maintain a continuous pressure on the catheter (not easy, because of the scarce support offered by the vein, as we discussed earlier) or place preventively a second catheter distal to the first that will stay in position during the coiling. This double catheter technique is quite interesting for the occlusion of major sinuses (see below), but it could be very hard to realize in small cortical veins, when navigation is usually very challenging.

Liquid materials, cyanoacrylates or dimethyl sulfoxide (DMSO) based (*), may also be used to occlude vessels. They are mostly used in the arterial compartment, but the injection at the venous side is becoming more and more popular. The disadvantage of the venous injection is of course that the material, behaving as contrast medium would, will run *away* from the fistula site, rather than *into* it, resulting in the occlusion of more veins than desired. It takes therefore quite a lot of expertise to obtain the correct placement of the embolic material. At times one can associate the liquids with coils: a few coils are deployed in the desired position forming a nest where the liquid will be subsequently trapped, completing the occlusion. The use of "gluing" liquids has one more potential danger, that is, gluing of the microcatheter in place. Retrieval could become impossible or at least very dangerous with the risk of tearing numerous

different veins along the way. With the advent of the recent detachable tip microcatheters, this occurrence is less of a problem, but it is still a possibility. In case it gets stuck, the microcatheter could be left in place. For that reason, some would prefer to access the intracranial veins from the jugular vein approach, rather than from the femoral vein, which would leave the microcatheter in the inferior vena cava, with the possibility of it curling up into the right atrium. Other occluding devices like detachable balloons or plugs have not been used in pial veins to our knowledge, the major difficulty being to navigate such devices against the direction of flow. The procedure ends when one has the **evidence** that the DAVF is completely obliterated. It does not suffice not seeing it any more when injecting contrast medium through the guiding catheter. It is almost always necessary to inject also all the other arteries, on both the same and the other side, both the anterior and the posterior circulation, both the meningeal and the pial arteries. More important is to well assure of the presence of a dense plug in the foot of the draining vein.

*DMSO-based liquid materials (DMSO-LM) are chemical solutions where the solvent is DMSO, which rapidly evaporates in contact with blood. The remaining solute will precipitate and solidify, behaving similarly to lava: it forms a crust around a liquid core, which under pressure will be later able to break the crust and flow in a new direction. The commercially available products are, in order of appearance on the market, Onyx (EV3, now Medtronic), Squid (Balt), and Phil (Microvention). In Onyx

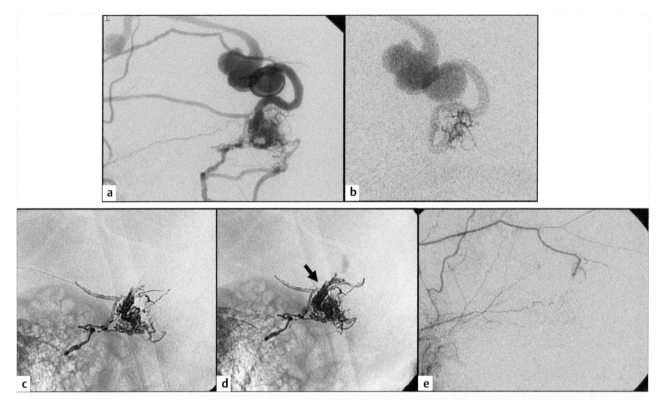

Fig. 22.5 (a) Dural arteriovenous fistula (DAVF) draining in a pial vein. (b) Superselective injection through a microcatheter. (c) Initial filling of the arterial network and part of the vein. (d) Final injection of the foot of the vein (*arrow*). (e) Complete DAVF occlusion.

and Squid, the precipitating agent is ethylene vinyl alcohol (EVOH), while in Phil the agent is hydroxyl ethyl methacrylate (HEMA).

The Arterial Approach

The treatment of DAVFs through the arterial route is probably the approach preferred by most operators, because it is usually safe and most successful. History tells us that it has not always been as successful as it is today. In the 1970s, 1980s, and 1990s, neurointerventionists could use particles (dura mater and polyvinyl alcohol) and glue (Histoacryl). Both proved to be ineffective for the same reason: they could not occlude the foot of the vein. Either they remained on the arterial side, trapped in the arterial network proximal to the A-V shunt, or they would pass into the vein, but then fly away with the high blood flow. In both cases, occasionally the cure could be randomly obtained by occluding most of the main arterial feeders, causing a major drop of the flow through the fistula and a spontaneous thrombosis of the vein. With glue, it was also possible that if some drops would remain lodged in the first segment of the draining vein, the inflammatory response of the vessel would go on to cause its complete occlusion. With the turn of the century, the advent of DMSO-LM allowed a different and more efficient approach. It is now possible to obtain a high rate of successful occlusions of DAFVs, whenever the catheter is located sufficiently close to the A-V shunt. The injection of the material obtains the progressive filling of most of the arterial network

and of the foot of the vein (▶ Fig. 22.5). The great advantage compared to cyanoacrylates is the fact that today's liquid embolic material does not fly away with flow but stays in the foot of the vein and it can be slowly and continuously injected so that it accumulates there. Most of the DAVFs draining in pial veins can today be cured in such a way (▶ Fig. 22.6).

22.2.2 DAVFs Draining in a Sinus

The EV options when the DAVF is draining into a sinus are much more complex and differentiated. On the other side, they are often a better option compared to surgery, more so than with DAVFs draining into pial veins, which may usually be as well cured by clipping, coagulating, or cutting the foot of the vein.

In this type of DAVF, the real challenge is to understand whether the sinus can be sacrificed or not. Of course it is always safer not to occlude a sinus, but at times it is the only or the best option. On angiographic images, it may be quite difficult to appreciate whether and how much the brain uses a sinus. The presence or absence of contrast medium in the target sinus when injecting the brain vessels is usually not a proof, due to many factors, but mostly to the dilution that comes from the noncontrasted A-V shunt. When the direction of flow in the sinus is orthodromic, that is, in the physiological direction, it is always better to keep the sinus patent. The occlusion of sinuses in such a situation has often led to complications due to venous infarctions. With the advent of DMSO-based liquids, it has

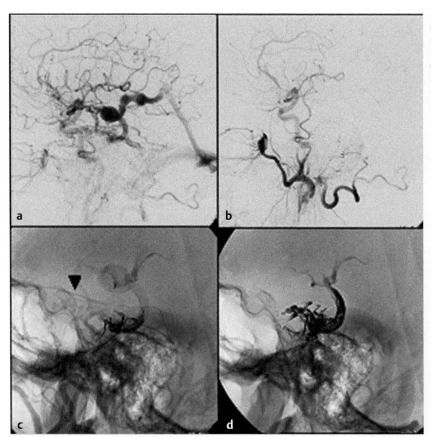

Fig. 22.6 **(a)** Dural arteriovenous fistula of the superior petrosal sinus: common carotid artery injection. **(b)** Cure post-transarterial injection of Onyx. **(c)** Microcatheter in the middle meningeal artery (MMA; *arrowhead*) and initial presence of Onyx in the foot of the vein. **(d)** Complete filling of the foot of the vein.

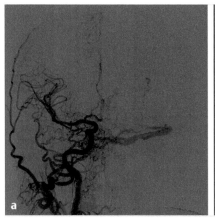
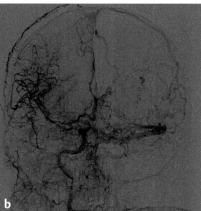

Fig. 22.7 **(a)** Sinus dural arteriovenous fistula at the torcular: right common carotid artery injection. The drainage is in the left transverse sinus, which is occluded on both sides. **(b)** Later phase of the same injection: from the sequestered sinus, there is a diffuse retrograde flow in most left hemispheric veins.

become possible to cure a sinus DAVF without having to sacrifice the sinus (see below).

Often though in DAVFs the sinus is already totally or partially thrombosed, causing a change in the direction of flow. When the flow in the sinus cannot go in the orthodromic direction, there is a reversal of flows that may involve not only the sinuses, but also the brain venous system. This is obviously true when a segment of sinus is occluded on both sides ("isolated" sinus; ▶ Fig. 22.7). Another peculiarity of sinus DAVFs is the possibility that all the A-V shunts are located on a very limited area, which at times may be even separated from the main lumen of the sinus, as in a natural or acquired segmentation. This possibility may be not clearly apparent on a superficial

evaluation of the angiographic images, but it could be very helpful when recognized, because the treatment could be limited to the occlusion of a much smaller segment of the sinus.

As with DAVF draining in a pial vein, the treatment of DAVF draining in a sinus can be performed through a venous or an arterial access.

The Venous Approach

Reaching a sinus through a venous access is usually not too complicated. Navigating upward from the internal jugular vein to the intracranial sinuses, the first potential difficulty is encountered at the jugular bulb, where at times the tortuous course and the bony structures oppose to a smooth advancement of the catheters. Advancing further, one has to well recognize the possible different intrasinus segmentations or parallel channels and has to avoid the openings of the cerebral veins. At the level of the torcular, the anatomic details are very variable: crossing from the right to the left transverse sinus may be at times very difficult. A common disposition is for the superior longitudinal sinus to continue into the right transverse sinus while the straight sinus continues into the left transverse sinus. The junction between the two transverse sinuses therefore may be more or less obvious, difficult to find, but it is rare to be missing. Navigating into the sinuses may be useful also when treating the DAVF through the arterial injection of liquids, when using a balloon to protect the lumen of the sinus (see below).

Once the final correct position inside the sinus is reached, it is possible to start the deployment of coils (usually large and long ones), and continue until the flow in the fistula is completely stopped. It commonly takes many coils and quite a long time to achieve the result, even if the sinus is not too big. It may also happen that during the deposition of coils the microcatheter is progressively pushed back separating from the initial correct position, risking on the one hand to interfere with the draining of normal veins into the sinus and on the other to have a suboptimal result on the fistula. Some neurointerventionists would therefore use two microcatheters in parallel, so that while one is used to place coils and may be thus pushed back, the other remains close to the fistula and can be utilized later to deploy more coils or to inject liquids.

The rate of success of the venous treatment of a DAVF with sinus occlusion is good, but not excellent. Some residual shunts may be visible in up to 10% of cases. In late years, we have therefore opted for the arterial approach as frequently as possible.

The Arterial Approach

A number of factors have contributed to the switch from the venous to the arterial approach: the venous approach is technically not simple, the exact features and details of the fistula are not well controlled, the results are at times disappointing, but mostly the limit of the venous approach is that it cannot be carried out in all instances when the sinus has to be preserved. The switch has come with the development of the DMSO-LM (Onyx was the first one), which has made it possible to reach all the feeders up to very fine arteries from one single injection point and to well control the deposition of the embolic material, avoiding unwanted diffusion. This was not possible with particles, nor usually with glue.

A few years later, the availability of large, long, and very compliant balloons (Copernic, Balt), which may be lodged in the sinus and inflated during Onyx injection, has further allowed high rates of complete DAVF cure, with preservation of the sinus (▶ Fig. 22.8). Today the treatment of a sinus DAVF is usually achieved by injection of the new liquids in one or two arterial feeders, contemporary or sequential, having positioned the balloon in the sinus and inflating it for a few minutes at a time. In some cases, the inflation of the balloon may be prolonged for a longer period of time, depending on the features of the normal venous drainage of the brain. When the desire is to occlude the sinus by filling it, as already described, coils may be deployed

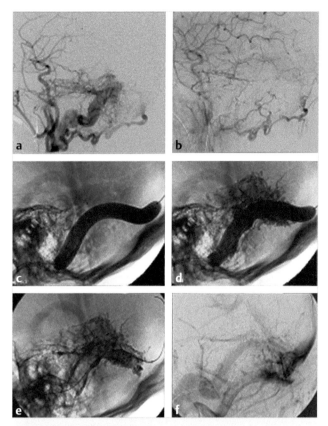

Fig. 22.8 (a) Dural arteriovenous fistula of the transverse-sigmoid sinus: lateral view. (b) Cure of the fistula post transarterial injection of Phil. (c) Protecting balloon in the sinus. (d) Phil and balloon final. (e) Transverse-sigmoid sinus remodeled by Phil and (f) still open and functioning.

from the vein, but one could also inject this material through an artery and from there push it into the sinus and fill it completely (▶ Fig. 22.9).

22.3 Results of Endovascular Treatment in DAVFs

The assessment of results is not a simple task in any sphere of medicine. It is especially true with vascular diseases of the brain. The parameters in play are multiple, variable, and often not known, plenty of *ifs* and *buts*, so that a simple and unanimous understanding is difficult to obtain. We will try to offer some numbers and explanations.

Since the introduction of new liquid embolics (Onyx) in 2007, we have treated over 250 DAVFs and achieved a rate of complete cure above 90% both when draining in the pial vein and when draining in the sinus. When the catheter is in a correct position, that is, close to the shunt, failures are really rare, and remnants or recurrences of DAVFs with drainage in a pial vein are below 5%. DAVFs draining in a sinus may have minor residual shunts more frequently both because the occlusion of the shunt is not desired and because they are often high-flow lesions where multiple different fistulous areas coexist (transverse-sigmoid sinus, torcular, and jugular bulb in the same patient are common). Also more frequently they require access

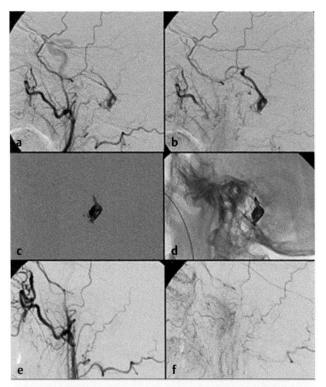

Fig. 22.9 (a,b) Early and late phase: dural arteriovenous fistula of a sequestered sigmoid sinus. **(c,d)** Intra-arterial injection of Onyx from the middle meningeal artery to fill completely the sinus. **(e,f)** Final cure.

from different arteries with multiple catheters in order to reach every compartment of the fistula. Notwithstanding these limitations, we believe the EVT is more successful than surgery also in this type of DAVF mainly because besides occluding most if not all incoming feeders, some material is often allowed to flow inside the sinus and laminate on its walls, occluding the shunts more effectively from the venous side.

Follow-up controls with an angiographic (digital subtraction angiography) complete check is mandatory in all cases. We usually prefer to do it 1 year after the intervention in order to be absolutely sure that if a very minimal residual shunt were present it would have had the time to become evident.

22.4 Complications

As with all other treatments of vascular diseases in the brain, there are morbidities and mortalities, but also failures. Complications may be the usual adverse events occurring in all EVTs: thromboembolism from catheters, arterial dissections, groin hematomas, X-ray alopecia, postprocedural fever or headaches.

There are also complications related specifically to this disease and to the underlying pathology. Catheterization of meningeal arteries is often difficult because of the small size, the frequent tortuosities, and the asperity of the angles and curves. It is not infrequent that rough maneuvers lead to the rupture of the artery with the possible formation of an extravasation or even a small A-V shunt. The injection of a small quantity of liquid embolics will immediately take care of the problem, but it will also bring about the occlusion of the route to access the

fistula. Catheterization of veins may also lead to ruptures, dissections, or occlusions, but the occurrence is much more rare in our experience.

More important are the complications related to the disease, even after a successful occlusion of the fistula.

22.4.1 Hemorrhagic Complications

Hemorrhagic complications are the most severe and the most frequent. They may be the consequence of different mechanisms.

Occlusion of Normal Drainage of the Brain (venous hemorrhagic infarction)

The brain can usually tolerate some venous occlusion or venous flow diversion. In some instances though, especially if large collectors are impaired, a venous infarct may follow the treatment of a DAVF. It is mandatory to pay great attention to the pretreatment images, trying to understand the ongoing pattern of the venous drainage of the brain. One common mistake is to consider the absence of contrast medium in the sinus after injection of the brain vessels as a proof of the possibility of sacrificing the sinus, while most of the times it is just a consequence of the dilution of the contrast medium due to the inflow of high quantities of noncontrasted blood from the fistula. In any case, it is always better to spare the intracranial sinuses whenever possible. Not only sinuses, but also the correct occlusion of the foot of a cortical vein drainage of a DAVF may also cause a venous infarct in adjacent territories, especially if the veins draining the fistula (and also brain tissue) are dilated. When the fistula is occluded, the flow decreases its volume and its speed: the vein will then thrombose unless the slow regular flow coming from normal tissue is sufficient to keep it going. But if the thrombosis is complete, a venous infarct may follow. We think that a few postprocedural days of anticoagulant therapy (usually low-molecular-weight heparin [LMWH]) is appropriate in most if not all DAVFs, starting toward the end of the procedure itself.

Rupture of an Especially Large Venous Dilatation, Following Its Thrombosis

This occurrence is unfortunately well known and has been experienced since the early times of neurointervention anytime a large volume of intravascular blood is forming a clot. Both in arteries (see the more recent experience in aneurysm treatment with flow diverters) and in veins the process may go on to burst the vessel and provoke a hemorrhage. It is frequently associated with a perivascular inflammatory reaction, hence the justification for a brief period of corticoid therapy, in cases where a complete cure of a DAVF is associated with sudden occlusion of a large venous dilatation.

Rupture of Small Pial Arterial Feeders, Once the Vein Is Successfully Occluded

As mentioned earlier, DAVFs may more often than not include pial arteries in the group of feeders. They are usually small and transverse the subarachnoid space and may rupture as feeders to a brain AVM would when the draining vein is occluded. Luckily this occurrence is rare, but it should be kept in mind if they are numerous and/or larger than usual. We have observed this outcome especially when retromesencephalic feeders participate to a high-flow fistula of the falcotentorial edge, draining in a vein of the Galen complex or in the straight sinus.

22.4.2 Cranial Nerves

Another complication related specifically to this disease is the damage to cranial nerves, usually due to ischemia following the embolization of the arterial supply to the nerves, in the context of the overall embolization of a certain region of the dura. Many different complications have been observed, but the most common ones are the following:

- Retinal or optic nerve ischemia during catheterization and embolization of ophthalmic arteries in cases of ethmoidal DAVFs, located close to the crista galli and draining into frontal veins directed upward toward the superior sagittal sinus (SSS). These DAVFs are fed mostly by ethmoidal branches of the ophthalmic artery. They can rarely be reached from an anterior branch of the middle meningeal artery that once on the midline descends along the SSS as an anterior meningeal artery retrogradely would. Only in this case would we suggest an arterial approach to the treatment of the DAVF. In cases where the only feeders come from the ophthalmic artery, we would prefer a venous approach or surgery.
- Oculomotor nerves may be damaged, causing a diplopia, when the arterial network of the walls of the cavernous sinus is injected. This happens usually in DAVFs of the cavernous sinus, which might at times be better treated with a venous approach occluding the sinus with coils. Occlusion of vessels in the same region may cause a trigeminal impairment.
- Connections between meningeal arteries and cerebellar arteries have only occasionally allowed the embolic material to occlude the supply to the acoustic nerve, but more frequently the facial nerve has been damaged injecting close to the foramen spinosum or into the mastoid arteries.
- The lower cranial nerves may be affected when occluding the jugular bulb or its feeding meningeal arteries.

Overall complications involving the cranial nerves are not infrequent (around 5% in the sensible locations) but have diminished with the introduction of DMSO-LM, compared with the former use of cyanoacrylates.

22.5 Failures and Redirection of Flow

Bad results may come from failing to occlude the A-V shunt, especially if occluding other vessels (arteries or veins) of the region.

If in the process of treating a DAVF the occluding device (liquid embolics, coils, balloons, plugs, etc.) is placed incorrectly, very serious consequences may arise. The occlusion of the feeders without the occlusion of the shunt may only expand the complexity of the problem: a whole new collateral arterial network will develop, which will be much more difficult to

navigate and to get eliminated. This is of course true for any A-V shunt, anywhere in the body. Oftentimes we have observed long-standing DAVFs where multiple treatment sessions had been performed, just by occluding surgically or endovascularly the arterial feeders, and that had become monstrous tangles of vessels, preventing any possibility of cure.

If the mistaken occlusion is on the venous side, a very dangerous flow redirection may follow, abruptly invading low-pressure venous systems with a blood torrent coming from the shunt. Impairment of brain functions, hemorrhages, and infarcts may be the final outcomes.

22.6 Advantages/Disadvantages Compared to Surgical Treatment

In our experience, the main advantages are the following:

- Better understanding of the venous compartment by sequential microcatheter subselective injection, that is, the exact location of the "foot" of the vein, which at a surgical exploration is often hidden and covered by the dura. The injection from the arterial side is by definition entering the very first part of the vein, while the venous occlusion (EV or surgical) might be a little distal to that.
- The possibility of occlusion of sinusal DAVFs without sacrificing the sinus, with better results than with sinus surgical skeletonization.
- The continuous and progressive control of the efficacy of the treatment during the intervention.
- In very high flow fistulas, the absence of blood loss, not having to cut the skin, the bone, and the meninges.
- The possibility to use heparin, even high dose, in the postprocedural days to avoid venous thrombosis.

The main disadvantage compared to surgery is possibly an inferior rate of cure, for failure of reaching the correct result. Surgery has also very limited risk of causing cranial nerve impairment.

22.7 Conclusion

The EVT of DAVFs has improved immensely since the early years of neurointervention. Most cranial DAVFs are today cured with high rate of success and low risks. Surgery is fortunately still a great support to the management of this fascinating disease.

References

[1] Djindjian R, Merland JJ. Superselective angiography of external carotid artery. New York, NY: Springer-Verlag; 1977

[2] Borden JA, Wu JK, Shucart WA. A proposed classification for spinal and cranial dural arteriovenous fistulous malformations and implications for treatment. J Neurosurg. 1995; 82(2):166–179

[3] Cognard C, Casasco A, Toevi M, Houdart E, Chiras J, Merland JJ. Dural arteriovenous fistulas as a cause of intracranial hypertension due to impairment of cranial venous outflow. J Neurol Neurosurg Psychiatry. 1998; 65(3):308–316

[4] Geibprasert S, Pereira V, Krings T, et al. Dural arteriovenous shunts: a new classification of craniospinal epidural venous anatomical bases and clinical correlations. Stroke. 2008; 39(10):2783–2794

23 Vein of Galen Aneurysmal Malformation

Lee-Anne Slater, Brian Drake, Peter Dirks, and Timo Krings

Abstract

Vein of Galen aneurysmal malformations (VGAM) are a challenging pediatric neurovascular shunting disease that require a multidisciplinary treatment approach in a specialized center accustomed to treating these rare malformations. Clinical and radiological features of VGAM, their association with outcome, and decision algorithms of when and how to treat are presented based on the pertinent literature and the authors' experience. In our experience, treatment is offered based on clinical presentation of the child and is typically done through a transarterial approach employing undiluted glue employing a staged approach to permit normal neurological development and a stepwise reduction of the shunt.

Keywords: pediatric vascular malformations, vein of Galen aneurysmal malformations, embolization, interventional neuroradiology, endovascular treatment

Key Points

- Vein of Galen aneurysmal malformations (VGAM) are arteriovenous fistulas involving the median vein of the prosencephalon.
- In our practice, children who are not presenting with heart failure or hydrocephalus are medically managed in the first weeks of life and endovascular treatment is performed when the child is around 3 months of age.
- Pretherapeutic clinical and imaging evaluation of the child is critical to determine both the appropriateness and timing of endovascular treatment.
- Melting brain and multi-organ failure are contraindications to treatment.

23.1 Introduction

Vein of Galen aneurysmal malformations (VGAM) are high-flow intracranial arteriovenous shunts that develop early in the embryonic period involving the choroidal circulation and the median prosencephalic vein (MPV), the embryonic precursor to the vein of Galen. They account for up to 37% of all pediatric vascular malformations. The use of routine antenatal ultrasound (US) for screening has resulted in an increase in the number of these cases being diagnosed in utero and as a result, physicians are now required to counsel parents regarding the condition and potential management strategies. Although overall VGAM are believed to be associated with poor outcomes, a better understanding of this disease, centralization of cases in high-volume centers, and better material have led to a significant number of patients with good clinical outcome. An understanding of the clinical, imaging, and angiographic features of this condition may assist in prediction of outcome and thus permit the physician to appropriately select patients that may benefit from treatment. Scoring systems have been proposed to try

and assist in predicting outcome and the appropriateness and best time for treatment if indicated.

This chapter aims to present the clinical and radiological features of VGAM and demonstrates how they can be used to predict outcome. In addition, the rationale for deciding if and when treatment is indicated will be presented along with an introduction to the management and endovascular treatment of this condition.

23.2 Materials and Methods

This chapter presents a combination of previously published articles, information obtained from institutional experience, and the personal experience of the authors. Clinical cases are used to illustrate the principles of treatment decision making as well as the endovascular management of VGAM.

23.3 Results

The analysis of previously published articles, institutional and personal experience, and clinical cases demonstrates the importance of recognizing VGAM and the clinical features and using them to help guide management decisions as well as the timing of treatment. In our practice, endovascular treatment of VGAM is performed, where possible, when the child is 3 months old with medical management and strict clinical follow-up of the child maintained in the interim. Failure of medical management, failure to thrive, a deviation in head circumference, or cognitive development should prompt earlier treatment. Conversely, if a child has a poor clinical score, or melting brain syndrome on magnetic resonance imaging (MRI), treatment should not be offered because in these patients intervention is likely futile.

23.4 Discussion

23.4.1 Introduction

VGAM account for up to 37% of all pediatric vascular malformations.[1] They occur early in the embryonic period and involve multiple shunts between the choroidal circulation and the MPV, the precursor to the vein of Galen. There are two types: the choroidal and mural types. The mural type is characterized by a few high-flow shunts into the anterior wall of the MPV. The choroidal type is characterized by multiple, often smaller, shunts through an arterial network prior to entering the MPV. Combinations of choroidal and mural types are possible.[2]

23.4.2 Presentation

With the widespread use of antenatal screening US, the prenatal diagnosis of VGAM is increasing. The diagnosis is made by identifying the dilated MPV; however, despite VGAM developing early in the embryonic stage at around 7 to 8 weeks of gestational age, there is usually insufficient dilatation to be detected until the third trimester.[3,4,5,6,7,8,9,10] There is no evidence that in the absence of multi-organ failure or brain parenchymal changes, an antenatal diagnosis of VGAM is more likely to be associated with a poor outcome and as such does not necessarily constitute an indication for therapeutic abortion. However, a prenatal diagnosis does permit preparation for appropriate neonatal postdelivery care. The most common presentation in the neonatal group is high-output cardiac failure.[8] Hydrodynamic disorders such as hydrocephalus and increasing head circumference are typically seen as the presenting feature in infancy.[2]

23.4.3 Natural History

VGAM, if left untreated, are associated with a poor outcome, and only a minority of untreated children with VGAM will do well.[3,11,12] Lasjaunias et al proposed a clinical scoring system to assist in determining the timing of treatment called the Bicêtre Neonatal Evaluation Score (▶ Table 23.1).[3,11,13] This scoring system assesses cardiac, cerebral, respiratory, hepatic, and renal systems with points lost for decreasing function in any of these categories. The maximum score is 21 and it is suggested that in neonates with scores less than 8, treatment should be withheld given they are unlikely to do well despite aggressive intervention. Subsequent to the development of this score, radiological and angiographic features suggested to be associated with poor outcome have included encephalomalacia, intraparenchymal calcifications, and angioarchitecture consisting of choroidal type nidus or jugular stenosis without cavernous drainage. Geibprasert et al evaluated clinical, imaging, and angiographic features that may predict outcome in VGAM patients and found that neurological symptoms at presentation, a medium to low overall neonatal score (< 12/21), a very poor score (< 2/5) in one or more categories of the Bicêtre neonatal evaluation score, focal parenchymal changes, calcifications, tonsillar herniation, arterial steal, or more than two groups of multiple arterial feeders were significantly associated with a poor outcome.[2]

23.4.4 Parenchymal Imaging

Parenchymal changes and calcifications were the most significant predictors of poor outcome on cross-sectional imaging findings.[12] Both these findings are indicators of irreversible damage accounting for their association with poor outcomes.

The parenchymal changes described include focal encephalomalacia that has been reported to relate to the presence of arterial steal and diffuse brain volume loss.[14] Detection of cerebral ischemia and infarction resulting from the steal phenomenon appears to be the etiology for the encephalomalacia. The use of diffusion-weighted imaging is particularly useful in detecting irreversible ischemic changes prior to the progression to encephalomalacia given the inherent high T2 signal intensity of the unmyelinated white matter can make it difficult to detect these changes on T2 or fluid attenuation inversion recovery weighted images.[15,16] Long-standing hydrocephalus is often seen in association with diffuse brain volume loss and more commonly seen in the older population. It is postulated that the diffuse volume loss results from either venous infarctions or a reduction in regional cerebral blood flow leading to arterial ischemia in the context of compromised periventricular venules secondary to high pressure from the hydrocephalus.[12] Computed tomography imaging is the best modality to detect calcifications. Parenchymal calcifications are an indicator of prolonged venous congestion.[17] Multiple factors contribute to the development of venous congestion and include extent of jugular bulb stenosis, lack of cavernous capture, and the presence of a high-flow shunt.

23.4.5 Angiography of Vein of Galen Aneurysmal Malformations

There are two forms of VGAM, the choroidal and mural types. Lasjaunias et al reported that patients with mural-type VGAM have a better clinical status; however, in the review by Geibprasert et al this was not found to be the case.[11,12] The arterial supply to VGAM arises from the anterior and posterior choroidal

Table 23.1 Bicêtre Neonatal Evaluation Score, maximum score = 21 (5 cardiac + 5 cerebral + 5 respiratory + 3 hepatic + 3 renal)

Points	Cardiac function	Cerebral function	Respiratory function	Hepatic function	Renal function
5	Normal	Normal	normal	–	–
4	Overload, no medical treatment	Subclinical, isolated EEG abnormalities	Tachypnea, finishes bottle	–	–
3	Failure; stable with medical treatment	Nonconvulsive intermittent neurologic signs	Tachypnea, does not finish bottle	No hepatomegaly, normal hepatic function	Normal
2	Failure; not stable with medical treatment	Isolated convulsion	Assisted ventilation, normal saturation $FiO_2 < 25\%$	Hepatomegaly, normal hepatic function	Transient anuria
1	Ventilation necessary	Seizures	Assisted ventilation, normal saturation $FiO_2 > 25\%$	Moderate or transient hepatic insufficiency	Unstable diuresis with treatment
0	Resistant to medical therapy	Permanent neurological signs	Assisted ventilation, desaturation	Abnormal coagulation, elevated enzymes	Anuria

Abbreviations: EEG, electroencephalogram; FiO_2, fraction of inspired oxygen.

Source: Data from Lasjaunias.[11]

arteries, the limbic arch, and subependymal branches from the basilar tip and proximal posterior cerebral arteries. Rarely, transdural supply is noted; however, this tends to be seen in older children with previous treatment and thought to result from partial thrombosis of the venous pouch. As previously mentioned, the venous drainage of VGAM is to the precursor to the vein of Galen, the MPV.

Vascular changes secondary to the increased flow include venous steno-occlusive disease; in particular, the jugular bulbs can demonstrate progressive narrowing with compensatory reflux into cortical veins. Venous varices can also develop in the context of outflow impairment. The presence of increased venous hypertension is associated with hydrocephalus and, if left untreated, venous congestive edema and cerebral volume loss.

23.4.6 Treatment

Prior to devising a management plan, the appropriateness of treatment needs to be determined. The Bicêtre neonatal evaluation score can be used to predict a neonate's chance of a good clinical outcome and thus select those suitable for active management. Neonates with scores less than 8 or a score of less than 2 in one or more categories are unlikely to do well and therefore withholding treatment is—in our group—believed to be the most appropriate course of action. Likewise, the presence of parenchymal changes and in particular melting brain indicate irreversible damage and signify contraindications to treatment (▶ Fig. 23.1).

In the patients that are likely to benefit from active management, the mainstay of treatment in the first instance is correction of high-flow cardiac and multiorgan failure and prevention of permanent neurological damage. When a neonate presents with high-output cardiac failure, medical management is the first line of treatment. The goal of treatment is to stabilize the child to delay endovascular treatment until the child is at least 3 months of age. At this age, treatment is technically somewhat easier and feasible due to the increased size and weight of the child making the vessels easier to navigate and allowing a greater volume of contrast per treatment. During this period, very careful clinical monitoring is required because any neurological decline should prompt immediate treatment. Similarly, if the neonate has high-output organ failure despite best medical therapy, endovascular treatment of the VGAM should be pursued.

The preferred method of endovascular treatment is via the transarterial route. Arterial access is obtained through either the umbilical artery when it remains patent or the common femoral artery. Microcatheters are guided to the site of the shunt and microcatheter injections are then used to confirm supply to the VGAM and to ensure no concurrent supply to eloquent structures such as the thalami. Once a suitable feeder has been identified, embolization can be performed using n-Butyl-cyanoacrylate (NBCA; ▶ Fig. 23.2). The concentration of glue as well as the positioning of the catheter is determined by how high flow the shunt is. For very fast flow and particularly direct shunts, a higher concentration of glue should be used and the catheter tip should be positioned against the wall of the vessel to promote rapid polymerization of the NBCA prior to it penetrating too far into the venous system. The NBCA should be mixed with tantalum powder to increase visibility when using high concentrations. In cases where there is an interposed network, more dilute glue is required to ensure penetration into the venous side.

Treatment is often staged. In the acute stage, the goal is to reduce the shunting volume sufficiently to improve high-output cardiac failure rather than to cure the entire vascular malformation. Treatment can then be performed weeks to months apart to gradually reduce the shunt until cure is achieved.

A transvenous approach can be used if there are no suitable arterial feeders available to access the shunt. Alternatively, if the shunt is very high flow, it is possible to use a combined approach with the venous approach used to deploy coils in the median prosencephalic vein to prevent migration of embolic material delivered from the arterial feeders to the pulmonary circulation. If a transvenous approach is to be pursued, imaging of the jugular bulbs and foramen needs to be performed to assess for stenosis or occlusion as this may affect access decisions.

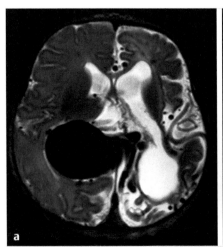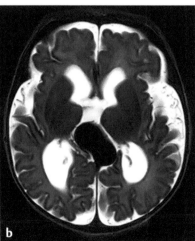

Fig. 23.1 **(a)** Axial T2 magnetic resonance imaging (MRI) showing left hemisphere encephalomalacia in a child whom no treatment was offered, contrasted with **(b)** axial T2 MRI without encephalomalacia in a child that subsequently underwent treatment.

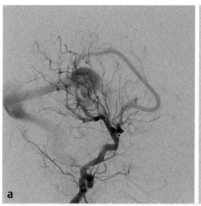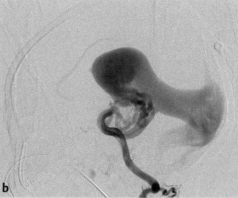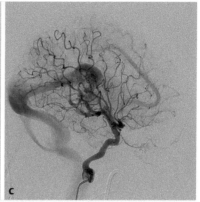

Fig. 23.2 Pre-embolization lateral internal carotid artery **(a)** and vertebral artery **(b)** angiogram showing anastomosis between pericallosal artery branches and posterior cerebral arteries branches shunting via fistulas into a dilated vein of Galen. **(c)** Postembolization lateral internal carotid angiogram showing improvement of the right cerebral hemisphere perfusion and reduction in the extent of the shunt.

23.5 Conclusion

VGAM is a rare vascular malformation. Thorough clinical and radiological assessment is required to determine if active management is appropriate and to determine the best timing of each stage of treatment. In the first instance, medical management to stabilize high-output cardiac failure is the treatment of choice with the aim being to delay endovascular treatment until the patient is 3 months of age. In cases of refractory, high-output cardiac failure or a clinical deterioration endovascular management should be performed.

References

[1] Berenstein A, Ortiz R, Niimi Y, et al. Endovascular management of arteriovenous malformations and other intracranial arteriovenous shunts in neonates, infants, and children. Childs Nerv Syst. 2010; 26(10):1345–1358

[2] Gailloud P, O'Riordan DP, Burger I, et al. Diagnosis and management of vein of Galen aneurysmal malformations. J Perinatol. 2005; 25(8):542–551

[3] Lasjaunias PL, Berenstein A, terBrugge K. Surgical Neuroangiography; Clinical and Interventional Aspects in Children. 2nd ed. Berlin: Springer; 2006

[4] Raybaud CA, Strother CM, Hald JK. Aneurysms of the vein of Galen: embryonic considerations and anatomical features relating to the pathogenesis of the malformation. Neuroradiology. 1989; 31(2):109–128

[5] Beucher G, Fossey C, Belloy F, Richter B, Herlicoviez M, Dreyfus M. Antenatal diagnosis and management of vein of Galen aneurysm: review illustrated by a case report [in French]. J Gynecol Obstet Biol Reprod (Paris). 2005; 34(6):613–619

[6] Fayyaz A, Qureshi IA. Vein of Galen aneurysm: antenatal diagnosis: a case report. J Pak Med Assoc. 2005; 55(10):455–456

[7] Nuutila M, Saisto T. Prenatal diagnosis of vein of Galen malformation: a multidisciplinary challenge. Am J Perinatol. 2008; 25(4):225–227

[8] Rodesch G, Hui F, Alvarez H, Tanaka A, Lasjaunias P. Prognosis of antenatally diagnosed vein of Galen aneurysmal malformations. Childs Nerv Syst. 1994; 10(2):79–83

[9] Ruano R, Benachi A, Aubry MC, Brunelle F, Dumez Y, Dommergues M. Perinatal three-dimensional color power Doppler ultrasonography of vein of Galen aneurysms. J Ultrasound Med. 2003; 22(12):1357–1362

[10] Santo S, Pinto L, Clode N, et al. Prenatal ultrasonographic diagnosis of vein of Galen aneurysms–report of two cases. J Matern Fetal Neonatal Med. 2008; 21(3):209–211

[11] Lasjaunias PL, Chng SM, Sachet M, Alvarez H, Rodesch G, Garcia-Monaco R. The management of vein of Galen aneurysmal malformations. Neurosurgery. 2006; 59(5) Suppl 3:S184–S194, discussion S3–S13

[12] Geibprasert S, Krings T, Armstrong D, Terbrugge KG, Raybaud CA. Predicting factors for the follow-up outcome and management decisions in vein of Galen aneurysmal malformations. Childs Nerv Syst. 2010; 26(1):35–46

[13] Mortazavi MM, Griessenauer CJ, Foreman P, et al. Vein of Galen aneurysmal malformations: critical analysis of the literature with proposal of a new classification system. J Neurosurg Pediatr. 2013; 12(3):293–306

[14] Grossman RI, Bruce DA, Zimmerman RA, Goldberg HI, Bilaniuk LT. Vascular steal associated with vein of Galen aneurysm. Neuroradiology. 1984; 26(5):381–386

[15] Baldoli C, Righini A, Parazzini C, Scotti G, Triulzi F. Demonstration of acute ischemic lesions in the fetal brain by diffusion magnetic resonance imaging. Ann Neurol. 2002; 52(2):243–246

[16] Guimiot F, Garel C, Fallet-Bianco C, et al. Contribution of diffusion-weighted imaging in the evaluation of diffuse white matter ischemic lesions in fetuses: correlations with fetopathologic findings. AJNR Am J Neuroradiol. 2008; 29(1):110–115

[17] Quisling RG, Mickle JP. Venous pressure measurements in vein of Galen aneurysms. AJNR Am J Neuroradiol. 1989; 10(2):411–417

24 Radiosurgical Basics for the Treatment of Arteriovenous Malformations: Indications and Techniques

Edward A. Monaco III, Andrew Faramand, Ajay Niranjan, and L. Dade Lunsford

Abstract

Arteriovenous malformations have been treated by stereotactic radiosurgery from its beginnings. As with many pathologies, the indications and techniques for the treatment of arteriovenous malformations by stereotactic radiosurgery have been refined over time with improvements in knowledge and technologies. The results of the controversial ARUBA trial have caused some to question the need to treat asymptomatic arteriovenous malformations. The purpose of this chapter is to introduce the indications for the treatment of arteriovenous malformations by stereotactic radiosurgery, explore the technique, and identify several of the areas in which this treatment has evolved.

Keywords: arteriovenous malformation, Gamma Knife, indications, stereotactic radiosurgery, techniques

Key Points

- Stereotactic radiosurgery (SRS) is one of several treatment options for arteriovenous malformations (AVMs).
- The indications for radiosurgery for AVMs include the following: surgically inaccessible or risky lesions, surgically low-risk lesions in medically infirm patients or those refusing surgery, limiting the risk of treating lesions in critical locations, treating residual nidus after previous failed treatments, and treating certain larger symptomatic lesions with no other treatment options.
- The ARUBA (unruptured brain arteriovenous malformations) trial does not conclusively aid in decision-making regarding unruptured AVMs and treatment by SRS due, in part, to a limited follow-up period.
- The Gamma Knife radiosurgical technique for AVM treatment involves stereotactic frame placement, image acquisition, target delineation, highly conformal dose planning, treatment execution, careful follow-up with serial magnetic resonance imaging studies, and confirmation of obliteration after the latency period with cerebral angiography.
- Various alterations to the radiosurgical technique like dose-staged treatment of larger AVMs and the avoidance of preradiosurgical endovascular nidus embolization allow for safer and more efficacious treatment.

24.1 Introduction

Arteriovenous malformations (AVMs) are congenital vascular abnormalities comprising feeding arteries that are directly connected with draining veins without the interposition of a capillary bed to dampen pressure. The basic structure of an AVM includes a nidus, which is a vascular mass that shunts the blood from the feeding arteries to the draining veins. AVMs are rare, with an estimated incidence of 1 in 100,000 persons per year and prevalence estimated at 18 per 100,000.[1,2] The primary concern in a patient harboring an AVM is the risk of rupture and the potential for devastating neurological sequelae or even death. In the absence of hemorrhage, AVMs can lead to intractable vascular headache syndromes or seizure disorders. In the era of modern imaging, an increasing proportion of patients are having AVMs identified incidentally with minimal to no symptoms. Cerebral angiography remains the "gold standard" for the diagnosis of AVMs given it provides detailed information about the topography of an AVM, identifies the presence of intranidal or feeding artery aneurysms, and delineates the venous drainage pattern. The main goals of AVM treatment are to reduce or eliminate the risk of hemorrhage, ameliorate nonhemorrhagic symptoms, avoid future neurological deficits, and to do so in a fashion that is associated with the fewest complications.

More than 50% of individuals with AVMs present with hemorrhage, most commonly an intraparenchymal hemorrhage or a subarachnoid hemorrhage.[3] Estimates on the overall risk of spontaneous AVM hemorrhage vary, but they typically range from around 2 to 4% per year and possibly less for unruptured AVMs.[4,5,6,7,8,9,10,11] After an initial hemorrhage, the risk of rebleeding is increased and ranges between 6 and 15% during the first year.[12,13,14,15] Myriad factors have been associated with an increased risk of hemorrhage including small volume, seizures at presentation, the presence of deep venous drainage, the presence of intranidal or feeding artery aneurysms, and AVM location.[16,17,18,19,20]

Four treatment options are available to patients with diagnosed AVMs: observation, surgical resection, endovascular embolization, or stereotactic radiosurgery (SRS). The latter three can be used alone or in combination. Surgical resection is the "gold standard" treatment for AVMs. Complete resection of an AVM results in immediate elimination of hemorrhage risk that must be counterbalanced with the risks of surgery (i.e., general anesthetic risks, infection, stroke, etc.). Spetzler and Martin, among others, defined nidus size, pattern of venous drainage, and location within highly functional brain regions as critical features of an AVM that serve as outcome predictors for surgical resection at centers of excellence.[21] These findings have been validated by various series and observational cohorts that indicate microsurgery is a safe and curative treatment strategy for low-grade AVMs.[22,23,24]

Endovascular embolization has been advocated as a primary treatment strategy for AVMs.[25] However, the curative potential of embolization alone is generally considered to be low.[26,27,28,29] Embolization using a variety of coil, particulate, or glue methods may be used as an adjunct prior to microsurgery to induce flow reduction, limit surgical bleeding, and occlude difficult-to-reach or deep-seated arterial feeders.[30] Complication rates during embolization procedures vary widely with morbidity ranging from 1.4 to 50% and mortality varying from 1 to 4%.[25,26,31,32,33,34,35,36,37] Given its lack of curative potential and its risk profile, a thoughtful evaluation of the role of embolization in each patient is necessary. One circumstance particularly suited to endovascular therapy may be treatment of aneurysms associated with AVMs.[38]

The role of observation in patients harboring AVMs has recently come into sharper focus.[39,40] Although the role of treatment in the setting of ruptured AVMs is generally agreed upon, the management of unruptured AVMs is controversial. The risks of spontaneous hemorrhage must be compared to treatment-associated morbidity and mortality. The unruptured brain arteriovenous malformations (ARUBA) trial was the first randomized trial regarding the management of unruptured AVMs.[39] The study was undertaken to further elucidate the natural history of unruptured AVMs and the treatment-associated risks. An exhaustive treatise on the results of ARUBA and its flaws, as pointed out by its many detractors, is beyond the scope of this chapter. However, a brief mention is useful. In the study, 109 patients were randomized to medical management, while 114 were assigned to receive intervention, either embolization, SRS, microsurgery, or a combination thereof. The primary outcome measures were the occurrence of stroke or death. During a follow-up period of 33 months, 30.7% of the patients undergoing intervention suffered a stroke or died, compared to only 10.1% in the medical management arm. Three times as many patients in the intervention cohort were clinically impaired (modified Rankin score of 2 or higher), 46.2 versus 15.1%. The authors concluded that medical management was superior to medical management plus intervention for unruptured AVMs in this population followed for less than 3 years. Some of the more pointed criticisms include the following: few screened patients were eventually randomized, microsurgery was little used in the setting of low-grade AVMs for which it is particularly suited, endovascular embolization was used in a disproportionate number of patients despite its lack of curative potential and notable risks, and the follow-up period of 33 months was not sufficiently long to detect the benefits of intervention.[41,42] Outside the realm of unruptured AVMs, there are patients who are simply too medically ill, too aged, or possessing very difficult to treat AVMs for which treatment risks are too high and for whom observation may be the only reasonable strategy.[43]

Radiation used to obliterate blood vessels in the brain as a treatment concept was first conceived of in the 1960s. Kjellberg advocated the proton Bragg peak stereotactic radiation approach in the 1970s and 1980s and more than 1,000 AVM patients were treated.[44,45] Only about 20% of patients experienced complete AVM obliteration using this technique. Lars Leksell treated the first patient harboring an AVM with the prototype Gamma Knife unit in Stockholm in 1970.[46] Target definition was based on the acquisition of biplane angiography performed during the procedure itself. Linear accelerator (LINAC) based technologies have been adapted for SRS for the treatment of AVMs at a number of centers worldwide.[47,48,49,50,51] The emphasis of this chapter will be on the use of the Gamma Knife given that it is the device with which the authors are most familiar and on which the abundance of the literature is based. As of 2015, more than 100,000 patients harboring AVMs have been treated using the Gamma Knife worldwide.

SRS can be defined as the targeting of a lesion in an imaging-defined stereotactic coordinate system with focused, highly selective, sharp dose fall-off radiation. SRS has become a well-established treatment modality for AVMs with myriad published reports documenting its safety and efficacy. Radiosurgery causes AVM obliteration by inducing vascular injury and fibrosis that eventually leads to vessel thrombosis and occlusion.[52] AVM obliteration rates vary widely and depend on the radiation dose administered and the volume of the AVM. The primary advantage of SRS for AVMs is risk avoidance, while the chief limitation is the latency period from the time of treatment to obliteration during which the risks of hemorrhage persist. This latency period is typically around 2 to 4 years, but can be longer. Patients who are not candidates for microsurgery due to advanced age, medical comorbidities, and surgical inaccessibility are often eligible for treatment with SRS. A complication unique to SRS treatment of AVMs is an adverse radiation effect (ARE). AREs can be transient or irreversible and can be defined as any new neurological symptom or sign that occurs after SRS in the absence of hemorrhage.[53] AREs reportedly occur in 3 to 11% of patients after SRS for AVMs.[54,55,56,57,58,59,60]

AVM treatment should be carefully tailored to each individual patient on the basis of his or her lesion, medical comorbidities, the risks and benefits of available options, and patient desires and expectations. A thorough understanding of the indications and techniques of AVM treatment greatly enhances the potential for patients to have excellent outcomes with minimal toxicity. The first objective of this chapter is to specifically delineate the indications for treatment of AVMs by SRS. The second objective is to explore various features of the radiosurgical technique.

24.2 Materials and Methods

A literature search of PubMed was performed to identify the relevant published literature regarding this topic. Institution experience from the University of Pittsburgh is included.

24.3 Results

24.3.1 Indications for Stereotactic Radiosurgery

In general, treatment of an AVM is indicated when the risks of the natural history are greater than the risks of treatment or when nonhemorrhagic symptoms are sufficiently incapacitating that accepting the risks of treatment is felt to be worth enduring to eliminate them (▶ Table 24.1).

The following factors are considered when determining a patient's suitability for SRS: age, medical comorbidities, history of AVM rupture, prior management, AVM volume and morphology, AVM location, presenting symptoms, angioarchitecture (i.e., diffuse vs. compact nidus), surgical candidacy, and the existence of feeding artery or intranidal aneurysms.

Table 24.1 Current roles for radiosurgical treatment of arteriovenous malformations (AVMs)

Indications for stereotactic radiosurgery treatment of AVMs

Deep-seated AVMs without surgical options

Small/medium sized AVMs

AVMs in critical locations with high surgical risk

Residual AVMs left after prior management

Select larger, symptomatic AVMs without treatment alternatives

One of the primary indications for SRS is when an AVM is not easily surgically accessible or its functional location has resulted in it being characterized a too high a risk for surgery.[21] For instance, AVMs within the brainstem are a particularly challenging entity wherein the often unacceptably high risks of surgery make SRS an attractive alternative.[61] In contrast, microsurgical resection for low-grade AVMs is the "gold standard," but SRS can be a gradually effective and relatively safe alternative for patients who are not candidates for surgery due to medical comorbidities or have declined it.[62]

SRS has a meaningful role in the treatment of residual AVM nidi that have been left after previous treatments. A meaningful number of patients reported on in radiosurgical series underwent prior attempts at microsurgical cure or endovascular embolization. Often in these cases, it is felt at the time of surgery that a remnant must be left to avoid harming a patient. One of the few published reports on the role of SRS for partially resected AVMs is by Ding et al.[63] In this case-matched analysis, no differences in the rates of obliteration and postradiosurgical hemorrhage were found between previously resected and unresected AVMs. Endovascular embolization may have been utilized in hopes of diminishing the nidus size, decreasing overall AVM flow, and potentially reducing the risk of subsequent hemorrhage. There are little data to support this hypothesis. SRS can also be repeated when it fails to achieve complete AVM obliteration.[64]

Finally, SRS is indicated for select patients with larger, symptomatic AVMs for whom no other treatment options are available. With the use of volume and dose staging, very challenging AVMs have a hope of meaningful rates of complete obliteration.

An important question regarding the indications for SRS is, How have the results of the ARUBA trial changed its indications for the treatment of unruptured AVMs? Because of its limited follow-up period of 33 months, and the latency of the treatment effect of SRS, the ARUBA study does not seem to aid in decision-making regarding SRS for AVMs at all. Several groups have specifically evaluated outcomes after SRS in ARUBA-eligible patients to offer more data. Ding et al reported on 509 ARUBA-eligible patients treated by SRS in a multicentered retrospective study with a mean follow-up period of 86 months.[42] This study suggests that on the basis of post-SRS hemorrhage rates and complications, a follow-up period of 15 to 20 years would be required to realize the benefits of SRS over conservative management. Using the same eligibility criteria as the ARUBA trial, Pollock et al retrospectively observed that the risk of stroke or death in 174 patients treated by SRS was 2% per year for the first 5 years after treatment and 0.2% thereafter.[65] They suggest that patients harboring small-volume AVMs may benefit from SRS when compared to the natural history over a period of 5 to 10 years. The lack of meaningful conclusions regarding SRS via the ARUBA trial, taken together with these data, supports a role for the treatment of unruptured AVMs in relatively young patients.

24.3.2 Gamma Knife Stereotactic Radiosurgery Technique

SRS with the Gamma Knife is a collaboration between a neurosurgeon, radiation oncologist, and medical physicist, and involves a multistep process (▶ Table 24.2). Under most

Table 24.2 Stereotypical radiosurgical treatment methods with the Gamma Knife

The steps of a typical Gamma Knife SRS procedure

Stereotactic head frame placement

Image acquisition (fine-cut axial contrasted and T2 MRI, stereotactic biplane angiography) and target definition

Dose selection and treatment planning

Treatment administration

Follow-up with serial MRI scans

Confirmation of obliteration by cerebral angiography

Abbreviations: MRI, magnetic resonance imaging; SRS, stereotactic radiosurgery.

circumstances, it is performed on an outpatient basis. We routinely use anticonvulsant therapy in patients harboring lobar AVMs in order to reduce the risk of periprocedural seizures. Traditionally, the procedure begins with the application of an imaging compatible stereotactic head frame to the patient. This is performed after the administration of local anesthetic to the scalp and often supplemented by intravenous sedation (fentanyl and midazolam). Children under the age of 12, or those who cannot tolerate the procedure otherwise, are often administered general endotracheal anesthesia. Prior to the introduction of the newest Gamma Knife, the Icon, the procedure was only very rarely performed in the absence of a head frame. The Icon device allows for mask-based immobilization when used in conjunction with the acquisition of stereotactic cone-beam computed tomography (CT) and real-time image-guidance movement tracking. Mask-based immobilization also allows for noninvasive fractionated or multisession treatments, although there are no data yet published regarding this technique.

Image acquisition is the next step. Since the early 1990s, the "gold standard" imaging studies obtained for treatment planning include high-resolution axial plane magnetic resonance imaging (MRI) coupled with biplane stereotactic cerebral angiography. Specifically, a contrast-enhanced three-dimensional volumetric study and a whole-head T2 fast-spin echo imaging sequence are acquired. Late arterial phase angiography images are typically selected for dose planning as they best demonstrate the AVM nidus and the early venous drainage. At times, MRI is contraindicated (i.e., pacemakers, paramagnetic metallic foreign objects), and contrast-enhanced CT angiography is performed. Catheter-based angiography is somewhat disadvantageous given that it is invasive and associated with a small risk of complications (i.e., groin hematoma, vascular injury, and stroke). Alternatives to catheter-based angiography like time-resolved CT angiography are few and in their infancy.[66] Imaging is collected with a fiducial apparatus attached to the head frame in order to delineate the target location in stereotactic space. Once collected, the stereotactic images are uploaded into the dose planning software. All imaging is carefully scrutinized to identify any intranidal or feeding artery aneurysms that may be present, given their presence is a risk factor for hemorrhage and may be an indication for endovascular embolization.[38]

The radiosurgical target includes the entire volume of the AVM nidus, defined as the shunt between the afferent arteries and the draining veins. Single or multiple isocenter plans are created in order to highly conform to the AVM nidus volume at

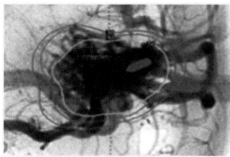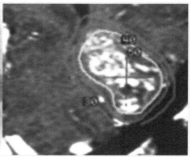

Fig. 24.1 Three-dimensional, highly conformal, multi-isocentric radiosurgical dose plan with a sharp dose fall-off as shown on corresponding stereotactic angiography (left) and fine-cut thin-sliced axial-contrasted magnetic resonance imaging (right).

the selected treatment isodose (typically the 50%; ▶ Fig. 24.1). Dose selection is made after consideration of factors such as of AVM volume, anatomic location, prior irradiation, and clinical history. An integrated logistic formula, which predicts a 3% risk of permanent radiation-induced complications, is used to select a margin dose. Doses sufficient to achieve the highest AVM obliteration rates are balanced against complication-associated risk factors. The minimal therapeutic margin dose ranges from 16 to 18 Gy, with increased obliteration rates achieved when doses of 20 to 23 Gy are administered. Depending on anatomic location, prescription dose formulae are modified. Immediately following the procedure, a single dose of intravenous methylprednisolone is administrated.

Follow-up after SRS is a critical component to the procedure's success. In our early experience, yearly angiograms were obtained to serially follow the obliterative response. Since the advent of MRI, scans are recommended at 6, 12, 24, and 36 months after SRS in the absence of new or unexpected symptoms to assess both the vascular and parenchymal response to treatment. If after 3 years the MRI scan indicates likely obliteration (diminished or absent contrast enhancement at the nidus site and lack of flow voids observed on T2 images), cerebral angiography is then generally recommended. Due to the invasive nature of angiography and potential complications, some patients may wish to avoid this test. However, Lee et al reported that MRI and MR angiography possess sensitivity and specificity for detecting obliteration of around 80 and 90%, respectively, suggesting the cerebral angiography remains an important confirmatory test for obliteration.[67] If complete obliteration or an isolated early draining is the result of the angiogram, no further treatment is recommended. Due to the persistent risk of AVM rupture in situations of residual AVM, an additional radiosurgical procedure is recommended to complete obliteration. After complete obliteration is confirmed on angiography, the risk of subsequent AVM rupture is less than 1% for a patient's entire remaining life expectancy. Even after obliteration is confirmed, patients should undergo serial MRI scan every few years to identify any long-term delayed SRS complications like cyst formation. This risk is typically low at around 1%, it but can be several folds higher in patients who undergo multiple SRS procedures.[68]

24.4 Discussion

A number of special considerations regarding nuances of the SRS technique are noteworthy (▶ Table 24.3). In patients who have suffered an AVM rupture and who are going to be treated

with SRS, it is preferable to wait until after the clot has been reabsorbed prior to treatment in order to prevent misidentification of the nidus. This time period is often 1 to 3 months and can be assessed on MRI or CT imaging.

Larger volume AVMs (> 10 cm³) are often challenging to treat. Single-stage SRS for these AVMs has been associated with low rates of obliteration and unacceptably high rates of AREs. In order to improve the safety and efficacy of treatment to these larger AVMs, volume staging was evaluated (▶ Fig. 24.2).[69] At the first treatment stage, the total volume of the AVM is outlined on the stereotactic MRI scans. This volume is then divided into approximately equal volumes using identified landmarks (i.e., major vessels). A dose plan is created for the entire AVM volume, after which isocenters are removed until around 50% of the volume remains covered. The first half of the AVM can then be treated with SRS, with a second stage performed 3 to 6 months later (the second half). With the current planning system, a stereotactic angiogram is not required at the second stage, given the MRI images from the first and second stages can be co-registered. More than two stages may be necessary to achieve complete obliteration depending on the nidus volume. A second strategy for large-volume AVMs is dose staging. Dose staging can be described as either a hypofractionated protocol or a repeat SRS. It is most often performed during LINAC-based treatments. Dosing and fractionation schedules vary widely. Moosa et al[70] compared outcomes after volume and dose staging of large (> 10 cm³) AVMs via a systematic literature review. Although complication rates were comparable, volume staging was twice as effective at achieving complete obliteration (47.5 vs. 22.8%, respectively).

Abla et al have proposed a unique approach whereby neoadjuvant volume-staged SRS is combined with delayed microsurgery to downgrade high-risk AVMs and offer an additional

Table 24.3 Select modifications to the SRS technique that have improved the safety and efficacy of the procedure

Adaptive modifications to the SRS technique for AVM treatment

Volume-staged AVM treatment

Volume-staged radiosurgical downgrading followed by microsurgery

Dose-staged AVM treatment (hypofractionation)

Repeat SRS

Avoidance of nidus-reducing endovascular embolization

Endovascular embolization of AVM-associated aneurysms

Abbreviations: AVM, arteriovenous malfunction; SRS, stereotactic radiosurgery.

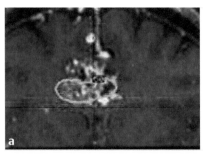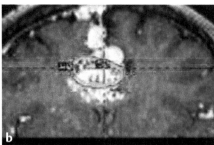

Fig. 24.2 Coronal-contrasted volumetric magnetic resonance imaging reconstructions showing the first (a) and second (b) stages of a volume-staged treatment for a larger deep-seated pericallosal arteriovenous malfunction.

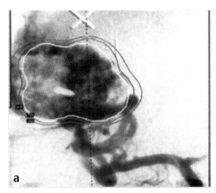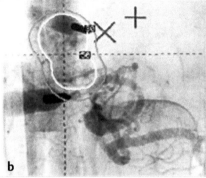

Fig. 24.3 Stereotactic angiographic images (a) at the time of first stereotactic radiosurgery (SRS) and (b) 4 years later at repeat SRS demonstrating a smaller persistent residual arteriovenous malfunction requiring additional treatment.

management strategy for select patients with very challenging AVMs.[71] In their retrospective series of 16 patients who underwent volume-staged SRS to high-risk surgical AVMs (Spetzler–Martin 4), SRS resulted in significantly downgrading the surgical risk (Spetzler–Martin 2.5). Fifteen of the AVMs were subsequently cured and 10 patients experience good outcomes. Such an approach has yet to be tested prospectively.

A repeat SRS procedure is often recommended if incomplete obliteration of an AVM nidus results after the initial treatment (▶ Fig. 24.3). Kano et al reported our repeat SRS protocol.[64] At the time of a repeat procedure, both high-definition MRI images and biplane stereotactic cerebral angiography are again obtained. Only the residual nidus is treated at the time of the repeat procedure. Similar prescription dose guidelines are followed at the repeat procedure. Margin doses may be increased by 1 to 2 Gy if the residual volume is smaller than the original volume, and they may be reduced by 1 to 2 Gy if the residual volume is larger than the original volume. Finally, in the setting of a patient who experienced a symptomatic ARE, a 1- to 2-Gy dose reduction was applied.

Endovascular embolization prior to SRS has been used to reduce the nidus size of larger AVMs in hopes of allowing for sufficient margin dosing to increase the benefit of treatment. This turns out not to be the case. Patients harboring AVMs without prior embolization are significantly more likely to experience complete obliteration than those who have had embolization.[72] Moreover, no significant protection from subsequent hemorrhage was detected in patients who underwent embolization. Several factors may contribute to the lower rates of obliteration seen after embolization plus SRS, including recanalization of previously occluded segments of AVM, more irregular dose planning, and obscuration of patent portions of AVM due to the presence of embolization material. At the present time, preradiosurgical embolization of AVMs is not preferred except in the presence of flow-related or intranidal aneurysms.

24.5 Conclusion

Radiosurgery is a powerful tool for the modern treatment of AVMs. AVMs represent a diverse and complex group of lesions that require tailored, individualized treatment strategies. Indications for radiosurgery have and will continue to evolve as our technologies improve and our understanding of the natural history and pathophysiology of AVMs increase. Radiosurgical techniques have changed to allow for the increased utility and safety of SRS in the treatment of AVMs. The initial results from the ARUBA trial did not meaningfully contribute to our knowledge on the role of SRS for the treatment of unruptured AVMs. Retrospective data from SRS-treated ARUBA-eligible patients suggest that in relatively younger patients the benefits of SRS may outweigh those of conservative treatment over the long term.

References

[1] Kim H, Su H, Weinsheimer S, Pawlikowska L, Young WL. Brain arteriovenous malformation pathogenesis: a response-to-injury paradigm. Acta Neurochir Suppl (Wien). 2011; 111:83–92

[2] Berman MF, Sciacca RR, Pile-Spellman J, et al. The epidemiology of brain arteriovenous malformations. Neurosurgery. 2000; 47(2):389–396, discussion 397

[3] Brown RD , Jr, Wiebers DO, Torner JC, O'Fallon WM. Frequency of intracranial hemorrhage as a presenting symptom and subtype analysis: a population-based study of intracranial vascular malformations in Olmsted Country, Minnesota. J Neurosurg. 1996; 85(1):29–32

[4] Brown RD , Jr, Wiebers DO, Forbes G, et al. The natural history of unruptured intracranial arteriovenous malformations. J Neurosurg. 1988; 68(3):352–357

[5] ApSimon HT, Reef H, Phadke RV, Popovic EA. A population-based study of brain arteriovenous malformation: long-term treatment outcomes. Stroke. 2002; 33(12):2794–2800

[6] Choi JH, Mast H, Sciacca RR, et al. Clinical outcome after first and recurrent hemorrhage in patients with untreated brain arteriovenous malformation. Stroke. 2006; 37(5):1243–1247

[7] Fults D, Kelly DL , Jr. Natural history of arteriovenous malformations of the brain: a clinical study. Neurosurgery. 1984; 15(5):658–662

[8] Halim AX, Johnston SC, Singh V, et al. Longitudinal risk of intracranial hemorrhage in patients with arteriovenous malformation of the brain within a defined population. Stroke. 2004; 35(7):1697–1702

[9] Ondra SL, Troupp H, George ED, Schwab K. The natural history of symptomatic arteriovenous malformations of the brain: a 24-year follow-up assessment. J Neurosurg. 1990; 73(3):387–391

[10] Stapf C, Mast H, Sciacca RR, et al. Predictors of hemorrhage in patients with untreated brain arteriovenous malformation. Neurology. 2006; 66(9):1350–1355

[11] Wedderburn CJ, van Beijnum J, Bhattacharya JJ, et al. SIVMS Collaborators. Outcome after interventional or conservative management of unruptured brain arteriovenous malformations: a prospective, population-based cohort study. Lancet Neurol. 2008; 7(3):223–230

[12] da Costa L, Wallace MC, Ter Brugge KG, O'Kelly C, Willinsky RA, Tymianski M. The natural history and predictive features of hemorrhage from brain arteriovenous malformations. Stroke. 2009; 40(1):100–105

[13] Hernesniemi JA, Dashti R, Juvela S, Väärt K, Niemelä M, Laakso A. Natural history of brain arteriovenous malformations: a long-term follow-up study of risk of hemorrhage in 238 patients. Neurosurgery. 2008; 63(5):823–829, discussion 829–831

[14] Itoyama Y, Uemura S, Ushio Y, et al. Natural course of unoperated intracranial arteriovenous malformations: study of 50 cases. J Neurosurg. 1989; 71(6):805–809

[15] Yamada S, Takagi Y, Nozaki K, Kikuta K, Hashimoto N. Risk factors for subsequent hemorrhage in patients with cerebral arteriovenous malformations. J Neurosurg. 2007; 107(5):965–972

[16] Graf CJ, Perret GE, Torner JC. Bleeding from cerebral arteriovenous malformations as part of their natural history. J Neurosurg. 1983; 58(3):331–337

[17] Waltimo O. The change in size of intracranial arteriovenous malformations. J Neurol Sci. 1973; 19(1):21–27

[18] Duong DH, Young WL, Vang MC, et al. Feeding artery pressure and venous drainage pattern are primary determinants of hemorrhage from cerebral arteriovenous malformations. Stroke. 1998; 29(6):1167–1176

[19] Marks MP, Lane B, Steinberg GK, Chang PJ. Hemorrhage in intracerebral arteriovenous malformations: angiographic determinants. Radiology. 1990; 176 (3):807–813

[20] Pollock BE, Flickinger JC, Lunsford LD, Bissonette DJ, Kondziolka D. Factors that predict the bleeding risk of cerebral arteriovenous malformations. Stroke. 1996; 27(1):1–6

[21] Spetzler RF, Martin NA. A proposed grading system for arteriovenous malformations. J Neurosurg. 1986; 65(4):476–483

[22] Davidson AS, Morgan MK. How safe is arteriovenous malformation surgery? A prospective, observational study of surgery as first-line treatment for brain arteriovenous malformations. Neurosurgery. 2010; 66(3):498–504, discussion 504–505

[23] Morgan MK, Rochford AM, Tsahtsarlis A, Little N, Faulder KC. Surgical risks associated with the management of Grade I and II brain arteriovenous malformations. Neurosurgery. 2004; 54(4):832–837, discussion 837–839

[24] Potts MB, Lau D, Abla AA, Kim H, Young WL, Lawton MT, UCSF Brain AVM Study Project. Current surgical results with low-grade brain arteriovenous malformations. J Neurosurg. 2015; 122(4):912–920

[25] Hartmann A, Pile-Spellman J, Stapf C, et al. Risk of endovascular treatment of brain arteriovenous malformations. Stroke. 2002; 33(7):1816–1820

[26] Gobin YP, Laurent A, Merienne L, et al. Treatment of brain arteriovenous malformations by embolization and radiosurgery. J Neurosurg. 1996; 85(1):19–28

[27] Ogilvy CS, Stieg PE, Awad I, et al. Special Writing Group of the Stroke Council, American Stroke Association. AHA Scientific Statement: recommendations for the management of intracranial arteriovenous malformations: a statement for healthcare professionals from a special writing group of the Stroke Council, American Stroke Association. Stroke. 2001; 32(6):1458–1471

[28] Ogilvy CS, Stieg PE, Awad I, et al. Stroke Council, American Stroke Association. Recommendations for the management of intracranial arteriovenous malformations: a statement for healthcare professionals from a special writing group of the Stroke Council, American Stroke Association. Circulation. 2001; 103(21):2644–2657

[29] Sinclair J, Kelly ME, Steinberg GK. Surgical management of posterior fossa arteriovenous malformations. Neurosurgery. 2006; 58(4) Suppl 2:ONS-189–ONS-201, discussion ONS-201

[30] Brown RD , Jr, Flemming KD, Meyer FB, Cloft HJ, Pollock BE, Link ML. Natural history, evaluation, and management of intracranial vascular malformations. Mayo Clin Proc. 2005; 80(2):269–281

[31] Debrun GM, Aletich V, Ausman JI, Charbel F, Dujovny M. Embolization of the nidus of brain arteriovenous malformations with n-butyl cyanoacrylate. Neurosurgery. 1997; 40(1):112–120, discussion 120–121

[32] Deruty R, Pelissou-Guyotat I, Amat D, et al. Complications after multidisciplinary treatment of cerebral arteriovenous malformations. Acta Neurochir (Wien). 1996; 138(2):119–131

[33] Frizzel RT, Fisher WS , III. Cure, morbidity, and mortality associated with embolization of brain arteriovenous malformations: a review of 1246 patients in 32 series over a 35-year period. Neurosurgery. 1995; 37(6):1031–1039, discussion 1039–1040

[34] Pasqualin A, Scienza R, Cioffi F, et al. Treatment of cerebral arteriovenous malformations with a combination of preoperative embolization and surgery. Neurosurgery. 1991; 29(3):358–368

[35] Paulsen RD, Steinberg GK, Norbash AM, Marcellus ML, Marks MP. Embolization of basal ganglia and thalamic arteriovenous malformations. Neurosurgery. 1999; 44(5):991–996, discussion 996–997

[36] Wikholm G, Lundqvist C, Svendsen P. Transarterial embolization of cerebral arteriovenous malformations: improvement of results with experience. AJNR Am J Neuroradiol. 1995; 16(9):1811–1817

[37] Taylor CL, Dutton K, Rappard G, et al. Complications of preoperative embolization of cerebral arteriovenous malformations. J Neurosurg. 2004; 100(5):810–812

[38] Kano H, Kondziolka D, Flickinger JC, et al. Aneurysms increase the risk of rebleeding after stereotactic radiosurgery for hemorrhagic arteriovenous malformations. Stroke. 2012; 43(10):2586–2591

[39] Mohr JP, Parides MK, Stapf C, et al. international ARUBA investigators. Medical management with or without interventional therapy for unruptured brain arteriovenous malformations (ARUBA): a multicentre, non-blinded, randomised trial. Lancet. 2014; 383(9917):614–621

[40] Al-Shahi Salman R, White PM, Counsell CE, et al. Scottish Audit of Intracranial Vascular Malformations Collaborators. Outcome after conservative management or intervention for unruptured brain arteriovenous malformations. JAMA. 2014; 311(16):1661–1669

[41] Rutledge WC, Abla AA, Nelson J, Halbach VV, Kim H, Lawton MT. Treatment and outcomes of ARUBA-eligible patients with unruptured brain arteriovenous malformations at a single institution. Neurosurg Focus. 2014; 37(3):E8

[42] Ding D, Starke RM, Kano H, et al. Radiosurgery for cerebral arteriovenous malformations in a randomized trial of unruptured brain arteriovenous malformations (ARUBA)-eligible patients: a multicenter study. Stroke. 2016; 47 (2):342–349

[43] Han PP, Ponce FA, Spetzler RF. Intention-to-treat analysis of Spetzler-Martin grades IV and V arteriovenous malformations: natural history and treatment paradigm. J Neurosurg. 2003; 98(1):3–7

[44] Kjellberg RN, Hanamura T, Davis KR, Lyons SL, Adams RD. Bragg-peak proton-beam therapy for arteriovenous malformations of the brain. N Engl J Med. 1983; 309(5):269–274

[45] Kjellberg RN. Stereotactic Bragg peak proton beam radiosurgery for cerebral arteriovenous malformations. Ann Clin Res. 1986; 18 Suppl 47:17–19

[46] Steiner L, Leksell L, Greitz T, Forster DM, Backlund EO. Stereotaxic radiosurgery for cerebral arteriovenous malformations. Report of a case. Acta Chir Scand. 1972; 138(5):459–464

[47] Betti OO, Munari C, Rosler R. Stereotactic radiosurgery with the linear accelerator: treatment of arteriovenous malformations. Neurosurgery. 1989; 24 (3):311–321

[48] Barcia-Salorio JL, Barcia JA, Soler F, Hernández G, Genovés JM. Stereotactic radiotherapy plus radiosurgical boost in the treatment of large cerebral arteriovenous malformations. Acta Neurochir Suppl (Wien). 1993; 58:98–100

[49] Colombo F, Benedetti A, Pozza F, Marchetti C, Chierego G. Linear accelerator radiosurgery of cerebral arteriovenous malformations. Neurosurgery. 1989; 24(6):833–840

[50] Loeffler JS, Alexander E , III, Siddon RL, Saunders WM, Coleman CN, Winston KR. Stereotactic radiosurgery for intracranial arteriovenous malformations using a standard linear accelerator. Int J Radiat Oncol Biol Phys. 1989; 17(3):673–677

[51] Friedman WA, Bova FJ, Mendenhall WM. Linear accelerator radiosurgery for arteriovenous malformations: the relationship of size to outcome. J Neurosurg. 1995; 82(2):180–189

[52] Schneider BF, Eberhard DA, Steiner LE. Histopathology of arteriovenous malformations after gamma knife radiosurgery. J Neurosurg. 1997; 87(3):352–357

[53] Kano H, Flickinger JC, Tonetti D, et al. Estimating the risks of adverse radiation effects after gamma knife radiosurgery for arteriovenous malformations. Stroke. 2017; 48(1):84–90

[54] Friedman WA, Bova FJ. Linear accelerator radiosurgery for arteriovenous malformations. J Neurosurg. 1992; 77(6):832–841

[55] Lunsford LD, Kondziolka D, Flickinger JC, et al. Stereotactic radiosurgery for arteriovenous malformations of the brain. J Neurosurg. 1991; 75(4):512–524

[56] Flickinger JC, Kondziolka D, Lunsford LD, et al. A multi-institutional analysis of complication outcomes after arteriovenous malformation radiosurgery. Int J Radiat Oncol Biol Phys. 1999; 44(1):67–74

[57] Flickinger JC, Kondziolka D, Pollock BE, Maitz AH, Lunsford LD. Complications from arteriovenous malformation radiosurgery: multivariate analysis and risk modeling. Int J Radiat Oncol Biol Phys. 1997; 38(3):485–490

[58] Flickinger JC, Lunsford LD, Kondziolka D, et al. Radiosurgery and brain tolerance: an analysis of neurodiagnostic imaging changes after gamma knife radiosurgery for arteriovenous malformations. Int J Radiat Oncol Biol Phys. 1992; 23(1):19–26

[59] Liscák R, Vladyka V, Simonová G, et al. Arteriovenous malformations after Leksell gamma knife radiosurgery: rate of obliteration and complications. Neurosurgery. 2007; 60(6):1005–1014, discussion 1015–1016

[60] Yamamoto Y, Coffey RJ, Nichols DA, Shaw EG. Interim report on the radiosurgical treatment of cerebral arteriovenous malformations. The influence of size, dose, time, and technical factors on obliteration rate. J Neurosurg. 1995; 83(5):832–837

[61] Kano H, Kondziolka D, Flickinger JC, et al. Stereotactic radiosurgery for arteriovenous malformations, Part 5: management of brainstem arteriovenous malformations. J Neurosurg. 2012; 116(1):44–53

[62] Kano H, Lunsford LD, Flickinger JC, et al. Stereotactic radiosurgery for arteriovenous malformations, Part 1: management of Spetzler-Martin Grade I and II arteriovenous malformations. J Neurosurg. 2012; 116(1):11–20

[63] Ding D, Xu Z, Shih HH, Starke RM, Yen CP, Sheehan JP. Stereotactic radiosurgery for partially resected cerebral arteriovenous malformations. World Neurosurg. 2016; 85:263–272

[64] Kano H, Kondziolka D, Flickinger JC, et al. Stereotactic radiosurgery for arteriovenous malformations, Part 3: outcome predictors and risks after repeat radiosurgery. J Neurosurg. 2012; 116(1):21–32

[65] Pollock BE, Link MJ, Brown RD. The risk of stroke or clinical impairment after stereotactic radiosurgery for ARUBA-eligible patients. Stroke. 2013; 44(2):437–441

[66] Turner RC, Lucke-Wold BP, Josiah D, et al. Stereotactic radiosurgery planning based on time-resolved CTA for arteriovenous malformation: a case report and review of the literature. Acta Neurochir (Wien). 2016; 158(8):1555–1562

[67] Lee CC, Reardon MA, Ball BZ, et al. The predictive value of magnetic resonance imaging in evaluating intracranial arteriovenous malformation obliteration after stereotactic radiosurgery. J Neurosurg. 2015; 123(1):136–144

[68] Pollock BE, Brown RD , Jr. Management of cysts arising after radiosurgery to treat intracranial arteriovenous malformations. Neurosurgery. 2001; 49(2):259–264, discussion 264–265

[69] Kano H, Kondziolka D, Flickinger JC, et al. Stereotactic radiosurgery for arteriovenous malformations, Part 6: multistaged volumetric management of large arteriovenous malformations. J Neurosurg. 2012; 116(1):54–65

[70] Moosa S, Chen CJ, Ding D, et al. Volume-staged versus dose-staged radiosurgery outcomes for large intracranial arteriovenous malformations. Neurosurg Focus. 2014; 37(3):E18

[71] Abla AA, Rutledge WC, Seymour ZA, et al. A treatment paradigm for high-grade brain arteriovenous malformations: volume-staged radiosurgical downgrading followed by microsurgical resection. J Neurosurg. 2015; 122(2):419–432

[72] Kano H, Kondziolka D, Flickinger JC, et al. Stereotactic radiosurgery for arteriovenous malformations after embolization: a case-control study. J Neurosurg. 2012; 117(2):265–275

25 Stereotactic Radiosurgery for Brain Arteriovenous Malformations

Or Cohen-Inbar, Dale Ding, and Jason P. Sheehan

Abstract

Brain arteriovenous malformations (AVMs) are rare, angioarchitecturally diverse vascular malformations that most frequently present with hemorrhage, seizure, headache, and focal neurological deficit. Left untreated, an AVM's rupture risk is approximately 2 to 4% annually, although certain factors, such as prior hemorrhage, deep location, deep venous drainage, and associated arterial aneurysms, have been shown to predispose AVMs to rupture. The management of AVMs is challenging and multifactorial, and a number of single-modality or multimodality therapies have been devised to treat these lesions. The primary goal of AVM treatment is complete obliteration of the nidus, which eliminates the risk of hemorrhage.

Stereotactic radiosurgery (SRS) is a minimally invasive alternative to resection and curative embolization for AVM intervention, and acts by inducing progressive endoluminal occlusion of nidal vasculature. Obliteration after SRS is achieved in approximately 70 to 80% of AVMs within 3 to 5 years of treatment, and is intimately related to nidus volume and SRS margin dose. Adverse radiation effects (ARE), defined as T2-weighted perinidal hyperintensities on magnetic resonance imaging, are radiologically evident in approximately one-third of patients after SRS. The rates of symptomatic and permanent ARE are approximately 10 and 2 to 3%, respectively. The risk of AVM hemorrhage persists during the latency period between SRS and nidal obliteration, and is comparable to or more benign than an untreated AVM's natural history. Large AVMs (diameter > 3 cm or volume > 12 cm^3) can be partially occluded with partial embolization prior to SRS, or treated with dose- or volume-staged SRS techniques. Pre-SRS embolization can also selectively occlude flow-related arterial aneurysms or intranidal arteriovenous fistulas.

Keywords: Gamma Knife, intracranial arteriovenous malformation, intracranial hemorrhages, radiosurgery, stroke, vascular malformations

- Stereotactic radiosurgery (SRS) is a minimally invasive alterative to microsurgical resection and curative embolization for the treatment of brain arteriovenous malformations (AVMs).
- The primary goal of SRS is obliteration of the AVM nidus; this can be achieved in approximately 70 to 80% of cases within 3 to 5 years of treatment, and obliteration is directly related to AVM volume and SRS margin dose.
- Adverse radiation effects (ARE) manifest as T2-weighted perinidal hyperintensities on magnetic resonance imaging, and they are radiologically evident in approximately one-third of patients after SRS; the rates of symptomatic and permanent ARE are approximately 10% and 2 to 3%, respectively.

- The risk of AVM hemorrhage persists during the latency period between SRS and nidal obliteration.
- Pre-SRS embolization can be employed to reduce the volume of large AVMs (diameter > 3 cm or volume > 12 cm^3) or to occlude associated arterial aneurysms or intranidal arteriovenous fistulas; however, embolized AVMs may have reduced the probability of SRS-induced obliteration.

25.1 Introduction

Cerebral arteriovenous malformations (AVMs) are rare congenital vascular malformations, consisting of an abnormal tangle of blood vessels within the intracranial space. AVM blood vessels shunt blood directly from arteries to veins without an intervening capillary bed, exposing the venous structures to abnormal hemodynamic forces.[1] The resultant abrupt transition from a high-pressure muscular arterial system to a low-pressure venous system results in venous dilatation and engorgement. Eventually, this process causes rupture of the AVM nidus, which is associated with significant morbidity and mortality.[2] Secondary processes evolving in time include vessel wall arterialization, with resultant edema and inflammation of the surrounding brain tissue.[3,4,5] Many patients suffer from the clinical manifestations of these pathological changes, such as focal neurological deficits and seizures.[6] The incidence of AVMs is similar for both genders, and they are typically diagnosed by early adulthood (third or fourth decades of life).[3] The incidence of cerebral AVMs is estimated to be in the order of 1.12 to 1.34 per 100,000 person-years.[7] Cerebral AVMs account for approximately 10% of subarachnoid hemorrhages and 1 to 2% of all strokes.[8] In the absence of treatment, the overall annual risk of a spontaneous hemorrhage from a cerebral AVM is approximately 2 to 4%, although this rate has been found to vary substantially depending on a number of patient- and AVM-specific factors.[3] In one study, the annual AVM hemorrhage rates ranged from 0.9% for low-risk patients (no history of prior AVM hemorrhage, superficial AVM location, AVM with a component of superficial venous drainage) to as high as 34.4% for high-risk patients (a history of prior AVM hemorrhage, deep AVM location, AVM with exclusively deep venous drainage).[5,6] The combination of a relatively young age at presentation and a nontrivial annual hemorrhage risk leads to a substantial lifetime risk of morbidity and mortality from untreated AVMs.[3,4]

AVMs continue to represent a significant clinical challenge, and expert opinions differ regarding the optimal management of AVMs.[9] Treatment goals also can vary among patients, and they might be directed toward reducing seizure activity, ameliorating symptomatic chronic "vascular steal," or alleviating neurological deficits caused by perinidal cerebral edema. However, the main goal of any intervention for AVMs is the complete obliteration of the nidus, thereby eliminating subsequent risk of hemorrhage. There currently exists significant controversy regarding the management of unruptured AVMs, with recent prospective studies reporting poorer short-term outcomes after intervention for unruptured AVMs compared to conservative management.[10,11] A randomized trial of unruptured brain arteriovenous malformations (ARUBA) reported significantly higher rates of symptomatic stroke and death in patients assigned to undergo intervention (31%) compared to those assigned to conservative management (10%) at a mean follow-up of 33 months.[10] The Scottish Audit of Intracranial Vascular Malformations prospective AVM cohort study similarly found that unruptured AVM patients who underwent intervention had significantly higher rates of death or sustained morbidity (defined as Oxford Handicap Scale ≥ 2 for ≥ 2 years at 4 years' follow-up and significantly higher rates of death or symptomatic stroke secondary to an AVM, associated aneurysm, or intervention at 12 years' follow-up).[11] A widely accepted view for the management of incidentally diagnosed AVMs is that the intervention is only justifiable if the risks of treatment-associated morbidity and mortality are less than those of the AVM's natural course.

Given its minimal invasiveness and favorable therapeutic profile, stereotactic radiosurgery (SRS) has emerged as an effective treatment for AVMs without immediate risk of hemorrhage.[12] Many small- or medium-sized (diameter < 3 cm or volume < 10–15 cm^3) AVMs that are deemed too risky for resection can be safely and completely obliterated by radiosurgery. Regardless of the SRS platform used (e.g., Gamma Knife, CyberKnife, Linear accelerator [LINAC] based system), AVM obliteration following radiosurgery ensues through progressive intimal thickening, thrombosis of irradiated vessels, and eventual occlusion of the vascular lumen.[13] The rate of obliteration, shown either on catheter cerebral angiography or magnetic resonance imaging (MRI), has been consistently reported to range from approximately 70 to 80% within 3 to 5 years of SRS in large, unselected cohorts.[9] Even for larger AVMs, some degree of AVM volume reduction typically occurs after SRS, thereby facilitating additional definitive treatment of the remaining nidus.[14] Additionally, some studies have suggested that SRS may confer partial protection from AVM hemorrhage during the latency period prior to complete obliteration.[15] The progressive thickening of vessel walls is postulated to reduce the tension within the vascular wall, acting to protect the nidus from rupture.[15]

25.1.1 Role of Pre-SRS AVM Embolization

Pre-SRS embolization is usually performed when an AVM nidus is too large (maximum diameter > 3 cm, volume > 10–15 cm^3) to treat with single-session SRS alone.[16] However, pre-SRS embolization has previously been reported to decrease the rate of AVM-nidus obliteration.[14,17] We found, in multivariate analysis, that pre-SRS embolization is an independent negative predictor of obliteration ($p < 0.001$).[6] One possible explanation is recanalization of the embolized portion of the nidus, which is not targeted with SRS.[18] Embolization can also make SRS more difficult if it treats parts of the nidus in multisegmented fashion rather than walling off a specific sector, transforming a compact nidus into a more diffuse one.

Some preclinical data suggest that embolic agents can scatter or absorb radiation, thereby reducing the effective radiosurgical dose to the targeted nidus.[19] However, Bing et al recently provided experimental data that contradict the notion of radiation beam scattering or absorption by embolic agents.[20] Another mechanism by which embolized AVMs are more susceptible to SRS treatment failure is embolization-induced angiogenesis, although the contribution of this biomolecular phenomenon to macroscopic outcomes is unknown.[21] In a matched cohort analysis of embolized and nonembolized AVMs treated with SRS, we found that, while the obliteration rate for the embolized AVM cohort was significantly lower than the nonembolized AVM cohort, the effect of prior embolization on post-SRS outcome was confounded by nidal angioarchitectural complexity (defined as the sum of the number of major feeding arteries and draining veins).[22] Finally, one should consider that inherent baseline differences between embolized and nonembolized AVMs may account for the disparities in outcomes after SRS.

25.1.2 Evaluation of Arteriovenous Malformation Obliteration

Catheter cerebral angiography continues to serve as the gold standard for confirming AVM obliteration after SRS, albeit its invasiveness makes it less ideal for routine follow-up. Consequently, most neurosurgeons prefer MRI for routine post-SRS follow-up, and use angiography to confirm obliteration after a lack of flow voids is observed on MRI. The authors previously conducted a study evaluating the sensitivity and specificity of MRI in evaluating AVM obliteration after SRS, compared to angiography.[23] The sensitivity was reported as 85 and 77% and the specificity was reported as 89 and 95% by two independent observers.[23] Therefore, MRI predicts AVM obliteration after SRS in the majority of patients and can be appropriately used in their follow-up.[23] Kano et al[24] suggested that the potential slight overestimation of obliteration rates as determined by MRI is balanced by the tendency to underestimate long-term obliteration rates based only on early follow-up examinations.[24] We advocate routine follow-up using MRI every 6 months for the first 2 years after SRS, unless there exists a clinical indication for more frequent evaluations (i.e., new or worsening neurological symptoms). Afterward, MRIs can be performed annually until obliteration is achieved, at which point we recommend angiography to confirm the lack of a residual nidus.

25.2 Results

25.2.1 Predicting Outcomes after SRS for AVMs

Arteriovenous Malformation Obliteration after SRS

The primary goal of SRS for AVMs is complete angiographic obliteration of the nidus. Nidal obliteration confers durable protection from future AVM hemorrhage. Flickinger et al performed a dose-response analysis for 197 AVM patients treated with SRS who had at least 3 years of post-treatment angiographic follow-up.[25] The median target volume was 4.1 cm^3, and the median treatment parameters were a minimum target dose (i.e., margin dose) of 20 Gy, maximum dose of 36 Gy, and isodose line of 50%, and two isocenters. AVM obliteration was achieved in 72% of cases. Of the 55 AVMs that did not undergo obliteration, 35 patients (64% of patent AVMs, 18% of overall study cohort) were determined to have a residual lesion due to persistent filling of untargeted portions of the original nidus. In the multivariate analysis for in-field obliteration, only margin dose ($p = 0.04$) was found to be an independent predictor.[1] Additionally, the authors constructed a sigmoid dose-response curve for obliteration, with margin doses of 13, 16, 20, and 25 Gy corresponding to obliteration rates of 50, 70, 90, and 98%, respectively. Margin dose was not significant in the multivariate analysis for overall AVM obliteration, in which only nidus volume ($p < 0.001$) was found to be predictive.

Spetzler–Martin Grade

Although the Spetzler–Martin (SM) grading system was originally devised with the intention of predicting outcomes after surgical resection of AVMs, it has also been shown to predict outcomes after SRS.[26] Andrade-Souza et al evaluated the outcomes of 136 AVMs treated with LINAC SRS and reported excellent outcome (complete AVM obliteration without new or worsening neurological deficit) in 89% of SM grade I AVMs, 70% of grade II AVMs, 62% of small grade III AVMs (diameter < 3 cm), and 45% of large grade III (diameter ≥ 3 cm) and grade IV AVMs.[27] Koltz et al analyzed a cohort of 102 AVM patients who underwent single session or dose-staged SRS and had at least 5 years of follow-up.[28] After a mean follow-up of 8.5 years, the obliteration rates, stratified by SM grade, were 100, 89, 86, 54, and 0% for grades I, II, III, IV, and V, respectively. The combined rate of major morbidity and mortality for SM grades I, II, III, IV, and V were 20, 11, 9, 18, and 75%, respectively.

In a cohort of 502 patients with SM grade I and II AVMs (median volume of 2.4 cm³) treated with SRS (median margin dose of 23 Gy) at our center with median radiologic and clinical follow-up durations of 48 and 62 months, obliteration was achieved in 76%, with actuarial rates of 41, 66, and 80% at 3, 5, and 10 years, respectively.[29] Radiologic, symptomatic, and permanent ARE developed in 37, 8, and 1%, respectively, and the annual rate of AVM hemorrhage during the post-SRS latency period was 1.4%. Kano et al reported the outcomes of 217 SM grade I and II AVMs (median volume of 2.3 cm³) treated with SRS (median margin dose of 22 Gy).[30] After a median follow-up of 64 months, the actuarial obliteration rate was 58, 90, and 93% at 3, 5, and 10 years, respectively. Symptomatic ARE developed in only 2% of patients, and all cases were transient. The annual post-SRS hemorrhage rate was 2.3%, and was significantly higher in AVMs with an associated arterial aneurysm.

In a cohort of 398 patients with SM grade III AVMs (median volume of 2.8 cm³) treated with SRS (median margin dose of 20 Gy) at our center with median radiologic and clinical follow-up durations of 54 and 68 months, obliteration was achieved in 69%, with actuarial rates of 38 and 60% at 3 and 5 years, respectively.[31] Radiologic, symptomatic, and permanent ARE developed in 35, 12, and 4%, respectively, and the annual rate of AVM hemorrhage during the post-SRS latency period was 1.7%. Kano et al analyzed the outcomes of 474 SM grade III AVMs (median volume of 3.8 cm³) treated with SRS (median margin dose of 20 Gy).[32] After a mean follow-up of 89 months, the actuarial obliteration rate was 48, 72, and 77% at 3, 5, and 10 years,

respectively. Symptomatic and permanent ARE developed in 6 and 3% of patients, respectively. The annual post-SRS hemorrhage rate was 2.7%.

In a cohort of 110 patients with SM grade IV and V AVMs (median volume of 5.7 cm³) treated with SRS (median margin dose of 19 Gy) at our center with median radiologic and clinical follow-up durations of 88 and 97 months, obliteration was achieved in 44%, with actuarial rates of 10 and 23% at 3 and 5 years, respectively.[33] Radiologic, symptomatic, and permanent ARE developed in 47, 12, and 3%, respectively, and the annual rate of AVM hemorrhage during the post-SRS latency period was 3.0%.

Radiosurgery-Based Arteriovenous Malformation Score

Pollock et al evaluated the outcomes of 220 AVM patients who underwent SRS.[34] Multivariate analysis found that smaller AVM nidus volume ($p = 0.003$), fewer number of draining veins ($p = 0.001$), younger patient age ($p = 0.0003$), hemispheric AVM location ($p = 0.002$), and lack of prior AVM embolization ($p = 0.02$) were independent predictors of excellent outcome, which was defined in this study as complete AVM obliteration without new neurological deficits. Based on this analysis, Pollock and Flickinger developed and externally validated the radiosurgery-based AVM score (RBAS), which comprised the variables AVM volume, patient age, and nidus location, to predict excellent outcome after AVM SRS.[35] The nidus location component of the RBAS was subsequently simplified into a two-tiered variable (deep vs. superficial) in the modified RBAS, wherein deep location comprised basal ganglia, thalamus, and brainstem.[36] The most recent version of the modified RBAS was described by Wegner et al and utilizes the same patient and AVM characteristics as the original RBAS, except the coefficient multiplier for the AVM location component was changed from 0.3 to 0.5.[37]

The RBAS has been shown to correlate with SRS outcomes in AVM cohorts from numerous centers.[27] Recently, Burrow et al analyzed the outcomes of 80 patients with an RBAS of 1 or lower (mean 0.76).[38] After a mean follow-up of 68 months, no patients experienced AVM hemorrhage, ARE, or a decline in modified Rankin scale (mRS) score. The obliteration rate for patients with at least 3 years of follow-up was 92%. The authors suggested that SRS may achieve comparable outcomes to resection for younger patients with superficial, small-volume AVMs who do not require surgical evacuation of a hematoma.[38]

However, the negative effect of patient age on AVM SRS outcomes, as suggested by the RBAS, is inconsistent. We performed a matched cohort study of 66 elderly AVM patients (age > 60 years) who underwent treatment with SRS and compared their outcomes to those of nonelderly patients, matched in a 1:1 ratio, with comparable AVMs.[39] The elderly AVM cohort had a significantly higher mean age (67 vs. 36 years, $p < 0.0001$), RBAS (1.70 vs. 1.11, $p < 0.0001$), and number of SRS isocenters (2.9 vs. 2.7, $p = 0.038$) compared to the nonelderly AVM cohort. Elderly age was not significantly associated with obliteration, ARE, or AVM hemorrhage after SRS. In summary, advanced age may not adversely affect AVM SRS outcomes, which contrasts with its negative impact on AVM surgical outcomes.[39]

Virginia Radiosurgery Arteriovenous Malformation Scale

We developed the Virginia Radiosurgery AVM Scale (VRAS) by analyzing our institutional Gamma Knife SRS experience of over 1,400 AVM patients treated over a period of 20 years.[6] Patients with at least 2 years of radiologic follow-up or those with less than 2 years of follow-up who developed treatment-related complications were selected, yielding 1,012 patients for analysis. Favorable outcome was defined as AVM obliteration, no post-SRS hemorrhage, and no permanently symptomatic ARE. The mean age was 34 years, and 56% had prior AVM hemorrhage. The mean AVM volume was 3.5 cm^3, including < 2 cm^3 in 20%, 2 to 4 cm^3 in 48%, and > 4 cm^3 in 32%. AVM location was eloquent in 67%, and 52% had a component of deep venous drainage. The SM grade was III or higher in 48%, and the mean RBAS was 1.35. The mean SRS margin dose was 21 Gy.

After a mean follow-up of 8 years, favorable outcome was achieved in 64% of patients. In the multivariate analysis of only patient and AVM variables (i.e., excluding SRS treatment parameters), age < 65 years (p = 0.041), smaller AVM volume (p < 0.001), noneloquent AVM location (p < 0.001), lack of prior AVM hemorrhage (p < 0.001), and lack of prior AVM embolization (p < 0.001) were found to be independent predictors of favorable outcome after SRS. Based on the significant factors in the multivariate model, the five-tiered VRAS was constructed, comprising AVM volume (< 2 cm^3 = 0 points, 2–4 cm^3 = 1 point, > 4 cm^3 = 2 points), eloquence of AVM location (noneloquent = 0 points, eloquent = 1 point), and history of AVM hemorrhage (unruptured = 0 points, ruptured = 1 point). The rates of favorable outcome for a VRAS of 0 to 1, 2, and 3 to 4 were 80, 70, and 45%, respectively.[6]

Since the VRAS is relatively new compared to the SM grading scale and RBAS, it has yet to be subjected to the same rigorous external testing as these two classification schemes. Recently, Huo et al analyzed a cohort of 162 patients with partially embolized AVMs who underwent SRS.[40] The VRAS was found be predictive of AVM obliteration (VRAS of 0–1, 2, 3, and 4 resulted in obliteration rates of 89, 68, 51, and 35%, respectively) and post-SRS complications, including hemorrhage, seizure, and headache (VRAS 0–2, 3, and 4 resulted in complication rates of 8, 24, and 29, respectively). We have performed an external validation of the VRAS in a multicenter cohort of over 2,000 AVM patients treated with SRS. The study was performed under the auspices of the International Gamma Knife Consortium, and the findings from this study demonstrate superiority of the VRAS over SM or RBAS systems in terms of predicting SRS outcomes in AVM patients. While SM grade and RBAS were significantly associated with AVM SRS outcomes, the VRAS was found to be the best predictor among the three grading systems.

25.2.2 Outcome of SRS for Different AVM Types

Primary Motor and Somatosensory Cortex AVMs

AVM nidus location carries tremendous prognostic significance when evaluating microsurgical or endovascular outcomes. Specific outcome data for primary motor or somatosensory cortex

(PMSC) AVMs is limited for all treatment modalities, including the radiosurgical literature.[41] We previously reported a series of 134 patients with PMSC AVMs who underwent SRS with median radiographic and clinical follow-up durations of 64 and 80 months, respectively.[41] The most common presenting symptoms were seizures (40%) and hemorrhage (28%), and 34% underwent pre-SRS embolization. The median AVM volume was 4.1 cm^3 (range: 0.1–22.6 cm^3), and the median margin dose was 20 Gy (range: 7–30 Gy).

The overall obliteration rate, determined by angiography or MRI, was 63%, stratified as 80% for small AVMs (volume < 3 cm^3) versus 55% for larger AVMs (volume > 3 cm^3). In the multivariate analysis, the lack of prior embolization (p = 0.002) and a single draining vein (p = 0.001) were found to be independent predictors of obliteration.[41] The cumulative obliteration rate for our cohort of PMSC AVMs was comparable to those of other series in the SRS literature (61–70%).[28,41,42] The obliteration rates, stratified by nidus size, were also similar to those of prior studies (83–87% for smaller AVMs with volume < 3 cm^3 and 50–56% for larger AVMs with volume > 3 cm^3).[28,41,42] The annual post-SRS hemorrhage risk of our PMSC AVM cohort was 2.5%, and SRS-related morbidity was transient and permanent in 14 and 6%, respectively. When we compared these PMSC AVMs to a matched cohort of noneloquent, lobar AVMs, we did not find statistically significant differences between the obliteration rates and clinical outcomes of the two cohorts.[41] SRS appears to offer a reasonable risk-to-benefit profile for these challenging lesions. Furthermore, eloquent location does not appear to confer the same negative prognostic value for SRS that it does for resection or embolization.[41] A literature review is given in ► Table 25.1.

SRS for Thalamic and Basal Ganglia AVMs

Deep-seated AVMs of the thalamus and basal ganglia constitute 4 to 11% of all cerebral AVMs,[4] and usually presenting at a younger age than AVMs in other locations.[43] The natural history of these AVMs tends to be more aggressive than that of lobar AVMs, with an annual hemorrhage risk approaching 10%.[5,43] A higher likelihood of rupture in these AVMs has been associated with the presence of deep venous drainage and a history of prior hemorrhage.[5] This predilection for hemorrhage is evident in the fact that up to 72 to 91% of basal ganglia and thalamic AVMs rupture prior to diagnosis.[43] The presence of adjacent critical neural pathways and nuclei results in significant morbidity and mortality associated with hemorrhage, steal phenomenon, or mass effect from these AVMs.

SRS has become the preferred therapy for small- to medium-sized AVMs of the basal ganglia and thalamus due to its minimally invasive nature and reasonable outcomes.[17,43,44,45] In a cohort of 60 patients with basal ganglia and thalamic AVMs, Sasaki et al[43] reported an 86% actuarial rate of complete obliteration at 2.5 years. Pollock et al[17] and Andrade-Souza et al[44] found lower obliteration rates. Pollock et al[17] analyzed a cohort of 56 patients with basal ganglia (n = 10), thalamic (n = 30), and brainstem (n = 16) AVMs, and reported complete obliteration in 43% after a median follow-up of 45 months. The actuarial obliteration rates at 3 and 4 years were 47 and 66%, respectively. These modest obliteration rates were attributed to a lower margin dose (median 18 Gy). Kano et al[46] reported a cohort of

Table 25.1 Stereotactic radiosurgery for arteriovenous malfunction review of major series

Authors	Year	N	Volume (cm³)	MD[a] (Gy)	Obliteration rate[b] (%)	Hemorrhage (%)	ARE (%)	M/M[c] (%)
Touboul et al[68]	1998	100	1.9	19	51	10	1[d]	8/NR
Chang et al[69]	2000	128	12.1	16	79	7	12,[e] 5,[f] 0.4[d]	5.4/NR
Schlienger et al[70]	2000	169	2.5	25	64	2	0.6[d]	2/NR
Massager et al[71]	2000	87	1.3	21.3	73[g]	3.4	5[d]	5/NR
Flickinger et al[72]	2002	351	5.7	20	75	NR	NR	NR
Friedman et al[73]	2003	269	8.4	NR	53	10	NR	5/NR
Bollet et al[74]	2004	118	7.4	18	54	1.7[h]	NR	7/NR
Shin et al[75]	2004	400	1.9	20	74,[g] 88[i]	1.9[h]	7,[f] 2[d]	NR
Liscák et al[76]	2007	330	3.9	20	92	2.1[h]	21,[e] 8[f]	3/1
Colombo et al[77]	2009	102	5.2	19	72	8	NR	1/1
Taeshineetanakul et al[78]	2012	139	3.8	19	66	NR	NR	NR
Fokas et al[79]	2013	164	4	19	61	1.3[h]	NR	5/NR
Franzin et al[80]	2013	127	2.7	22	69	2.1[h]		7/4
Starke et al[6]	2013	1,012	3.5	21	69	1.1[h]	38,[e] 10[f], 2[d]	NR
Hattangadi-Gluth et al[81]	2014	248	3.5	15	65	5	NR	1/1
Missios et al[82]	2014	152	6.3	18	46	4	23,[f] 2[d]	2/2
Paúl et al[83]	2014	662	3.6	19	75	1.2[h]	NR	4/2
Wang et al[84]	2014	116	4.7	NR	82	1.9[h]	5[f]	7
Cheng et al[85]	2012	182	3.4	21.3	57.7	11.5/2.9[h]	4.9[f]	4.9/NR
Kano et al[46]	2012	133	2.7	20	72[j]	11/6.3[h]	4.5[f]	4.5/NR

Abbreviations: ARE, adverse radiation effects (perinidal T2-weighted hyperintensities on follow-up magnetic resonance imaging [MRI]); NR, not reported.

Note: Predictors based on multivariate analysis, when available. Unknown if significant factors were derived from univariate or multivariate analysis.

[a]MD, margin dose. Mean values were preferentially reported; when a mean value was not available, the median was reported.

[b]Included obliteration determined by MRI alone and confirmed by angiography.

[c]Morbidity/mortality.

[d]Permanent.

[e]Radiologic.

[f]Symptomatic.

[g]Actuarial obliteration rate at 3 years.

[h]Annual hemorrhage rate.

[i]Actuarial obliteration rate at 5 years.

[j]Actuarial obliteration rate at 4 years.

133 patients with basal ganglia and thalamic AVMs, 85% of which had a prior hemorrhage. The actuarial obliteration rates at 3 and 5 years were 57 and 72%, respectively. Factors significantly associated with obliteration were basal ganglia AVM location, smaller nidus volume, and higher margin dose. The actuarial post-SRS hemorrhage rates at 1, 2, 3, 5, and 10 years were 4.5, 6.2, 9.0, 11.2, and 15.4%, respectively, with an annual post-SRS hemorrhage rate of 4.7%. Permanently symptomatic ARE developed in 4.5%.[46] A literature review is given in ▶ Table 25.1.

Stereotactic Radiosurgery for Brainstem Arteriovenous Malformations

Brainstem AVMs constitute 2 to 6% of cerebral AVMs.[47] Similar to basal ganglia and thalamic AVMs, posterior fossa (brainstem and cerebellum) AVMs have a significantly higher rate of hemorrhagic presentation than supratentorial lobar AVMs.[48] The natural history untreated brainstem AVMs is associated with a high risk of major morbidity or mortality secondary to hemorrhage.[3,24,44,48] Kiran et al[49] reported an 81% incidence of hemorrhagic presentation in patients with deep-seated AVMs of the basal ganglia, thalamus, and brainstem. No single management option is applicable to all brainstem AVMs.[45] However, most of the SRS literature for brainstem AVMs supports a lower rate of treatment-related morbidity than surgical resection, ranging from 5 to 12%.[17,47,50]

Many authors reported a significantly higher obliteration rate when employing a margin dose of at least 20 Gy.[45,47,50] In one study, the actuarial obliteration rate at 3 years was reported to be 69% in nidi treated with a margin dose of 18 to 20 Gy versus 14% in nidi receiving < 18 Gy.[50] The radiation tolerance limit of the brainstem remains controversial, despite the development of numerous predictive models.[50] A higher margin dose, albeit more effective in attaining obliteration, may cause severe symptomatic ARE in patients with brainstem AVMs, and thus the dose should be carefully selected. We analyzed a cohort of

85 brainstem AVMs treated with SRS.[45] The median AVM volume and margin dose were 1.4 cm[3] (range: 0.1–8.9 cm[3]) and 20 Gy, respectively. The median follow-up duration was 102 months (range: 24–252 months). Repeat SRS for residual nidi was performed in 21% of patients. Two patients underwent a third SRS session 7 and 16 years after a failed repeat SRS procedure. Obliteration was noted in 59%, with actuarial obliteration rates of 46 and 61% at 3 and 5 years, respectively. In congruence with other reports, higher margin dose ($p = 0.001$) and smaller nidus volume ($p = 0.026$) were found to be significantly associated with obliteration. Asymptomatic ARE were radiologically evident in 28%, and permanent neurological deficits occurred in 11%.[45] A literature review is given in ▸ Table 25.1.

Stereotactic Radiosurgery for Large Arteriovenous Malformations

The optimal management of large (> 10–15 cm[3]) AVMs is controversial. High rates of morbidity and mortality plague all treatment modalities, including surgical resection,[51] embolization,[52] and SRS. Large and SM grade IV and V AVMs continue to present management challenges for intervention with SRS due to their longer latency periods and lower obliteration rates.[33,52] While the obliteration rate remains intimately related to the total radiation dose administered to the nidus,[53] treating large AVMs with traditionally effective margin doses frequently results in an unacceptable high risk of ARE.[51,53] Modern treatment strategies for large-volume AVMs employ the delivery of the radiation doses in multiple fractions, with either dose- or volume-staged SRS.

Dose-staged SRS is performed by administering several smaller doses of radiation (typically 5–6 Gy) to the entire AVM nidus over a period of a few weeks. Volume-staged SRS divides the AVM nidus into distinct geometric sections, and each section is then treated separately with a substantially higher those than can be safely administered to the entire AVM nidus. Each volume-staged treatment is separated by 3 to 6 months. Both hypofractionated (i.e., dose-staged) and volume-staged SRS have been shown to be as effective as single-session SRS for large AVMs, with reduced rates of complication.[51] Pollock et al[54] compared volume-staged to single-session SRS procedures and found that volume staging resulted in less radiation exposure to the adjacent brain.[54]

A systematic review of dose- and volume-staged SRS for the treatment of large (volume > 10 cm[3]) AVMs was recently performed.[51] The mean complete obliteration rates for dose- and volume-staged SRS were 23 and 48%, respectively. Obliteration was achieved in 19 and 49% of patients in the dose- and volume-staged groups, respectively. Symptomatic radiosurgery imaging changes (RICs) were reported in 13.5% and 13.6% in the dose-staged and volume-staged SRS cohorts, respectively. The mean rates of post-SRS latency period hemorrhage were 12 and 18% for the dose- and volume-staged SRS cohorts, respectively.[51] Based on that analysis, it appears that volume-staged SRS affords higher obliteration rates and similar complication rates compared to dose-staged SRS, and thus, volume staging may be the superior approach for large AVMs that are not amenable to single-session SRS.[51]

Another potential approach, recently reported by Abla et al,[55] is the use of upfront volume-staged SRS to downgrade large AVMs so that the shrunken nidus can be definitively treated with resection. The authors treated a cohort of 16 supratentorial AVMs with this combined approach. The mean initial SM and supplemented SM grades were 4 and 7.1, respectively. The mean number of volume-staged SRS sessions was 2.7 (range: 2–5), and the mean time interval between first SRS session and microsurgical resection was 5.7 years. The mean SM and supplemented SM grades were reduced to 2.5 and 5.6, respectively; volume-staged SRS resulted in a downgrading of 1.5 grades for each classification system. The maximum median AVM diameter was reduced by 3.0 cm (reduced by 2.9 cm). Therefore, volume-staged SRS can reduce the size of large AVMs, transforming high-grade, inoperable AVMs into low- and intermediate-grade, operable lesions with acceptable surgical risks.[55] A literature review is given in ▸ Table 25.1. An example patient is shown in ▸ Fig. 25.1.

25.2.3 Role of SRS in the Management of Unruptured AVMs

The management of unruptured AVMs is controversial. While some experts recommend therapeutic intervention, others endorse conservative management.[5,42] Furthermore, for incidentally diagnosed AVMs that are asymptomatic, any intervention is prophylactic and, therefore, only justifiable if the risks of treatment-related morbidity and mortality do not exceed those of the AVM's natural history. Such controversy led to ARUBA, which attempted to evaluate the difference in outcome between unruptured AVM patients randomized to medical therapy with or without intervention. Medically managed patients were found to have a significantly lower short-term risk of death or symptomatic stroke based on the interim analysis (mean follow-up duration of 33 months). These conclusions have been extensively disputed based on methodological flaws inherent to ARUBA's study design and analysis. Although unruptured AVMs have a more favorable natural history than ruptured lesions, their annual hemorrhage risk is not negligible, and it was noted to be 2.2% in the medical arm of ARUBA.[4] Thus, depending on an AVM's angioarchitecture and location, it may still cause significant long-term morbidity and mortality, even the absence of prior hemorrhage.

We analyzed a cohort of 444 unruptured AVMs treated with SRS.[42] The mean AVM volume was 4.2 cm[3], 14% of nidi were in a deep location, and the SM grade was III or higher in 44%. The median margin dose was 20 Gy. After mean radiologic and clinical follow-up durations of 76 and 86 months, respectively, obliteration was achieved in 62%, with actuarial obliteration rates of 30 and 53% at 3 and 5 years, respectively. In the multivariate analysis, a lack of prior embolization ($p < 0.001$), a single draining vein ($p < 0.001$), lower SM grade ($p = 0.016$), higher margin dose ($p < 0.001$), and the development of radiologic ARE ($p = 0.004$) were found to be independent predictors of obliteration. The annual post-SRS hemorrhage rate was 1.6%. ARE were radiologically evident, symptomatic, and permanent in 49, 14, and 2%, respectively.[42] SRS appears to offer a reasonable risk-to-benefit profile for the treatment of unruptured AVMs.[42]

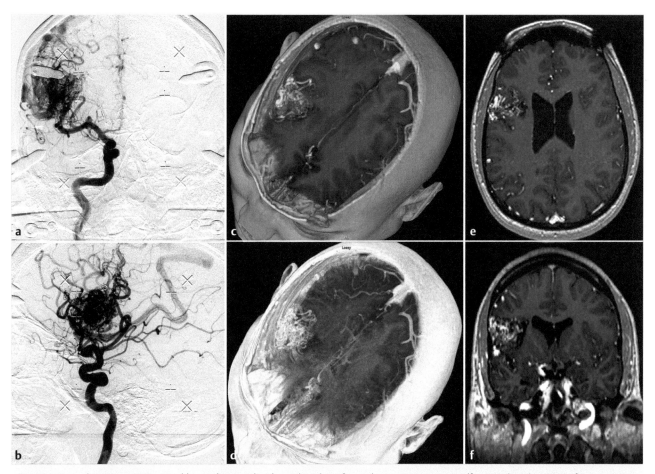

Fig. 25.1 Example patient. A 38-year-old man diagnosed with a right Sylvian fissure large arteriovenous malfunction (AVM) in 2006 after presenting with seizures and related hemorrhage. He underwent several embolizations that did not result in obliteration. **(a–f)** Images taken at the time of stereotactic radiosurgery. GKRS 2012. **(a,b)** Angiography in anteroposterior (AP) and lateral views, respectively, showing a large AVM. **(c,d)** 3D reconstruction of the magnetic resonance angiography. **(e,f)** T1WI in axial and coronal views (*continued*).

However, there is no high level of evidence that the outcomes of any AVM treatment are superior to conservative management for unruptured AVMs. A literature review is given in ▶ Table 25.1.

25.2.4 SRS for Intracranial Dural Arteriovenous Fistulas

The management of intracranial dural arteriovenous fistulas (DAVFs) differs from that of intraparenchymal AVMs, and thus, the role of SRS in the treatment of DAVFs is also different.[56] When intervention for a DAVF is indicated (i.e., presence of venous reflux into a dural venous sinus, cortical venous reflux, direct cortical venous drainage (CVD), or cortical venous ectasia), the first-line treatment is embolization from a transvenous or transarterial endovascular approach in most cases. Generally, only DAVFs that have failed initial treatment with embolization and/or surgical ligation are referred for SRS. Due to the uncommon occurrence of DAVFs and primary use of SRS as a salvage therapy in many cases, the literature regarding DAVF SRS outcomes is relatively sparse compared to that of AVMs. We

analyzed a cohort of 55 patients with DAVFs treated at our center, with a 36% incidence of hemorrhagic presentation.[57] The Borden grade was I, II, and III in 29, 22, and 49%, respectively. Prior interventions included embolization in 65% and microsurgery in 20%. The median margin dose was 21 Gy. Follow-up angiography was available in 83% of patients, and obliteration was achieved in 65%. Post-SRS hemorrhage occurred in 5%, but none resulted in permanent neurological deficits.

We recently performed a systematic review of SRS outcomes for DAVFs, which yielded 19 studies comprising 729 patients and 743 DAVFs.[58] The mean obliteration rate was 63% (95% confidence interval [CI]: 52–74%). The rates of post-SRS hemorrhage, new or worsened neurological symptoms, and mortality were 1.2, 1.3, and 0.3%, respectively. Compared to cavernous sinus (CS) DAVFs, non-CS DAVFs had a lower obliteration rate (73 vs. 58%, respectively) and a higher post-SRS hemorrhage rate (0 vs. 1.3%, respectively), although these differences were not statistically significant. Compared to DAVFs without CVD, DAVFs with CVD had significantly lower obliteration rates (75 vs. 56%, respectively; $p = 0.03$). The post-SRS hemorrhage rates of DAVFs with and without CVD were 4.2 and 0%, respectively.

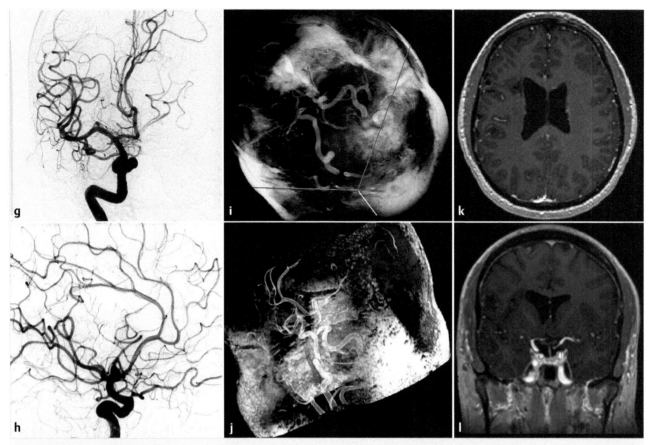

Fig. 25.1 (*continued*) (**g–l**) Images taken 3 years after SRS showing complete obliteration. (**g,h**) Angiography in AP and lateral views, respectively, showing complete obliteration. (**i,j**) 3D reconstruction of the MRA. (**k,l**) T1WI in axial and coronal views.

25.3 Discussion

25.3.1 Complications after SRS for AVMs

Adverse Radiation Effects

The most common SRS-induced complication is radiologically evident ARE, otherwise known as RICs. ARE are common after AVM radiosurgery, and occur in approximately one-third of patients. Most radiologic ARE are asymptomatic. Symptomatic ARE occur in approximately 10% of patients, and those with permanent symptoms comprise only 2 to 3% of patients.

Flickinger et al analyzed the ARE profile of 307 AVM patients treated with SRS who had at least 24 months of follow-up (median duration 44 months).[59] Radiologic and symptomatic ARE were evident in 30 and 9% of patients, respectively. The development of post-SRS ARE typically precedes obliteration, and the median time to onset of radiologic and symptomatic ARE in this cohort was 12 and 14 months, respectively. Only 3% of patients in this study had radiologic ARE that failed to resolve after 2 years. The actuarial resolution rate of radiologic ARE was 81% at 3 years, with a median time to resolution of 12 months. Notably, the actuarial radiologic ARE resolution rate at 3 years was significantly lower in symptomatic compared to asymptomatic patients (95 vs. 53%, respectively; $p = 0.03$). In the multivariate analysis, only the 12-Gy volume ($p < 0.0001$) was

independently associated with radiologic ARE. In a separate multivariate analysis for predictors of symptomatic ARE, both 12-Gy volume (V12; $p = 0.001$) and brainstem location ($p = 0.007$) were significant.[59]

Latency Period Hemorrhage

Two aspects of latency period hemorrhage are controversial in the AVM SRS literature. The first is how the latency period hemorrhage rate compares to that of the natural history hemorrhage risk prior to SRS. Specifically, is the post-SRS hemorrhage rate higher, lower, or the same as the AVM's natural history hemorrhage risk? The second is whether the risk of AVM hemorrhage persists after complete angiographic AVM obliteration.

Maruyama et al analyzed a cohort of 500 AVM patients treated with SRS, with a median observation period of 7.8 years, including a median of 0.4 years from diagnosis to SRS, 2.0 years from SRS to obliteration, and 5.4 years after obliteration.[60] The frequency of hemorrhage was 8.4% from diagnosis to SRS, 5.0% from SRS to obliteration, and 2.4% after obliteration. Follow-up angiography in all six patients with postobliteration hemorrhage did not show evidence of AVM recanalization. The mortality rate of those who suffered post-SRS hemorrhage was 24% (7/29 patients). Compared to the pre-SRS hemorrhage risk, the risk of hemorrhage was reduced by 54% after SRS (hazard ratio: 0.46; 95% CI: 0.26–0.80; $p = 0.006$) and by 88% after obliteration (hazard ratio: 0.12; 95% CI: 0.05–0.29; $p < 0.001$). Compared to latency period hemorrhage risk between SRS and obliteration, the risk of hemorrhage was reduced by 74% after obliteration (hazard ratio: 0.26; 95% CI: 0.10–0.68; $p = 0.006$). Patients with ruptured AVMs had significantly greater reductions in hemorrhage risk after SRS compared to those with unruptured AVMs. Among ruptured AVMs ($N = 310$), the annual post-SRS hemorrhage rates at 1, 2, 3, and greater than 3 years were 6.3, 6.8, 6.4, and 6.3%, respectively.

We analyzed a cohort of 1,204 AVM patients treated with SRS at our center.[15] The annual pre-SRS hemorrhage risk from birth to SRS was 2.0%, including 3.7% for patients with prior hemorrhage. The annual pre-SRS hemorrhage risk from diagnosis to SRS was 6.6%, including 10.4 and 3.9% for patients with and without prior hemorrhage, respectively. The annual post-SRS hemorrhage rate was 2.5%, including 2.8 and 2.2% for patients with and without prior hemorrhage, respectively. In the multivariate analysis, only lower margin dose ($p = 0.046$) was found to be an independent predictor of postradiosurgery hemorrhage.

Kano et al evaluated a cohort of 407 patients with ruptured AVMs who underwent SRS, with a median follow-up of 66 months (range: 2–274 months).[61] The annual hemorrhage risks from birth to SRS and from diagnosis to SRS were 3.4 and 16.5%, respectively. The annual post-SRS hemorrhage rate was 1.3%. Of the 29 patients with a single post-SRS hemorrhage, 12 died (mortality rate: 41%) at a median follow-up of 22 months. All three patients with two post-SRS hemorrhages died (mortality rate: 100%). In the multivariate analysis, the presence of a patent AVM-associated arterial aneurysm ($p < 0.0001$) and lower margin dose ($p < 0.0005$) were found to be independent predictors of post-SRS hemorrhage. AVMs with a patent prenidal or intranidal aneurysm had a significantly higher post-SRS hemorrhage rate than AVMs an associated aneurysm, which was occluded (i.e., by surgical clipping or embolization) prior to SRS (6.4 vs. 0.8% per year, $p = 0.033$). In this cohort, there were no hemorrhages after obliteration.

25.3.2 Repeat Stereotactic Radiosurgery for AVM's Residuals

As long as the AVM nidus remains patent, the risk of hemorrhage persists, and further management is warranted. Generally repeat SRS should be considered if the AVM is patent 3 to 4 years after a prior SRS. There is limited evidence regarding the efficacy of repeat SRS for AVMs. Rates of complete obliteration after repeat SRS previously reported by our group have been lower than from the initial SRS procedure, although this approach remains a reasonable treatment option for residual AVMs.[45] Additionally, in many cases, the first SRS procedure that fails to obliterate the AVM still results in volume reduction of the nidus, which may facilitate the success of a second SRS procedure. The role, safety, and efficacy of repeat SRS or microsurgical resection for incompletely obliterated AVMs have yet to be completely defined.[62]

25.3.3 Seizure Outcomes after Stereotactic Radiosurgery for AVMs

Seizures are the second most frequent presentation of brain AVMs, following hemorrhage, and are the most common presentation of unruptured AVMs. Although the primary goal of AVM treatment is obliteration of the nidus to eliminate the risk of hemorrhage, seizure outcomes also affect a patient's long-term neurological function and quality of life. Baranoski et al performed a meta-analysis of seizure outcomes stratified by treatment modality.[63] AVMs treated with microsurgery had the highest rates of seizure control (78%; 95% CI: 70–86%), followed by SRS (63%; 95% CI: 55–70%) and embolization (49%; 95% CI: 32–67%). However, SRS-treated patients with AVM obliteration had a higher rate of seizure control than surgically treated AVMs (85%; 95% CI: 79–91%). The rates of de novo seizures after treatment were highest for embolization (39%; 95% CI: 8–68%), followed by microsurgery (9%; 95% CI: 5–13%) and SRS (5%; 95% CI: 3–8%).[63]

Wang et al compared the seizure outcomes of AVMs treated with resection versus SRS, and found divergent seizure outcomes based on preoperative seizure status.[64] Patients with preoperative seizures were significantly more likely to have seizure recurrence (overall rate of 60%) after SRS (odds ratio of 4.3; 95% CI: 1.2–15.0; $p = 0.021$). However, patients without preoperative seizures were significantly more likely to have de novo seizures (overall rate of 18%) after resection (odds ratio of 8.7; 95% CI: 3.1–24.5; $p < 0.001$). In this cohort, AVM obliteration was significantly associated with seizure freedom ($p = 0.002$). We performed a systematic review of seizure outcomes in AVM patients treated with SRS reviewing 19 studies and 3,971 patients.[65] The incidence of seizure presentation was 28%, and the rates of seizure freedom and seizure control after SRS were 44 and 69%, respectively. Seizure freedom was significantly more common in obliterated AVMs than patent AVMs (82 vs. 41%, respectively; $p = 0.0007$).

We analyzed a cohort of 1,007 AVM patients who underwent SRS at our center for factors associated with seizure presentation and seizure outcomes. The incidence of seizure presentation was 23%, which was significantly higher for cortical compared to noncortical AVMs (33 vs. 6%, respectively; $p < 0.0001$).[66] Of cortical locations, seizure presentation was significantly less common in occipital AVMs (22%; $p = 0.0012$) compared to those located in the frontal (37%), temporal (38%), and parietal (34%) lobes. In the multivariate analysis, a lack of prior AVM hemorrhage ($p < 0.0001$), larger nidus diameter ($p < 0.0001$), and cortical location ($p < 0.0001$) were independent predictors of seizure presentation. In patients with seizure presentation ($N = 229$), the rates of seizure improvement and remission were 57 and 20%, respectively.[67] In the multivariate analysis, prior AVM hemorrhage ($p = 0.015$), longer follow-up duration ($p < 0.0001$), and a lack of post-SRS hemorrhage ($p = 0.048$) were independent predictors of seizure improvement. In this analysis, AVM obliteration was not predictive of seizure improvement. Based on the low risk of de novo seizures after SRS for AVM patients without a history of seizures, the administration of prophylactic anticonvulsants does not appear warranted.

25.4 Conclusion

SRS affords predictable treatment outcomes for AVM patients, with a reasonable risk-to-benefit profile for most lesions, and yields favorable results with respect to obliteration, hemorrhage risk, and seizure control. It is a preferred therapeutic modality for small- to medium-sized AVMs located in deep or eloquent brain regions. The SM grade, RBAS, and VRAS can be utilized to predict radiologic and clinical outcomes after AVM SRS. The SRS outcomes for large AVMs (diameter > 3 cm or volume > 10–15 cm^3) are less optimal. For these lesions, pre-SRS embolization to achieve volume reduction, hypofractionated (dose-staged) SRS, or volume-staged SRS may be viable approaches to achieve acceptable obliteration rates while limiting treatment-related morbidity. Residual AVMs that remain patent 3 to 4 years after the initial SRS procedure can be managed with repeat SRS or resection.

References

[1] Atkinson RP, Awad IA, Batjer HH, et al. Joint Writing Group of the Technology Assessment Committee American Society of Interventional and Therapeutic Neuroradiology; Joint Section on Cerebrovascular Neurosurgery a Section of the American Association of Neurological Surgeons and Congress of Neurological Surgeons; Section of Stroke and the Section of Interventional Neurology of the American Academy of Neurology. Reporting terminology for brain arteriovenous malformation clinical and radiographic features for use in clinical trials. Stroke. 2001; 32(6):1430–1442

[2] Hartmann A, Mast H, Mohr JP, et al. Morbidity of intracranial hemorrhage in patients with cerebral arteriovenous malformation. Stroke. 1998; 29(5):931–934

[3] Ondra SL, Troupp H, George ED, Schwab K. The natural history of symptomatic arteriovenous malformations of the brain: a 24-year follow-up assessment. J Neurosurg. 1990; 73(3):387–391

[4] Brown RD , Jr, Wiebers DO, Forbes G, et al. The natural history of unruptured intracranial arteriovenous malformations. J Neurosurg. 1988; 68(3):352–357

[5] Stapf C, Mast H, Sciacca RR, et al. Predictors of hemorrhage in patients with untreated brain arteriovenous malformation. Neurology. 2006; 66(9):1350–1355

[6] Starke RM, Yen CP, Ding D, Sheehan JP. A practical grading scale for predicting outcome after radiosurgery for arteriovenous malformations: analysis of 1012 treated patients. J Neurosurg. 2013; 119(4):981–987

[7] Al-Shahi R, Bhattacharya JJ, Currie DG, et al. Scottish Intracranial Vascular Malformation Study Collaborators. Scottish Intracranial Vascular Malformation Study (SIVMS): evaluation of methods, ICD-10 coding, and potential sources of bias in a prospective, population-based cohort. Stroke. 2003; 34 (5):1156–1162

[8] Perret G, Nishioka H. Report on the cooperative study of intracranial aneurysms and subarachnoid hemorrhage. Section VI. Arteriovenous malformations. An analysis of 545 cases of cranio-cerebral arteriovenous malformations and fistulae reported to the cooperative study. J Neurosurg. 1966; 25 (4):467–490

[9] Cohen-Inbar O, Lee CC, Xu Z, Schlesinger D, Sheehan JP. A quantitative analysis of adverse radiation effects following Gamma Knife radiosurgery for arteriovenous malformations. J Neurosurg. 2015; 123(4):945–953

[10] Mohr JP, Parides MK, Stapf C, et al. international ARUBA investigators. Medical management with or without interventional therapy for unruptured brain arteriovenous malformations (ARUBA): a multicentre, non-blinded, randomised trial. Lancet. 2014; 383(9917):614–621

[11] Al-Shahi Salman R, White PM, Counsell CE, et al. Scottish Audit of Intracranial Vascular Malformations Collaborators. Outcome after conservative management or intervention for unruptured brain arteriovenous malformations. JAMA. 2014; 311(16):1661–1669

[12] Yen CP, Ding D, Cheng CH, Starke RM, Shaffrey M, Sheehan J. Gamma Knife surgery for incidental cerebral arteriovenous malformations. J Neurosurg. 2014; 121(5):1015–1021

[13] Chang SD, Shuster DL, Steinberg GK, Levy RP, Frankel K. Stereotactic radiosurgery of arteriovenous malformations: pathologic changes in resected tissue. Clin Neuropathol. 1997; 16(2):111–116

[14] Pollock BE, Meyer FB. Radiosurgery for arteriovenous malformations. J Neurosurg. 2004; 101(3):390–392, discussion 392

[15] Yen CP, Sheehan JP, Schwyzer L, Schlesinger D. Hemorrhage risk of cerebral arteriovenous malformations before and during the latency period after GAMMA knife radiosurgery. Stroke. 2011; 42(6):1691–1696

[16] Sirin S, Kondziolka D, Niranjan A, Flickinger JC, Maitz AH, Lunsford LD. Prospective staged volume radiosurgery for large arteriovenous malformations:

[17] Pollock BE, Gorman DA, Brown PD. Radiosurgery for arteriovenous malformations of the basal ganglia, thalamus, and brainstem. J Neurosurg. 2004; 100 (2):210–214

[18] Saatci I, Geyik S, Yavuz K, et al. Endovascular treatment of brain arteriovenous malformations with prolonged intranidal Onyx injection technique: long-term results in 350 consecutive patients with completed endovascular treatment course. J Neurosurg. 2011; 115(1):78–88

[19] Andrade-Souza YM, Ramani M, Beachey DJ, et al. Liquid embolisation material reduces the delivered radiation dose: a physical experiment. Acta Neurochir (Wien). 2008; 150(2):161–164, discussion 164

[20] Bing F, Doucet R, Lacroix F, et al. Liquid embolization material reduces the delivered radiation dose: clinical myth or reality? AJNR Am J Neuroradiol. 2012; 33(2):320–322

[21] Buell TJ, Ding D, Starke RM, Webster Crowley R, Liu KC. Embolization-induced angiogenesis in cerebral arteriovenous malformations. J Clin Neurosci. 2014; 21(11):1866–1871

[22] Oermann EK, Ding D, Yen CP, et al. Effect of prior embolization on cerebral arteriovenous malformation radiosurgery outcomes: a case-control study. Neurosurgery. 2015; 77(3):406–417, discussion 417

[23] Lee CC, Reardon MA, Ball BZ, et al. The predictive value of magnetic resonance imaging in evaluating intracranial arteriovenous malformation obliteration after stereotactic radiosurgery. J Neurosurg. 2015; 123(1):136–144

[24] Kano H, Kondziolka D, Flickinger JC, et al. Stereotactic radiosurgery for arteriovenous malformations, Part 5: management of brainstem arteriovenous malformations. J Neurosurg. 2012; 116(1):44–53

[25] Flickinger JC, Pollock BE, Kondziolka D, Lunsford LD. A dose-response analysis of arteriovenous malformation obliteration after radiosurgery. Int J Radiat Oncol Biol Phys. 1996; 36(4):873–879

[26] Spetzler RF, Martin NA. A proposed grading system for arteriovenous malformations. J Neurosurg. 1986; 65(4):476–483

[27] Andrade-Souza YM, Zadeh G, Ramani M, Scora D, Tsao MN, Schwartz ML. Testing the radiosurgery-based arteriovenous malformation score and the modified Spetzler-Martin grading system to predict radiosurgical outcome. J Neurosurg. 2005; 103(4):642–648

[28] Koltz MT, Polifka AJ, Saltos A, et al. Long-term outcome of Gamma Knife stereotactic radiosurgery for arteriovenous malformations graded by the Spetzler-Martin classification. J Neurosurg. 2013; 118(1):74–83

[29] Ding D, Yen CP, Xu Z, Starke RM, Sheehan JP. Radiosurgery for low-grade intracranial arteriovenous malformations. J Neurosurg. 2014; 121(2):457–467

[30] Kano H, Lunsford LD, Flickinger JC, et al. Stereotactic radiosurgery for arteriovenous malformations, Part 1: management of Spetzler-Martin Grade I and II arteriovenous malformations. J Neurosurg. 2012; 116(1):11–20

[31] Ding D, Yen CP, Starke RM, Xu Z, Sun X, Sheehan JP. Radiosurgery for Spetzler-Martin Grade III arteriovenous malformations. J Neurosurg. 2014; 120(4):959–969

[32] Kano H, Flickinger JC, Yang HC, et al. Stereotactic radiosurgery for Spetzler-Martin Grade III arteriovenous malformations. J Neurosurg. 2014; 120(4):973–981

[33] Ding D, Yen CP, Starke RM, Xu Z, Sun X, Sheehan JP. Outcomes following single-session radiosurgery for high-grade intracranial arteriovenous malformations. Br J Neurosurg. 2014; 28(5):666–674

[34] Pollock BE, Flickinger JC, Lunsford LD, Maitz A, Kondziolka D. Factors associated with successful arteriovenous malformation radiosurgery. Neurosurgery. 1998; 42(6):1239–1244, discussion 1244–1247

[35] Pollock BE, Flickinger JC. A proposed radiosurgery-based grading system for arteriovenous malformations. J Neurosurg. 2002; 96(1):79–85

[36] Pollock BE, Flickinger JC. Modification of the radiosurgery-based arteriovenous malformation grading system. Neurosurgery. 2008; 63(2):239–243, discussion 243

[37] Wegner RE, Oysul K, Pollock BE, et al. A modified radiosurgery-based arteriovenous malformation grading scale and its correlation with outcomes. Int J Radiat Oncol Biol Phys. 2011; 79(4):1147–1150

[38] Burrow AM, Link MJ, Pollock BE. Is stereotactic radiosurgery the best treatment option for patients with a radiosurgery-based arteriovenous malformation score ≤ 1? World Neurosurg. 2014; 82(6):1144–1147

[39] Ding D, Xu Z, Yen CP, Starke RM, Sheehan JP. Radiosurgery for cerebral arteriovenous malformations in elderly patients: effect of advanced age on outcomes after intervention. World Neurosurg. 2015; 84(3):795–804

[40] Huo X, Jiang Y, Lv X, et al. Gamma Knife surgical treatment for partially embolized cerebral arteriovenous malformations. J Neurosurg. 2016; 124(3):767–776

[41] Ding D, Yen CP, Xu Z, Starke RM, Sheehan JP. Radiosurgery for primary motor and sensory cortex arteriovenous malformations: outcomes and the effect of eloquent location. Neurosurgery. 2013; 73(5):816–824, 824

[42] Ding D, Yen CP, Xu Z, Starke RM, Sheehan JP. Radiosurgery for patients with unruptured intracranial arteriovenous malformations. J Neurosurg. 2013; 118(5):958–966

[43] Sasaki T, Kurita H, Saito I, et al. Arteriovenous malformations in the basal ganglia and thalamus: management and results in 101 cases. J Neurosurg. 1998; 88(2):285–292

[44] Andrade-Souza YM, Zadeh G, Scora D, Tsao MN, Schwartz ML. Radiosurgery for basal ganglia, internal capsule, and thalamus arteriovenous malformation: clinical outcome. Neurosurgery. 2005; 56(1):56–63, discussion 63–64

[45] Yen CP, Steiner L. Gamma knife surgery for brainstem arteriovenous malformations. World Neurosurg. 2011; 76(1–2):87–95, discussion 57–58

[46] Kano H, Kondziolka D, Flickinger JC, et al. Stereotactic radiosurgery for arteriovenous malformations, Part 4: management of basal ganglia and thalamus arteriovenous malformations. J Neurosurg. 2012; 116(1):33–43

[47] Kurita H, Kawamoto S, Sasaki T, et al. Results of radiosurgery for brain stem arteriovenous malformations. J Neurol Neurosurg Psychiatry. 2000; 68(5):563–570

[48] Stefani MA, Porter PJ, terBrugge KG, Montanera W, Willinsky RA, Wallace MC. Angioarchitectural factors present in brain arteriovenous malformations associated with hemorrhagic presentation. Stroke. 2002; 33(4):920–924

[49] Kiran NAS, Kale SS, Kasliwal MK, et al. Gamma knife radiosurgery for arteriovenous malformations of basal ganglia, thalamus and brainstem–a retrospective study comparing the results with that for AVMs at other intracranial locations. Acta Neurochir (Wien). 2009; 151(12):1575–1582

[50] Koga T, Shin M, Terahara A, Saito N. Outcomes of radiosurgery for brainstem arteriovenous malformations. Neurosurgery. 2011; 69(1):45–51, discussion 51–52

[51] Moosa S, Chen CJ, Ding D, et al. Volume-staged versus dose-staged radiosurgery outcomes for large intracranial arteriovenous malformations. Neurosurg Focus. 2014; 37(3):E18

[52] Yang SY, Kim DG, Chung HT, Paek SH, Park JH, Han DH. Radiosurgery for large cerebral arteriovenous malformations. Acta Neurochir (Wien). 2009; 151(2):113–124

[53] Flickinger JC, Kondziolka D, Lunsford LD, et al. Arteriovenous Malformation Radiosurgery Study Group. Development of a model to predict permanent symptomatic postradiosurgery injury for arteriovenous malformation patients. Int J Radiat Oncol Biol Phys. 2000; 46(5):1143–1148

[54] Pollock BE, Kline RW, Stafford SL, Foote RL, Schomberg PJ. The rationale and technique of staged-volume arteriovenous malformation radiosurgery. Int J Radiat Oncol Biol Phys. 2000; 48(3):817–824

[55] Abla AA, Rutledge WC, Seymour ZA, et al. A treatment paradigm for high-grade brain arteriovenous malformations: volume-staged radiosurgical downgrading followed by microsurgical resection. J Neurosurg. 2015; 122(2):419–432

[56] Yen CP, Lanzino G, Sheehan JP. Stereotactic radiosurgery of intracranial dural arteriovenous fistulas. Neurosurg Clin N Am. 2013; 24(4):591–596

[57] Cifarelli CP, Kaptain G, Yen CP, Schlesinger D, Sheehan JP. Gamma knife radiosurgery for dural arteriovenous fistulas. Neurosurgery. 2010; 67(5):1230–1235, discussion 1235

[58] Chen CJ, Lee CC, Ding D, et al. Stereotactic radiosurgery for intracranial dural arteriovenous fistulas: a systematic review. J Neurosurg. 2015; 122(2):353–362

[59] Flickinger JC, Kondziolka D, Pollock BE, Maitz AH, Lunsford LD. Complications from arteriovenous malformation radiosurgery: multivariate analysis and risk modeling. Int J Radiat Oncol Biol Phys. 1997; 38(3):485–490

[60] Maruyama K, Kawahara N, Shin M, et al. The risk of hemorrhage after radiosurgery for cerebral arteriovenous malformations. N Engl J Med. 2005; 352(2):146–153

[61] Kano H, Kondziolka D, Flickinger JC, et al. Aneurysms increase the risk of rebleeding after stereotactic radiosurgery for hemorrhagic arteriovenous malformations. Stroke. 2012; 43(10):2586–2591

[62] Yen CP, Varady P, Sheehan J, Steiner M, Steiner L. Subtotal obliteration of cerebral arteriovenous malformations after gamma knife surgery. J Neurosurg. 2007; 106(3):361–369

[63] Baranoski JF, Grant RA, Hirsch LJ, et al. Seizure control for intracranial arteriovenous malformations is directly related to treatment modality: a meta-analysis. J Neurointerv Surg. 2014; 6(9):684–690

[64] Wang JY, Yang W, Ye X, et al. Impact on seizure control of surgical resection or radiosurgery for cerebral arteriovenous malformations. Neurosurgery. 2013; 73(4):648–655, discussion 655–656

[65] Chen CJ, Chivukula S, Ding D, et al. Seizure outcomes following radiosurgery for cerebral arteriovenous malformations. Neurosurg Focus. 2014; 37(3):E17

[66] Ding D, Starke RM, Quigg M, et al. Cerebral arteriovenous malformations and epilepsy, part 1: predictors of seizure presentation. World Neurosurg. 2015; 84(3):645–652

[67] Ding D, Quigg M, Starke RM, et al. Cerebral arteriovenous malformations and epilepsy, part 2: predictors of seizure outcomes following radiosurgery. World Neurosurg. 2015; 84(3):653–662

[68] Touboul E, Al Halabi A, Buffat L, et al. Single-fraction stereotactic radiotherapy: a dose-response analysis of arteriovenous malformation obliteration. Int J Radiat Oncol Biol Phys. 1998; 41(4):855–861

[69] Chang JH, Chang JW, Park YG, Chung SS. Factors related to complete occlusion of arteriovenous malformations after gamma knife radiosurgery. J Neurosurg. 2000; 93 Suppl 3:96–101

[70] Schlienger M, Atlan D, Lefkopoulos D, et al. Linac radiosurgery for cerebral arteriovenous malformations: results in 169 patients. Int J Radiat Oncol Biol Phys. 2000; 46(5):1135–1142

[71] Massager N, Régis J, Kondziolka D, Njee T, Levivier M. Gamma knife radiosurgery for brainstem arteriovenous malformations: preliminary results. J Neurosurg. 2000; 93 Suppl 3:102–103

[72] Flickinger JC, Kondziolka D, Maitz AH, Lunsford LD. An analysis of the dose-response for arteriovenous malformation radiosurgery and other factors affecting obliteration. Radiother Oncol. 2002; 63(3):347–354

[73] Friedman WA, Bova FJ, Bollampally S, Bradshaw P. Analysis of factors predictive of success or complications in arteriovenous malformation radiosurgery. Neurosurgery. 2003; 52(2):296–307, discussion 307–308

[74] Bollet MA, Anxionnat R, Buchheit I, et al. Efficacy and morbidity of arc-therapy radiosurgery for cerebral arteriovenous malformations: a comparison with the natural history. Int J Radiat Oncol Biol Phys. 2004; 58(5):1353–1363

[75] Shin M, Maruyama K, Kurita H, et al. Analysis of nidus obliteration rates after gamma knife surgery for arteriovenous malformations based on long-term follow-up data: the University of Tokyo experience. J Neurosurg. 2004; 101(1):18–24

[76] Liscák R, Vladyka V, Simonová G, et al. Arteriovenous malformations after Leksell Gamma Knife radiosurgery: rate of obliteration and complications. Neurosurgery. 2007; 60(6):1005–1014, discussion 1015–1016

[77] Colombo F, Cavedon C, Casentini L, Francescon P, Causin F, Pinna V. Early results of CyberKnife radiosurgery for arteriovenous malformations. J Neurosurg. 2009; 111(4):807–819

[78] Taeshineetanakul P, Krings T, Geibprasert S, et al. Angioarchitecture determines obliteration rate after radiosurgery in brain arteriovenous malformations. Neurosurgery. 2012; 71(6):1071–1078, discussion 1079

[79] Fokas E, Henzel M, Wittig A, Grund S, Engenhart-Cabillic R. Stereotactic radiosurgery of cerebral arteriovenous malformations: long-term follow-up in 164 patients of a single institution. J Neurol. 2013; 260(8):2156–2162

[80] Franzin A, Snider S, Boari N, et al. Evaluation of prognostic factors as predictor of AVMS obliteration after Gamma Knife radiosurgery. Acta Neurochir (Wien). 2013; 155(4):619–626

[81] Hattangadi-Gluth JA, Chapman PH, Kim D, et al. Single-fraction proton beam stereotactic radiosurgery for cerebral arteriovenous malformations. Int J Radiat Oncol Biol Phys. 2014; 89(2):338–346

[82] Missios S, Bekelis K, Al-Shyal G, Rasmussen PA, Barnett GH. Stereotactic radiosurgery of intracranial arteriovenous malformations and the use of the K index in determining treatment dose. Neurosurg Focus. 2014; 37(3):E15

[83] Paúl L, Casasco A, Kusak ME, Martínez N, Rey G, Martínez R. Results for a series of 697 arteriovenous malformations treated by gamma knife: influence of angiographic features on the obliteration rate. Neurosurgery. 2014; 75(5):568–583, 582–583, quiz 583

[84] Wang YC, Huang YC, Chen HC, et al. Linear accelerator stereotactic radiosurgery in the management of intracranial arteriovenous malformations: long-term outcome. Cerebrovasc Dis. 2014; 37(5):342–349

[85] Cheng CH, Crowley RW, Yen CP, Schlesinger D, Shaffrey ME, Sheehan JP. Gamma Knife surgery for basal ganglia and thalamic arteriovenous malformations. J Neurosurg. 2012; 116(4):899–908

26 Radiosurgery for Dural Arteriovenous Fistulas: Indications and Outcomes

Cheng-Chia Lee, Huai-Che Yang, Hsiu-Mei Wu, Wen-Yuh Chung, Wan-Yuo Guo, and David H.C. Pan

Abstract

Stereotactic radiosurgery using the Gamma Knife or other radiosurgical devices is a safe and effective alternative treatment for dural arteriovenous fistulas (DAVFs). This method provides a minimally invasive therapeutic modality for patients who harbor less aggressive DAVFs, but who suffer from intolerable headache, pulsatile tinnitus, or ocular symptoms. For aggressive DAVFs with extensive cortical venous drainage, immediate risks of hemorrhage, progressive neurological deficits, or severe venous hypertension, initial treatment with endovascular procedure, including embolization and angioplasty, or surgery is suggested. In such cases, radiosurgery may serve as a secondary treatment for further management of the residual fistulas. The latent period for the effects of radiation to occur and the longer time for cure compared to surgery and endovascular therapy remains a major drawback for radiosurgery. However, the gradual obliteration of a DAVF after radiosurgery can avoid immediate risk of aggravated venous hypertension or infarction, which sometimes complicates endovascular embolization and surgery. It is believed that using a multidisciplinary approach to DAVF management yields better results.

Keywords: dural arteriovenous fistula, Gamma Knife, stereotactic, radiosurgery

Key Points

- For Borden type I (Cognard type I, IIa) dural arteriovenous fistulas (DAVFs) with persistent benign symptoms (pulsatile tinnitus or ocular symptoms), radiosurgery may be indicated as an initial treatment.
- For Borden type II/III (Cognard type IIa + b, IIb, III) DAVFs with asymptomatic cortical venous drainage (CVD; headache, pulsatile tinnitus, or ocular symptoms), endovascular procedure may be the first-line management. Radiosurgery can be considered an initial treatment alternatively for patients who are elderly, medically frail, or harboring complicated angioarchitecture.
- For Borden type II/III (Cognard type IIa + b, IIb, III) DAVFs with severe symptomatic CVD (hemorrhage or progressive neurological deficits), surgery or endovascular procedures are indicated for the initial treatment.
- An obliteration rate of 70% is expected for the cavernous sinus DAVFs, and 60% for the noncavernous sinus DAVFs. Few complications are reported.

26.1 Introduction

Intracranial dural arteriovenous fistulas (DAVFs) are abnormal arteriovenous communications within the dura, in which meningeal arteries shunt blood directly into the dural sinus or leptomeningeal veins.[1,2] DAVF is considered an acquired disease, although the exact pathophysiology was not well established. DAVFs with anterograde cortical venous drainage (CVD) have been clinically regarded as benign, whereas DAVFs with retrograde CVD are considered aggressive in behavior. For DAVFs without CVD or DAVFs with asymptomatic CVD, radiosurgery may be indicated as an initial treatment. An obliteration rate of 70% is expected for the cavernous sinus (CS) DAVFs, and 60% for the noncavernous sinus (NCS) DAVFs. For aggressive DAVFs with extensive CVD, harboring severe venous hypertension, progressive neurological deficits, or immediate risks of hemorrhage, initial treatment with endovascular intervention, including embolization and angioplasty, or surgery is suggested.

26.1.1 Epidemiology

The incidence of DAVFs has been estimated at 5 to 20% of all intracranial vascular malformations.[1,3,4,5] DAVFs comprise only 6% of supratentorial vascular malformations, whereas they are 35% of infratentorial malformations.[6] The median age of presentation for a DAVF is 50 to 60 years of age with no sex preference, though there is a wide range seen.[7,8] Unlike the more common intracerebral or parenchymal arteriovenous malformations (AVMs), DAVFs most commonly occur in the regions of the CS, transverse/sigmoid sinuses, tentorium/torcula, or cerebral convexities with drainage to superior sagittal sinus (▶ Fig. 26.1, ▶ Table 26.1)[1,9,10]

The underlying etiology and natural course of DAVF are not yet very well understood, and the magnitude of the risk varies considerably between studies.[11,12,13,14] Söderman et al reported an 85-patient series with 25-year follow-up that demonstrated approximately 1.5% annual hemorrhage rate among the patients without previous hemorrhage and 7.4% among those with previous hemorrhage.[13]

26.1.2 Clinical Manifestations

The clinical presentation of a DAVF is dependent on its location and pattern of the venous drainage (▶ Fig. 26.1). The most common locations are the CS, followed by transverse-sigmoid sinus, which together account for about 80% of the cases.[4] Patients with CS DAVFs often have ocular manifestations (exophthalmos, chemosis, visual impairment, and diplopia). In the transverse-sigmoid sinus (TSS) DAVFs, pulsatile tinnitus and throbbing headache were the most common symptoms.[4]

Similar to other cerebral AVMs, DAVFs can hemorrhage, with an estimated annual risk of approximately 1.5 to 1.8%.[13] van Dijk et al in 2002 reported that persistence of the cortical venous reflux in DAVFs yields an annual hemorrhage rate of 8.1% and a mortality rate of 10.4%.[14] Duffau et al reported a high risk of early rebleeding (35% within 2 weeks) after the first episode of hemorrhage, with graver consequence from the second

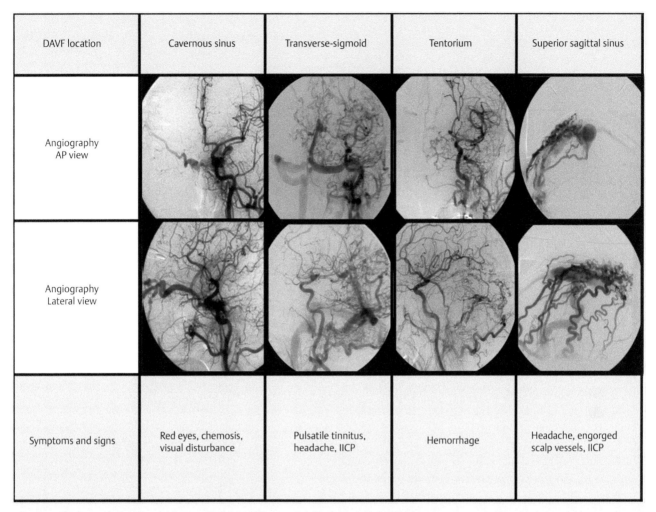

DAVF location	Cavernous sinus	Transverse-sigmoid	Tentorium	Superior sagittal sinus
Angiography AP view				
Angiography Lateral view				
Symptoms and signs	Red eyes, chemosis, visual disturbance	Pulsatile tinnitus, headache, IICP	Hemorrhage	Headache, engorged scalp vessels, IICP

Fig. 26.1 The common locations and symptoms/signs of intracranial dural arteriovenous fistulas.

Table 26.1 Incidence of intracerebral hemorrhage (ICH) and nonhemorrhagic neurological deficit (NHND) before GKRS in 321 patients with DAVFs

	Number	ICH	(Percentage)	NHND	(Percentage)
Cavernous sinus	206	7	(3.4)	9	(4.4)
Transverse–sigmoidal sinus	72	8	(11.1)	27	(37.5)
Petrosal sinus	9	1	(11.1)	4	(44.4)
Superior sagittal sinus	8	0	–	3	(37.5)
Tentorium	9	2	(22.2)	4	(44.5)
Frontal base (anterior fossa)	6	3	(50.0)	3	(50)
Sphenoparietal	4	2	(50.0)	0	–
Vein of Galen	2	0	–	1	(50)
Jugular foramen	2	0	–	0	–
Clivus	2	0	–	0	–
Foramen magnum	1	0	–	1	(100)
Total	321	23	(7.2)	52	(16.2)

Abbreviations: DAVFs, dural arteriovenous fistulas; GKRS, Gamma Knife radiosurgery.

Note: Nonhemorrhagic neurological deficits include hemiparesis, hemiparesthesia, cerebellar sign, dementia, and mental confusion.

bleed.[12] Söderman et al in 2008 evaluated hemorrhage rate in their 85 cases of DAVFs with retrograde CVD. They found a lower hemorrhage rate compared to those of the other previous reports. In their patients already presenting with an intracranial hemorrhage, the annual risk for the recurrent hemorrhage was 7.4%, while in those patients not presenting with a hemorrhage, the bleeding rate was approximately 1.5% per year.[13] Pan et al in 2013[4] reported a Gamma Knife radiosurgery (GKRS) series of 321 DAVF patients; 7 of the 206 CS DAVF patients (3.4%) experienced a hemorrhage and 16 of the 115 NCS DAVF patients (13.9%) had a hemorrhagic event prior to diagnosis. The report also demonstrated that arteriovenous shunts involving the anterior skull base, tentorium, or sphenoparietal sinus harbored a higher risk of hemorrhage[4] (▶ Table 26.1).

Beyond hemorrhagic episodes, some patients suffered persistent or slowly progressive neurological deficits, including symptoms of hemiparesis, hemiparesthesia, cerebellar sign, dementia, and mental confusion. From the authors' experience in analysis of 321 DAVF patients, the incidence of nonhemorrhagic neurological deficits (NHND) is 4.4% (9 of 206 cases) in CS DAVFs and 37.4% (43 of 115 cases) in NCS DAVFs (▶ Table 26.1).

26.1.3 Pathophysiology

DAVFs are thought to be acquired due to inflammation, thrombosis, or trauma of the dural sinus. However, the exact etiology and underlying disease are difficult to trace in many cases and the DAVFs are considered idiopathic.[15,16] A thorough understanding of a DVAF morphology requires a detailed cerebral angiographic investigation. Drainage of the venous flow from DAVF can be antegrade or retrograde through a dural sinus, through a cortical vein, or both. The pattern of the venous drainage is not necessary static though. Gradual alternation in the venous flow from antegrade to retrograde and delayed recruitment of arterial feeders into the nidus (sump effect) have been observed in some patients.[8,17,18] This is hypothesized to occur as a result of progressive sinus hypertension with redirection of the blood flow into cortical veins.[2,9,19] The gradual venous hypertension and reflux of the cortical veins may eventually predispose to the risks of cerebral hemorrhage and/or other neurological deficits.[1]

Not all DAVFs demonstrate such a progressive clinical course though. Although not frequently seen, some DAVFs can regress and thrombose gradually, resulting in a spontaneous cure.[20,21] The factors predisposing to DAVF progression or involution have not been clearly clarified.

26.1.4 Angioarchitecture and Classifications of DAVF

There are at least three classifications for intracranial DAVFs (▶ Table 26.2, ▶ Table 26.3, ▶ Table 26.4). The most popularly used classifications in DAVFs are Cognard classification and Borden–Shucart system.[9,19] Both systems classify the DAVFs based on their angiographic venous drainage pattern However, owing to the unique clinical characteristics of DAVFs involving the CS, Barrow's classification, which describes the feeding arteries to the CS DAVFs, is also commonly used to classify this particular type of DAVFs.[22]

Table 26.2 Cognard classification for dural arteriovenous fistulas

Cognard type	Description
I	Confined to sinus wall with normal anterograde flow
IIa	Confined to sinus with cortical veins reflux
IIb	Retrograde drains into sinus with cortical veins reflux
IIa + b	Retrograde drains into sinus + cortical veins
III	Drains direct into cortical veins (not to sinus) drainage
IV	Drains direct into cortical veins (not to sinus) drainage with venous ectasia
V	Spinal perimedullary venous drainage, associated with progressive myelopathy

Table 26.3 Borden classification for dural arteriovenous fistulas

Borden type	Description
I	Drains anterograde into venous sinus
II	Drains retrograde into venous sinus + cortical vein
III	Drains retrograde into cortical vein only

Table 26.4 Barrow classification for the CS DAVFs

Barrow type	Description
A	Direct high-flow shunts between ICA and CS
B	Indirect low-flow shunts meningeal branches of ICA and CS
C	Indirect low-flow shunts meningeal branches of ECA and CS
D	Indirect low-flow shunts meningeal branches of both ICA and ECA and CS

Abbreviations: CS, cavernous sinus; DAVFs, dural arteriovenous fistulas; ECA, external carotid artery; ICA, internal carotid artery.

The system of Cognard similarly separates DAVFs depending on the site of drainage and the presence of CVD, and also considers the direction of flow through the draining vein as well as the presence of cortical venous ectasia[9] (▶ Table 26.2). Cognard type I DAVFs have solely antegrade sinus drainage, similar to the Borden–Shucart system. Cognard type II DAVFs demonstrate retrograde drainage and are subdivided depending on whether drainage is through the sinus (IIa), cortical vein (IIb), or both (IIa + b). Cognard type III DAVFs drain directly into cortical veins similar to the Borden–Shucart system, but Cognard gives lesions with venous ectasia a separate designation of type IV. DAVFs that drain into spinal perimedullary veins are designated type V by Cognard. Cognard et al present their series of 258 patients and demonstrate a strong correlation between DAVF type and rate of aggressive clinical symptoms and risk of hemorrhage.

The Borden–Shucart system distinguishes DAVFs depending on the site of drainage and the presence of CVD[19] (▶ Table 26.3). Tape I DAVFs drain directly into the sinus or meningeal veins with antegrade flow, whereas type II DAVFs have retrograde flow through the sinus into the subarachnoid veins. Type III DAVFs directly drain into the subarachnoid veins in a retrograde fashion.

According to Barrow's classification,[22] CS DAVFs are classified into direct (type A) and indirect (types B–D) types (▶ Table 26.4). Direct CS DAVFs are high-flow shunts between the cavernous portion of the internal carotid artery and the CS, usually caused by a traumatic laceration of the internal carotid artery or rupture of an intracavernous carotid aneurysm. Indirect CS DAVFs are dural fistulas between the CS and meningeal branches of the internal carotid artery (type B), the external carotid artery (type C), or both (type D).

26.1.5 Treatment Options

The recommended therapeutic intervention for a DAVF is dependent on the anticipated natural history and hemodynamic change of the lesion. For lesions with antegrade sinus drainage (Borden type I or Cognard type I) and benign clinical manifestations, intervention is usually palliative or observational unless the patient's symptoms are intolerable.[5,8] For patients with throbbing headache, pulsatile tinnitus, ophthalmological deterioration, progressive neurological deficits, increased intracranial pressure, or elevated risk of hemorrhage, therapeutic intervention is recommended.[9,19,23,24]

Advances in the field of interventional neuroradiology have increased treatment options for patients with DAVFs. Obliteration of the fistula can be attempted through a transarterial or transvenous route. Transarterial embolization alone rarely leads to a complete obliteration of the DAVF, because there are usually numerous arterial feeders to the nidus. The purpose of a transarterial approach is mainly for reduction of arterial feeders and the palliative symptomatic relief.[23] For curative treatment, additional treatment through a retrograde transvenous approach may be necessary. In transvenous embolization, superselective disconnection of the refluxing vein is preferred over sacrifice of the dural sinus, although this sometimes becomes necessary to achieve a cure.[23] Endovascular therapy can also be combined with surgery or radiosurgery when it is not feasible to completely obliterate a DAVF alone.

An open surgical approach is indicated for DAVFs with aggressive features that are not amenable to comprehensive endovascular treatment. Typically, lesions involving the anterior cranial fossa or tentorial incisura are often associated with hemorrhage; thus, surgical intervention is indicated. Surgical strategies include ligation of the fistula at the junction with the drainage vein, interruption of arterial feeders, coagulation and/or excision of the fistula in the dura, and resection of the involved sinus.[25,26,27] Recent studies have suggested that disconnection of the draining vein alone without resection of the sinus is equally efficacious as resection of the fistula. The former can avoid risks of venous hypertension associated with the sinus removal, particularly where the sinus is patent.[28,29,30,31] Reported morbidity and mortality of surgical intervention has ranged from 0 to 13%.[31]

Stereotactic radiosurgery (SRS) has long been used for treatment of intraparenchymal AVMs, and treatment of DAVFs would be a natural extension of this. In 1993, Chandler and Friedman first reported a case in which a DAVF located in the anterior fossa was successfully treated with radiosurgery.[32] Since then, radiosurgical treatment has been delivered for DAVFs in various locations including CS, transverse-sigmoid sinus, superior sagittal sinus, tentorium, and other locations.[33,34,35,36,37,38,39,40,41] Radiosurgery is often combined with endovascular therapy to provide immediate relief of symptoms and possibly reduction of the hemorrhage risk.[10,33,35,36,42,43,44] In some reports, DAVF obliteration rates using radiosurgery alone are comparable to those using the combined method, as the rates of symptomatic improvement.[34,36,38] Complications directly related to the radiosurgical procedure are only uncommonly found.

26.1.6 Treatment Strategy for a Dural Arteriovenous Fistula

The management for a DAVF should be individualized, taking into consideration the clinical presentation of the patient, the anticipated natural history of the lesion based on location and angioarchitecture of the DAVFs, and the benefit and inherent risk of the treatment modality. It is generally agreed that DAVFs presenting with hemorrhage, progressive neurological deficits, or increased intracranial pressure require prompt treatment by endovascular embolization, surgery, or a combination of these procedures, to provide immediate relief of the venous congestion.

For Borden type II–III (or Cognard type IIb, IIa + b, III, IV, and V) lesions with a single or few CVDs, or DAVFs with an isolated dural sinus and CVDs, complete obliteration of the lesion may be achieved effectively by surgery or endovascular intervention.[45,46,47] However, when DAVFs involve dural sinuses with multiple complex feeders and CVDs, surgical and endovascular treatment can be technically challenging. Lucas et al in 1997 reported a meta-analysis and concluded that even with combined therapy of surgery and embolization, over 30% of DAVFs involving transverse-sigmoid sinus will demonstrate residual filling or persistent symptoms.[48] The current application of SRS can provide an additional therapeutic method to improve the treatment result.

When a treatment is indicated for Borden type I DAVF (or Cognard type I and IIa), the therapeutic benefit should outweigh the risks of the treatment. Evidence had shown that injury or increased pressure in the dural sinus could trigger the development of DAVFs or cause neurologic deficits secondary to venous hypertension.[2] Thus, sacrificing a functioning dural sinus in Borden type I DAVFs by transvenous intervention or surgery may not be justified. Furthermore, it is difficult to achieve a complete obliteration of Borden type I DAVF by transarterial embolization alone due to the frequently complex and torturous course of the arterial supply.[23] Studies had shown that local ischemia caused by incomplete closure of the DAVFs after endovascular and/or surgical intervention can increase expression of various vascular growth factors, which can recruit new collaterals resulting in recanalization of the DAVFs.[49,50,51,52] Thus, the use of endovascular intervention or surgery as a first-line treatment for Borden type I DAVFs with the intention of palliation rather than cure should carefully balance the risks and benefits of the procedure. Our study and others' have shown that DAVFs with benign venous drainage can be safely treated using radiosurgery with a high angiographic complete obliteration rate with preservation of functioning dural sinuses.[5,34,38,41]

Currently, our strategy of treatment for DAVF patients is as follows:

- For Borden type I (Cognard type I, IIa) DAVFs with persistent benign symptoms (headache, pulsatile tinnitus, or eye symptoms), radiosurgery may be indicated as an initial treatment.
- For Borden type II/III (Cognard type IIa + b, IIb, III) DAVFs with retrograde CVD the following strategy is adopted:
  - For symptomatic CVD[24] (with hemorrhage, increased intracranial pressure, or progressive neurological deficits), surgery or endovascular procedures are indicated for the initial treatment.
  - For symptomatic CVD[24] (with only headache, pulsatile tinnitus, or eye symptoms, but without hemorrhage or increased intracranial pressure), endovascular procedure may be the first-line management. Alternatively, radiosurgery can be considered as an initial treatment for patients who are elderly, medically frail, or harboring complex DAVFs.

26.1.7 Principle and Dosage of Stereotactic Radiosurgery

SRS is characterized by a steep dose fall-off of radiation to the target margin, thereby relatively sparing the radiation exposure to surrounding normal tissues. Its application has been improved by many neurosurgeons, neuroradiologists, radiation oncologists, and physicists to advance the treatment for intracranial vascular or neoplastic lesions. Although SRS facilities change over the ensuing decades, the basic concepts have not changed: the radiobiological effects of radiosurgery on vascular lesions is due to an endothelial damage, undulation of internal elastic membrane, proliferative vasculopathy with narrowing the lumen, subendothelial cell proliferation, and, finally, complete lumen obliteration.[53]

Target localization of the DAVF is performed by integrating imaging data from a stereotactic noncontrast magnetic resonance imaging (MRI), a thin-cut axial view time-of-flight magnetic resonance angiography (MRA), and a cerebral X-ray angiogram. Our goal of the treatment is to occlude the fistulous shunts completely. Proper delineation of the treatment target to include all abnormal arteriovenous shunts on the dural sinus wall is crucial for a successful treatment (▶ Fig. 26.2, ▶ Fig. 26.3) The target volume is defined along the involved dural sinus wall where the true arteriovenous fistula occurs.[2,17,38,54,55] The remote arterial feeders and drainage veins distal to the sinus are excluded from the treatment volume, as they are not considered a part of the true nidus.

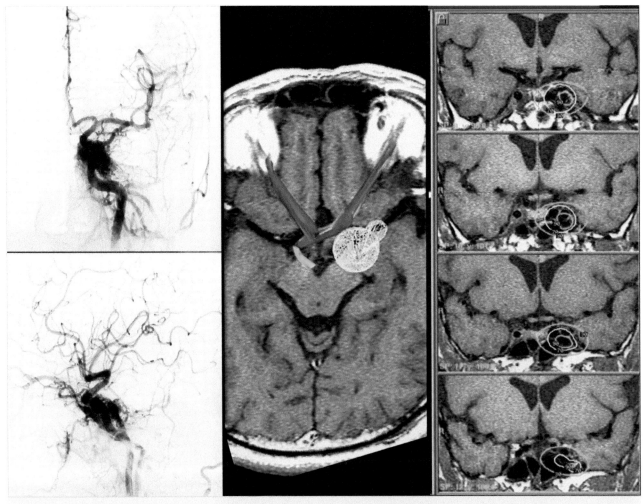

Fig. 26.2 Dosing plan for a cavernous sinus dural arteriovenous fistula. Red: optic apparatus. Green: the oculomotor nerve. Yellow: the radiation volume.

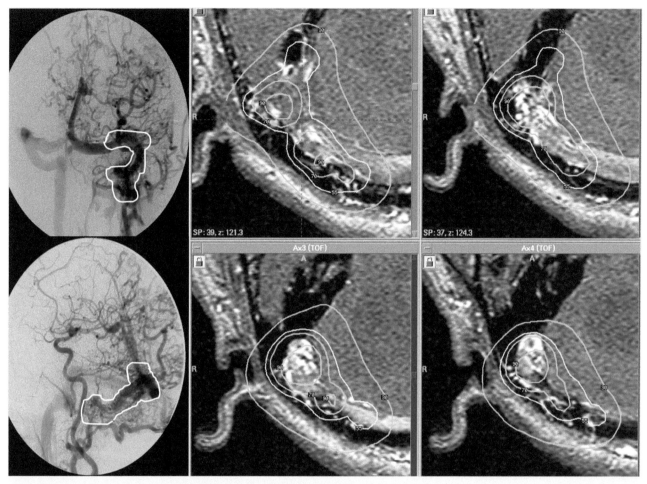

Fig. 26.3 Dosing plan for a transverse-sigmoid sinus dural arteriovenous fistula.

Usually, the prescribed margin dose for DAVF radiosurgery is around 18 to 20 Gy (range of 15–25 Gy). The target coverage is within a 50 to 70% isodose line. For the treatment of CS DAVFs, using a large (14 or 18 mm in type C and 16 mm in Perfexion Gamma Knife) collimator to cover the margin of the CS is preferred (▶ Fig. 26.2). For the NCS DAVFs, a greater number of isocenters (several large and many 8-mm small shots) were used to cover the treatment volume (▶ Fig. 26.3). Care is taken to protect the adjacent critical structures such as the optic nerve and brainstem to receive radiation doses less than 8 to 10 Gy.

After GKRS, both a clinical neurological examination and a radiographic imaging study (MRI with MRA) are performed at 6-month intervals. Cerebral X-ray angiography is usually performed between 1 and 3 years after GKRS, if complete regression of the lesion has been shown on the MRI. For CS DAVFs, a noninvasive color Doppler ultrasonography (CDU) examined through eyeballs is performed every 3 months to evaluate flow direction and velocity in the superior ophthalmic vein (SOV). Frequently, normalization of the CDU is associated with concomitant findings of complete obliteration of DAVF on the MRI and cerebral angiography.[56]

Patient outcomes after radiosurgery are grouped into four categories: (1) complete improvement, indicating complete symptomatic relief with complete obliteration of the DAVF on cerebral angiogram and/or MRA; (2) partial improvement, indicating partial resolution of clinical symptoms with greater than 50% regression of the DAVF nidus on MRA; (3) stationary, indicating no change of the DAVF nidus on the follow-up MRI; and (4) progression, indicating enlargement or aggressive change of the DAVF nidus on MRA.

26.1.8 Outcome of Dural Arteriovenous Fistula Radiosurgery

In the authors' series at the Taipei Veterans General Hospital, post-GKRS follow-up studies were available in 156 (76%) of 206 patients with CS DAVFs and in 108 (94%) of 115 patients with NCS DAVFs. The median follow-up period for CS group was 20.8 months (range of 1–149 months), while for NCS group it was 28 months (range of 2–141 months).

▶ Table 26.5 summarizes the clinical outcomes in our 264 DAVF patients with follow-ups. For the CS DAVFs, 109 of the 156 patients (70%) showed complete improvement, while 47 (30%) were partially improved. No lesions were stationary or progressed after radiosurgery. For the NCS DAVFs, 64 of the 108 (59%) patients showed complete improvement, 40 (37%) were partially improved, 2 (2%) were stationary, 1 (1%) showed progression, and 1(1%) died. The illustrative cases are showed in ▶ Fig. 26.4 and ▶ Fig. 26.5.

Table 26.5 Clinical outcomes after GKRS in 264 patients with DAVFs available for neurological and imaging follow-ups

	CS	NCS
Complete obliteration	109 (70%)	64 (59%)
Partial obliteration	47 (30%)	40 (37%)
Stationary (no charge)	–	2 (2%)
Progression	–	1 (1%)
Death	–	1 (1%)
Total	156	108

Abbreviations: CS, cavernous sinus; DAVFs, dural arteriovenous fistulas; GKRS, Gamma Knife radiosurgery; NCS, noncavernous sinus.

In order to evaluate the response to GKRS in DAVFs with different venous drainage patterns, we further analyzed treatment results of the 108 patients with NCS DAVFs based on the Cognard and Borden classification systems, respectively (▶ Table 26.6, ▶ Table 26.7). The results show that radiosurgery was effective in treating Cognard type I and IIa lesions (benign lesions) with complete obliteration rates of 77 and 68%, respectively. However, for Cognard type IIb and IIa + b lesions, a lower cure rate was observed: 57% and 32%, respectively. Of the Cognard type III, IV, and V patients, complete obliteration was observed in 80, 50, and 33% patients, respectively (▶ Table 26.6).

On the other hand, the results are similar when using Borden classification. For the Borden type I lesions, complete obliteration was achieved in 72% of the patients, while the other 28% had partial improvement. However, for Borden type II and III lesions, a lower cure rate was observed. Of the 48 Borden type II and III patients, complete obliteration was observed in 21 (44%) patients, with another 48% showing partial improvement, 4% stationary, and 2% progression. There was 1 late mortality (2%) in the group of type II–III DAVF patients (▶ Table 26.7).

For patients with CS DAVFs, the median obliteration time is 21.4 months in MRI/MRA and 24.2 months in cerebral angiography. For patients with NCS DAVFs, the median obliteration time is 31.1 months in MRI/MRA and 32.8 months in cerebral angiography. However, the symptom relief usually comes before

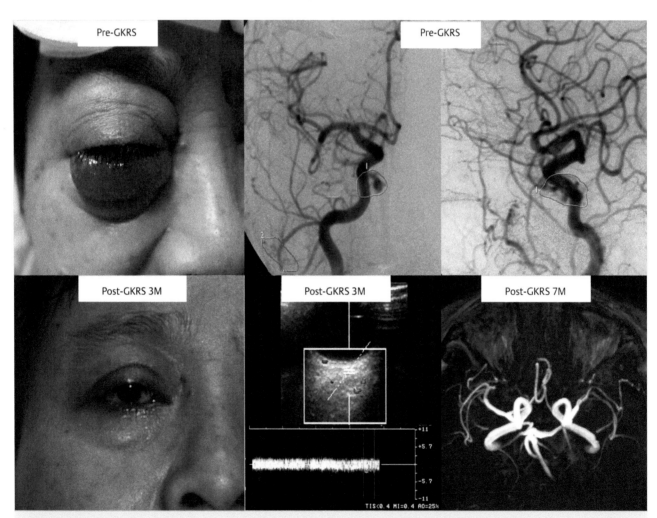

Fig. 26.4 Case illustration for a cavernous sinus (CS) dural arteriovenous fistula (DAVF). A 50-year-old female patient had a right CS DAVF with proptosis, chemosis, red eye, and bruits. The visual acuity and field were normal. The cerebral angiography showed a Barrow's type D DAVF. The margin dose of 17.5 Gy was delivered to the nidus of DAVF via single fraction of Gamma Knife radiosurgery (GKRS). Three months after GKRS, the ocular symptoms and signs were cured with no visual complications. The magnetic resonance angiography showed a total obliteration 7 months after GKRS.

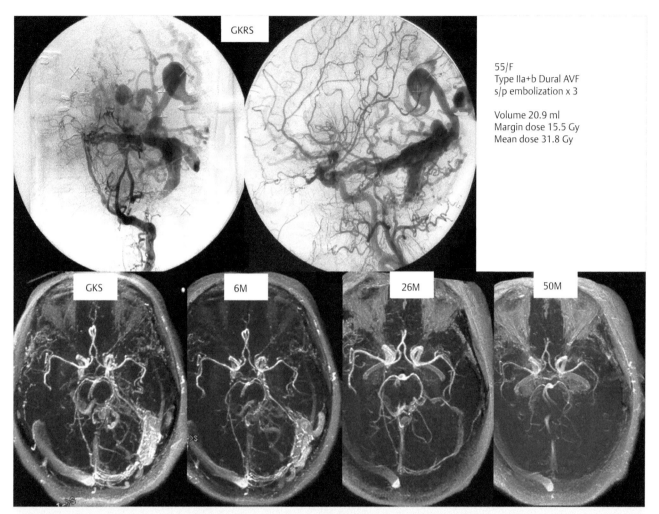

55/F
Type IIa+b Dural AVF
s/p embolization x 3

Volume 20.9 ml
Margin dose 15.5 Gy
Mean dose 31.8 Gy

Fig. 26.5 Case illustration for a noncavernous sinus dural arteriovenous fistula (DAVF). A 55-year-old female patient had a right transverse-sigmoid DAVF with pulsatile tinnitus. She underwent three times transarterial embolization, but the symptom persisted. Cognard type IIa + b with cortical venous drainage was impressed before GKRS. The margin dose of 17.5 Gy was delivered to the nidus of DAVF via single fraction of Gamma Knife radiosurgery (GKRS). The radiation volume was 20.9 mL. The shunting portion of DAVF was closed on the 26 months after GKRS, accompanying with the annoying symptoms. The 50th magnetic resonance angiography showed a total obliteration.

Table 26.6 Clinical outcomes after GKRS in 108 patients with NCS DAVFs stratified by Cognard classification

Cognard type	Complete obliteration	Partial obliteration	Stationary	Progression	Death	Total	Total obliteration (%)
I	17	5	0	0	0	22	77
II	26	12	0	0	0	38	68
IIb	4	3	0	0	0	7	57
IIa + b	8	14	1	1	1	25	32
III	4	1	0	0	0	5	80
IV	4	3	1	0	0	8	50
V	1	2	0	0	0	3	33
Total	64	40	2	1	1	108	59

Abbreviations: DAVFs, dural arteriovenous fistulas; GKRS, Gamma Knife radiosurgery; NCS, noncavernous sinus.

Table 26.7 Clinical outcomes after GKRS in 108 patients with NCS DAVFs stratified by Borden classification

Borden type	Complete obliteration	Partial obliteration	Stationary	Progression	Death	Total	Total classification (%)
I	43	17	0	0	0	60	72
II	12	18	1	1	0	32	38
III	9	5	1	0	1	16	56
Total	64	40	2	1	1	108	59

Abbreviations: DAVFs, dural arteriovenous fistulas; GKRS, Gamma Knife radiosurgery; NCS, noncavernous sinus.

neuroimaging obliteration. For the CS DAVFs, the estimated clinical/symptomatic cure rates are 70% at the first-year follow-up and 90% at the second-year follow-up (▶ Fig. 26.6). It takes more time for the non-CS DAVFs, but the estimated clinical/symptomatic cure rates are 60 and 80% in the first- and second-year follow-ups, respectively (▶ Fig. 26.7). Several reports including the authors' have noted that the time span between radiosurgery and DAVF obliteration in some cases can be as short as within 6 months.[5,34,57,58,59] Because the fistulous vessels of DAVFs that lie along the sinus wall are usually small, DAVFs seem to respond more promptly to radiosurgery, compared with intracerebral AVMs.[38]

As mentioned earlier, for the CS or non-CS DAVFs, most ocular symptoms and signs were regressed before total obliteration. ▶ Table 26.8 demonstrates the various ocular presentations in 156 CS DAVF patients with regular clinical follow-up. After SRS, almost all patients had partial, subtotal, or complete recovery from red eye, chemosis, proptosis, bruits, headache, ocular pain, visual impairment, and diplopia. Only two patients with proptosis had no any improvement. Several patients had temporary worsening of visual acuity and field before the onset of clinical improvement. We believed that a gradual change of the velocity and direction of the venous flow occurred immediately after SRS, and it took 3 to 9 months to normalize the reverse pulsatile flow in SOV.[56] The details will be described in the section of complications below (▶ Table 26.9).

In the literature, cumulative reports have proven the efficacy of GKRS in treating DAVFs. ▶ Table 26.10 summarizes the SRS series for DAVFs since 1994. Guo et al[34] and Pollock et al[39] have separately reported an approximately 80% obliteration rate for CS DAVFs treated by Gamma Knife alone or combined with embolization. In Koebbe's University of Pittsburgh (UPMC) series published in 2005, all 18 patients had complete or near-complete resolution of their presenting symptoms.[10] Söderman et al in 2006 reported on 49 patients with 52 DAVFs, with a 68% obliteration rate and another 24% with flow regression at 2 years.[5] More recently, at the University of Virginia, Cifarelli et al in 2010 reported a 65% obliteration rate in a series of 55 DAVF patients.[60] O'Leary achieved a 77% complete obliteration rate with improvement in another 15% of patients.[43] Yang et al in 2010 reported a series of 40 DAVF patients treated at the UPMC. They found an 83% obliteration rate for patients who had upfront radiosurgery with embolization and a 67% obliteration rate in patients who underwent radiosurgery alone at a median follow-up of 45 months (range of 23–116 months).[61] Cavernous carotid fistulas were associated with higher rates of occlusion

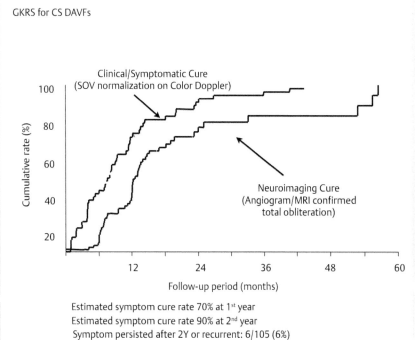

Fig. 26.6 Kaplan-Meier plot for cavernous sinus (CS) dural arteriovenous fistulas. For the CS, most ocular symptoms and signs were regressed before total obliteration.

GKRS for CS DAVFs

Clinical/Symptomatic Cure (SOV normalization on Color Doppler)

Neuroimaging Cure (Angiogram/MRI confirmed total obliteration)

Cumulative rate (%)

Follow-up period (months)

Estimated symptom cure rate 70% at 1st year
Estimated symptom cure rate 90% at 2nd year
Symptom persisted after 2Y or recurrent: 6/105 (6%)

GKRS for non-CS DAVFs

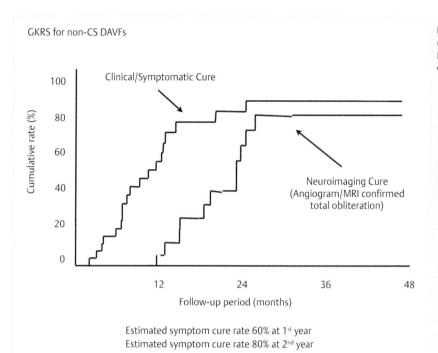

Fig. 26.7 Kaplan-Meier plot for non-CS (noncavernous sinus) dural arteriovenous fistulas. For the CS, most ocular symptoms and signs were regressed before total obliteration.

Estimated symptom cure rate 60% at 1st year
Estimated symptom cure rate 80% at 2nd year

Table 26.8 Cavernous sinus DAVFs: symptoms/signs and results after GKRS (n = 156)

Improvement	Red eye	Chemosis	Proptosis	Bruit	Headache/eye pain	Visual impairment	Diplopia
Complete	78	39	29	23	21	20	31
Subtotal	17	10	2	2	5	8	105
Partial	11	3	3	4	8	10	5
None	–	–	2	–	–	–	–
Total	106	52	36	29	34	39	49

Abbreviations: DAVFs, dural arteriovenous fistulas; GKRS, Gamma Knife radiosurgery.

(p = 0.012) and symptom improvement (p = 0.010) than were transverse-sigmoid sinus-related fistulas[61] (▶ Table 26.11). Although some of the patients in these publications had been treated with surgical resection or endovascular embolization prior to radiosurgery, they were referred for radiosurgery for further management of the residual DAVFs. From these studies, we can estimate an overall success rate of complete obliteration associated with radiosurgery of DAVFs at 65 to 77%, with a

Table 26.9 Complications after GKRS for DAVFs

Cavernous sinus (n = 156)	N	%
• Diplopia with cranial nerve palsy	2	1.3
• Vision deterioration	0	0
Noncavernous sinus (n = 108)	**N**	**%**
• Venous hemorrhage (ICH)	2	1.9
• Radiation-induced focal edema	6	5.5
• Cranial nerve deficits	1	0.9
• Clinical silent dural sinus occlusion	10	9
• Chronic encapsulated hematoma	4	3.7

Abbreviations: DAVFs, dural arteriovenous fistulas; GKRS, Gamma Knife radiosurgery; ICH, intracerebral hemorrhage.

greater number of patients gaining symptomatic relief from the radiosurgical treatment.

Several studies had noted that the period between radiosurgery and DAVF obliteration in some cases could be short, as compared to results of AVM radiosurgery.[5,34,57,58,59] Different opinions might exist regarding the extent to which obliteration after radiosurgery could be attributed to the treatment, or the natural course of the disease, especially when there are several case reports showing spontaneous DAVF obliteration.[21,62,63,64] Nevertheless, a fast closure of the fistulas will shorten the period that the patient suffers from throbbing headache, tinnitus, or ophthalmological symptoms. In addition, for the cases with cortical venous reflux, multimodal treatment including radiosurgery and endovascular procedure may reduce the exposed time at risk of intracerebral hemorrhage or disease progression.

26.1.9 Complications

The potential complications after radiosurgery include persistent venous hypertension, intracranial hemorrhage, cranial nerve dysfunction, sinus stenosis with thrombus formation, late cystic expanding hematoma, and focal radiation-induced brain edema.

Table 26.10 Summary of the SRS series for intracranial DAVFs

Author (year)	Patients (n)	Age (y)	SRS modality	Previous embolization (n/n)	Previous microsurgery (n/n)	Margin dose (Gy)	Radiation volume (mL)	F/U (m)	Complete obliteration (n/n)	Post-SRS hemorrhage (n)	Post-SRS NHND (n)	Mortality (n)
Pan et al (2013)[4]	321	58	GKRS	41/321	13/321	17.2	4.7 for CS 16.9 for NCS	21 for CS 28 for NCS	173/264	2	0	1
Söderman et al (2013)[73]	65	–	GKRS	10/67	3/67	20–25	–	–	37/63	2	2	0
Piippo et al (2013)[74]	16	–	LINAC	13/17	0/17	18	–	–	9/17	0	0	0
Oh et al (2012)[75]	43	–	GKRS	30/43	0/43	19	6.9	–	32/43	1	1	0
Hanakita et al (2012)[76]	22	57	GKRS	10/22	2/22	21	1.5	27	12/22	0	0	0
Gross et al (2012)[77]	8	57	LINAC	4/9	0/9	17.7	1	35	8/9	0	0	0
Cifarelli et al (2010)[60]	55	50	GKRS	36/55	11/55	21	–	36	30/46	3	1	0
Yang et al (2010)[61]	40	69	GKRS	19/44	0/44	20	2	45	32/44	1	0	1
Kida (2009)[78]	13	54	GKRS	7/13	0/13	18.9	–	24	5/13	0	0	0
Söderman et al (2006)[5]	49	–	GKRS	7/52	3/52	22	–	–	28/41	2	1	0
Koebbe et al (2005)[10]	18	65	GKRS	13/23	0/23	20	2.16	46	15/18	0	1	0
Pan et al (2002)[38]	20	53	GKRS	–	–	16.5–19	1.7–40.7	19	11/19	0	0	0
O'Leary et al (2002)[43]	16	56	GKRS	–	–	25	–	24	10/13	0	1	0
Chung et al (2002)[79]	8	56	GKRS	3/8	1/8	20	–	17	1/8	0	1	0
Friedman et al (2001)[33]	23	57	GKRS	2/23	0/23	18	9.6	21	7/17	0	0	0
Shin et al (2000)[40]	2	65	GKRS	0/2	0/2	20	–	28	2/2	0	0	0
Pollock et al (1999)[39]	20	67	GKRS	2/20	0/20	20	2.8	12	13/15	0	1	0
Link et al (1996)[36]	29	61	GKRS	2/29	1/29	19.2	3.3	–	13/18	0	0	0
Lewis et al (1994)[35]	7	61	LINAC	7/7	0/7	15.6	–	24	3/7	0	1	0

Abbreviation: CS, cavernous sinus; DAVFs, dural arteriovenous fistulas; F/U, follow-up; GKRS, Gamma Knife radiosurgery; Gy, Gray; LINAC, linear-accelerator-based radiosurgery; m, month; n, number; NCS, noncavernous sinus; NHND, nonhemorrhage neurological deficits; SRS, stereotactic radiosurgery; y, years.

Table 26.11 Factors associated with DAVF obliteration via SRS

Author (year)	Favorable associated with DAVF obliteration	Unfavorable associated with DAVF obliteration	Not associated with DAVF obliteration
Yang et al (2013)[80]	CS DAVFs	–	–
Cifarelli (2010)[60]	Borden type I DAVFs	Any DAVFs with CVD	Gender Prior endovascular therapy for DAVF Prior craniotomy for DAVF Location of DAVF Size of DAVF Multihole versus single-hole DAVF
Hanakita et al (2012)[76]	Hemorrhage at presentation Target volume < 1.5 mL Cognard types III or IV DAVF	Any DAVFs with CVD	Age Gender Location of DAVF Prior therapy
Söderman et al (2006)[5]	–	–	Minimal radiation dose to DAVF

Abbreviations: CS, cavernous sinus; CVD, cortical venous drainage; DAVF, dural arteriovenous fistula; SRS, stereotactic radiosurgery.

For a DAVF with retrograde CVD, the risk of intracranial hemorrhage after radiosurgery continues until such venous reflux has ceased, which is equivalent to the closure of the arteriovenous fistula. Although the hemorrhage risk after radiosurgery in the latency period before DAVF obliteration is low, Söderman et al showed a 2.5% annual hemorrhage rate after GKRS,[5] and our data showed a 0.8% (n = 2/264) hemorrhage rate[4] (► Table 26.9).

In CS DAVFs, the normalization of the reverse pulsatile flow in SOV is usually observed at 3 to 9 months after GKRS,[56] indicating a gradual change of the velocity and direction of the venous flow. After the treatment, thrombosis of the SOV may be sometimes observed by MRI in patients with temporary worsening of symptoms and signs before the onset of clinical improvement.[65] Lau et al reported such a case of concurrent thrombus formation in the SOV and anterior CS 1 month after radiosurgery. Barcia-Salorio et al also reported that 2 of their 25 patients had experienced a temporary worsening of symptoms as the shunt occluded.[57]

For the non-CS DAFs, some complications such as venous hemorrhage, radiation-induced brain edema, new-onset cranial nerve deficits, and chronic encapsulated expanding hematoma may occur. Clinical silent dural sinus occlusion sometimes happened, but interventions were not necessary for these complications (► Table 26.9).

Other radiation-related complications are rare. Until now, there is no report of temporal lobe radiation necrosis, hypothalamic–pituitary axis dysfunction, or radiation-induced secondary brain tumor for DAVF patients treated with SRS.

26.1.10 The Role of Combining Sinus Recanalization and SRS for Complicated DAVFs

Two hypotheses have been proposed for the initial pathophysiology of DAVFs. One is physiological arteriovenous shunts are open due to an increment of the sinus and venous pressure.[2] The other one is angiogenesis when venous hypertension is induced by an obstruction of the venous outflow may reduce

cerebral perfusion and lead to hypoxia with de novo formation of DAVFs.[66] Based on these theories, a correction of the venous hypertension in the sinus should reduce cerebral venous edema and reverse vicious cycle of creating DAVFs. Using endovascular balloon angioplasty or stent implantation inside the sinus may correct such venous hypertension.

This is especially important when facing the patients with complicated DAVFs, such as multiple DAVFs, poor normal venous drainage (e.g., bilateral transverse-sigmoid sinus nearly occluded or superior sagittal sinus nearly occluded), diffuse cortical vein drainage with venous congestion, or repeated recurrent DAVFs. Sinus occlusion by embolization or resection sometimes carries the risk of further damaging the venous drainage and cause disastrous results. Unpredictable flow change may shut down the driving force of functional intracranial flow. Any therapeutic intervention of DAVFs in these conditions should be performed carefully after recognizing that the fistulous portion of the sinus does not have a drainage function.

In these difficult conditions, recanalization of the sinus combined with SRS could be the possible option to restore venous outflow and correct venous hypertension. Recently, we began to use balloon inflation or stent placement combined with GKRS to treat some DAVFs with partially obstructed sinuses. The idea of angioplasty is also proposed in some authors' reports.[67,68,69,70,71,72] In 2000, Murphy et al reported a case of TSS DAVF treated with transluminal angioplasty and stent placement in a partially thrombosed fistulous sinus.[48,71] Other authors subsequently described that stent placement for DAVFs as a promising technique and that it should be considered a first-line treatment.[68,69]

In the authors' experience, the use of balloon dilation or stent implantation did improve the direction and flow of venous return, and might facilitate DAVF obliteration if subsequent GKRS was performed (► Fig. 26.8). Venous angioplasty can reduce elevated venous pressure and decrease venous reflux. Stenting in dural sinus may reconstruct the venous channel and outlet, and restore physiological venous drainage system. Adjuvant SRS may offer gradual fistula obliteration time for self-adaptation. After SRS, medical treatment such as anticoagulants may be necessary for a period of time. The treatment for a

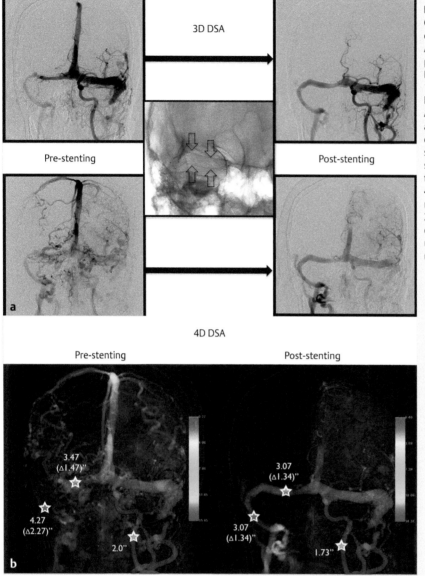

Fig. 26.8 (a) Combining sinus recanalization and Gamma Knife radiosurgery (GKRS) for a complicated dural arteriovenous fistula (DAVF). A 63-year-old female patient had left-side pulsatile tinnitus and bilateral red eye (Rt > Lt). Progressive declined memory was found in recent 1 year. A left Cognard type IIa + b DAVF with bilateral occlusive sinus disorder was impressed. A total occlusion was found in left sigmoid sinus, and the antegrade venous drainage was partially obstructed on the middle level of right transverse sinus. The patient underwent angioplasty with stenting for the right transverse sinus, to keep the patency of intracranial drainage. **(b)** On the 4D digital subtraction angiography, the more rapid transit time was noted after stenting (from 2.27 to 1.43 ms), and reduced the number of cortical vein reflux. One week later, the patient underwent GKRS for the residual left DAVFs (arrow: the location of stent).

complicated DAVF is skillful, and the study on the efficacy and safety of the angioplasty combined with SRS is still ongoing. More case population is needed for consolidating the clinical result.

References

[1] Awad IA, Little JR, Akarawi WP, Ahl J. Intracranial dural arteriovenous malformations: factors predisposing to an aggressive neurological course. J Neurosurg. 1990; 72(6):839–850

[2] Hamada Y, Goto K, Inoue T, et al. Histopathological aspects of dural arteriovenous fistulas in the transverse-sigmoid sinus region in nine patients. Neurosurgery. 1997; 40(3):452–456, discussion 456–458

[3] Newton TH, Cronqvist S. Involvement of dural arteries in intracranial arteriovenous malformations. Radiology. 1969; 93(5):1071–1078

[4] Pan DH, Wu HM, Kuo YH, Chung WY, Lee CC, Guo WY. Intracranial dural arteriovenous fistulas: natural history and rationale for treatment with stereotactic radiosurgery. Prog Neurol Surg. 2013; 27:176–194

[5] Söderman M, Edner G, Ericson K, et al. Gamma knife surgery for dural arteriovenous shunts: 25 years of experience. J Neurosurg. 2006; 104(6):867–875

[6] Aminoff MJ. Vascular anomalies in the intracranial dura mater. Brain. 1973; 96(3):601–612

[7] Goto K, Sidipratomo P, Ogata N, Inoue T, Matsuno H. Combining endovascular and neurosurgical treatments of high-risk dural arteriovenous fistulas in the lateral sinus and the confluence of the sinuses. J Neurosurg. 1999; 90(2): 289–299

[8] Satomi J, van Dijk JM, Terbrugge KG, Willinsky RA, Wallace MC. Benign cranial dural arteriovenous fistulas: outcome of conservative management based on the natural history of the lesion. J Neurosurg. 2002; 97(4):767–770

[9] Cognard C, Gobin YP, Pierot L, et al. Cerebral dural arteriovenous fistulas: clinical and angiographic correlation with a revised classification of venous drainage. Radiology. 1995; 194(3):671–680

[10] Koebbe CJ, Singhal D, Sheehan J, et al. Radiosurgery for dural arteriovenous fistulas. Surg Neurol. 2005; 64(5):392–398, discussion 398–399

[11] Brown RD , Jr, Wiebers DO, Nichols DA. Intracranial dural arteriovenous fistulae: angiographic predictors of intracranial hemorrhage and clinical outcome in nonsurgical patients. J Neurosurg. 1994; 81(4):531–538

[12] Duffau H, Lopes M, Janosevic V, et al. Early rebleeding from intracranial dural arteriovenous fistulas: report of 20 cases and review of the literature. J Neurosurg. 1999; 90(1):78–84

[13] Söderman M, Pavic L, Edner G, Holmin S, Andersson T. Natural history of dural arteriovenous shunts. Stroke. 2008; 39(6):1735–1739

[14] van Dijk JM, terBrugge KG, Willinsky RA, Wallace MC. Clinical course of cranial dural arteriovenous fistulas with long-term persistent cortical venous reflux. Stroke. 2002; 33(5):1233–1236

[15] Chaudhary MY, Sachdev VP, Cho SH, Weitzner I , Jr, Puljic S, Huang YP. Dural arteriovenous malformation of the major venous sinuses: an acquired lesion. AJNR Am J Neuroradiol. 1982; 3(1):13–19

[16] Houser OW, Campbell JK, Campbell RJ, Sundt TM , Jr. Arteriovenous malformation affecting the transverse dural venous sinus–an acquired lesion. Mayo Clin Proc. 1979; 54(10):651–661

[17] Awad IA. The diagnosis and management of intracranial dural arteriovenous malformations. Contemporary Neurosurgery. 1991; 13(4):1–5

[18] Cognard C, Houdart E, Casasco A, Gabrillargues J, Chiras J, Merland JJ. Long-term changes in intracranial dural arteriovenous fistulae leading to worsening in the type of venous drainage. Neuroradiology. 1997; 39(1):59–66

[19] Borden JA, Wu JK, Shucart WA. A proposed classification for spinal and cranial dural arteriovenous fistulous malformations and implications for treatment. J Neurosurg. 1995; 82(2):166–179

[20] Davies MA, Ter Brugge K, Willinsky R, Wallace MC. The natural history and management of intracranial dural arteriovenous fistulae. Part 2: aggressive lesions. Interv Neuroradiol. 1997; 3(4):303–311

[21] Luciani A, Houdart E, Mounayer C, Saint Maurice JP, Merland JJ. Spontaneous closure of dural arteriovenous fistulas: report of three cases and review of the literature. AJNR Am J Neuroradiol. 2001; 22(5):992–996

[22] Barrow DL, Spector RH, Braun IF, Landman JA, Tindall SC, Tindall GT. Classification and treatment of spontaneous carotid-cavernous sinus fistulas. J Neurosurg. 1985; 62(2):248–256

[23] Sarma D, ter Brugge K. Management of intracranial dural arteriovenous shunts in adults. Eur J Radiol. 2003; 46(3):206–220

[24] Zipfel GJ, Shah MN, Refai D, Dacey RG , Jr, Derdeyn CP. Cranial dural arteriovenous fistulas: modification of angiographic classification scales based on new natural history data. Neurosurg Focus. 2009; 26(5):E14

[25] Kawaguchi T, Hosoda K, Shibata Y, Kidoguchi K, Koyama J, Tamaki N. Direct surgical removal of the dural arteriovenous fistulas involving transverse-sigmoid sinuses. J Clin Neurosci. 2002; 9 Suppl 1:16–18

[26] Liu JK, Dogan A, Ellegala DB, et al. The role of surgery for high-grade intracranial dural arteriovenous fistulas: importance of obliteration of venous outflow. J Neurosurg. 2009; 110(5):913–920

[27] Sundt TM , Jr, Piepgras DG. The surgical approach to arteriovenous malformations of the lateral and sigmoid dural sinuses. J Neurosurg. 1983; 59(1):32–39

[28] Collice M, D'Aliberti G, Talamonti G, et al. Surgical interruption of leptomeningeal drainage as treatment for intracranial dural arteriovenous fistulas without dural sinus drainage. J Neurosurg. 1996; 84(5):810–817

[29] Hoh BL, Choudhri TF, Connolly ES , Jr, Solomon RA. Surgical management of high-grade intracranial dural arteriovenous fistulas: leptomeningeal venous disruption without nidus excision. Neurosurgery. 1998; 42(4):796–804, discussion 804–805

[30] Thompson BG, Doppman JL, Oldfield EH. Treatment of cranial dural arteriovenous fistulae by interruption of leptomeningeal venous drainage. J Neurosurg. 1994; 80(4):617–623

[31] van Dijk JM, TerBrugge KG, Willinsky RA, Wallace MC. Selective disconnection of cortical venous reflux as treatment for cranial dural arteriovenous fistulas. J Neurosurg. 2004; 101(1):31–35

[32] Chandler HC , Jr, Friedman WA. Successful radiosurgical treatment of a dural arteriovenous malformation: case report. Neurosurgery. 1993; 33(1):139–141, discussion 141–142

[33] Friedman JA, Pollock BE, Nichols DA, Gorman DA, Foote RL, Stafford SL. Results of combined stereotactic radiosurgery and transarterial embolization for dural arteriovenous fistulas of the transverse and sigmoid sinuses. J Neurosurg. 2001; 94(6):886–891

[34] Guo WY, Pan DH, Wu HM, et al. Radiosurgery as a treatment alternative for dural arteriovenous fistulas of the cavernous sinus. AJNR Am J Neuroradiol. 1998; 19(6):1081–1087

[35] Lewis AI, Tomsick TA, Tew JM , Jr. Management of tentorial dural arteriovenous malformations: transarterial embolization combined with stereotactic radiation or surgery. J Neurosurg. 1994; 81(6):851–859

[36] Link MJ, Coffey RJ, Nichols DA, Gorman DA. The role of radiosurgery and particulate embolization in the treatment of dural arteriovenous fistulas. J Neurosurg. 1996; 84(5):804–809

[37] Maruyama K, Shin M, Kurita H, Tago M, Kirino T. Stereotactic radiosurgery for dural arteriovenous fistula involving the superior sagittal sinus. Case report. J Neurosurg. 2002; 97(5) Suppl:481–483

[38] Pan DH, Chung WY, Guo WY, et al. Stereotactic radiosurgery for the treatment of dural arteriovenous fistulas involving the transverse-sigmoid sinus. J Neurosurg. 2002; 96(5):823–829

[39] Pollock BE, Nichols DA, Garrity JA, Gorman DA, Stafford SL. Stereotactic radiosurgery and particulate embolization for cavernous sinus dural arteriovenous fistulae. Neurosurgery. 1999; 45(3):459–466, discussion 466–467

[40] Shin M, Kurita H, Tago M, Kirino T. Stereotactic radiosurgery for tentorial dural arteriovenous fistulae draining into the vein of Galen: report of two cases. Neurosurgery. 2000; 46(3):730–733, discussion 733–734

[41] Wu HM, Pan DH, Chung WY, et al. Gamma Knife surgery for the management of intracranial dural arteriovenous fistulas. J Neurosurg. 2006; 105 Suppl:43–51

[42] Brown RD , Jr, Flemming KD, Meyer FB, Cloft HJ, Pollock BE, Link ML. Natural history, evaluation, and management of intracranial vascular malformations. Mayo Clin Proc. 2005; 80(2):269–281

[43] O'Leary S, Hodgson TJ, Coley SC, Kemeny AA, Radatz MW. Intracranial dural arteriovenous malformations: results of stereotactic radiosurgery in 17 patients. Clin Oncol (R Coll Radiol). 2002; 14(2):97–102

[44] Pan HC, Sun MH, Yang DY, et al. Multidisciplinary treatment of cavernous sinus dural arteriovenous fistulae with radiosurgery and embolization. J Clin Neurosci. 2005; 12(7):744–749

[45] Heros RC. Gamma knife surgery for dural arteriovenous fistulas. J Neurosurg. 2006; 104(6):861–863, discussion 865–866

[46] Jiang C, Lv X, Li Y, Zhang J, Wu Z. Endovascular treatment of high-risk tentorial dural arteriovenous fistulas: clinical outcomes. Neuroradiology. 2009; 51 (2):103–111

[47] van Rooij WJ, Sluzewski M, Beute GN. Dural arteriovenous fistulas with cortical venous drainage: incidence, clinical presentation, and treatment. AJNR Am J Neuroradiol. 2007; 28(4):651–655

[48] Lucas CdeP, Caldas JG, Prandini MN. Do leptomeningeal venous drainage and dysplastic venous dilation predict hemorrhage in dural arteriovenous fistula? Surg Neurol. 2006; 66 Suppl 3:S2–S5, discussion S5–S6

[49] Klisch J, Kubalek R, Scheufler KM, Zirrgiebel U, Drevs J, Schumacher M. Plasma vascular endothelial growth factor and serum soluble angiopoietin receptor sTIE-2 in patients with dural arteriovenous fistulas: a pilot study. Neuroradiology. 2005; 47(1):10–17

[50] Kojima T, Miyachi S, Sahara Y, et al. The relationship between venous hypertension and expression of vascular endothelial growth factor: hemodynamic and immunohistochemical examinations in a rat venous hypertension model. Surg Neurol. 2007; 68(3):277–284, discussion 284

[51] Terada T, Tsuura M, Komai N, et al. The role of angiogenic factor bFGF in the development of dural AVFs. Acta Neurochir (Wien). 1996; 138(7):877–883

[52] Zhu Y, Lawton MT, Du R, et al. Expression of hypoxia-inducible factor-1 and vascular endothelial growth factor in response to venous hypertension. Neurosurgery. 2006; 59(3):687–696, discussion 687–696

[53] Schneider BF, Eberhard DA, Steiner LE. Histopathology of arteriovenous malformations after Gamma Knife radiosurgery. J Neurosurg. 1997; 87(3):352–357

[54] Graeb DA, Dolman CL. Radiological and pathological aspects of dural arteriovenous fistulas. Case report. J Neurosurg. 1986; 64(6):962–967

[55] Nishijima M, Takaku A, Endo S, et al. Etiological evaluation of dural arteriovenous malformations of the lateral and sigmoid sinuses based on histopathological examinations. J Neurosurg. 1992; 76(4):600–606

[56] Chiou HJ, Chou YH, Guo WY, et al. Verifying complete obliteration of carotid artery-cavernous sinus fistula: role of color Doppler ultrasonography. J Ultrasound Med. 1998; 17(5):289–295

[57] Barcia-Salorio JL, Soler F, Barcia JA, Hernández G. Stereotactic radiosurgery for the treatment of low-flow carotid-cavernous fistulae: results in a series of 25 cases. Stereotact Funct Neurosurg. 1994; 63(1–4):266–270

[58] Hasuo K, Mizushima A, Matsumoto S, et al. Type D dural carotid-cavernous fistula. Results of combined treatment with irradiation and particulate embolization. Acta Radiol. 1996; 37(3, Pt 1):294–298

[59] Onizuka M, Mori K, Takahashi N, et al. Gamma knife surgery for the treatment of spontaneous dural carotid-cavernous fistula. Neurol Med Chir (Tokyo). 2003; 43(10):477–482, discussion 482–483

[60] Cifarelli CP, Kaptain G, Yen CP, Schlesinger D, Sheehan JP. Gamma knife radiosurgery for dural arteriovenous fistulas. Neurosurgery. 2010; 67(5):1230–1235, discussion 1235

[61] Yang HC, Kano H, Kondziolka D, et al. Stereotactic radiosurgery with or without embolization for intracranial dural arteriovenous fistulas. Neurosurgery. 2010; 67(5):1276–1283, discussion 1284–1285

[62] Olutola PS, Eliam M, Molot M, Talalla A. Spontaneous regression of a dural arteriovenous malformation. Neurosurgery. 1983; 12(6):687–690

[63] Pritz MB, Pribram HF. Spontaneous closure of a high-risk dural arteriovenous malformation of the transverse sinus. Surg Neurol. 1991; 36(3):226–228

[64] Saito A, Furuno Y, Nishimura S, Kamiyama H, Nishijima M. Spontaneous closure of transverse sinus dural arteriovenous fistula: case report. Neurol Med Chir (Tokyo). 2008; 48(12):564–568

[65] Lau LI, Wu HM, Wang AG, Yen MY, Hsu WM. Paradoxical worsening with superior ophthalmic vein thrombosis after gamma knife radiosurgery for dural arteriovenous fistula of cavernous sinus: a case report suggesting the mechanism of the phenomenon. Eye (Lond). 2006; 20(12):1426–1428

[66] Tirakotai W, Bertalanffy H, Liu-Guan B, Farhoud A, Sure U. Immunohistochemical study in dural arteriovenous fistulas and possible role of local hypoxia for the de novo formation of dural arteriovenous fistulas. Clin Neurol Neurosurg. 2005; 107(6):455–460

[67] Choi BJ, Lee TH, Kim CW, Choi CH. Reconstructive treatment using a stent graft for a dural arteriovenous fistula of the transverse sinus in the case of hypoplasia of the contralateral venous sinuses: technical case report. Neurosurgery. 2009; 65(5):E994–E996, discussion E996

[68] Levrier O, Métellus P, Fuentes S, et al. Use of a self-expanding stent with balloon angioplasty in the treatment of dural arteriovenous fistulas involving the transverse and/or sigmoid sinus: functional and neuroimaging-based outcome in 10 patients. J Neurosurg. 2006; 104(2):254–263

[69] Liebig T, Henkes H, Brew S, Miloslavski E, Kirsch M, Kühne D. Reconstructive treatment of dural arteriovenous fistulas of the transverse and sigmoid sinus: transvenous angioplasty and stent deployment. Neuroradiology. 2005; 47(7):543–551

[70] Malek AM, Higashida RT, Balousek PA, et al. Endovascular recanalization with balloon angioplasty and stenting of an occluded occipital sinus for treatment of intracranial venous hypertension: technical case report. Neurosurgery. 1999; 44(4):896–901

[71] Murphy KJ, Gailloud P, Venbrux A, Deramond H, Hanley D, Rigamonti D. Endovascular treatment of a grade IV transverse sinus dural arteriovenous fistula by sinus recanalization, angioplasty, and stent placement: technical case report. Neurosurgery. 2000; 46(2):497–500, discussion 500–501

[72] Yeh PS, Wu TC, Tzeng WS, Lin HJ. Endovascular angioplasty and stent placement in venous hypertension related to dural arteriovenous fistulas and venous sinus thrombosis. Clin Neurol Neurosurg. 2010; 112(2):167–171

[73] Söderman M, Dodoo E, Karlsson B. Dural arteriovenous fistulas and the role of gamma knife stereotactic radiosurgery: the Stockholm experience. Prog Neurol Surg. 2013; 27:205–217

[74] Piippo A, Niemela M, van Popta J, et al. Characteristics and long-term outcome of 251 patients with dural arteriovenous fistulas in a defined population. J Neurosurg. 2013; 118(5):923–934

[75] Oh JT, Chung SY, Lanzino G, et al. Intracranial dural arteriovenous fistulas: clinical characteristics and management based on location and hemodynamics. J Cerebrovasc Endovasc Neurosurg. 2012; 14(3):192–202

[76] Hanakita S, Koga T, Shin M, Shojima M, Igaki H, Saito N. Role of Gamma Knife surgery in the treatment of intracranial dural arteriovenous fistulas. J Neurosurg. 2012; 117 Suppl:158–163

[77] Gross BA, Ropper AE, Popp AJ, Du R. Stereotactic radiosurgery for cerebral dural arteriovenous fistulas. Neurosurg Focus. 2012; 32(5):E18

[78] Kida Y. Radiosurgery for dural arteriovenous fistula. Prog Neurol Surg. 2009; 22:38–44

[79] Chung WY, Shiau CY, Wu HM, et al. Staged radiosurgery for extra-large cerebral arteriovenous malformations: method, implementation, and results. J Neurosurg. 2008; 109 Suppl:65–72

[80] Yang HC, Kano H, Kondziolka D, et al. Stereotactic radiosurgery with or without embolization for intracranial dural arteriovenous fistulas. Neurosurgery. 2010; 67(5):1276–1283; discussion 1284-1275

27 Multidisciplinary Management of Arteriovenous Malformations

Federico Cagnazzo, Thomas J. Sorenson, and Giuseppe Lanzino

Abstract

The contemporary management of complex brain arteriovenous malformations (AVMs) often requires a multidisciplinary approach, including embolization, microsurgical resection, and stereotactic radiosurgery (SRS). The current literature regarding the multimodality treatment of AVMs was explored with the aim to report the results of various combinations of these treatment modalities. The combined management usually allows four options. Preoperative embolization can be considered for high-grade AVMs, or as a targeted treatment for portions of the AVM difficult to deal with at surgery. Similarly, presurgical SRS is a feasible option to reduce nidus size, blood flow, and deep/eloquent nidus for easier microsurgical resection. However, surgical approach after radiation should be appropriately timed, considering the fact that during the 3-year latency period necessary to maximize the histological changes incited by SRS, the patient is exposed to a higher risk of hemorrhage. Contrariwise, the real effectiveness of pre-SRS endovascular embolization remains uncertain, and a lower occlusion rate is often reported in the literature. In addition, there is a lack of convincing studies that report the real effectiveness of triplicate treatment, and the sum of procedural risks of each treatment should be carefully considered. Furthermore, target endovascular treatment of brain AVMs associated aneurysms is safe and effective, and can be performed using coils or liquid embolic agents depending on location and size. Several treatment modalities are currently available for the management of complex brain AVMs. However, multidisciplinary approach should be accurately individualized while considering the sum of procedural risks of each treatment.

Keywords: arteriovenous malformations, multidisciplinary management, surgical treatment, stereotactic radiosurgery, endovascular embolization, aneurysms associated with AVMs

- High-grade arteriovenous malformations are complex lesions that require a multidisciplinary decision-making.
- Microsurgical resection, endovascular embolization, and stereotactic radiosurgery can be used in a multimodal strategy.
- Patients amenable to treatment with a multidisciplinary approach should be meticulously selected with consideration of the summative procedural risks of each treatment.
- Presurgical embolization and radiosurgery are often used to reduce the size of larger AVMs and to allow a safer and effective surgical resection.
- Embolization before stereotactic radiosurgery is controversial, but can be used to increase the rate of total obliteration.
- Endovascular-targeted treatment of the aneurysms associated with AVMs is safe and effective.

27.1 Introduction and General Principles

Making the decision to treat a patient with a cerebral arteriovenous malformation (AVM) involves an understanding of the complex balance between the risks of rupture and the risks associated with treatment. Because of this fine line, the contemporary management of brain AVMs often requires a multidisciplinary approach and the coordination of several treatment modalities, including embolization, microsurgical resection, and stereotactic radiosurgery (SRS). However, these treatment options alone are not optimal for complex AVMs as microsurgical resection is associated with higher morbidity, but SRS and endovascular treatment are associated with low obliteration rates. To minimize the disadvantages of each treatment modality, a multidisciplinary approach should be evaluated for certain lesions, including high-grade AVMs with complex angioarchitecture that are large, deep, and located in eloquent brain areas.

27.2 Materials and Methods

The current literature regarding the multimodality treatment of AVMs was explored. In this chapter, we report the results of published series that utilized various combinations of microsurgical resection, endovascular embolization, and SRS.

27.3 Results and Discussion

The combined management of patients with high-grade AVMs usually allows four options:
- Endovascular treatment before microsurgical resection.
- Endovascular embolization before SRS.
- Radiosurgery before microsurgical resection.
- Radiosurgery, endovascular embolization, and microsurgical resection.

Because each individual treatment option and each combination therapy carry a specific cure and complication rate, the first decision is whether treatment is indicated.

27.3.1 Multimodal Strategy: Presurgical Endovascular Embolization

In high-grade Spetzler–Martin (SM) AVMs with complex angioarchitecture, complete obliteration is often impractical with endovascular embolization or surgical resection alone, making a combined approach valuable.[1] For this combined approach, embolization is often used as the first modality to allow for an easier, safer, and more thorough subsequent microsurgical resection as preliminary embolization can reduce AVM blood flow, reduce intraoperative blood loss, and facilitate

Table 27.1 Recent series of embolization as adjunctive treatment for microsurgical arteriovenous malformation resection

Author/year	Number of patients	Embolized patients (%)	Grade (SM)	Permanent morbidity (%)	Mortality (%)	Postsurgical obliteration (%)
Lawton (2003)[5]	76	98.6	III	3.9	3.9	97.4
Hartmann et al (2005)[1]	119	100	I–V	5	0	NA
Weber (2007)[6]	47	100	I–V	7.1	0	97.8
Natarajan et al (2008)[2]	28	100	I–V	3.6	3.6	96.4
Bradac (2013)[28]	76	35.5	I–V	3.9	0	97.1
Nataraj et al (2014)[4]	265	38	I–V	6	1	99
Theofanis et al (2014)[3]	264	38.3	I–V	1.9	2.7	100
Korja (2014)[7]	562	9.3	I–III	7.7	1.4	NA
Potts (2015)[8]	232	42.7	I–II	3	0.4	100

Abbreviation: SM, Spetzler–Martin.

surgical manipulation.[2] Furthermore, the progressive reduction of blood flow may produce a gradual adaptation of the surrounding parenchyma to the hemodynamic changes, decreasing the risk of normal perfusion pressure breakthrough.

As another complementary technique to surgical resection, embolization can also be used to target specific components of a complex AVM. Targeted embolization may facilitate the recognition and occlusion of deep feeding arteries that are often encountered in a late phase of AVM resection and can be otherwise difficult to manage during surgery.[2] Additionally, endovascular therapy is a safe and effective strategy for treating AVM-associated aneurysms, which are often the source of intracranial hemorrhage.[3]

However, these combined approaches can also be associated with higher rates of complication. Partial occlusion of an AVM by embolization can modify the hemodynamic status of the AVM and the surrounding parenchyma with decreased and increased blood flow areas into the nidus and cerebral vasculature. Similarly, obstruction and/or slowing of venous outflow can increase the risk of rupture. To minimize these risks, timely surgical treatment after embolization is recommended.[4] The results of presurgical embolization appear inhomogeneous in different clinical series (▶ Table 27.1).

Theofanis et al reported a higher rate of complications in a group of patients treated with multiple presurgical embolization attempts. Of the 264 AVMs treated with microsurgery, preoperative embolization was used in 38.3%. Complications were seen in 7.2% and were associated with multiple embolization attempts (odds ratio [OR]: 1.6) on multivariate analysis. Seven patients experienced a hemorrhage related to embolization treatment before surgery.[3]

Comparable results were found by Natarajan et al. Despite a high occlusion rate after combined endovascular and surgical treatment, the authors reported a higher postoperative complication rate (14%) compared to presurgical embolization. Twenty-eight AVMs (average size/volume 3.56 cm/13.03 mL) were embolized preoperatively in 55 sessions with Onyx. The average final percentage of endovascular nidal obliteration was 74.11%. The long-term radiological follow-up showed residual AVM in only one patient who was treated with radiosurgery.[2]

However, the higher rate of treatment-related complications in combined endovascular and surgical treatment can be potentially related to the more complex angioarchitecture of treated

AVMs. Nataraj et al treated 101 patients with presurgical embolization. Of these patients, 100 (99%) had complete occlusion of the AVM at the end of the treatment cycle, and 87 (86%) had a favorable outcome. In all, 37% of SM grade IV–V AVMs were treated with both embolization and surgery, compared to 7% of high-grade AVMs treated with surgery alone. Taking into account the higher SM grade in the combined group, the morbidity rate was slightly higher in the combined group (6% of new severe deficits), compared to the surgical group (0% of new severe deficits).[4]

The aforementioned series show the efficacy of combined treatment, despite the higher rate of complications than surgery alone. When considering treatment options, preoperative embolization should be considered for high-grade SM AVMs or as a targeted treatment for portions of the AVM more difficult to deal with at surgery or to target associated aneurysms.[9] Preoperative embolization should rarely be indicated for AVMs smaller than 3 cm because of their low rate of surgical morbidity.

27.3.2 Multimodal Strategy: Presurgical Stereotactic Radiosurgery

As stated earlier, the surgical resection of many large, high-grade AVMs is often correlated with a high procedural risk, and many lesions are considered inoperable for their size and angioarchitecture. For these challenging lesions, the use of presurgical SRS can be evaluated to reduce the size and/or to target deeper areas of the AVM, allowing for a safer and more effective subsequent surgical resection.[10]

There are two methods of SRS delivery: single session (SS) and volume staged (VS). In SS, a single, high dose of irradiation is applied. This option is best indicated for small AVMs; SS-SRS is not effective for nidal volumes greater than 3 cm in diameter, because the treatment requires reduction of the marginal dose below an acceptable amount. Under this range of radiation dose, the obliteration rate is less than 70%.[11]

VS SRS is the other strategy that is best indicated for large AVMs. This approach divides a large AVM into smaller portions, and each portion is treated separately with a high-dose radiation and an acceptably low rate of post-SRS complications.[12,13]

Recently, Abla et al reported a series of high-grade AVMs that were treated with VS-SRS followed by surgical resection of the

Table 27.2 Principal series of combined radiosurgery and surgical treatment

Author/year	Number of patients	Patients treated with SRS	Grade (SM)	Time before surgery (y)	Hemorrhage during period before surgery (%)	Occlusion (%)	Good clinical outcome (%)
Asgari (2009)[14]	8	8	III–IV	7	25	100	62
Sanchez-Mejia et al (2009)[15]	42	21	I–IV	4.7	33	NA[a]	NA[b]
Abla et al (2015)[11]	16	16	III–V	5.7	56	93.8	62
Tong et al (2016)[10]	42	42	II–IV	5.1	40	100	81

Abbreviation: SM, Spetzler–Martin; SRS, stereotactic radiosurgery.

[a]The incidence of residual arteriovenous malformation was lower in pre-irradiated patients.

[b]All patients (irradiated and nonirradiated) had a worsening in neurological function between diagnosis and resection.

residual (after SRS) nidus (► Table 27.2). Sixteen AVMs (mean SM grade: 4; mean diameter: 5.9 cm) underwent treatment, and the average SM grade was reduced to 2.5 and the average maximum AVM size was reduced to 3 cm. The lesions were surgically resected after a mean interval of 5.7 years. Postoperative angiography confirmed curative AVM resection in 15 patients (93.8%).[11]

Tong et al compared two groups of radiated and nonradiated patients, who underwent surgical resection for AVMs. In 42 patients treated with SRS, the mean AVM volume, size, and SM grade were reduced, respectively, by 76.8, 41, and 61.9%. Additionally, the operative time, blood loss, and perioperative neurological deterioration were all significantly lower in the pretreated group. The authors conclude that presurgical SRS treatment can facilitate AVM resection.[10]

Other authors demonstrated the usefulness and the efficacy of presurgical irradiation. Sanchez-Mejia et al reported 21 previously irradiated grade III–IV AVMs, and compared these patients with the nonirradiated group. Patients that underwent radiosurgical treatment had lower blood loss, lower surgical times, and a lesser rate of preoperative embolization.[15] Reduced blood loss is likely because SRS causes progressive luminal thrombosis with consequent narrowing or vessel obliteration. Thus, blood flow through the AVM is reduced and the coagulation of the sclerotic arteries becomes easier, especially for the perforating arteries, which are usually weak and thin.[10,11,15,16]

Despite the theoretical utility of SRS before AVM resection, the beneficial effects are not immediate. In fact, a 3-year latency period is necessary to maximize the histological changes incited by SRS.[15] During this period, the patient is exposed to the risk of hemorrhage, which should be factored into the estimation of treatment risks.

Presurgical SRS can be considered in selected cases of large AVMs, aiming to reduce nidus size, blood flow, and deep/eloquent nidus for easier subsequent microsurgical resection. However, surgical resection after radiation should be appropriately timed to find the optimal balance between beneficial SRS-induced changes and hemorrhage risk related to the latency period.

27.3.3 Multimodal Strategy: Pre-SRS Endovascular Embolization

In selected AVM cases, SRS has been established as an effective individual treatment. However, large AVMs require high doses of radiation that result in low obliteration rates and frequent adverse radiation effects.[3,4] For these cases, SRS can be used as an adjuvant treatment with endovascular embolization. These therapies in theory should work together by allowing embolization to reduce the size of large AVMs and SRS treatment to fully occlude the shrunken lesion. This approach is also beneficial because high bleed-risk components of AVM, such as intranidal aneurysms or high-flow fistulas, are usually less sensitive to radiosurgery. Thus, initially targeting these specific portions of the AVM with embolization can be used to make the AVM more amenable to subsequent SRS therapy. Finally, embolization of high-flow fistulas can reduce the venous pressure into the AVM nidus, decreasing the risk of hemorrhage and SRS-induced vasogenic edema.[9] Zabel-du Bois et al[17] reported 78% rate of complete obliteration at 4-year follow-up for AVMs treated with pre-SRS embolization therapy. Complete obliteration was obtained in 90% of SM grade I–II and in 59% of SM grade III–IV AVMs.

However, the real effectiveness of AVM embolization combined with SRS remains uncertain as the literature is controversial. Many series suggest that pre-SRS embolization of AVMs is actually associated with lower obliteration rates and worse outcome. Andrade-Souza et al[18] reported a lower obliteration rate (47 vs. 70%) in 47 patients treated with pre-SRS glue embolization compared to 47 patients treated with SRS alone.[10] Additionally, Schwyzer et al[19] showed the results of 215 patients that underwent partial endovascular embolization followed by SRS. Angiographic results of combined treatments were worse (33% total obliteration) compared with patients in whom SRS was used alone (60.9% total obliteration). Furthermore, treatment-related complications were higher (2.7%) in the pre-SRS embolization group, compared with patients treated with SRS alone (1.3%).[13]

Similar results were found by Xu et al[20] in a large systematic meta-analysis of 10 studies including 1,988 patients, which compared SRS effectiveness in patients with and without pre-SRS embolization therapy AVM obliteration rates at 3 years were significantly lower in the pre-SRS embolization group (41%), compared to patients who had undergone radiosurgery alone (59%). No significant differences between these groups of treatments were found regarding the rates of hemorrhage and permanent deficits from radiation-induced changes. Other authors have underlined the lower complete occlusion of pre-SRS embolization compared with SRS therapy alone (Schlienger: 54 vs. 71%[21]; Kano: 59 vs. 76%[16]; ► Table 27.3).

Several mechanisms have been suggested to explain the lower efficacy of pre-SRS embolization. Recanalization of the

Table 27.3 Principal series of combined endovascular embolization with stereotactic radiosurgery

Author/year	Number of patients	Embolized patients (%)	Grade (SM)	Permanent morbidity (%)	Mortality (%)	Post-SRS obliteration (%)
Gobin (1996)[22]	125	100	I–V	12.8	1.6	69
Zabel-du Bois et al (2007)[17]	50	100	I–IV	0	0	78
Andrade-Souza et al (2007)[18]	244	25	I–IV	6	0	47
Blackburn (2011)[23]	21	100	II–V	14	0	81
Schwyzer et al (2012)[19]	215	100	I–IV	7.9	1.9	33
Kano et al (2012)[12]	120	100	I–V	2.5	5.8	59
Xu et al (2014)[20]	1,988	30	NA	3.3	NA	41
Oermann (2015)[24]	1,010	24	I–IV	2.5	NA	49

Abbreviations: SM, Spetzler–Martin; SRS, stereotactic radiosurgery.

nidus after embolization and enhanced hypoxia-induced angiogenesis with subsequent lower radiosensitivity are some of the theories proposed.[9] Alternatively, embolization may obscure the targeting of the nidus with a suboptimal dose planning for radiosurgery[25,26]

Before pre-SRS embolization therapy is completely abandoned, it is important to point out that combined treatment is often used to treat more complex AVMs than radiosurgery alone. As such, the lower obliteration rate may be related to a selection bias, and not to the therapy itself.[26] However, few studies report good results of pre-SRS embolization therapy and, as such, it is currently not recommended.

27.3.4 Complex Brain Arteriovenous Malformations: Multimodality Treatment Integration

Deep-seated, high-grade SM, and complex angioarchitecture (arterial feeders and venous drainage) AVMs represent a challenge for all invasive therapeutic approaches. Many giant AVMs (nidus diameter > 6 cm) have deep components within the basal ganglia, thalamus, or other eloquent areas. Based on their size and location, these lesions are often considered "untreatable."

During the past two decades, the improvement of microsurgical techniques, electrophysiological monitoring, preoperative embolization, and SRS now allows for the possibility of safely resecting some of these lesions, often with a multimodal approach.[27] Due to procedural risks, unruptured SM grade IV–V AVMs may be considered for simple observation. However, some of these lesions, especially in young patients and after rupture may be considered for a multimodal approach.[28]

In the literature, the rate of combination of all treatments is variable in different series. In the ARUBA (a randomized trial of unruptured brain arteriovenous), 28 (25%) patients randomized to intervention received multimodality treatment.[29] Embolization was used as a surgical adjunct in 12 patients and was combined with SRS in 15 patients. Only 1 patient was treated with a combination of all three modalities. Similarly, in the multicenter Scottish Audit of Intracranial Vascular Malformations, only 1 patient underwent all types of treatments, among 35 (34%) patients who underwent multimodality treatment.[30]

Theofanis et al reported 10 patients (3.8%), among the 264 patients that were treated with a combination of all modalities. In all patients, microsurgical resection resulted in complete obliteration and cure of the AVM.[3]

Chang et al described a large series of 53 patients with giant AVMs (nidus > 6.8 cm). Most patients received multimodality treatment, with 23 patients treated with a combination of embolization, radiosurgery, and surgery. The overall outcome was excellent in 27 patients, good in 15 patients, and poor in 3 patients. The long-term complication rate in surviving patients was 15%, mostly deriving from the summative complications of each individual treatment.[26] This series suggests that selected giant AVMs in symptomatic patients can be treated with a multimodal approach with good outcomes and acceptable risks profile.

Nataraj et al reported a considerable series of 265 AVMs treated with a single or combined approach. Fourteen patients (5.3%) underwent all three modalities. Among these, there was one SM grade II, six SM grade III, and seven SM grade IV AVMs. The SM grade was found to correlate negatively with a cure. There was a favorable outcome in 13 (93%) patients treated with all three modalities. The authors were able to cure 92% of SM grade I–IV lesions treated with a multimodality approach. Alternatively, only 53% of treated SM grade V lesions were cured.[4]

Posterior fossa AVMs are relatively uncommon (5–18% of brain AVMs) and are often difficult to treat. Hemorrhage is more frequent in this location compared to its supratentorial counterpart. Kelly et al presented their series with a multimodality treatment of 48 patients with SM grade III–IV AVMs located in the posterior fossa. There were 13 patients with cerebellar AVMs, 29 with brainstem AVMs, and 6 with AVMs in both locations. Twenty-three patients underwent multimodality treatment with a combination of surgery and embolization, with or without radiosurgery. The author underlined the concept that multimodality treatment in this series allowed better clinical outcomes (81%) with acceptable complication rates.[31]

In cases of complex AVMs, the combination of endovascular embolization, SRS, and microsurgery should be evaluated. While the combination of two modality treatments is well described in the literature, there is a lack of convincing studies that report the actual effectiveness of triplicate treatment.

Patients amenable to treatment with triple strategy should be carefully selected while considering the sum of procedural risks of each treatment.

27.3.5 Management of Aneurysms Associated with Arteriovenous Malformations

The management of AVM-associated aneurysms depends on different factors. There is a general agreement for initial treatment of the source of bleeding. For this reason, it is important to determine whether the source of hemorrhage is the aneurysm or the nidus.

Aneurysms are classified as intranidal (within the nidus and fill early during angiography), flow related (located on the arterial feeders, proximal or distal), and unrelated (arteries unrelated to AVM flow). Their pathogenesis is not completely understood, but the importance of hemodynamic factors and hyperdynamic circulation is generally agreed upon. This theory is supported by the fact that aneurysms associated with AVMs are often present on the feeding arteries supplying the lesion and spontaneous regression of the aneurysm after AVM resection has been observed.[32]

The prevalence of arterial aneurysms in patients with brain AVMs is estimated to be between 5 and 20%.[32,33] AVM-associated intracranial aneurysms lead to a higher AVM bleeding risk and pose important therapeutic challenges.[32] The incidence of pretreatment rebleeding of AVM-associated aneurysms has been reported to range between 6 and 16% within 1 year.[34] Considering the frequent poor functional outcome after aneurysm rebleeding, endovascular embolization of the ruptured aneurysm should be performed early using coils or liquid embolic agents depending on location and size

The treatment of associated aneurysms depends on different factors. In ruptured AVMs, there is general agreement that if an associated flow-related aneurysm is the source of the hemorrhage, then the aneurysm should be treated similarly to isolated berry aneurysms presenting with subarachnoid hemorrhage. In patients with an unruptured AVM, associated aneurysms can be managed with a strategy similar to the one adopted for incidental aneurysms in general. The exception are distal flow-related aneurysms that often regress spontaneously after treatment of the AVM.[32,35] Redekop et al reported an 80% rate of complete regression of distal flow-related aneurysms following AVM obliteration, and 67% regression after incomplete AVM treatment with resultant reduction in the size of the nidus by more than 50%. Based on these considerations, conservative management of small distal flow-related aneurysms should be considered if the AVM is treated.

27.4 Conclusion

Brain AVMs are often complex lesions that require a multidisciplinary decision-making. Several treatment modalities are currently available for the management of these lesions, including microsurgical resection, embolization, and SRS. Patients amenable to a multidisciplinary approach should be accurately selected considering the sum of procedural risks of each treatment.

References

[1] Hartmann A, Mast H, Mohr JP, et al. Determinants of staged endovascular and surgical treatment outcome of brain arteriovenous malformations. Stroke. 2005; 36(11):2431–2435

[2] Natarajan SK, Ghodke B, Britz GW, Born DE, Sekhar LN. Multimodality treatment of brain arteriovenous malformations with microsurgery after embolization with onyx: single-center experience and technical nuances. Neurosurgery. 2008; 62(6):1213–1225, discussion 1225–1226

[3] Theofanis T, Chalouhi N, Dalyai R, et al. Microsurgery for cerebral arteriovenous malformations: postoperative outcomes and predictors of complications in 264 cases. Neurosurg Focus. 2014; 37(3):E10

[4] Nataraj A, Mohamed MB, Gholkar A, et al. Multimodality treatment of cerebral arteriovenous malformations. World Neurosurg. 2014; 82(1–2):149–159

[5] Lawton MT. Spetzler-Martin grade III arteriovenous malformations: Surgical results and a modification of the grading scale. Neurosurgery. 2003; 52:740–749

[6] Weber W, Kis B, Siekmann R, et al. Preoperative embolization of intracranial arteriovenous malformations with Onyx. Neurosurgery. 2007; 61:244–252; discussion 252-254

[7] Korja M, Bervini D, Assaad N, et al. Role of surgery in the management of brain arteriovenous malformations: prospective cohort study. Stroke. 2014; 45:3549–3555

[8] Potts MB, Lau D, Abla AA, et al. Current surgical results with low-grade brain arteriovenous malformations. J Neurosurg. 2015; 122:912–920

[9] Morgan MK, Zurin AA, Harrington T, Little N. Changing role for preoperative embolisation in the management of arteriovenous malformations of the brain. J Clin Neurosci. 2000; 7(6):527–530

[10] Tong X, Wu J, Pan J, et al. Microsurgical resection for persistent arteriovenous malformations following Gamma Knife radiosurgery: a case-control study. World Neurosurg. 2016; 88:277–288

[11] Abla AA, Rutledge WC, Seymour ZA, et al. A treatment paradigm for high-grade brain arteriovenous malformations: volume-staged radiosurgical downgrading followed by microsurgical resection. J Neurosurg. 2015; 122(2): 419–432

[12] Kano H, Kondziolka D, Flickinger JC, et al. Stereotactic radiosurgery for arteriovenous malformations, Part 6: multistaged volumetric management of large arteriovenous malformations. J Neurosurg. 2012; 116(1):54–65

[13] Pollock BE, Kline RW, Stafford SL, Foote RL, Schomberg PJ. The rationale and technique of staged-volume arteriovenous malformation radiosurgery. Int J Radiat Oncol Biol Phys. 2000; 48(3):817–824

[14] Asgari S, Bassiouni H, Gizewski E, et al. AVM resection after radiation therapy–clinico-morphological features and microsurgical results. Neurosurg Rev. 2010; 33:53–61

[15] Sanchez-Mejia RO, McDermott MW, Tan J, Kim H, Young WL, Lawton MT. Radiosurgery facilitates resection of brain arteriovenous malformations and reduces surgical morbidity. Neurosurgery. 2009; 64(2):231–238, discussion 238–240

[16] Yen CP, Schlesinger D, Sheehan JP. Natural history of cerebral arteriovenous malformations and the risk of hemorrhage after radiosurgery. Prog Neurol Surg. 2013; 27:5–21

[17] Zabel-du Bois A, Milker-Zabel S, Huber P, et al. Risk of hemorrhage and obliteration rates of LINAC-based radiosurgery for cerebral arteriovenous malformations treated after prior partial embolization. Int J Radiat Oncol Biol Phys. 2007; 68:999–1003

[18] Andrade-Souza YM, Ramani M, Scora D, et al. Embolization before radiosurgery reduces the obliteration rate of arteriovenous malformations. Neurosurgery. 2007; 60:443–451; discussion 451-452

[19] Schwyzer L, Yen CP, Evans A, et al. Long-term results of gamma knife surgery for partially embolized arteriovenous malformations. Neurosurgery. 2012; 71:1139–1147; discussion 1147-1148

[20] Xu F, Zhong J, Ray A, et al. Stereotactic radiosurgery with and without embolization for intracranial arteriovenous malformations: a systematic review and meta-analysis. Neurosurg Focus. 2014; 37:E16

[21] Schlienger M, Atlan D, Lefkopoulos D, et al. Linac radiosurgery for cerebral arteriovenous malformations: results in 169 patients. Int J Radiat Oncol Biol Phys. 2000; 46:1135–1142

[22] Gobin YP, Laurent A, Merienne L, et al. Treatment of brain arteriovenous malformations by embolization and radiosurgery. J Neurosurg. 1996; 85:19–28

[23] Blackburn SL, Ashley WW, Jr., Rich KM, et al. Combined endovascular embolization and stereotactic radiosurgery in the treatment of large arteriovenous malformations. J Neurosurg. 2011; 114:1758–1767

[24] Oermann EK, Ding D, Yen CP, et al. Effect of prior embolization on cerebral arteriovenous malformation radiosurgery outcomes: A case-control study. Neurosurgery. 2015; 77:406–417; discussion 417

[25] Lunsford LD, Niranjan A, Kondziolka D, Sirin S, Flickinger JC. Arteriovenous malformation radiosurgery: a twenty year perspective. Clin Neurosurg. 2008; 55:108–119

[26] Chang SD, Marcellus ML, Marks MP, Levy RP, Do HM, Steinberg GK. Multimodality treatment of giant intracranial arteriovenous malformations. Neurosurgery. 2003; 53(1):1–11, discussion 11–13

[27] Chang SD, Lopez JR, Steinberg GK. The usefulness of electrophysiological monitoring during resection of central nervous system vascular malformations. J Stroke Cerebrovasc Dis. 1999; 8(6):412–422

[28] Bradac O, Charvat F, Benes V. Treatment for brain arteriovenous malformation in the 1998–2011 period and review of the literature. Acta Neurochir (Wien). 2013; 155(2):199–209

[29] Mohr JP, Parides MK, Stapf C, et al. international ARUBA investigators. Medical management with or without interventional therapy for unruptured brain arteriovenous malformations (ARUBA): a multicentre, non-blinded, randomised trial. Lancet. 2014; 383(9917):614–621

[30] Al-Shahi Salman R, White PM, Counsell CE, et al. Scottish Audit of Intracranial Vascular Malformations Collaborators. Outcome after conservative management or intervention for unruptured brain arteriovenous malformations. JAMA. 2014; 311(16):1661–1669

[31] Kelly ME, Guzman R, Sinclair J, et al. Multimodality treatment of posterior fossa arteriovenous malformations. J Neurosurg. 2008; 108(6):1152–1161

[32] Redekop G, TerBrugge K, Montanera W, Willinsky R. Arterial aneurysms associated with cerebral arteriovenous malformations: classification, incidence, and risk of hemorrhage. J Neurosurg. 1998; 89(4):539–546

[33] Lv X, Wu Z, Li Y, et al. Endovascular treatment of cerebral aneurysms associated with arteriovenous malformations. Eur J Radiol. 2012; 81(6):1296–1298

[34] Gross BA, Du R. Rate of re-bleeding of arteriovenous malformations in the first year after rupture. J Clin Neurosci. 2012; 19(8):1087–1088

[35] Meisel HJ, Mansmann U, Alvarez H, Rodesch G, Brock M, Lasjaunias P. Cerebral arteriovenous malformations and associated aneurysms: analysis of 305 cases from a series of 662 patients. Neurosurgery. 2000; 46(4):793–800, discussion 800–802

28 Treatment of Inoperable Cerebral Arteriovenous Malformations

Marshall C. Cress, Jason M. Davies, and Elad I. Levy

Abstract

This chapter on the treatment of "inoperable" arteriovenous malformations (AVMs) critically evaluates what constitutes an "inoperable" AVM and how to best manage patients with this pathology. Due to continued technological and technical advances, "inoperable" AVMs constitute a shrinking subset of an already uncommon pathology. There are two types of inoperable AVMs. Type 1 lesions are not amenable to microneurosurgical resection because of a prohibitively high-risk profile, but they may be readily treatable by radiosurgery and/or endovascular neurosurgery. Type 2 lesions are too risky for treatment by any modality unless the patient is experiencing severe neurologic dysfunction or has suffered a hemorrhage. This chapter explores not just the evidence, but also the nuances involved in making safe decisions about how to optimize the care of these patients.

Keywords: inoperable arteriovenous malformations, radiosurgery, endovascular therapy, arteriovenous malformation treatment, lesion anatomy

- The successful treatment of "inoperable" arteriovenous malformations (AVMs) requires that a neurosurgeon shift away from the classic paradigms applied in a traditional, open microneurosurgical approach.
- Continual advances in technology and surgical technique, as well as the dynamic nature of lesions, necessitate constant reevaluations of patients with "inoperable" AVMs to ensure that their lesion has not shifted into the classification of a treatable AVM.
- Multimodality treatment of an "inoperable" AVM may provide a cure without subjecting a patient to the same risk that they would incur with treatment by microneurosurgical techniques or an isolated endovascular or radiosurgical approach.

28.1 Introduction

Open neurosurgical resection has been the gold standard for durable obliteration of arteriovenous malformations (AVMs) since inception of the specialty. Although open techniques have evolved somewhat with technological innovations, including the surgical microscope, improved noninvasive and angiographic imaging, and neuronavigation, the tenets have remained relatively constant. It is the standard for which newer treatment modalities (i.e., radiosurgery and endovascular therapy) are compared—with regard to both risk profile and treatment outcomes. These newer therapies have armed neurosurgeons with less invasive treatment options. The decision

points for the surgeon then become more complex: not only *should* an AVM be treated, but also *how.*

The Spetzler–Martin AVM grading scale uses anatomical considerations to assess risk for surgical treatment of AVMs (▶ Table 28.1).[1] Although widely used to describe AVMs in general, its applicability to treatment with radiosurgery and/or endovascular surgery is less clear, and the morbidity and mortality considerations associated with open resection do not apply with non-microsurgical options.[2,3]

What truly constitutes an "inoperable" AVM? Is there a subset of patients who might be appropriate for treatment (by any modality) despite what might classically be seen as having a prohibitive risk profile? Certain AVMs might be considered "inoperable" upon first evaluation. However, patients suffering devastating or recurrent hemorrhage or developing neurologic deficits can quickly force the issue and tip the balance toward moving forward with treatment in spite of a high-risk profile. Therefore, it behooves the vascular neurosurgeon to have a sense of how to manage these difficult AVMs. This chapter presents the evidence for considering treatment of AVMs that might otherwise be considered "inoperable" and describes less conventional approaches to treatment that may be particularly germane to these lesions.

28.2 Materials and Methods

When approaching an intricate topic such as the treatment of "inoperable" AVMs, one must incorporate a number of aspects into their knowledge base to ensure an adequate understanding of the subject. The information provided in this chapter is based on published articles, editorials, and case-specific examples. The remainder of this chapter is devoted to providing a concise summary of this information and how it pertains to the management of "inoperable" AVMs.

Table 28.1 Spetzler–Martin classification of cerebral arteriovenous malformations

Graded feature	Points assigned
Size	
Small (<3 cm)	1
Medium (3–6 cm)	2
Large (>6 cm)	3
Eloquence of adjacent brain	
Noneloquent	0
Eloquent	1
Venous drainage pattern	
Superficial only	0
Deep	1

Source: Adapted from Spetzler and Martin.[1]

Note: AVM Grade = [size] + [eloquence] + [venous drainage]; that is, [1, 2, or 3] + [0 or 1] + [0 or 1].

28.3 Results

28.3.1 Developing a Frame of Reference for "Inoperable" AVMs

Simply proceeding to write about how "inoperable" AVMs should be treated is putting the cart before the horse. "Inoperable" is a hazy categorization that would likely create significant discussion among even the most experienced surgeons. Neurosurgeons are acutely aware that almost any surgery could be performed if outcomes were to be disregarded, but we also recognize that to do so would be an entirely unacceptable reality. Therefore, we must reconcile what we consider an "inoperable" AVM before discussing how to treat the pathology.

The mental hurdle vascular neurosurgeons must overcome when managing "inoperable" AVMs relates to the juxtaposition of the terms treatment and inoperable. It is critical to stress that observation, although not a proactive form of treatment, should be considered a valid management option; and expectant management of lesions that are felt to have more risk associated with intervention (by any modality) than with observation is entirely reasonable. We urge readers to keep this management option in mind as they proceed through this chapter.

The A Randomized trial of Unruptured Brain Arteriovenous malformations (ARUBA) trial[4] has created considerable dissent among physicians regarding the best course of treatment for patients with AVMs by reporting that medical management is superior to intervention. However, it is important to point out that this trial's results should not be extrapolated to the patient with an "inoperable" AVM for several reasons. Firstly, the trial was stopped prematurely, and as such, long-term results are as of yet unknown. Many feel that the report of medical superiority may erode with time, and it is possible that quite different conclusions may become apparent upon completion of the 10-year follow-up period. Secondly, several issues have been raised with the study's methodology. These issues have been outlined in editorials and evaluated by further studies. Some of the major points are as follows: the disease process is very heterogeneous, which stresses the rigid constraints of the purported randomized controlled trial; there was a bias toward nonsurgical therapy and no data published on cure rates. Furthermore, among patients undergoing intervention, only a small minority of cases involved surgical resection, with the remainder split among alternatives that are known to be noncurative in the short term. This suggests that the proportion of incompletely obliterated AVMs was high and, hence, even "treated" lesions continued to contribute to ongoing ruptures; centers only had to manage 10 patients with AVMs per year to be eligible for enrollment, and there were no minimum requirements for the treating neurosurgeons, which calls into question the microneurosurgical expertise applied to this population.[5,6,7] ARUBA included no patients with a Spetzler–Martin grade higher than IV. In fact, most patients (62%) had scores of 2 or less, and, in accordance with their inclusion criteria, all patients had a modified Rankin scale score of 1 or lower.[4] Finally, ARUBA, being a trial aimed at unruptured lesions, excluded AVMs with evidence (symptomatic or not) of hemorrhage. Hemorrhage is one of the factors that may shift the risk–benefit equation for patients with "inoperable" AVMs and lead the neurosurgeon to reconsider treatments that convey some risk. For these reasons, completely dismissing the initiation of the treatment of a patient with an "inoperable" AVM on the basis of the ARUBA trial would be a miscalculation.

We posit that AVMs with a severe treatment risk profile should only be considered for surgical intervention if they have failed conservative management in one of two ways:

- The patient is suffering severe, progressive symptoms attributable to the AVM that, when compared to the risk profile for treatment, make continued observation unacceptable.
- The patient experiences an AVM rupture that portends a riskier course for continued observation. There is significant nuance to this point that will be discussed below.

The fear of intracranial hemorrhage and its sequelae is a driving force behind decision-making for both patients and their treating surgeons. AVM-associated hemorrhage alone is not grounds for moving forward with treatment. There is evidence that patients who suffer AVM hemorrhage (in the form of either a primary or a recurrent bleed) may not have as poor a neurologic outcome as matched cohorts who experience spontaneous intracranial hemorrhage without an associated vascular anomaly.[8,9] There is also evidence, though, that higher grade AVMs (such as our "inoperable" cases) may have a more aggressive course and catastrophic outcome when they bleed primarily or recurrently.[10] However, we also know that patients who experience AVM ruptures have a higher risk of recurrent hemorrhage than those patients in whom the AVM remains unruptured.[8,11] Therefore, we maintain that rupture is a valid reason to proceed with treatment of an "inoperable" AVM *only if* the surgeon has weighed the patient's status and risk of future hemorrhage, neurologic morbidity, and mortality appropriately against the great risk that will be incurred with treatment of the AVM.

28.3.2 Salient Points for Radiosurgical or Endovascular Treatment

There are certain considerations that a treating physician must weigh if a patient is not a surgical candidate, but their AVM is felt to be amenable to endovascular therapies, radiosurgery, or a combination of the two. If intervention and/or radiosurgery are/is being considered, the surgeon must exquisitely understand the anatomy of the lesion. We feel that a vital part of this endeavor is performing a diagnostic cerebral angiogram before making any formal treatment decisions. At times, the lesion's complexity may even justify microcatheter exploration (without treatment) at the time of the initial angiogram so that the anatomy of specific feeding pedicles can be elucidated. This anatomy can then be used to evaluate the risk of treatment based on the type of therapy that is being considered and provide time for the treatment team to formulate a thoughtful treatment plan that is tailored to the specifics of the patient and his/her lesion.

As mentioned earlier, the classically applied Spetzler–Martin grading scale, although more widely understood and therefore useful for discussion, is not ideal for evaluating the treatment risk of an AVM if the intended modality is radiosurgery or endovascular embolization. To address this need, several modality-specific scores have been developed.

The Pollock–Flickinger score[3,12] evaluates factors that are more specific/critical to radiosurgery than those evaluated in the Spetzler–Martin grade. Volume, age, and location (superficial vs. deep) can be used to predict the likelihood of AVM obliteration as well as functional decline.[12] In a more contemporary approach, the University of Virginia AVM grading system has also been shown to be very predictive of stereotactic radiosurgery outcome of AVM patients. Stereotactic radiosurgery has been applied to the treatment of large, inoperable AVMs by using either hypofractionated dosing or volume staging, with the literature suggesting that the latter technique may be more effective.[13,14,15,16] Another technique describes the use of volume-staged radiosurgery to obliterate or downsize AVMs so that the residual lesion can be operated in a safe manner.[16]

Radiosurgery is an attractive option for inoperable AVMs, but it is not without its own risks. It is well known that the risk of hemorrhage remains during the time that it takes for the occurrence of AVM obliteration. The literature raises several other concerns in regard to stereotactic radiosurgery. A recent meta-analysis of large AVMs treated with radiosurgery found that the mortality rate from hemorrhage was 40.08% with a 6.1% annual risk of re-hemorrhage for patients who presented with rupture.[17] Furthermore, the medical community's understanding of secondary harms from stereotactic radiosurgery continues to evolve, and yet, for younger patients being considered for treatment, physicians do not fully know the risks they incur over a long expected lifespan. One such issue is that of secondary neoplasms. The supportive evidence is far from certain, but even the possibility of an association between radiation and secondary tumorigenesis should be enough to at least create a moment of pause when contemplating proceeding with therapeutic radiation in children and young adults.[18,19,20,21,22,23] Other more clearly defined sequelae of stereotactic radiosurgery include radiation necrosis, perilesional ischemic strokes, and cyst development.[24,25,26] For AVM treatment in particular, occlusion of draining veins may increase the likelihood of post-radiosurgery hemorrhage.[27,28] This speaks to the need to understand anatomy and consider whether a large AVM with isolated drainage is appropriate for radiosurgery, and, if it is deemed appropriate, ensure that the treatment plan reflects this understanding. Overall, reported rates for radiosurgical cures are encouraging, but cure is not certain. Therefore, we feel that initiating a treatment plan that involves radiation should be weighed particularly carefully.

Endovascular practitioners have similarly developed grading schemes specific to their treatment modality. It is now understood that the Spetzler–Martin grade is not a good predictor of complications when undertaking endovascular treatment. Two recently published scales used to predict outcome for endovascular treatment of AVMs are the Buffalo score[2] and the arteriovenous malformation embocure score (AVMES;[29] ▶ Table 28.2). Neither system has been externally validated, and they have significant differences.

The AVMES is designed to stratify the risk associated with a curative embolization of cerebral AVMs. It assigns numerical values to the size of the nidus, the number of feeding pedicles, the number of draining veins, and vascular eloquence. The last variable is a corollary to the concept of eloquence evaluated by the Spetzler–Martin grade that attempts to define risk incurred by embolizations performed near critical structures. The AVMES

Table 28.2 Summary of the Buffalo score and the arteriovenous malformation embocure score (AVMES)

Buffalo score[a]		AVMES[b]	
Graded feature	Points assigned	Graded feature	Points assigned
Number of arterial pedicles		Number of arterial particles	
1 or 2	1	1–3	1
3 or 4	2	4–6	2
5 or more	3	7 or more	3
Diameter of arterial pedicle		Size of the nidus	
Most > 1 mm	0	< 3 cm	1
Most ≤ 1 mm	1	3–6 cm	2
		> 6 cm	3
Nidus location		Vascular eloquence	
Noneloquent	0	Noneloquent	0
Eloquent	1	Eloquent	1

[a]Data from Dumont et al.[2]
[b]Data from Lopes et al.[29]

defines vascular eloquence as a pedicle that is less than 20 mm from the internal carotid artery or the first segments of cerebral arteries that are too small for catheterization. The authors report that the AVMES has good discriminative ability for complications and complete obliteration, with increasing scores showing higher complication rates and lower obliteration rates.[29]

The Buffalo score also stratifies the risk of endovascular treatment of AVMs regardless of whether the intent is complete obliteration by endovascular or multimodality treatment. It scores the number of arterial pedicles, the diameter of the pedicles, and the eloquence of the nidus location. The authors directly compared the abilities of the Buffalo score and Spetzler–Martin grade to predict complication rates and found that increasing Buffalo score (but not increasing Spetzler–Martin grade) was strongly correlated with an increased complication rate. The Buffalo score does not correlate with complete endovascular obliteration, which is an important differentiation with the AVMES.[2]

If the goal of treatment is to achieve complete obliteration of an AVM in the safest possible way, stand-alone embolization is often not the correct decision. Although the AVMES does correlate with complications, untoward outcomes still occurred in a patient population that underwent endovascular treatment with the stated goal of cure rather than as an adjunctive therapy. This potentially leads to more aggressive embolizations than those that might be undertaken if the goal is not necessarily an isolated embocure but rather a multimodality cure. In this sense, the Buffalo score is more nimble and may provide a more practical way of assessing the portion of risk associated with AVM embolization when a multimodality treatment is planned from the outset.

28.3.3 Defining and Classifying "Inoperable" Arteriovenous Malformations

On the basis of the points raised above, it behooves us to crystallize how we define an "inoperable" AVM so that readers fully understand our frame of reference when deciding on treatment. There are two types of AVMs that we will consider for the purposes of "inoperable" AVMs.

The first subtype is a lesion that, by any surgical standard and for any reason (such as location and complexity), is not amenable to treatment by microneurosurgical resection (either primarily or in concert with preoperative embolization) but that may be appropriate for treatment by endovascular embolization alone, radiosurgery alone, or a combination of embolization and radiosurgery. This subtype should *not* be viewed to include a lesion that may be reasonable for microneurosurgery but is felt to be better suited for embolization or radiosurgery—it should only include lesions that are felt to be truly unsuitable for open resection. Treatment may still be appropriate to undertake regardless of presentation (i.e., inclusive of both asymptomatic and symptomatic/hemorrhagic AVMs) if a non-microneurosurgical intervention provides a reasonable chance for cure. To simplify the ensuing discussion, we will refer to this entity as a "type 1 inoperable AVM."

A "type 2 inoperable AVM" is a lesion that, at least if it presents in an asymptomatic fashion, would be judged unsuitable for treatment regardless of modality. In these cases, the patient would only receive treatment if his/her symptoms were to have failed conservative management in one of the two ways previously described—progressive, severe symptoms, or hemorrhage.

This classification relies on the premise that, despite a plethora of data and classification schemes, sometimes physicians are left to approach a treatment decision based on a gestalt of the patient's status, the anatomy of the AVM, and the ability of one's surgical/interventional skills. In the case of many patients' AVMs, physicians' choices for management could vary widely on the basis of the surgeon's skills and biases. However, we still feel that there are lesions that would generally be judged to fall into the subtypes outlined earlier, regardless of which surgeon evaluates the patient.

In the following section, we present several case examples to outline lesions that we feel would almost uniformly be judged to fit into the described subtypes and that are managed with various non-microneurosurgical treatments. Where appropriate, we will also provide references and evidence for treatment modalities in regard to how they relate to the case examples.

28.3.4 Case Examples for the Treatment of "Inoperable" AVMs

Type 1 Inoperable AVMs

Case 1—A 48-year-old man presented with seizures. Imaging workup revealed an unruptured left frontoparietal Spetzler–Martin grade V AVM with left middle cerebral artery (MCA), lenticulostriate, pericallosal, and callosal marginal arterial feeding pedicles. The lesion was deemed too risky for operative intervention due to proximity to the motor, premotor, and speech cortex. After discussion of treatment options, the patient decided to undergo multiple rounds of angiographic embolization (angioembolization). A total of 10 rounds of embolization with Onyx-18 (Covidien, Irvine, CA, United States) and Trufill (Trufill *n*-BCA [n-butyl cyanoacrylate] Liquid Embolic System; Codman Neuro, Raynham, MA, United States) were performed with near-complete obliteration of the lesion. (We sometimes choose to perform embolizations with *n*-BCA if the target vessels are too fine to allow distal catheterization.) After these

embolizations, only a small anterior remnant fed by lenticulostriate pedicles remained (▶ Fig. 28.1). Over the course of the embolizations, the patient experienced transient episodes of sensory dysfunction in his right arm and leg, as well as dysarthria and hair loss, but these symptoms improved significantly with time.

Given that the nidus obliteration reduced the grade of the AVM, assumptions about proximity to eloquence and implications for treatment options were reconsidered. The patient was offered options to treat the remnant with either stereotactic radiosurgery or open craniotomy for resection. He elected to undergo surgical resection.

A left frontoparietal craniotomy was performed using neuronavigation and motor- and sensory-evoked potential monitoring. Direct cortical stimulation was performed to identify the motor strip, and the AVM nidus was resected anterior to eloquent areas that were identified by intraoperative mapping. Although previously embolized portions of the lesion were intentionally left in situ to avoid neurological deficit, all residual flow through the AVM was abolished, as demonstrated by no residual AVM detected on the postoperative angiogram. The patient recovered well from surgery and has remained free from hemorrhage on subsequent follow-up.

This case example illustrates the dynamic nature of the decision-making process. Although the lesion was initially judged to be too risky for surgical resection based on involvement of both motor and speech cortex in the dominant hemisphere, these risks were largely neutralized by undertaking extensive targeted angioembolizations. Although complete cure was not achieved through nonsurgical means, the lesion was transformed from one wherein surgery was too dangerous into one wherein surgery was perfectly appropriate and resulted in complete cure without long-term morbidity. At each follow-up, the treatment plan must be critically reconsidered to evaluate if the initial premises still hold, and if not, what might be appropriate next steps to help the patient achieve the best possible outcome.

Type 2 Inoperable AVMs

Brainstem Arteriovenous Malformation

Case 2—A 28-year-old man presented with blurred/double vision, left facial numbness, and subjective left-sided weakness. Imaging (computed tomography [CT] and magnetic resonance imaging [MRI]) demonstrated hemorrhage in the posterior midbrain (▶ Fig. 28.2a–c). A digital subtraction angiogram (DSA) identified a Spetzler–Martin grade III AVM supplied by fine basilar artery apex perforators (▶ Fig. 28.2d–f) and draining into the deep venous system through the straight sinus. The patient was discharged without intervention 8 days later with only a residual internuclear ophthalmoplegia (INO).

Given the midbrain hemorrhage and his long life expectancy, we felt that treatment should be undertaken. This was done in delayed fashion to allow the patient to recover from his neurologic insult. Furthermore, given that it is not unusual for the angioarchitecture to be obscured by acute hemorrhage, a delayed angiogram may more accurately delineate the extent of the lesion. Stereotactic radiosurgery was considered—two series that describe radiosurgical treatment of brainstem AVMs report final obliteration rates of 59 and 76% with associated adverse radiation effects of 6 and 10%, respectively.[24,30] Three

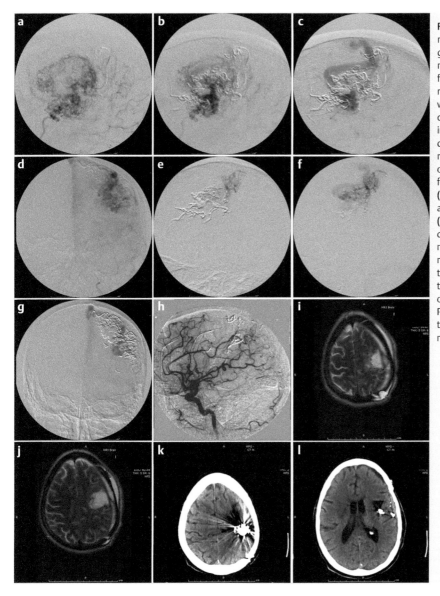

Fig. 28.1 Case 1: This patient underwent 10 rounds of embolization of a Spetzler–Martin grade V left frontoparietal arteriovenous malformation (AVM). **(a–c)** Sequential images from a lateral angiogram demonstrating the residual AVM after four rounds of embolization with Onyx-18 and Trufill (Trufill *n*-BCA [n-butyl cyanoacrylate]). **(d)** Anteroposterior (AP) injection of middle cerebral artery (MCA) pedicle demonstrating residual AVM nidus following six rounds of embolization. **(e,f)** Sequential images of a microcatheterization and injection of a MCA feeding pedicle prior to round 8 of embolization. **(g)** AP angiogram demonstrating residual nidus after 10 rounds of embolization. **(h)** Intraoperative angiogram in lateral projection demonstrating complete obliteration of AVM nidus. Postoperative T2-weighted magnetic resonance imaging **(i,j)** with two slices through the AVM resection cavity and computed tomography **(k,l)** images at similar levels showing obliteration of AVM with no residual flow voids. Previously embolized vessels are noted posterior to the resection cavity where intraoperative mapping revealed eloquence.

concerns were raised that ultimately pushed us toward other options. First, the patient presented with hemorrhage, so there would be a continued hemorrhage risk until involution. Second, the patient was relatively young, so there was hesitancy to expose his midbrain to radiation. Lastly, careful evaluation of the angioarchitecture left us confident that there was a reasonable chance at an endovascular cure if (1) the main vascular pedicle could be catheterized and (2) adequate nidal penetration could be achieved, thereby indirectly occluding the remaining fine perforators feeding the nidus.

The patient returned 2 months later for follow-up angiography and possible embolization. The major feeding pedicle could be catheterized, and the patient had no symptoms after performing a superselective Wada test.[31] Embolization with Onyx was performed, and there was excellent nidal penetration. The AVM appeared to be cured on the completion angiogram (▶ Fig. 28.3a–d). The patient was discharged home on postprocedure day 1 with no new complaints or deficits.

He returned 8 days later with increasingly slurred speech and dysmetria that had developed over the past 2 days. He did not have weakness or new visual disturbances. Noninvasive imaging showed changes consistent with the previous embolization without sign of hemorrhage. DSA identified new filling of the AVM through fine perforating vessels off of the basilar artery apex with the same pattern of venous drainage as on previous studies (▶ Fig. 28.3e,f).

Because of the continued AVM filling and progressive symptoms, further treatment was required. Microneurosurgery had an unacceptable risk profile. Stereotactic radiosurgery was considered once more, but hesitancy remained for the same reasons as discussed previously. Then how to attempt a cure endovascularly? Again, the key lies in studying the AVM's anatomy. The patent feeding pedicles were now too fine to catheterize. This led us to consider a transvenous embolization procedure. There have been descriptions of cases where AVMs unsuitable for arterial embolization were cured with this

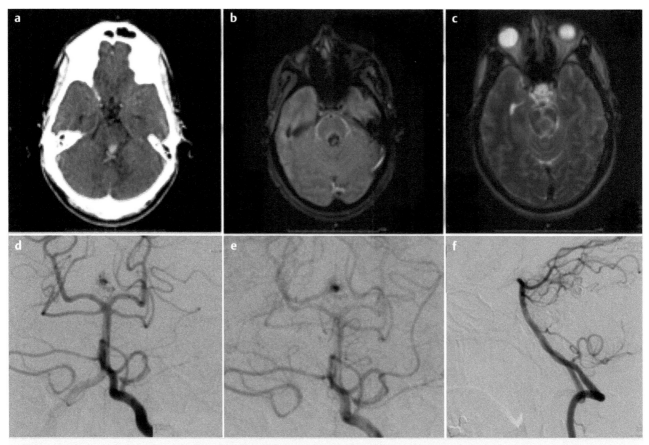

Fig. 28.2 Case 2: This patient presented with hemorrhage and the radiographic findings shown here. **(a)** Noncontrast head computed tomography scan showing hemorrhage in the posterior midbrain. **(b)** Gradient echo heme and **(c)** T2 magnetic resonance imaging sequences showing the same hemorrhage with better detail. **(d)** Early arterial anteroposterior angiogram showing the arteriovenous malformation (AVM) filling from basilar artery perforators. **(e)** Late arterial phase showing an early draining vein. **(f)** Early arterial lateral angiogram showing the AVM.

technique.[32,33,34,35,36] Typically, these lesions have a single draining vein, as did our patient's lesion.

On the basis of this analysis, we elected to attempt transvenous embolization. We generally perform AVM embolizations at our institution while the patient is under conscious sedation so that the clinical examination can be easily and reliably monitored throughout the case. We have published articles on multiple techniques for which the outcomes are satisfactory compared with those relative to general anesthesia, and we believe that conscious sedation actually adds a level of safety to the procedure.[37,38,39,40,41] However, in this case, the patient was placed under general anesthesia with neuromonitoring so that a transvenous embolization could be performed. The anesthesiologist was prepared in case adenosine-induced flow arrest was necessary to allow adequate transnidal penetration. The venous system was catheterized, and the microcatheter was navigated to the proximal portion of the vein just as it emerged from the AVM. An arterial run confirmed adequate catheter position (▸ Fig. 28.3g–i). As an attempt was made to move the venous catheter forward to optimize the chance of nidal penetration without venous reflux, the microcatheter shifted to a point on the roadmap that was inferior to the vein's trajectory. A microinjection confirmed that the microcatheter was outside the vessel. The anesthesiologist immediately initiated flow

arrest with adenosine. Onyx embolization was initiated in the subarachnoid space to occlude the vascular injury, and the catheter was slowly withdrawn into the vessel to continue embolization of the AVM. Flow arrest was maintained until the embolization had been completed (approximately 1 minute). Completion angiograms demonstrated no residual filling of the AVM (▸ Fig. 28.3j, k).

The patient's neuromonitoring showed no changes, and he was extubated immediately. Before leaving the angiography suite, he was able to count fingers and move all extremities. His examination continued to improve from his preprocedure baseline, and physical/occupational therapy cleared him for discharge by postprocedure day 5. At the time of discharge, his pupils were large but reactive to light bilaterally. He had a disconjugate gaze, but his INO had improved. He had full strength in all extremities. Follow-up DSA at 3 months confirmed continued complete obliteration of the AVM.

Large Bilateral Thalamic and Basal Ganglia AVM[42]

A 12-year-old boy presented to his primary care physician with a 3-month history of progressive gait abnormality. An MRI of the brain (▸ Fig. 28.4) showed bilateral basal ganglia and thalamic AVMs with evidence of hemorrhage and a small area of

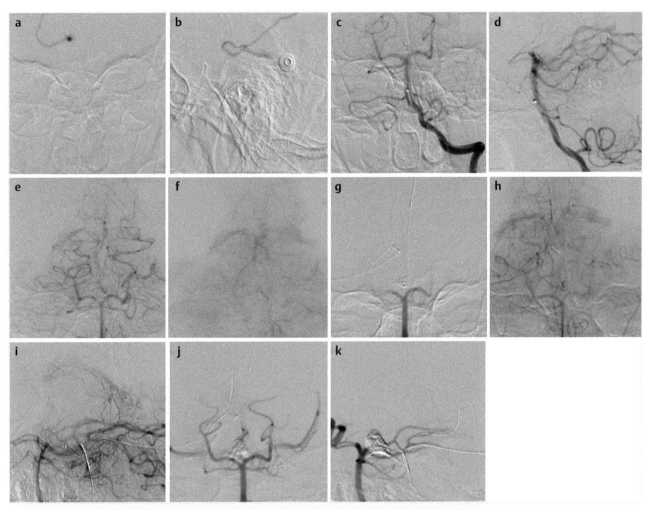

Fig. 28.3 Case 2: The patient underwent two embolizations (each with Onyx)—one arterial and one venous. (a) Anteroposterior (AP) angiogram of microcatheter injection showing filling of the arteriovenous malformation (AVM) with drainage into an early vein. (b) Lateral angiogram of microcatheter injection showing filling of the AVM with drainage into an early vein. (c) AP angiogram after arterial embolization showing no filling of the AVM or early venous drainage. (d) Lateral angiogram after arterial embolization showing no filling of the AVM or early venous drainage. (e,f) AP angiogram after patient returned with worsening symptoms. (e) The early arterial phase showing filling of the residual AVM nidus. (f) The capillary phase capturing an early draining vein. (g,h) AP angiogram prior to transvenous embolization. The microcatheter has been navigated into the proximal portion of the draining vein (g), which is no longer filling in (h) because it is occluded by the microcatheter. (i) Lateral angiogram prior to transvenous embolization. The microcatheter has been navigated into the proximal portion of the draining vein. (j) AP angiogram after transvenous embolization. There is no filling of the AVM. The Onyx cast has conformed to the shape of the interpeduncular cistern. (k) Lateral angiogram after transvenous embolization. There is no filling of the AVM. The Onyx cast has conformed to the shape of the interpeduncular cistern.

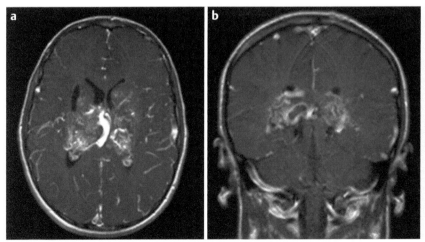

Fig. 28.4 Case 3: Magnetic resonance imaging at initial presentation. (a) T1-weighted, axial, gadolinium-enhanced image at the level of the foramen of Monro. (b) T1-weighted, coronal, gadolinium-enhanced image posterior to the third ventricle. (Reproduced with permission of Lee et al.[42] Released under a Creative Commons Attribution License.)

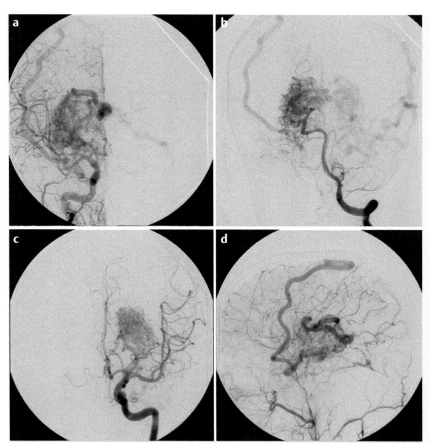

Fig. 28.5 Case 3: Diagnostic cerebral angiogram at initial presentation. (a) Anteroposterior (AP) right carotid injection. (b) AP left vertebral injection. (c) AP left carotid injection. (d) Lateral right carotid injection. (Reproduced with permission of Lee et al.[42] Released under a Creative Commons Attribution License.)

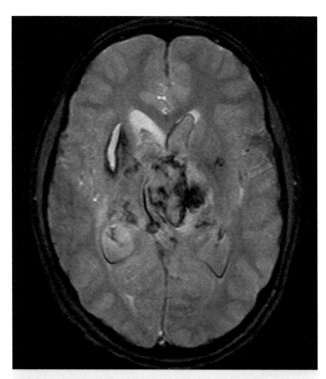

Fig. 28.6 Case 3: Axial gradient echo heme sequence magnetic resonance imaging 8 months after diagnosis, during presentation with status epilepticus. (Reproduced with permission of Lee et al.[42] Released under a Creative Commons Attribution License.)

encephalomalacia adjacent to the AVM on the right. DSA confirmed bilateral thalamic and basal ganglia Spetzler–Martin grade IV AVMs that were supplied by the right posterior communicating artery, the P2 and P3 posterior cerebral artery segments, and the left anterior choroidal artery. Drainage of the AVM was into the superior sagittal sinus on the right and the superior sagittal sinus, inferior petrosal sinus, and transverse sinus on the left (▶ Fig. 28.5). Ultimately, the decision was made to observe the patient, and he was placed on levetiracetam for seizure prophylaxis.

The decision to manage the patient medically is prudent in this situation since the patient is minimally symptomatic and the lesions are anatomically complex. Both AVMs have a complex arterial supply. There would likely be vessels that are difficult to catheterize as well as en passage pedicles. We did not recommend radiosurgery to the bilateral deep gray structures in an asymptomatic 12-year-old. In fact, perilesional strokes have actually been described in patients who received radiosurgery for deep-seated AVMs.[25] Therefore, we would advocate observation in this setting.

Eight months later, the patient was readmitted for evaluation of seizure activity, but continuous electroencephalographic monitoring was negative. The patient was discharged home, and the levetiracetam was discontinued at that time. Three days after returning home, he presented to the hospital in status epilepticus with a Glasgow Coma Scale score of 4. After intubation and initiation of antiepileptic medication, an MRI of the brain showed evidence of intraventricular hemorrhage with hydrocephalus (▶ Fig. 28.6). A ventriculostomy was placed and

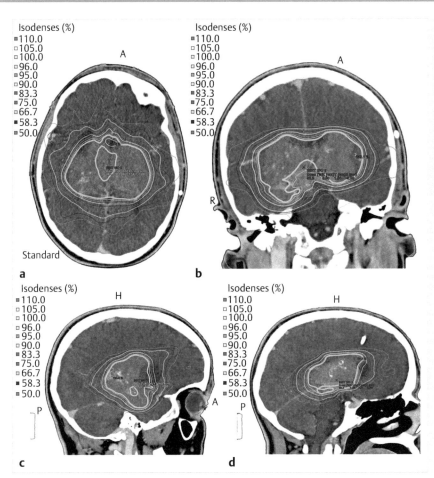

maintained for approximately 2 weeks to manage elevated intracranial pressures. Ultimately, the patient developed post-hemorrhagic hydrocephalus requiring ventriculoperitoneal shunt placement.

The patient was discharged to an inpatient rehabilitation unit 1 week later. He improved to the point that he was awake and alert and could answer some questions with short phrases and follow commands. He had a diffuse, symmetric quadriparesis, but he could ambulate with a gait belt and assistance.

The patient's parents were very concerned about re-hemorrhage and further neurological decline. After much discussion, the family was offered hypofractionated stereotactic radiosurgery. As mentioned previously, endovascular treatment was unlikely to result in cure. However, considering the radiosurgery as an adjunct for volume reduction may have allowed more favorable radiosurgical planning. Given the complexity and volume of the AVMs, preradiosurgery endovascular treatment (if possible) would likely require multiple sessions to minimize the risk of acute hemorrhage.[43] This delay could be problematic, because the patient had already experienced a debilitating hemorrhage. Therefore, it is sensible to limit the risk and delay that would be incurred from staged interventions by proceeding directly to stereotactic radiosurgery.

Two months after his discharge to an inpatient rehabilitation facility, the patient underwent frameless stereotactic radiosurgery using the Trilogy radiosurgery unit (Varian Medical Systems, Palo Alto, CA). A total of 30 Gy was delivered in doses of five fractions on an every-other-day schedule for the first four fractions and a 1-week break before the fifth fraction due to hospitalization for a seizure. Radiation was delivered with nine static beams using mini-multileaf collimation with intensity-modulated radiation therapy due to the complex shape of the bilateral target (▶ Fig. 28.7). The patient tolerated the procedure well.

The patient was followed closely and had several admissions over the next year for seizure activity. He developed lower extremity contractures requiring Achilles tendon releases. In addition, he developed dystonia and spasticity that was eventually treated with an intrathecal baclofen pump. Repeat DSA (▶ Fig. 28.8) 10 months after radiosurgery showed obliteration of the nidus and absence of filling of the AVMs. The MRI (▶ Fig. 28.9) continued to show cavitary microcystic changes in the area of the previous AVMs.

Two years after treatment, the patient was able to sit with minimal support and had 4+/5 to 5/5 strength bilaterally. He participated in home schooling and was able to play simple songs on the piano. He continued to have dystonic movements,

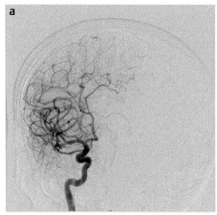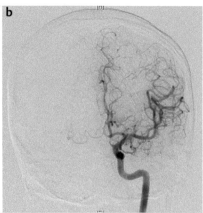

Fig. 28.8 Case 3: Diagnostic cerebral angiogram 10 months after radiation treatment. **(a)** Anteroposterior (AP) right carotid injection. **(b)** AP left carotid injection. (Reproduced with permission of Lee et al.[42] Released under a Creative Commons Attribution License.)

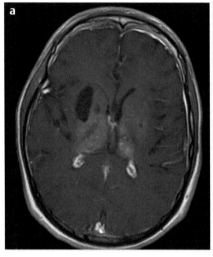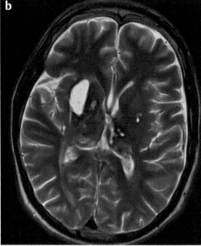

Fig. 28.9 Case 3: Magnetic resonance imaging 10 months after radiation treatment. **(a)** T1-weighted, axial, gadolinium-enhanced image at the level of the foramen of Monro. **(b)** T2-weighted, axial image at the same level. (Reproduced with permission of Lee et al.[42] Released under a Creative Commons Attribution License.)

and verbal interactions were limited to single words. He had not experienced any further hemorrhage.

28.4 Conclusion

Due to the lack of treatment options previously available to neurosurgeons, the treatment of "inoperable" AVMs is still in its infancy. However, given access to modern techniques, we are now able to offer concrete treatment options with reasonable chances of cure to patients with "inoperable" AVMs. This is especially true for patients with type 1 inoperable AVMs. These patients can now receive a non-microneurosurgical treatment that affords them a cure without having to wait for a devastating event that subsequently commits them to the morbidity of a craniotomy or worse—waiting for another hemorrhage. Type 1 inoperable AVMs often lend themselves to treatment with radiosurgery and/or endovascular surgery. In these situations, the Spetzler–Martin grade will be unlikely to correlate with the risk of treatment, so applying a newer grading scheme, such as the Buffalo, University of Virginia, or Pollock–Flickinger scores, to predict the chance of complications will often be more appropriate. This allows for a more modality-specific evaluation of risks and outcomes for patients with high Spetzler–Martin grade AVMs who might have a classically "inoperable" AVM.

For the time being, there are still patients who are better suited to remain under observation than receive treatment. Patients with type 2 inoperable AVMs do have the benefit of access to multiple treatment modalities should the need arise. As technology continues to evolve and current therapies become better understood, recommendations for type 2 inoperable lesions may change from observation to some form of intervention.

Unfortunately, AVMs are an uncommon pathology, of which "inoperable" AVMs are becoming a smaller subset with each passing year. As such, evidence guiding their management is limited. The evidence presented in this chapter is low level—essentially retrospective reviews, case series, and expert opinions. It is still vitally important to keep the lessons of others in mind so that our future patients do not fall victim to unnecessary complications. There are important questions that remain to be answered in the treatment of "inoperable" AVMs. Initial results for AVMs treated by endovascular therapy and/or radiosurgery suggest that complete occlusion, when achieved, is durable. Longer follow-up will be critical to validate these treatments relative to microneurosurgery. Also, because many patients with AVMs are children and young adults, the long-term consequences of radiosurgery will need to be better understood to both prevent unintended consequences and understand if there are situations where radiosurgery is safe in this population.

In conclusion, successful management of "inoperable" AVMs requires a neurosurgeon who is well versed in more than just microneurosurgery. It also requires an understanding of the strengths and weaknesses of radiosurgical and endovascular approaches. Continual advances in technology and treatment techniques obligate surgeons to continually reassess patients with "inoperable" AVMs to make certain that they are afforded an opportunity for treatment if their AVM is amenable to newer, safer treatments. Regardless of how the field progresses, one thing will remain certain—AVMs are a heterogeneous pathology that can be remarkably humbling to treat. Therefore, the most successful surgeons will always be the ones whose technical prowess is heavily tempered by a respectful understanding of the formidable foe and of all the therapeutic tools available.

References

[1] Spetzler RF, Martin NA. A proposed grading system for arteriovenous malformations. J Neurosurg. 1986; 65(4):476–483

[2] Dumont TM, Kan P, Snyder KV, Hopkins LN, Siddiqui AH, Levy EI. A proposed grading system for endovascular treatment of cerebral arteriovenous malformations: Buffalo score. Surg Neurol Int. 2015; 6:3

[3] Pollock BE, Flickinger JC. A proposed radiosurgery-based grading system for arteriovenous malformations. J Neurosurg. 2002; 96(1):79–85

[4] Mohr JP, Parides MK, Stapf C, et al. international ARUBA investigators. Medical management with or without interventional therapy for unruptured brain arteriovenous malformations (ARUBA): a multicentre, non-blinded, randomised trial. Lancet. 2014; 383(9917):614–621

[5] Conger A, Kulwin C, Lawton MT, Cohen-Gadol AA. Endovascular and microsurgical treatment of cerebral arteriovenous malformations: current recommendations. Surg Neurol Int. 2015; 6:39

[6] Day AL, Dannenbaum M, Jung S. A randomized trial of unruptured brain arteriovenous malformations trial: an editorial review. Stroke. 2014; 45(10):3147–3148

[7] Lawton MT. The role of AVM microsurgery in the aftermath of a randomized trial of unruptured brain arteriovenous malformations. AJNR Am J Neuroradiol. 2015; 36(4):617–619

[8] Choi JH, Mast H, Sciacca RR, et al. Clinical outcome after first and recurrent hemorrhage in patients with untreated brain arteriovenous malformation. Stroke. 2006; 37(5):1243–1247

[9] van Beijnum J, Lovelock CE, Cordonnier C, Rothwell PM, Klijn CJ, Al-Shahi Salman R, SIVMS Steering Committee and the Oxford Vascular Study. Outcome after spontaneous and arteriovenous malformation-related intracerebral haemorrhage: population-based studies. Brain. 2009; 132 (Pt 2):537–543

[10] Laakso A, Dashti R, Juvela S, Isarakul P, Niemelä M, Hernesniemi J. Risk of hemorrhage in patients with untreated Spetzler-Martin grade IV and V arteriovenous malformations: a long-term follow-up study in 63 patients. Neurosurgery. 2011; 68(2):372–377, discussion 378

[11] Al-Shahi R, Warlow C. A systematic review of the frequency and prognosis of arteriovenous malformations of the brain in adults. Brain. 2001; 124(Pt 10):1900–1926

[12] Pollock BE, Flickinger JC. Modification of the radiosurgery-based arteriovenous malformation grading system. Neurosurgery. 2008; 63(2):239–243, discussion 243

[13] Hattangadi JA, Chapman PH, Bussière MR, et al. Planned two-fraction proton beam stereotactic radiosurgery for high-risk inoperable cerebral arteriovenous malformations. Int J Radiat Oncol Biol Phys. 2012; 83(2):533–541

[14] Fogh S, Ma L, Gupta N, et al. High-precision volume-staged Gamma Knife surgery and equivalent hypofractionation dose schedules for treating large arteriovenous malformations. J Neurosurg. 2012; 117 Suppl:115–119

[15] AlKhalili K, Chalouhi N, Tjoumakaris S, Rosenwasser R, Jabbour P. Staged-volume radiosurgery for large arteriovenous malformations: a review. Neurosurg Focus. 2014; 37(3):E20

[16] Seymour ZA, Sneed PK, Gupta N, et al. Volume-staged radiosurgery for large arteriovenous malformations: an evolving paradigm. J Neurosurg. 2016; 124 (1):163–174

[17] Mau CY, Sabourin VM, Gandhi CD, Prestigiacomo CJ. SLAM: Stereotactic radiosurgery of Large Arteriovenous Malformations: meta-analysis of hemorrhage in high-grade Pollock-Flickinger AVMs. World Neurosurg. 2016(85):32–41

[18] Yu JS, Yong WH, Wilson D, Black KL. Glioblastoma induction after radiosurgery for meningioma. Lancet. 2000; 356(9241):1576–1577

[19] Strojan P, Popović M, Jereb B. Secondary intracranial meningiomas after high-dose cranial irradiation: report of five cases and review of the literature. Int J Radiat Oncol Biol Phys. 2000; 48(1):65–73

[20] Kaido T, Hoshida T, Uranishi R, et al. Radiosurgery-induced brain tumor. Case report. J Neurosurg. 2001; 95(4):710–713

[21] Akamatsu Y, Murakami K, Watanabe M, Jokura H, Tominaga T. Malignant peripheral nerve sheath tumor arising from benign vestibular schwannoma treated by gamma knife radiosurgery after two previous surgeries: a case report with surgical and pathological observations. World Neurosurg. 2010; 73 (6):751–754

[22] You SH, Lyu CJ, Kim DS, Suh CO. Second primary brain tumors following cranial irradiation for pediatric solid brain tumors. Childs Nerv Syst. 2013; 29 (10):1865–1870

[23] Marta GN, Murphy E, Chao S, Yu JS, Suh JH. The incidence of second brain tumors related to cranial irradiation. Expert Rev Anticancer Ther. 2015; 15(3):295–304

[24] Yen CP, Steiner L. Gamma Knife surgery for brainstem arteriovenous malformations. World Neurosurg. 2011; 76(1–2):87–95, discussion 57–58

[25] Kim DH, Kang DH, Park J, Hwang JH, Park SH, Son WS. Delayed perilesional ischemic stroke after Gamma-Knife radiosurgery for unruptured deep arteriovenous malformation: two case reports of radiation-induced small artery injury as possible cause. J Cerebrovasc Endovasc Neurosurg. 2015; 17(1):36–42

[26] Herbert C, Moiseenko V, McKenzie M, et al. Factors predictive of symptomatic radiation injury after linear accelerator-based stereotactic radiosurgery for intracerebral arteriovenous malformations. Int J Radiat Oncol Biol Phys. 2012; 83(3):872–877

[27] Celix JM, Douglas JG, Haynor D, Goodkin R. Thrombosis and hemorrhage in the acute period following Gamma Knife surgery for arteriovenous malformation. Case report. J Neurosurg. 2009; 111(1):124–131

[28] Yen CP, Khaled MA, Schwyzer L, Vorsic M, Dumont AS, Steiner L. Early draining vein occlusion after gamma knife surgery for arteriovenous malformations. Neurosurgery. 2010; 67(5):1293–1302, discussion 1302

[29] Lopes DK, Moftakhar R, Straus D, Munich SA, Chaus F, Kaszuba MC. Arteriovenous malformation embocure score. J Neurointerv Surg. 2016; 8(7):685–691

[30] Kano H, Kondziolka D, Flickinger JC, et al. Stereotactic radiosurgery for arteriovenous malformations, part 5: management of brainstem arteriovenous malformations. J Neurosurg. 2012; 116(1):44–53

[31] Tawk RG, Tummala RP, Memon MZ, Siddiqui AH, Hopkins LN, Levy EI. Utility of pharmacologic provocative neurological testing before embolization of occipital lobe arteriovenous malformations. World Neurosurg. 2011; 76(3–4):276–281

[32] Nguyen TN, Chin LS, Souza R, Norbash AM. Transvenous embolization of a ruptured cerebral arteriovenous malformation with en-passage arterial supply: initial case report. J Neurointerv Surg. 2010; 2(2):150–152

[33] Consoli A, Renieri L, Nappini S, Limbucci N, Mangiafico S. Endovascular treatment of deep hemorrhagic brain arteriovenous malformations with transvenous onyx embolization. AJNR Am J Neuroradiol. 2013; 34(9):1805–1811

[34] Martínez-Galdámez M, Saura P, Saura J, Muñiz J, Albisua J, Pérez-Higueras A. Transvenous onyx embolization of a subependymal deep arteriovenous malformation with a single drainage vein: technical note. BMJ Case Rep. 2013; 2013:bcr2012010603

[35] Mendes GA, Silveira EP, Caire F, et al. Endovascular management of deep arteriovenous malformations: single institution experience in 22 consecutive patients. Neurosurgery. 2016; 78(1):34–41

[36] Iosif C, Mendes GA, Saleme S, et al. Endovascular transvenous cure for ruptured brain arteriovenous malformations in complex cases with high Spetzler-Martin grades. J Neurosurg. 2015; 122(5):1229–1238

[37] Abou-Chebl A, Lin R, Hussain MS, et al. Conscious sedation versus general anesthesia during endovascular therapy for acute anterior circulation stroke: preliminary results from a retrospective, multicenter study. Stroke. 2010; 41 (6):1175–1179

[38] Chamczuk AJ, Ogilvy CS, Snyder KV, et al. Elective stenting for intracranial stenosis under conscious sedation. Neurosurgery. 2010; 67(5):1189–1193, discussion 1194

[39] Ogilvy CS, Yang X, Jamil OA, et al. Neurointerventional procedures for unruptured intracranial aneurysms under procedural sedation and local anesthesia: a large-volume, single-center experience. J Neurosurg. 2011; 114 (1):120–128

[40] Kan P, Jahshan S, Yashar P, et al. Feasibility, safety, and periprocedural complications associated with endovascular treatment of selected ruptured aneurysms under conscious sedation and local anesthesia. Neurosurgery. 2013; 72(2):216–220, discussion 220

[41] Rangel-Castilla L, Cress MC, Munich SA, et al. Feasibility, safety, and periprocedural complications of pipeline embolization for intracranial aneurysm treatment under conscious sedation: university at buffalo neurosurgery experience. Neurosurgery. 2015; 11 Suppl 3:426–430

[42] Lee J, Tanaka T, Westgate S, Nanda A, Cress M, Litofsky NS. Hypofractionated stereotactic radiosurgery in a large bilateral thalamic and basal ganglia arteriovenous malformation. Case Rep Neurol Med. 2013; 2013:631028

[43] Ovalle F, Shay SD, Mericle RA. Delayed intracerebral hemorrhage after uneventful embolization of brain arteriovenous malformations is related to volume of embolic agent administered: multivariate analysis of 13 predictive factors. Neurosurgery. 2012; 70(2) Suppl Operative:313–320

29 Considerations for Pediatric Ateriovenous Malformations

Ameet V. Chitale, David M. Sawyer, Ricky Medel, Aaron S. Dumont, and Peter S. Amenta

Abstract

Pediatric arteriovenous malformations (AVMs) differ significantly from those that present in the adult population. Children more frequently present with intracranial hemorrhage, though it is controversial whether there is an increased rate of rupture in these patients. Pediatric AVM patients are faced with a high cumulative lifetime morbidity and, due to plasticity of the still-developing brain, appear to tolerate invasive therapy to a greater degree than adults. Patient- and lesion-specific factors necessitate a multidisciplinary approach to treatment, including surgical resection, radiosurgery, and/or embolization. Surgical resection provides the highest rate of obliteration and is considered the definitive treatment when AVM size, location, and morphology are amenable. The appearance of recurrent AVMs after complete obliteration has been documented in children. The nature of these recurrences is not known, but the risks conferred by them lead many clinicians to perform radiographic follow-up for a longer period of time than in adult patients.

Keywords: pediatric AVM, arteriovenous malformation, congenital AVM, rupture risk, complete obliteration, recurrence, radiographic surveillance

- Arteriovenous malformations (AVMs) are the most common cause of intracranial hemorrhage in children, leading to high rates of morbidity and mortality.
- The morbidity of pediatric AVMs is secondary to the high lifetime hemorrhage risk, seizures, mass effect, and/or hydrocephalus.
- Management options include observation and medical control of seizures, surgical resection, endovascular embolization, radiosurgery, or a combination of these modalities.
- Size, location, and angioarchitecture are important factors in determining the most effective treatment strategy for an individual lesion.
- There is a risk of recurrence after successful obliteration of AVMs in children, which warrants longitudinal radiographic follow-up.

29.1 Introduction

Arteriovenous malformations (AVMs) are considered congenital lesions, with pediatric AVMs representing a subset that present particularly early in life. However, there is evidence to suggest that AVMs presenting in childhood are a qualitatively distinct group. These lesions appear to differ from AVMs diagnosed in adulthood in their clinical presentation, morphologic characteristics, and potential to evolve over time.

About 60 to 85% of pediatric patients present with a hemorrhage,[1,2] and most authors agree that children presenting with AVMs are more likely to do so with a hemorrhage as their initial event than are adults.[2,3,4] However, it is difficult to determine with any precision the actual risk of hemorrhage in pediatric AVM patients, because the baseline prevalence of the disease has not been adequately elucidated.[2] Estimations of the annual risk of hemorrhage in children harboring AVMs have been derived from retrospective studies, and this value ranges from 2 to 10% per year depending on definition of onset as either the time of diagnosis or birth.[5] It is therefore unclear whether the risk is greater than the accepted value of 2 to 4% per year in adults. Importantly, there is evidence to suggest AVM rupture in the pediatric population may be more severe and result in higher morbidity and mortality, due to the prevalence of deep-seated AVMs in children.[3,6]

Pediatric AVMs may be more prone to rupture compared to their adult counterparts for a number of reasons. Multiple series have demonstrated AVM volume to be inversely proportional to the risk of hemorrhage, with smaller lesions showing a greater tendency for hemorrhage.[6,7,8] AVMs have been observed to enlarge over time, thereby possibly conferring increasing protection against hemorrhage. However, some studies have reported the opposite relationship between volume and risk of bleeding.[9,10,11] The immaturity of the cerebral vasculature in the pediatric population plays a role in the risk of rupture. Autoregulation of cerebral blood flow is impaired in pediatric patients, leading to labile hemodynamics. In turn, significant fluctuations in flow result in frequent and stronger stresses to the walls of an AVM and increased likelihood of rupture.[2] An infratentorial location of the AVM, which is associated with an increased risk of bleeding, is also frequent in the pediatric population.[12]

Less commonly, pediatric patients with AVMs will present with a constellation of symptoms, including headache, seizures, and a progressive neurologic deficit. Newborns with large AVMs and vein of Galen malformations have a unique clinical presentation of high-output heart failure as a result of shunting through the lesion.[13,14]

29.2 Management of Pediatric Arteriovenous Malformations

29.2.1 Surgery

Complete microsurgical resection of AVMs represents the definitive treatment option and plays a particularly important role in the management of pediatric AVMs (▶ Fig. 29.1). The prolonged expected lifespan in this population increases the cumulative risk of rupture over a lifetime. Furthermore, the propensity for recurrence or growth of partially treated lesions stresses the importance of complete obliteration when possible. Finally, the high frequency of hemorrhagic presentations results in an

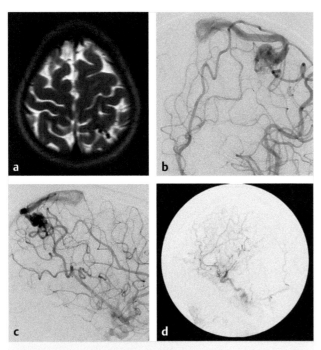

Fig. 29.1 A 13-year-old neurologically intact female patient presenting with headaches. **(a)** Axial T2-weighted magnetic resonance imaging demonstrating a 1.4 × 1.5 cm left parietal arteriovenous malformation (AVM) with the nidus centered in the postcentral gyrus. **(b)** Left anterior oblique angiogram shows a relatively compact nidus fed by distal branches of the left middle cerebral artery and anterior cerebral artery. A single large superficial draining vein drains to the superior sagittal sinus. **(c)** Lateral angiogram demonstrating the AVM. **(d)** Intraoperative angiogram of the left internal carotid arteries circulation demonstrating complete resection of the AVM. The patient was discharged with mild right hemianesthesia. At 6-month follow-up, the hemianesthesia had resolved; however, the patient complained of persistent right lower extremity diminished proprioception.

increased number of emergent clinical situations, in which open surgery is required to remove space-occupying hematomas and resect the ruptured AVM.

Recent retrospective studies have reported on the efficacy and safety of surgical treatment of AVMs in children. Successful treatment is often judged as complete obliteration of the lesion on postoperative angiography. Multiple series pertaining to microsurgical resection demonstrate AVM obliteration rates, as confirmed with angiography, in the range of 65 to 100%, with many studies reporting complete resection in over 80% of cases.[15] Importantly, surgical resection results in immediate obliteration of the lesion and removal of risk of future rupture. The importance of this definitive treatment is amplified in those presenting with rupture, as they have a significant risk of suffering a second bleed within 1 year.[15,16] Deep venous drainage seems to contribute to incomplete obliteration of the AVM.[15]

Another approach to quantifying outcomes after AVM treatment in children involves comparing preoperative and postoperative neurologic disability by utilizing the modified Rankin scale (mRS). In a series reported by Sanchez-Mejia et al comparing surgical results in children and adults, pediatric patients had mRS values of 0 to 2 (living independently) in 90.6% of

cases versus 71.4% in adults. Additionally, 93.8% of pediatric patients had an improvement in mRS compared to 69.8% of adults.[17] This effect was unexplained by measureable differences in the characteristics of the patients or their lesions, leading the authors to suggest that recovery from surgical AVM resection is augmented in children by neural plasticity. Other investigators have noted that the additional benefit of fewer comorbidities in pediatric patients makes them more capable than adults of recovering from catastrophic hemorrhages when treated surgically, reinforcing this notion.[18]

Surgical resection of AVMs in children does carry significant morbidity, and complication rates range from 5 to 33%. In particular, questions about the safety of AVM surgery often center on the immediate risk of blood loss and the long-term risk of neurologic deficit. In children, intraoperative blood loss is a particular concern because of their relatively small intravascular volume.[18] However, recent series have shown that intraoperative blood loss can be consistently controlled at acceptable levels under the appropriate conditions.[15] Meticulous hemostasis is maintained during the entire operation and preoperative embolization has a role in obliterating arterial pedicles that are anticipated to be problematic.[18] Additionally, it is important to closely monitor the patient's hemodynamics and cerebral perfusion during surgery by means of central venous and arterial lines and neurophysiological monitoring.[18]

Resection of the entire AVM must be performed to eliminate the risk of rupture, and confirmatory imaging is required to prove that no residual lesion has been left behind. Angiography is the imaging gold standard and intraoperative angiography has been shown to increase the rate of complete microsurgical obliteration.[19] At the conclusion of the resection, angiography can be performed in the operating room or in the angiography suite while the patient remains under general anesthesia. Evidence of residual AVM prompts immediate re-resection and additional angiography until the entire lesion is removed.

Neurologic deficits caused by the resection of brain parenchyma are a known complication of open microsurgery, and can to a certain extent be predicted based on the anatomy of the lesion and the planned surgical approach. Many AVMs can be successfully removed with no permanent deficit or only an expected loss of a visual field, but operating on lesions that reside in eloquent cortex is more likely to produce lasting deficits affecting the functional status of the patient.[15] An important consideration in very young patients is the inability to fixate the head, precluding the use of frameless stereotactic navigation and making resection of complex lesions more difficult.[18] However, newer navigation systems that do not require rigid head fixation may at least overcome some of the historical challenges with navigation.

29.2.2 Radiosurgery

Radiosurgery is used as the primary modality in a select group of pediatric patients with AVMs. In particular, it allows treatment of lesions that would be unsafe to surgically resect, due to either their deep location or proximity to eloquent cortex (▶ Fig. 29.2).

A significant body of literature has examined the efficacy and safety of radiosurgery as a treatment for pediatric AVMs. Obliteration rates are favorable, ranging from 51 to 90% in published

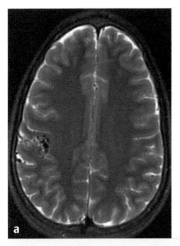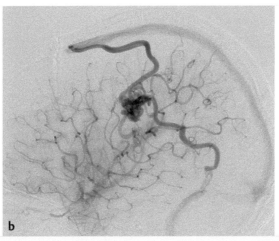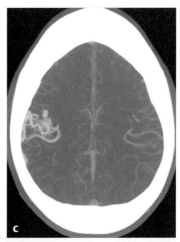

Fig. 29.2 A 14-year-old neurologically intact male patient presenting with seizures. **(a)** Axial T2-weighted magnetic resonance imaging demonstrating an unruptured 2.1 × 2.6 cm right frontal arteriovenous malformation (AVM) with a nidus centered in the primary motor strip. **(b)** Lateral angiogram shows the nidus to be fed by multiple distal right middle cerebral artery branches. Drainage is through superficial draining veins that empty into the superior sagittal sinus and right transverse sinus. **(c)** Computed tomography angiography used for stereotactic radiosurgery planning.

reports.[20] Nicolato et al reported that the probability of obliteration by single-session radiosurgery is significantly reduced by nidus volumes > 10 mL. Additionally, these patients had higher probability of hemorrhage and neurologic sequelae.[20] Radiation dose is an important factor that influences obliteration rates, re-hemorrhage rates, and acute radiation toxicity. When possible, children should be treated with the same dose as adult patients with AVMs,[21] as optimal prescription dose is associated with improved obliteration and reduced bleeding during the latency period. Staged radiosurgical treatment may be necessary in large volume AVMs or when optimal doses cannot otherwise be achieved in a single session.[20,22,23,24]

Importantly, radiosurgical obliteration is a slow process, with involution of the lesion occurring on average 2 years after the completion of treatment.[20] This latency period raises concern because of the potential for hemorrhage prior to complete obliteration—bleeding during the latency period occurs at a rate of 0.0 to 22.7% in the literature.[20] There is some evidence that this rate does not differ from the natural history risk in the absence of treatment initiation,[5] but it nonetheless represents a period of vulnerability that is not present in patients treated surgically.

Reported rates of permanent complications from radiosurgery in children are generally low (0.0–17.6%),[20] but some concern still exists regarding the long-term effects of radiation in the brains of children.[25] Increased rates of malignancy have been hypothesized,[26] but to date there has been no study establishing radiosurgery for AVMs as a causative agent for malignancy.[21] More subtle and diffuse effects on cognitive ability have also been considered, with some data showing school performance deficits in children treated for AVMs with radiosurgery.[27]

29.2.3 Embolization

Endovascular embolization plays a significant role in the treatment of pediatric AVMs and carries a relatively low complication rate. Small lesions with a limited number of arterial feeding vessels are potential targets for curative embolization,[12] but

most studies report an obliteration rate of around 20%.[28,29,30,31] Furthermore, there is a greater potential for children with AVMs to experience recurrence,[27,32] leading some to advocate surgical resection of lesions that are completely obliterated with embolization.[15]

This therapeutic profile allows embolization to occupy an important position as an adjunctive treatment, often complementing surgery or radiosurgery. Embolization is commonly performed preoperatively in order to increase the safety of microsurgical resection. Embolization of an AVM can significantly reduce the vascularity of the lesion,[12] allowing for resection that tightly hugs the nidus and spares normal parenchyma. Additionally, embolization reduces the risk of hemorrhage during surgery by obliterating arterial feeding vessels, especially those that would be difficult to access surgically.[15] Another use of embolization is to reduce the size of AVMs such that they are appropriate targets for radiosurgery.[21,33,34] For large lesions located in eloquent cortex, this has the potential to reduce the nidus size and allow higher radiation doses, offering a higher chance of cure. Reyns et al noted prior embolization as a negative predictive factor for complete embolization after radiosurgery; however, it is likely that preradiosurgery embolization was performed in lesions with larger niduses.[21]

29.2.4 Multimodality Treatment

Surgical resection offers the highest rate of obliteration and many authors agree that it should be employed for any lesion that can be safely excised.[15,20] Radiosurgery can be used as a primary treatment modality in lesions that are difficult to access surgically, but there is controversy regarding how many AVMs meet this description. Proponents of radiosurgery suggest that a high number of pediatric malformations are deep seated or located in eloquent cortex and are appropriate targets for radiosurgery.[20,21] Other authors believe that most AVMs being treated with radiosurgery could instead be safely resected with immediate obliteration and better outcomes.[15] In reality, the risk–benefit profile of surgery and radiosurgery for any given AVM is influenced by institutional expertise and experience, precluding the delineation of strict criteria.

29.3 Recurrence and Surveillance of Pediatric AVMs

Traditionally, AVMs are considered congenital malformations that form during early embryogenesis, resulting in lesions that have achieved their final anatomic configuration at the time of birth. However, growth of AVMs has been observed in both children and adults and may lead to progressive neurologic symptoms. AVM expansion is thought to be due to persistent hemodynamic stress, which enlarges the existing abnormal vasculature. There is also evidence supporting the evolution of the immature pediatric cerebral vasculature over time.

AVM recurrence refers to the presentation of a new lesion, either symptomatically or on follow-up imaging, after the original malformation was confirmed to be completely obliterated on delayed imaging.[5] This is considered to be a rare event in adult patients, but appears to occur with greater frequency in children. Whereas less than a fifth of AVMs present in pediatric patients, the majority of recurrent lesions reported in the literature have occurred in this population. Moderately sized cohort studies have suggested that the rate of recurrence in pediatric patients is in the range of 4.2 to 15%,[35,36,37] and recurrences have been documented up to 19 years after obliteration.[38] The reason for the increased incidence of recurrence in children is unknown, but some authors have suggested that the immaturity of the cerebral vasculature in these patients may allow angiogenesis to occur after surgical resection, resulting in continued evolution of the lesion over time.[32] Others infer that the recurrences in fact originate from angiographically occult residual lesions. The significant risks posed by recurrence should be addressed by following patients clinically and radiographically in a longitudinal fashion. However, there is no clear consensus on how this should be accomplished.

There are a number of imaging options available for use in following these patients, including digital subtraction angiography (DSA) and magnetic resonance imaging and angiography (MRI/MRA). DSA is the gold standard for the evaluation of AVMs. However, magnetic resonance studies are the predominant modality used for evaluating AVM patients of any age as they progress through multistage therapy or radiosurgery, and are also commonly used in longitudinal surveillance of children after obliteration of the lesion. MRI offers an advantage over DSA in avoiding ionizing radiation, although both techniques usually require conscious sedation or general anesthesia in younger pediatric patients. Some authors have questioned the sensitivity of MRI in detecting recurrent lesions in children, given that recurrence has been documented by DSA following recent negative MRI/MRA evaluation, suggesting that the incidence of recurrent AVMs may be higher than reported since most patients are followed by MRI.[37,39]

When AVMs recur in pediatric patients, they do so with a mean latency after confirmed obliteration of 33.6 to 108 months, with a few occurring much later.[32,35,37,40] This raises the question of how often and for how long patients should be evaluated for the presence of recurrence after treatment. Most authors recommend follow-up periods of at least 6 to 12 months,[6,32,36,41] with

some suggesting that longer surveillance (consisting of repeat imaging at 5 years or more) is necessary.[2,37,40]

It is likely that long-term radiographic surveillance of pediatric AVM patients is beneficial, with the risks of obtaining imaging outweighed by the possibility of detecting an early recurrence. Currently, follow-up protocols are based mainly on institutional and individual clinician preference. Additional investigation is needed to delineate the optimal modality, frequency, and duration of radiographic screening to benefit these patients.

29.4 Conclusion

AVMs present disproportionately with hemorrhage in children, with worse outcomes than in adults. Considering the significant risks of hemorrhage or re-hemorrhage over the long expected lifespan of pediatric patients, aggressive treatment of AVMs is warranted. Surgical resection offers the highest rate of obliteration and should be employed when it is expected to be safe and efficacious. Special considerations regarding blood loss and intraoperative monitoring must be made in children. Radiosurgery is effective and should be used to treat lesions that present unacceptable surgical risk. The latency period between treatment and obliteration, which can be expected to last 2 years, leaves patients vulnerable to initial or recurrent hemorrhage. The long-term effect of radiosurgery on the brain of a child is not well defined. Embolization has poor rates of primary obliteration, but is useful as an adjuvant therapy to reduce the size of an AVM and eliminate arterial feeders prior to surgery or radiosurgery. Pediatric patients should receive longitudinal radiographic follow-up even after successful obliteration due to the risk of recurrence.

References

[1] Blount JP, Oakes WJ, Tubbs RS, Humphreys RP. History of surgery for cerebrovascular disease in children. Part III. Arteriovenous malformations. Neurosurg Focus. 2006; 20(6):E11

[2] Bristol RE, Albuquerque FC, Spetzler RF, Rekate HL, McDougall CG, Zabramski JM. Surgical management of arteriovenous malformations in children. J Neurosurg. 2006; 105(2) Suppl:88–93

[3] Kondziolka D, Humphreys RP, Hoffman HJ, Hendrick EB, Drake JM. Arteriovenous malformations of the brain in children: a forty year experience. Can J Neurol Sci. 1992; 19(1):40–45

[4] Fullerton HJ, Achrol AS, Johnston SC, et al. UCSF BAVM Study Project. Long-term hemorrhage risk in children versus adults with brain arteriovenous malformations. Stroke. 2005; 36(10):2099–2104

[5] Darsaut TE, Guzman R, Marcellus ML, et al. Management of pediatric intracranial arteriovenous malformations: experience with multimodality therapy. Neurosurgery. 2011; 69(3):540–556, discussion 556

[6] Niazi TN, Klimo P , Jr, Anderson RC, Raffel C. Diagnosis and management of arteriovenous malformations in children. Neurosurg Clin N Am. 2010; 21(3): 443–456

[7] Celli P, Ferrante L, Palma L, Cavedon G. Cerebral arteriovenous malformations in children. Clinical features and outcome of treatment in children and in adults. Surg Neurol. 1984; 22(1):43–49

[8] Waltimo O. The relationship of size, density and localization of intracranial arteriovenous malformations to the type of initial symptom. J Neurol Sci. 1973; 19(1):13–19

[9] Hernesniemi JA, Dashti R, Juvela S, Väärt K, Niemelä M, Laakso A. Natural history of brain arteriovenous malformations: a long-term follow-up study of risk of hemorrhage in 238 patients. Neurosurgery. 2008; 63(5):823–829, discussion 829–831

[10] Stapf C, Mast H, Sciacca RR, et al. Predictors of hemorrhage in patients with untreated brain arteriovenous malformation. Neurology. 2006; 66(9):1350–1355

[11] Stefani MA, Porter PJ, terBrugge KG, Montanera W, Willinsky RA, Wallace MC. Large and deep brain arteriovenous malformations are associated with risk of future hemorrhage. Stroke. 2002; 33(5):1220–1224

[12] Zheng T, Wang QJ, Liu YQ, et al. Clinical features and endovascular treatment of intracranial arteriovenous malformations in pediatric patients. Childs Nerv Syst. 2014; 30(4):647–653

[13] Merritt C, Feit LR, Valente JH. A neonate with high-outflow congestive heart failure and pulmonary hypertension due to an intracranial arteriovenous malformation. Pediatr Emerg Care. 2011; 27(7):645–648

[14] Mascarenhas MI, Moniz M, Ferreira S, Goulão A, Barroso R. High-output heart failure in a newborn. BMJ Case Rep. 2012; 2012:bcr2012006289

[15] Gross BA, Storey A, Orbach DB, Scott RM, Smith ER. Microsurgical treatment of arteriovenous malformations in pediatric patients: the Boston Children's Hospital experience. J Neurosurg Pediatr. 2015; 15(1):71–77

[16] Blauwblomme T, Bourgeois M, Meyer P, et al. Long-term outcome of 106 consecutive pediatric ruptured brain arteriovenous malformations after combined treatment. Stroke. 2014; 45(6):1664–1671

[17] Sanchez-Mejia RO, Chennupati SK, Gupta N, Fullerton H, Young WL, Lawton MT. Superior outcomes in children compared with adults after microsurgical resection of brain arteriovenous malformations. J Neurosurg. 2006; 105(2) Suppl:82–87

[18] Rubin D, Santillan A, Greenfield JP, Souweidane M, Riina HA. Surgical management of pediatric cerebral arteriovenous malformations. Childs Nerv Syst. 2010; 26(10):1337–1344

[19] Kotowski M, Sarrafzadeh A, Schatlo B, et al. Intraoperative angiography reloaded: a new hybrid operating theater for combined endovascular and surgical treatment of cerebral arteriovenous malformations: a pilot study on 25 patients. Acta Neurochir (Wien). 2013; 155(11):2071–2078

[20] Nicolato A, Longhi M, Tommasi N, et al. Leksell Gamma Knife for pediatric and adolescent cerebral arteriovenous malformations: results of 100 cases followed up for at least 36 months. J Neurosurg Pediatr. 2015; 16(6):736–747

[21] Reyns N, Blond S, Gauvrit JY, et al. Role of radiosurgery in the management of cerebral arteriovenous malformations in the pediatric age group: data from a 100-patient series. Neurosurgery. 2007; 60(2):268–276, discussion 276

[22] Potts MB, Sheth SA, Louie J, et al. Stereotactic radiosurgery at a low marginal dose for the treatment of pediatric arteriovenous malformations: obliteration, complications, and functional outcomes. J Neurosurg Pediatr. 2014; 14(1):1–11

[23] Smyth MD, Sneed PK, Ciricillo SF, et al. Stereotactic radiosurgery for pediatric intracranial arteriovenous malformations: the University of California at San Francisco experience. J Neurosurg. 2002; 97(1):48–55

[24] Zabel-du Bois A, Milker-Zabel S, Huber P, Schlegel W, Debus J. Pediatric cerebral arteriovenous malformations: the role of stereotactic linac-based radiosurgery. Int J Radiat Oncol Biol Phys. 2006; 65(4):1206–1211

[25] Zadeh G, Andrade-Souza YM, Tsao MN, et al. Pediatric arteriovenous malformation: University of Toronto experience using stereotactic radiosurgery. Childs Nerv Syst. 2007; 23(2):195–199

[26] Wilkins RH. Natural history of intracranial vascular malformations: a review. Neurosurgery. 1985; 16(3):421–430

[27] Yeon JY, Shin HJ, Kim JS, Hong SC, Lee JI. Clinico-radiological outcomes following gamma knife radiosurgery for pediatric arteriovenous malformations. Childs Nerv Syst. 2011; 27(7):1109–1119

[28] Fournier D, TerBrugge KG, Willinsky R, Lasjaunias P, Montanera W. Endovascular treatment of intracerebral arteriovenous malformations: experience in 49 cases. J Neurosurg. 1991; 75(2):228–233

[29] Valavanis A, Yaşargil MG. The endovascular treatment of brain arteriovenous malformations. Adv Tech Stand Neurosurg. 1998; 24:131–214

[30] van Rooij WJ, Jacobs S, Sluzewski M, Beute GN, van der Pol B. Endovascular treatment of ruptured brain AVMs in the acute phase of hemorrhage. AJNR Am J Neuroradiol. 2012; 33(6):1162–1166

[31] Yu SC, Chan MS, Lam JM, Tam PH, Poon WS. Complete obliteration of intracranial arteriovenous malformation with endovascular cyanoacrylate embolization: initial success and rate of permanent cure. AJNR Am J Neuroradiol. 2004; 25(7):1139–1143

[32] Kader A, Goodrich JT, Sonstein WJ, Stein BM, Carmel PW, Michelsen WJ. Recurrent cerebral arteriovenous malformations after negative postoperative angiograms. J Neurosurg. 1996; 85(1):14–18

[33] Gobin YP, Laurent A, Merienne L, et al. Treatment of brain arteriovenous malformations by embolization and radiosurgery. J Neurosurg. 1996; 85(1):19–28

[34] Pollock BE, Gorman DA, Coffey RJ. Patient outcomes after arteriovenous malformation radiosurgical management: results based on a 5- to 14-year follow-up study. Neurosurgery. 2003; 52(6):1291–1296, discussion 1296–1297

[35] Klimo P , Jr, Rao G, Brockmeyer D. Pediatric arteriovenous malformations: a 15-year experience with an emphasis on residual and recurrent lesions. Childs Nerv Syst. 2007; 23(1):31–37

[36] Lang SS, Beslow LA, Bailey RL, et al. Follow-up imaging to detect recurrence of surgically treated pediatric arteriovenous malformations. J Neurosurg Pediatr. 2012; 9(5):497–504

[37] Morgenstern PF, Hoffman CE, Kocharian G, Singh R, Stieg PE, Souweidane MM. Postoperative imaging for detection of recurrent arteriovenous malformations in children. J Neurosurg Pediatr. 2015:1–7

[38] Higuchi M, Bitoh S, Hasegawa H, Obashi J, Hiraga S. Marked growth of arteriovenous malformation 19 years after resection: a case report. No Shinkei Geka. 1991; 19(1):75–78

[39] Ali MJ, Bendok BR, Rosenblatt S, Rose JE, Getch CC, Batjer HH. Recurrence of pediatric cerebral arteriovenous malformations after angiographically documented resection. Pediatr Neurosurg. 2003; 39(1):32–38

[40] Andaluz N, Myseros JS, Sathi S, Crone KR, Tew JM , Jr. Recurrence of cerebral arteriovenous malformations in children: report of two cases and review of the literature. Surg Neurol. 2004; 62(4):324–330, discussion 330–331

[41] Weil AG, Li S, Zhao JZ. Recurrence of a cerebral arteriovenous malformation following complete surgical resection: a case report and review of the literature. Surg Neurol Int. 2011; 2:175

30 Management of Residual and Recurrent Arteriovenous Malformations

Daniel Raper, David M. Sawyer, Peter S. Amenta, and Ricky Medel

Abstract

Incompletely obliterated arteriovenous malformations are encountered in clinical practice due to either failure of the primary treatment strategy, latency in treatment effect for radiosurgery, or lesion recurrence. Partial treatment in most circumstances does not confer a protective benefit and generally increases the rate of hemorrhage over the natural history. These lesions must be evaluated based on grade, angioarchitecture, location, previous treatments, and any existing neurological deficits at presentation. For those lesions that are amenable, surgical resection should be undertaken. Lesions that are deemed unsuitable for surgery should be evaluated for radiosurgery. Embolization is generally only useful as part of a multimodal treatment strategy, but may be beneficial in isolation for those patients with associated aneurysms, vascular steal, or the minority in whom a cure can be obtained. Patients must be counseled regarding the natural history, as well as the risks and benefits of any proposed treatment. High-grade (Spetzler–Martin IV and V) lesions are generally best managed conservatively.

Keywords: recurrent AVM, residual AVM, arteriovenous malformation, hidden compartment, incomplete obliteration, partial resection, staged treatment, radiographic surveillance, risk assessment, multimodality treatment

Key Points

- Residual and recurrent brain arteriovenous malformations (AVMs) are commonly encountered in clinical practice due to the complex nature of many lesions, the extended time course of radiosurgical treatment, and the prevalence of staged treatment strategies.
- Incomplete obliteration, in almost all circumstances, confers no benefit and may even increase the rate of hemorrhage.
- Ongoing radiographic surveillance is essential to assess residual and recurrent AVMs, and for any suspected change a diagnostic cerebral angiogram (DSA) should be performed.
- Surgical excision remains the "gold standard" for patients with low-grade lesions (Spetzler–Martin grades I and II) in noneloquent locations.
- In any patient undergoing surgical intervention, DSA should be performed intraoperatively or immediately postoperatively to ensure complete excision.

30.1 Introduction

Treatment of recurrent and residual arteriovenous malformations (AVMs) remains a difficult clinical problem. Treatment options for AVMs include planned staged procedures, procedures that are aimed at reducing the volume of the AVM to potentiate other treatments, and procedures whose efficacy is delayed over multiple years. The natural history of residual and recurrent AVMs is not well defined. Flow dynamics in these lesions can change over time, and the risk of hemorrhage or rehemorrhage after partial treatment is not well understood. Furthermore, the risks of treating residual or recurrent AVMs depend on the initial treatment modality and on a number of lesion-specific factors.

The natural history of untreated AVMs suggests an annual hemorrhage rate of 2.2% for unruptured lesions and 4.5% for those with previous rupture lesions.[1] Features such as exclusively deep venous drainage and associated aneurysms further increase this risk.[1] When considering younger patients, this portends a substantial lifetime risk of hemorrhage. Should this occur, the morbidity and mortality vary from 16 to 45% and 1 to 20%, respectively,[2,3,4] and up to 45% of patients will not return to functional independence.[5] Recently, a randomized trial of unruptured brain arteriovenous malformations (ARUBA) was conducted and halted early with the conclusion that medical therapy was superior to interventional management of unruptured lesions.[6] This result has been criticized, primarily because of the methods utilized for intervention. Specifically, out of 116 people randomized to interventional management, only 18 (15%) were treated surgically.[6] Furthermore, 73 patients (53 ongoing treatment and 20 treatment pending) at the time of analysis had yet to undergo definitive management.[6] This highlights the importance of treatment modality in the management of AVMs, with microsurgical resection remaining the gold standard when feasible.

A comprehensive literature review from 2011 assessing outcomes in more than 13,000 patients demonstrated that incomplete obliteration is a common finding after initial treatment for AVMs.[7] This further highlights the importance of treatment planning and emphasizes that the clinician taking care of patients with AVMs will often be confronted with patients harboring incompletely treated or recurrent lesions.

Similar to those with a de novo presentation, assessment and treatment of recurrent or residual AVMs relies on a thorough assessment of the angiographic anatomy, categorization of the risk of hemorrhage, and tailoring of an individual treatment plan based on a multidisciplinary consideration of the risks and benefits of treatment.

30.2 Methods

In addition to utilizing the authors' own experience, a PubMed search was conducted using the keywords "incomplete obliteration brain arteriovenous malformations," "incomplete resection brain arteriovenous malformations," "residual brain arteriovenous malformations," "residual cerebral arteriovenous malformations," and "recurrent brain arteriovenous malformations." Articles published within the last 15 years were considered. The senior author reviewed all articles for relevance. The American Heart Association (AHA) guidelines as well as key publications were also employed.

30.3 Presentation

Staged therapy has been used for many years in the management of complex AVMs,[8,9] and so the presentation of recurrent or residual AVMs is less often an acute symptomatic occurrence and more often a radiologic diagnosis or one made on routine follow-up. On the other hand, residual or recurrent AVMs can still cause an array of symptoms. These include hemorrhage (intracerebral, subarachnoid, or intraventricular), seizure, and neurologic change from steal phenomena. In pediatric patients, recurrent or breakthrough seizures, worsening hydrocephalus, or progressive heart failure may be an indication of failure of prior treatment.

30.4 Radiographic Surveillance

Among patients with AVMs that have been previously treated (either with an intent to cure or as part of a multistage treatment plan), follow-up imaging plays an important role in monitoring AVM progression. In asymptomatic patients, magnetic resonance imaging (MRI) and MR angiography provide satisfactory anatomical detail and are noninvasive. FLAIR (fluid attenuation inversion recovery) sequences can demonstrate mass effect on surrounding brain as well as radiation-induced parenchymal changes, and susceptibility- or gradient-weighted imaging can detect hemorrhages in the area of the AVM. Modern MR angiography approaches the resolution of computed tomography (CT) angiography and gives a satisfactory means of following these lesions over time. However, for cases that remain indeterminate or in which there is a question of planning an additional treatment, the gold standard imaging modality remains cerebral angiography. Intraoperative angiography is often useful to confirm complete obliteration of an AVM.[10] Cerebral angiography is essential in the evaluation of recurrent or residual AVMs in order to characterize any changes to the lesion size, arterial supply, or development of concerning features such as intranidal aneurysms, venous ectasia, or strictures.

30.5 Recurrent Arteriovenous Malformations

The traditional understanding of the natural history of AVMs states that following complete resection, there is no risk of recurrence. This has been supported in several large series in adult patients.[11,12,13] Recurrent AVMs after complete resection have, however, been reported in the pediatric population.[14,15,16,17] Yasargil first reported recurrent AVM in a pediatric patient who had undergone surgical resection of a right frontal AVM with subsequent angiographic confirmation of obliteration of the nidus and early venous drainage.[17] In one series, angiographic recurrence was seen in 14.3% of patients and occurred 4 to 5 years after the primary treatment (surgical resection) in all cases.[15] A second series reported a 5.5% recurrence rate by angiography at a mean of 9 years after complete surgical resection.[16] In a review of pediatric series in which follow-up was performed with MRI, recurrence occurred at an average of 5.5 years after initial resection (range: 1–9 years).[14] Recurrent AVMs have been reported even following multiple complete resections with angiographic cure,[18] or following complete resection with intraoperative angiographic confirmation.[10] Recurrences in adults are much rarer than in children, though they have been reported.[10,19] The explanation for these cases may be related to a "hidden compartment" in certain AVMs, in which internal steal causes some portion of a residual AVM to remain angiographically occult.[20] Alternately, the immature cerebrovascular system in the pediatric patient may contribute to the capacity to form another AVM.[10] Early postoperative angiography can miss residual AVM due to vasospasm, transient thrombus within an AVM nidus, or edema.[10] In the largest series of AVMs investigating recurrence, young age and deep venous drainage were the most important factors predicting recurrence.[19] Nevertheless, due to the overall low rate of recurrence, these authors advise that, in the case of adult patients with complete resection and a negative postoperative angiogram, regular angiographic surveillance is not necessary.

30.6 Treatment Modalities

30.6.1 Stereotactic Radiosurgery

Stereotactic radiosurgery (SRS) may be useful in a large proportion of AVMs, either as a treatment with intent to cure for patients with surgically or endovascularly inaccessible lesions, or as part of a multimodality treatment strategy. The radiobiological response to SRS can take 2 years or longer to become fully apparent. The most important factor in assessing the ability of SRS to provide a cure is the volume, with nidal volumes less than 3 mL being the best candidates. A number of grading scales have been proposed to assess the radiosurgical response of AVMs.[21]

A number of factors have been associated with incomplete radiosurgical treatment or recurrence after SRS. Hemorrhage has been associated with incomplete obliteration of the AVM nidus.[22] Incomplete obliteration is seen in 42% of patients with high-flow fistulas after radiotherapy.[23] In a retrospective series of 139 patients treated with SRS, lower rates of obliteration were associated with angioarchitectural characteristics indicative of higher flow such as perinidal angiogenesis and arterial enlargement.[24] A systematic review of 14 studies in 733 patients with incompletely treated AVMs that were treated with repeat radiosurgery yielded an obliteration rate of 61% with risk of AVM-related hemorrhage of 7.6% and radiation-induced changes of 7.4%.[25] The type of initial treatment also influences the efficacy of subsequent SRS. Among a series of 169 patients treated with radiosurgery, those who had been previously treated with embolization had a lower obliteration rate than those with primary SRS treatment.[26]

For patients with large AVMs, staged-volume radiosurgery is a strategy in which the AVM volume is divided into smaller "parcels" to target in individual treatment sessions.[27] In this way, a residual AVM is progressively treated over time. Treatment sessions may be staged at 3- to 9-month intervals. In a small series of patients, this strategy yielded a 10-year complete angiographic occlusion rate of 89%, but with a 27.8% hemorrhage rate.[28] In series of multistaged SRS for AVMs, 5-year total obliteration rates were 62%, but the cumulative hemorrhage rates after SRS were 4.3, 8.6, 13.5, and 36% at 1, 2, 5, and 10 years, respectively.[27] It is difficult to accurately define the risk in these lesions, which were deemed "unsuitable for surgery," but these results likely represent an improvement on their natural history. It is important to note that the planning method and type of imaging used for radiosurgical planning may have an effect on obliteration rates achieved due to a potentially better ability to visualize the AVM nidus.[29]

Any recurrence after initial treatment may change the drainage pattern of the AVM, effectively creating a new lesion. In those with an angiographically identifiable nidus, the hemorrhage rate is generally regarded as identical to untreated AVMs. However, there does exist evidence to suggest that radiosurgically treated lesions with subtotal obliteration have a lower rate of hemorrhage.[30] In the series by Abu-Salma et al including 121 patients with subtotal obliteration, defined as obliteration of the nidus with persistence of an early draining vein, there were no instances of hemorrhage over a mean follow-up of 44 months.[30,31] This does represent a select group of patients, but suggests that this group may not require further intervention. Importantly, this angioarchitecture may represent a stage during the evolution to obliteration or an endpoint in itself.[32,33]

30.6.2 Embolization

Embolization alone has the potential to offer a cure in only a small proportion of AVMs, typically those supplied by one or two arterial feeders, located at a safe distance from other branch arteries supplying normal parenchyma. To the extent that an initial treatment leaves an AVM nidus incompletely embolized, recurrence can be expected; this may be accompanied by development of new arterial feeders or recanalization of the initial feeding arteries, depending on the AVM angioarchitecture and the embolizate used initially.

N-butylcyanoacrylate (NBCA) is a fast-drying liquid adhesive, which has traditionally been used for embolization of AVMs either with a view to cure or as part of a multimodality strategy of treatment. Onyx, a newer liquid embolic agent, has also been widely used for embolization of AVMs. It is available in two concentrations, 6.0% (Onyx 18) and 8.0% (Onyx 34), with different viscosities, and has more of a "lava-like" passage through embolized blood vessels. Onyx and NBCA were investigated in a randomized trial that demonstrated equivalent safety and efficacy, with both agents having the potential to reduce AVM volume by greater than 50%.[34] Even in cases of complete AVM obliteration, however, there have been cases of recanalization due to Onyx resorption.[9] A series of cases treated with presurgical embolization demonstrated evidence of canalization in almost 15% of cases.[35]

More importantly, lesions that are initially treated with embolization may cause an AVM to alter its hemodynamic properties. Usually, if the largest arterial feeder is embolized, this results in a decrease in the rate and amount of arteriovenous shunting, thus decreasing the risk of hemorrhage. However, there remains a risk of collateralization after embolization of other arteries that were not previously angiographically visible. For this reason, any AVM that is embolized with intent to cure must be followed closely, ideally with serial angiography.

The strategy of targeted embolization, with a view to subsequent radiosurgery, although initially associated with increased risk of complications,[7,36] has been proposed as a means to reduce interim hemorrhage risk and increase GKRS (gamma knife radiosurgery) efficacy.[37] This remains controversial and

likely increases the risk of incomplete obliteration following radiosurgery.[38] The use of this strategy is dependent upon the angioarchitecture of the lesion, with it possessing the ability to potentially afford a lower side effect profile than with radiosurgery alone.[38] Embolization has also been employed to complete a partial treatment after SRS.[39] In both cases, the same principles of occlusion of the nidus depend on accurate identification of the nidus on cerebral angiography, and accessibility of the nidus via the endovascular route for embolization.

Embolization has also been used in isolation to palliatively treat large, unresectable AVMs without the expectation of complete obliteration. In the literature, AVMs chosen for this manner of treatment are typically large lesions located in eloquent cortex that are not amenable to either surgical or radiosurgical therapy. These large malformations are often associated with progressive neurologic deficits, which may be the result of a vascular steal phenomenon that induces adjacent cerebral hypoperfusion, mass effect, or repeated hemorrhage.[40,41] The intention of palliative embolization is to reduce these progressive neurologic deficits.

Benefit has previously been reported for palliative embolization in some small patient series, with some indication of improvement in adjacent cerebral perfusion after treatment.[42] However, more robust studies have indicated that the risk–benefit profile for this strategy is not favorable.[43] Specifically, it has been repeatedly shown that the risk of subsequent hemorrhage in patients with large, unresectable AVMs is actually increased significantly after palliative or incomplete embolization.[44,45,46] Conservative medical management is generally the most appropriate therapy for patients who present with lesions that are deemed unsuitable for surgical or radiosurgical intervention.[47] The exception to this philosophy is in those patients with perinidal aneurysms that are amenable to embolization. The presence of associated aneurysms increases the risk of hemorrhage, up to 10% in some series;[48] therefore, these should be treated if possible.[49,50]

30.6.3 Surgery

Surgical resection has been shown to be a safe and effective treatment for many AVMs and remains the recommended initial treatment strategy for low-grade (Spetzler–Martin grades I, II, and some grade III) lesions.[47,51] Many small, hemispheric lesions can be cured with low morbidity with a surgical management strategy.[52] Potts et al[53] recently published their series of 232 (120 ruptured) grade I (33%) and II (67%) malformations undergoing surgical excision. Ninety-seven percent of patients were improved or unchanged from their baseline, with unruptured patients having the best outcomes. There was an overall surgical morbidity of 3%. Importantly, partial surgical resection confers no benefit and may increase the risk of subsequent hemorrhage. One study in high-grade AVMs that underwent partial resection demonstrated a 10-fold risk of hemorrhage after partial resection, compared with those without surgical treatment.[46,52] The risk of incomplete resection varies by grade and surgeon experience, but rates between 1 and 18% have been published in the literature.[54] In order to eliminate this occurrence, surgical intervention should include either intraoperative or immediate postoperative angiography to ensure complete excision of the lesion. Should residual lesion be

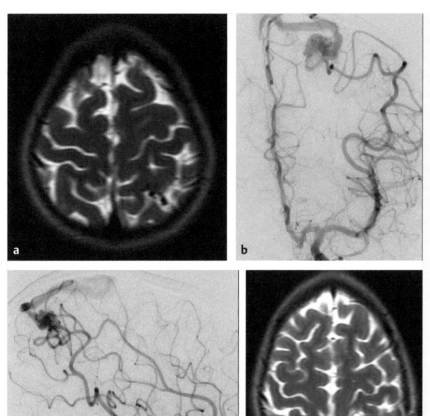

Fig. 30.1 A 13-year-old female patient with severe headaches found to have a left parietal arteriovenous malformation (AVM) on magnetic resonance imaging (MRI; **a**). Cerebral angiogram demonstrated a 2.1 × 2 × 1.7 cm left parietal AVM (**b,c**). Intraoperative angiogram demonstrated a small area of residual nidus that was subsequently excised. Postoperative angiogram and MRI (**d**) confirmed complete excision.

identified, the patient must be taken for re-exploration and excision.[55] ▶ Fig. 30.1 depicts a patient treated by the authors in whom residual intraoperative angiography demonstrated a residual nidus that was then completely excised.

30.7 Management Strategy

Assessment of the risk of intervention in residual or recurrent AVMs can be more complex than for previously untreated lesions and the simple application of grading scales such as the Spetzler–Martin scale (to assess surgical risk),[51] the Virginia Radiosurgery AVM scale (to assess the radiosurgical risk),[21] or other scoring systems assessing endovascular treatment risks[56] is likely less accurate. For Spetzler–Martin grade I or II lesions in noneloquent cortex, surgical excision remains the "gold standard." Again, excision must be confirmed by DSA and re-exploration undertaken if any residual is identified. Radiosurgery is effective for lesions that are not amenable to surgical excision, but there remains a risk of rupture until obliteration is obtained. The only exception is in those with subtotal obliteration as previously defined. Staged radiosurgery also represents a treatment alternative for larger lesions that are inappropriate for single-session therapy. Concerning endovascular embolization, this should only be performed for cure in the minority of cases where there is a high likelihood of success. It may be performed as part of a multimodal treatment strategy to address a particular feature of the lesion (i.e., perinidal

aneurysms). In most circumstances, it should not be performed for "palliative" purposes.

Those patients harboring grade IV and V lesions are generally afforded better outcomes by natural history than through intervention.[46] The hemorrhage rate in this group may be lower than for patients with grade I–III lesions.[46] Indications for treatment of this population include associated aneurysms and steal phenomenon. Isolated cases may be candidates for attempted cure, but this should only be performed by surgeons with significant experience in the management of AVMs.

30.8 Conclusion

Residual and recurrent brain AVMs are commonly encountered in clinical practice due to the complex nature of many lesions, the extended time course of radiosurgical treatment, and the prevalence of staged treatment strategies. Depending on the angioarchitecture and flow characteristics of the residual/recurrent lesion, the risk associated with these lesions may be equivalent to, or greater than, the original lesion. Only in the minority of situations is the risk of hemorrhage lowered through partial treatment. For this reason, when considering intervention for a patient with a residual or recurrent AVM, a similar treatment approach should be taken as toward a naive lesion. Faced with an AVM that demonstrates residual early venous filling or recurrence, it should be remembered that after radiosurgery, ongoing treatment effect occurs over time. Thus, evaluating the risks and benefits of intervention for AVM must take into account the changing risk profile of these lesions. Ongoing radiographic surveillance is essential to assess residual and recurrent AVMs, and for any suspected change, a diagnostic cerebral angiogram should be performed.

References

[1] Gross BA, Du R. Natural history of cerebral arteriovenous malformations: a meta-analysis. J Neurosurg. 2013; 118(2):437–443

[2] Hartmann A, Mast H, Mohr JP, et al. Morbidity of intracranial hemorrhage in patients with cerebral arteriovenous malformation. Stroke. 1998; 29(5):931–934

[3] Brown RD , Jr, Wiebers DO, Torner JC, O'Fallon WM. Frequency of intracranial hemorrhage as a presenting symptom and subtype analysis: a population-based study of intracranial vascular malformations in Olmsted Country, Minnesota. J Neurosurg. 1996; 85(1):29–32

[4] Al-Shahi R, Warlow C. A systematic review of the frequency and prognosis of arteriovenous malformations of the brain in adults. Brain. 2001; 124(Pt 10):1900–1926

[5] Majumdar M, Tan L, Chen M. Critical assessment of the morbidity associated with ruptured cerebral arteriovenous malformations. J Neurointerv Surg. 2016; 8(2):163–167

[6] Mohr JP, Parides MK, Stapf C, et al. international ARUBA investigators. Medical management with or without interventional therapy for unruptured brain arteriovenous malformations (ARUBA): a multicentre, non-blinded, randomised trial. Lancet. 2014; 383(9917):614–621

[7] van Beijnum J, van der Worp HB, Buis DR, et al. Treatment of brain arteriovenous malformations: a systematic review and meta-analysis. JAMA. 2011; 306(18):2011–2019

[8] Andrews BT, Wilson CB. Staged treatment of arteriovenous malformations of the brain. Neurosurgery. 1987; 21(3):314–323

[9] Bauer AM, Bain MD, Rasmussen PA. Onyx resorbtion with AVM recanalization after complete AVM obliteration. Interv Neuroradiol. 2015; 21(3):351–356

[10] Gaballah M, Storm PB, Rabinowitz D, et al. Intraoperative cerebral angiography in arteriovenous malformation resection in children: a single institutional experience. J Neurosurg Pediatr. 2014; 13(2):222–228

[11] Drake CG. Cerebral arteriovenous malformations: considerations for and experience with surgical treatment in 166 cases. Clin Neurosurg. 1979; 26:145–208

[12] Heros RC, Korosue K, Diebold PM. Surgical excision of cerebral arteriovenous malformations: late results. Neurosurgery. 1990; 26(4):570–577, discussion 577–578

[13] Jomin M, Lesoin F, Lozes G. Prognosis for arteriovenous malformations of the brain in adults based on 150 cases. Surg Neurol. 1985; 23(4):362–366

[14] Kader A, Goodrich JT, Sonstein WJ, Stein BM, Carmel PW, Michelsen WJ. Recurrent cerebral arteriovenous malformations after negative postoperative angiograms. J Neurosurg. 1996; 85(1):14–18

[15] Lang SS, Beslow LA, Bailey RL, et al. Follow-up imaging to detect recurrence of surgically treated pediatric arteriovenous malformations. J Neurosurg Pediatr. 2012; 9(5):497–504

[16] Andaluz N, Myseros JS, Sathi S, Crone KR, Tew JM , Jr. Recurrence of cerebral arteriovenous malformations in children: report of two cases and review of the literature. Surg Neurol. 2004; 62(4):324–330, discussion 330–331

[17] Yaşargil M. Microneurosurgery. Stuttgart: Thieme; 1987:182–189

[18] Nagm A, Horiuchi T, Ichinose S, Hongo K. Unique double recurrence of cerebral arteriovenous malformation. Acta Neurochir (Wien). 2015; 157(9):1461–1466

[19] Morgan MK, Patel NJ, Simons M, Ritson EA, Heller GZ. Influence of the combination of patient age and deep venous drainage on brain arteriovenous malformation recurrence after surgery. J Neurosurg. 2012; 117(5):934–941

[20] Pellettieri L, Svendsen P, Wikholm G, Carlsson CA. Hidden compartments in AVMs–a new concept. Acta Radiol. 1997; 38(1):2–7

[21] Starke RM, Yen CP, Ding D, Sheehan JP. A practical grading scale for predicting outcome after radiosurgery for arteriovenous malformations: analysis of 1012 treated patients. J Neurosurg. 2013; 119(4):981–987

[22] Izawa M, Hayashi M, Chernov M, et al. Long-term complications after gamma knife surgery for arteriovenous malformations. J Neurosurg. 2005; 102 Suppl:34–37

[23] Yuki I, Kim RH, Duckwiler G, et al. Treatment of brain arteriovenous malformations with high-flow arteriovenous fistulas: risk and complications associated with endovascular embolization in multimodality treatment. Clinical article. J Neurosurg. 2010; 113(4):715–722

[24] Taeshineetanakul P, Krings T, Geibprasert S, et al. Angioarchitecture determines obliteration rate after radiosurgery in brain arteriovenous malformations. Neurosurgery. 2012; 71(6):1071–1078, discussion 1079

[25] Awad AJ, Walcott BP, Stapleton CJ, Ding D, Lee CC, Loeffler JS. Repeat radiosurgery for cerebral arteriovenous malformations. J Clin Neurosci. 2015; 22(6):945–950

[26] Schlienger M, Atlan D, Lefkopoulos D, et al. Linac radiosurgery for cerebral arteriovenous malformations: results in 169 patients. Int J Radiat Oncol Biol Phys. 2000; 46(5):1135–1142

[27] Kano H, Kondziolka D, Flickinger JC, et al. Stereotactic radiosurgery for arteriovenous malformations, Part 6: multistaged volumetric management of large arteriovenous malformations. J Neurosurg. 2012; 116(1):54–65

[28] Huang PP, Rush SC, Donahue B, et al. Long-term outcomes after staged-volume stereotactic radiosurgery for large arteriovenous malformations. Neurosurgery. 2012; 71(3):632–643, discussion 643–644

[29] Amponsah K, Ellis TL, Chan MD, et al. Retrospective analysis of imaging techniques for treatment planning and monitoring of obliteration for gamma knife treatment of cerebral arteriovenous malformation. Neurosurgery. 2012; 71(4):893–899

[30] Abu-Salma Z, Nataf F, Ghossoub M, et al. The protective status of subtotal obliteration of arteriovenous malformations after radiosurgery: significance and risk of hemorrhage. Neurosurgery. 2009; 65(4):709–717, discussion 717–718

[31] Abecassis IJ, Xu DS, Batjer HH, Bendok BR. Natural history of brain arteriovenous malformations: a systematic review. Neurosurg Focus. 2014; 37(3):E7

[32] Yen CP, Varady P, Sheehan J, Steiner M, Steiner L. Subtotal obliteration of cerebral arteriovenous malformations after gamma knife surgery. J Neurosurg. 2007; 106(3):361–369

[33] Steiner L, Lindquist C, Adler JR, Torner JC, Alves W, Steiner M. Clinical outcome of radiosurgery for cerebral arteriovenous malformations. J Neurosurg. 1992; 77(1):1–8

[34] Loh Y, Duckwiler GR, Onyx Trial Investigators. A prospective, multicenter, randomized trial of the Onyx liquid embolic system and N-butyl cyanoacrylate embolization of cerebral arteriovenous malformations. Clinical article. J Neurosurg. 2010; 113(4):733–741

[35] Natarajan SK, Ghodke B, Britz GW, Born DE, Sekhar LN. Multimodality treatment of brain arteriovenous malformations with microsurgery after embolization with onyx: single-center experience and technical nuances. Neurosurgery. 2008; 62(6):1213–1225, discussion 1225–1226

[36] Pollock BE, Flickinger JC, Lunsford LD, Maitz A, Kondziolka D. Factors associated with successful arteriovenous malformation radiosurgery. Neurosurgery. 1998; 42(6):1239–1244, discussion 1244–1247

[37] Xiaochuan H, Yuhua J, Xianli L, Hongchao Y, Yang Z, Youxiang L. Targeted embolization reduces hemorrhage complications in partially embolized cerebral AVM combined with gamma knife surgery. Interv Neuroradiol. 2015; 21(1):80–87

[38] Oermann EK, Ding D, Yen CP, et al. Effect of prior embolization on cerebral arteriovenous malformation radiosurgery outcomes: a case-control study. Neurosurgery. 2015; 77(3):406–417, discussion 417

[39] Hodgson TJ, Kemeny AA, Gholkar A, Deasy N. Embolization of residual fistula following stereotactic radiosurgery in cerebral arteriovenous malformations. AJNR Am J Neuroradiol. 2009; 30(1):109–110

[40] Batjer HH, Devous MD , Sr, Seibert GB, et al. Intracranial arteriovenous malformation: relationships between clinical and radiographic factors and ipsilateral steal severity. Neurosurgery. 1988; 23(3):322–328

[41] Choi JH, Mast H, Hartmann A, et al. Clinical and morphological determinants of focal neurological deficits in patients with unruptured brain arteriovenous malformation. J Neurol Sci. 2009; 287(1–2):126–130

[42] Al-Yamany M, Terbrugge KG, Willinsky R, Montanera W, Tymianski M, Wallace MC. Palliative embolisation of brain arteriovenous malformations presenting with progressive neurological deficit. Interv Neuroradiol. 2000; 6(3):177–183

[43] Başkaya MK, Heros RC. Indications for and complications of embolization of cerebral arteriovenous malformations. J Neurosurg. 2006; 104(2):183–186, discussion 186–187

[44] Miyamoto S, Hashimoto N, Nagata I, et al. Posttreatment sequelae of palliatively treated cerebral arteriovenous malformations. Neurosurgery. 2000; 46(3):589–594, discussion 594–595

[45] Kwon OK, Han DH, Han MH, Chung YS. Palliatively treated cerebral arteriovenous malformations: follow-up results. J Clin Neurosci. 2000; 7 Suppl 1:69–72

[46] Han PP, Ponce FA, Spetzler RF. Intention-to-treat analysis of Spetzler-Martin grades IV and V arteriovenous malformations: natural history and treatment paradigm. J Neurosurg. 2003; 98(1):3–7

[47] Baskaya MK, Jea A, Heros RC, Javahary R, Sultan A. Cerebral arteriovenous malformations. Clin Neurosurg. 2006; 53(1):114–144

[48] da Costa L, Wallace MC, Ter Brugge KG, O'Kelly C, Willinsky RA, Tymianski M. The natural history and predictive features of hemorrhage from brain arteriovenous malformations. Stroke. 2009; 40(1):100–105

[49] Platz J, Berkefeld J, Singer OC, et al. Frequency, risk of hemorrhage and treatment considerations for cerebral arteriovenous malformations with associated aneurysms. Acta Neurochir (Wien). 2014; 156(11):2025–2034

[50] Flores BC, Klinger DR, Rickert KL, et al. Management of intracranial aneurysms associated with arteriovenous malformations. Neurosurg Focus. 2014; 37(3):E11

[51] Sisti MB, Kader A, Stein BM. Microsurgery for 67 intracranial arteriovenous malformations less than 3 cm in diameter. J Neurosurg. 1993; 79(5):653–660

[52] Sisti MB, Kader A, Stein BM. Microsurgery for 67 intracranial arteriovenous malformations less than 3 cm in diameter. J Neurosurg. 1993; 79(5):653–660

[53] Potts MB, Lau D, Abla AA, Kim H, Young WL, Lawton MT, UCSF Brain AVM Study Project. Current surgical results with low-grade brain arteriovenous malformations. J Neurosurg. 2015; 122(4):912–920

[54] Hoh BL, Carter BS, Ogilvy CS. Incidence of residual intracranial AVMs after surgical resection and efficacy of immediate surgical re-exploration. Acta Neurochir (Wien). 2004; 146(1):1–7, discussion 7

[55] Hoh BL, Carter BS, Ogilvy CS. Incidence of residual intracranial AVMs after surgical resection and efficacy of immediate surgical re-exploration. Acta Neurochir (Wien). 2004; 146(1):1–7, discussion 7

[56] Bell DL, Leslie-Mazwi TM, Yoo AJ, et al. Application of a novel brain arteriovenous malformation endovascular grading scale for transarterial embolization. AJNR Am J Neuroradiol. 2015; 36(7):1303–1309

31 Epilepsy Management for Arteriovenous Malformation

Mark Quigg

Abstract

About one-third of patients with arteriovenous malformation (AVM) present with seizures, and about 40% of those will have AVM-related epilepsy (AVMRE). Seizures will persist despite best antiepileptic drug (AED) therapy in about 15 to 20% of those with AVMRE. Risk factors for development of AVMRE described by most studies include superficial cortical location—usually in frontotemporal regions—and previous hemorrhage. Intervention for AVM is primarily undertaken for risks of hemorrhage, but surgery, embolization, or stereotactic radiosurgery (SRS) have all demonstrated reasonably high rates of sustained seizure remission in those with AVMRE. Comparative studies suggest that open surgery may have more beneficial effects in seizure remission than other treatment modalities in patients with AVMRE. Conversely, SRS has fewer problems associated with de novo, postoperative AVMRE than surgery in those patients with AVM and without preoperative seizures. Modern practice with multiple modalities with embolization, SRS, and open surgery in a staged fashion has demonstrated efficacy in seizure remission that correlates with obliteration of the AVM nidus, regardless of intervention.

Keywords: epilepsy, anticonvulsant medication, seizure remission, arteriovenous malformation, sudden unexpected death in epilepsy, subarachnoid hemorrhage, radiosurgery, embolization

Key Points

- About one-third of patients with arteriovenous malformation (AVM) present with seizures, and about 40% of those will have AVM-related epilepsy (AVMRE).
- Seizures will persist despite best antiepileptic drug therapy in about 15 to 20% of those with AVMRE.
- Risk factors for development of AVMRE described by most studies include superficial cortical location—usually in frontotemporal regions—and previous hemorrhage.
- Surgery, embolization, or stereotactic radiosurgery and combinations of interventions have all demonstrated reasonably high rates of sustained seizure remission in those with AVMRE.
- Efficacy in seizure remission correlates with obliteration of the AVM nidus, regardless of the mode of intervention.

31.1 Introduction

Many patients with arteriovenous malformation (AVM) present with seizures and can be considered as having epilepsy; an important minority remains with recurring seizures despite maximal therapy. Although intracranial hemorrhage and its attendant morbidity and mortality remain appropriate foci of study of AVM, epilepsy adds to the risks of AVM and merits additional consideration in the overall care of the patient with AVM-related epilepsy (AVMRE).

The prevalence, characteristics, and responses to treatment of epilepsy associated with AVM (AVMRE) will be outlined placing this specific disorder in the context of epilepsy in general. The mechanisms of epileptogenesis will also be briefly discussed.

31.2 Definitions, Morbidity, and Mortality of Epilepsy

A practical definition of epilepsy is "at least two unprovoked seizures occurring more than 24 hours apart" or "one unprovoked seizure and a [high] probability of further seizures."[1] Seizures are considered "medically intractable" when a patient has failed to become seizure free with trials of at least two anticonvulsant medications (antiepileptic drugs [AED]).[2] Rather than layering on two or more AED, most epileptologists recommend serial trials of single AED since side effects and teratogenicity of AED rise rapidly, and seizures may paradoxically worsen, with polypharmacy.[3]

A recent review by Laxer et al lays out the epidemiology and risks of epilepsy.[4] The incidence of epilepsy in developed countries is approximately 50 per 100,000 individuals per year. The prevalence of epilepsy in developed countries ranges between 4 and 10 per 1,000 individuals per year. About 20 to 30% of patients with epilepsy can be expected to be "medically intractable," and only 4% of adult patients can expect to remit per year even taking into account all current therapies.[4] About 50% of patients can be expected to achieve sustained seizure freedom with the introduction of a single, well-tolerated AED; a trial of a second AED brings that proportion to about 65%.[5]

The most common scheme for rating seizure outcomes after epilepsy surgery is the "Engels criteria" that classify outcome 2 years after surgery into four grades and subgrades: Ia: seizure-free; Ib: free from all disabling seizures (effectively no seizures except for simple partial seizures or auras); II: rare disabling seizures; III: worthwhile improvement, and IV: no worthwhile improvement.[6] Quality of life (QOL) or functional outcomes after "lesionless" epilepsy surgery show meaningful or durable improvements only in the case of class I outcomes.[7,8,9] In other words, improvements in epilepsy do not occur linearly; a 50% improvement in seizure frequency, for example, does not translate into a 50% improvement in cognition, driving, or employment. Most benefits in epilepsy treatment accrue to those who are truly seizure free (Engels Class I) rather than to those whose seizures have merely improved (Engels Class II or worse).

Accordingly, burdens of intractable epilepsy are considerable. In a comparative study from 2011, the global burden of epilepsy for women was greater than that of breast cancer, and was nearly four times greater than that of prostate cancer for men.[10] Because this comparison omits epilepsy's effects of stigma and social exclusion, the actual burdens may be even higher. People with epilepsy, in comparison to matched U.S. Census bureau norms, receive less education, are less likely to be married, employed, or driving, and are more likely to have diverse psychosocial problems and subjectively worse lifestyles.[11]

Dysfertility, sexual dysfunction, and other consequences of hormonal and sleep dysregulation worsen overall QOL.[12]

Many studies of AVM center on expected rates of death or major disability from hemorrhage. Epilepsy itself, in addition, carries an additional risk of early death. Mortality is greater for those with epilepsy than for those without for many reasons, including sudden unexpected death in epilepsy (SUDEP), accidents, suicide, vascular disease, pneumonia, and factors directly related to underlying causes (e.g., AVM, but also including brain tumors, neurodegenerative disease, and cerebral vascular disease, among others). Overall, people with epilepsy have a 1.6 to 11.4 times greater mortality rate than expected.[4,13] Many centers now focus on SUDEP, especially given its higher-than-expected incidence in placebo-controlled arms in standard randomized, controlled AED trials.[14] The average incidence of SUDEP is 1 per 1,000 patients with epilepsy per year. SUDEP is more common in those with medically intractable epilepsy. In adults with refractory epilepsy, the incidence is 6 per 1,000 patients per year, and the lifetime incidence is 7 to 35%.[15]

Therefore, epilepsy is a common and important disorder with psychiatric, psychological, and medical consequences. The information available on AVMRE should be evaluated in this context.

31.3 Prevalence, Incidence, and Characteristics of AVMRE

One shortcoming that quickly becomes evident when reviewing the literature on the intersections between AVM and seizures is that authors, especially in earlier studies, often fail to explicitly distinguish among "presenting seizures," recurring seizures, or medically intractable epilepsy.

31.3.1 Seizures as Presenting Sign in Arteriovenous Malformation

Some studies focus on the initial presenting sign or symptom of AVMs as opposed to other possible symptoms or signs. For example, a large multicenter study by Hofmeister et al gathered 1,289 patients with AVM from three centers and evaluated the broad demographics of AVM.[16] The initial presenting symptoms were, in order, hemorrhage (54%), seizures (40%), chronic headache (14%), and focal neurological deficits of varying time courses (persisting, progressive, or transient, totaling to 20%). Some studies of AVMRE excluded patients with hemorrhage. In the studies of unruptured AVM, Al-Shahi Salman et al[17] and Garcin et al,[18] the largest group of patients, about 50%, presented with "incidental" AVMs. Initial seizures comprised 29 to 41% of presenting signs.

31.3.2 Prevalence of AVM-Related Epilepsy

▶ Table 31.1 summarizes the results of studies that report the occurrence of AVMRE beyond the initial presentation; most of these studies do not clearly distinguish between presenting seizures and preoperative continuing seizures. Given that limitation, the average prevalence of AVMRE before surgical intervention is 32% (range: 18–57%).

Table 31.1 Incidence of "presenting seizures" and epilepsy in studies of arteriovenous malformation–related epilepsy

First author (year)	N	Overall (N, %)	Single seizure (N, %)	Epilepsy (N, %)
Murphy (1985)[22]	115	66 (57)	57 (86)	9 (14)
Crawford (1986)[21]	343	61 (18)	–	–
Heikkinen (1989)[28]	129	29 (22)	–	–
Steiner (1992)[29]	247	98 (40)	–	–
Sutcliffe (1992)[30]	160	48 (30)	–	–
Piepgras (1993)[25]	280	117 (42)	–	–
Turjman (1995)[23]	100	47 (47)	–	–
Gerszten (1996)[31]	72	15 (21)	–	–
Osipov (1997)[26]	328	92 (28)	57 (62)	35 (38)
Falkson (1997)[32]	101	24 (24)	–	–
Hoh (2002)[24]	424	141 (33)	–	–
Schäuble (2004)[27]	285	70 (25)	13 (19)	57 (81)
Englot (2012)[19]	440	130 (30)	98 (81)	23 (5)
Galletti (2014)[20]	101	31 (31)	6 (19)	25 (81)
Al-Shahi Salman (2014)[17]	204	85 (42)	41 (48)	44 (52)
Total	3329	1054 (32)	272 (58)	193 (42)

Estimates of the severity and medical intractability of AVMRE are difficult because of variations in definitions and study designs. Three studies focused on presurgery seizures with definitions clearly stated regarding medical intractability. Osipov et al described the characteristics of seizures before surgical treatment of unruptured AVMs in a prospective cohort of 328 patients, of which 92 (28%) presented with seizures unrelated to hemorrhage. Of these 92 patients, 62% of this sample had only a single seizure at presentation; 11% continued to have weekly, 19% monthly, and 9% annual seizures. Since all patients were treated with AED, the incidence of medically intractable AVMRE was 35% of the sample of those who presented with seizures and 11% of the total sample who presented with unruptured AVMs.

Englot et al defined preoperative and postoperative outcomes in terms of "medical intractability" using the rigorous definition of failure of two AED trials.[19] Out of 440 patients with AVM, a total of 130 (30%) experienced preoperative seizures. Of these individuals, 98 (75%) had seizures as their presenting symptom, and 23 (18%) progressed to medically refractory AVMRE. It should be noted that this estimate derived from a rigorous definition falls under the average prevalence obtained from ▶ Table 31.1 and occupies the lower range commonly accepted as medically intractable epilepsy in general.

A prospective study by Josephson et al evaluated the longitudinal risk of development of epilepsy after presenting with a first AVM-related seizure in a sample that included those patients who experienced hemorrhage as well as those with unruptured AVMs.[33] The 5-year risk of developing epilepsy was 58% (95th confidence interval: 40–76%). The proportion of patients with unruptured AVMs who achieved a 2-year span of seizure freedom was 45% of those with epilepsy. Therefore, in this sample of unruptured AVMs, 55% remained with continuing seizures.

31.3.3 Types and Severity of AVM-Related Seizures

Some studies define the severity of seizures as "disabling" or "severe" seizures, based on frequency, intractability, or type without providing clear definitions. This is not a judgment against authors: "disabling" in Engel's criteria is stated without definition as well.[6] To paraphrase Potter Stewart in his Supreme Court concurrence, disability, like pornography, may be hard to define, but we know it when we see it. Many physicians equate the loss or alteration of consciousness as the primary consideration in defining disabling (i.e., as experienced with complex partial seizures). Although simple partial seizures spare consciousness, their interruptive and anxiety-provoking aspects may disproportionately affect QOL, an opinion supported by evaluations of QOL by seizure type.[34]

The types of seizures that occur with AVMs should, theoretically, be confined to focal seizures with or without secondary generalization, presuming that an AVM causes a discrete epileptic focus, or at most a limbus of adjacent epileptic tissue. Since secondarily generalized seizures can appear to witnesses as primary generalized seizures (especially those that propagate rapidly from the focus), listings of seizure types unsupported by electroencephalographic (EEG) findings should be viewed cautiously. Many reports feature a surprisingly high distribution of "generalized tonic–clonic" seizures with an across-study average of 63% (range: 5–81%; ▶ Table 31.2). In our subspecialty epilepsy clinic, simple partial seizures both before and after intervention are the predominant seizure type in AVMRE, an experience reflected by the proportions reported by a most recent study[20] as well as one of the more thorough early studies.[21] The across-study average of simple partial seizures is 25% of all seizure types (▶ Table 31.2).

31.3.4 EEG Assessment of Preoperative AVM-Related Epilepsy

EEG is a commonly used tool in assessment of epilepsy, but few studies of AVMRE report EEG findings, and only one appears to have evaluated EEGs uniformly across their samples. In a case series in which all patients underwent epilepsy surgery for intractable AVMRE and in which all underwent routine EEG

recorded from the scalp, 37% of patients had interictal epileptiform discharges[37] (IEDs; the principal abnormality predictive of epilepsy present in patients with epilepsy in between seizures).

Other studies report the incidence of IEDs of those for whom EEG results were available. A recent case series of AVMRE documented that 13% had focal interictal epileptiform discharges.[20] Earlier studies show sensitivity of routine EEG between 38 and 86%.[38,39] In comparison, the best estimates of sensitivity of a single, routine EEG for patients with known epilepsy of any cause range between 29 and 55%.[40,41,42] Therefore, the rate of IEDs found preoperatively in AVMRE is within ranges reported for epilepsy in general.

Long-term video EEG, as opposed to routine EEG, is used to localize the epileptogenic zone before epilepsy surgery by capturing seizures rather than just IED. However, no studies are available to describe findings with this standard preoperative technique. The closest report with uniform EEG use was Yeh et al who used a combination of preoperative chronic EEG to capture "EEG abnormalities" and intraoperative electrocorticography (ECoG) to evaluate the location of the epileptic focus in relation to AVM.[43] They documented that in 46% of subjects, with the use of these combined techniques, an epileptic focus was found. Although generalized seizures were not seen, in 44% of those with IEDs, remote foci in the mesial temporal structures—supposedly regions of secondary epileptogenesis—were seen beyond the regions of AVM.

31.3.5 Risk Factors of AVM-Related Epilepsy

Demographic or AVM characteristics that may place patients at higher risk of presenting with seizures or continuing with AVMRE vary among reports (▶ Table 31.3).[18,19,20,21,22,23,24,33,35,44,45] Regarding demographics, a minority of studies found that male sex[18,19,24] and younger age[24] carried higher risks for AVMRE. Two studies contradicted each other over prior AVM surgery.[21,24] Ding et al noted that prior AVM embolization worsened the likelihood of AVMRE.[45] Patients with neurological deficits associated with their AVM were found to have higher rates of AVMRE in two studies.[22,46]

The possible contribution of hemorrhage to the development of AVMRE was nearly uniformly evaluated in those studies that included patients with ruptured AVM. The majority of studies found that prior hemorrhage of AVM contributed to the likelihood of developing or presenting with AVMRE.[19,21,46] By virtue of its prospective acquisition and careful longitudinal follow-up, the study by Josephson et al may be considered the most rigorous.[33] The 5-year risk of first-ever seizure after presentation was higher for AVMs presenting with intracranial hemorrhage or focal neurologic deficit (23%) than for incidental AVMs (8%). An early study of a cohort of 343 patients followed longitudinally similarly found that development of epilepsy was confined to those with hemorrhage at a rate of 1% per year in absence of surgical treatment.[21] Englot et al, more recently, found that 43% of those with prior hemorrhage had AVMRE as opposed to 13% without hemorrhage.[19] Counter to the above studies, a retrospective study by Ding et al found that those patients without prior hemorrhage before undergoing SRS were 22 times more likely to have preoperative AVMRE than those with hemorrhage.[45]

Table 31.2 Distribution in seizure types reported in arteriovenous malformation–related epilepsy

First author (year)	Simple partial	Complex partial	Partial (total)	Generalized
Crawford (1986)[21]	45%	13%	58%	42%
Turjman (1995)[23]	25%	1%	26%	74%
Osipov (1997)[26]	31%	29%	60%	40%
Kurita (1998)[35]	31%	14%	44%	56%
Hoh (2002)[24]	9%	10%	19%	81%
Schäuble (2004)[27]	48%	14%	62%	38%
Yang (2012)[36]	19%	10%	29%	71%
Garcin (2012)[18]	18%	21%	39%	61%
Galletti (2014)[20]	74%	21%	95%	5%
Total	25%	12%	37%	63%

Table 31.3 Factors associated with development of arteriovenous malformation–related epilepsy. Studies noted by first author and year of publication[47]

Sex	Male	Not significant	Female
	Hoh (2002)[24] Garcin (2012)[18] Englot (2012)[19]	Crawford (1986)[21] Kurita (1998)[35] Josephson (2011)[33] Galletti (2014)[20] Ding 2015[4,5]	
Age	Younger	Not significant	Older
	Crawford (1986)[21] Hoh (2002)[24]	Crawford (1986)[21] Kurita (1998)[35] Josephson (2011)[33] Englot (2012)[19] Galletti (2014)[20] Ding 2015[4,5]	
Neuro deficit	Present	Not significant	Not present
	Murphy (1985)[22] Josephson (2011)[33]		
Prior surgery	Present	Not significant	Not present
	Crawford (1986)[21]		Ding (2015)[45]
Prior embolization	Present	Not significant	Not present
	Ding (2015)[45]		
Prior hemorrhage	Present	Not significant	Not present
	Crawford (1986)[21] Josephson (2011)[33] Englot (2012)[19]	Murphy (1985)[22] Hoh (2002)[24]	Ding (2015)[45]
Size/volume	Larger	Not significant	Smaller
	Crawford (1986)[21] Eisenschenk (1998)[24] Hoh (2002)[24] Englot (2012)[19] Garcin (2012)[18] Ding (2015)[45]	Turjman (1995)[23] Kurita (1998)[35] Josephson (2011)[33] Galletti (2014)[20]	
Location	Cortical/ superficial	Not significant	Deep/ subtentorial
	Crawford (1986)[21] Turjman (1995)[23] Hoh (2002)[24] Englot (2012)[19] Ding (2015)[45]	Kurita (1998)[35]	
	More likely	Not significant	Less likely
Frontal	Turjman (1995)[23] Eisenschenk (1998)[24] Englot (2012)[19] Garcin (2012)[18] Galletti (2014)[20]	Kurita (1998)[35]	

Table 31.3 continued

Sex	Male	Not significant	Female
Temporal	Turjman (1995)[23] Hoh (2002)[24] Josephson (2011)[33] Englot (2012)[19] Galletti (2014)[20]	Kurita (1998)[35]	
Parietal			
Occipital			Galletti (2014)[20] Ding (2015)[45]
Pseudoa- neurysm	Present	Not significant	Not present
		Kurita (1998)[35] Ding (2015)[45]	Turjman (1995)[23]
Single draining vein (n)	Present	Not significant	Not present
		Kurita (1998)[35]	Ding (2015)[45]
Venous drain (n)	Deep	Not significant	Superficial
		Kurita (1998)[35]	Turjman (1995)[23] Garcin (2012)[18] Galletti (2014)[20] Ding (2015)[45]
Spetzler– Martin grade	More severe	Not significant	Less severe
		Englot (2012)[19] Ding (2015)[45]	

Studies differ in the effects of AVM characteristics in association with epilepsy. Studies split almost evenly finding that larger AVMs have higher rates of AVMRE. Notably, the prospective incidence study by Josephson et al found that AVM size had no significant risks for AVMRE.[46] The location of AVM is a more consistent predictor of AVMRE; most studies determined that frontal, temporal, or frontotemporal locations were particularly susceptible to AVMRE.[18,19,20,23,24,44,46] Supporting these findings were Galletti et al and Ding et al who found, in a complementary fashion, that AVMs in the occipital region were particularly less susceptible to AVMRE.[20,48] Other facets of AVM morphology such as pseudoaneurysms, a single draining vein, superficial versus deep venous drainage, and Speltzer-Martin grade carried mixed associations with AVMRE.

31.3.6 Morbidity and Mortality of Preoperative AVMRE

Few studies have evaluated preoperative morbidity or mortality of AVMRE as a factor distinct from that of AVM in general. Regarding perceived morbidity, one study of SRS-treated patients surveyed them early in the latency period after SRS but before the emergence of radiosurgical or clinical changes. "Irreversible physical disabilities" had the most unfavorable effect on QOL compared to "reversible" symptoms such as epilepsy, headache, or transient physical symptoms.[49]

Prospective studies on the natural history of AVM may have data pertinent to seizure-related mortality hidden within causes of death. For example, the comparison of intervention versus conservative therapy for AVM by Al-Shahi Salman et al found that the overall risk of mortality over a 12-year follow-up period due to AVM was higher after intervention than for conservative management.[17] Forty-one deaths occurred across both arms; the cause of death was listed as "other" for 26 (62%) compared to an AVM- or intervention-related death. Certainly, SUDEP, seizure-associated trauma, or other complications of epilepsy could lay hidden in "other" deaths in this cohort.

31.4 Outcomes of Treatment for AVM-Related Epilepsy

AVMRE is merely one reason among several—future hemorrhage, worsening neurological deficits, etc.—to proceed with interventions. Several prospective comparisons of intervention versus conservative management, patients—who are not randomized—usually are younger and more likely to have AVMRE than patients followed in the conservative arms.[17,46] Thus, patients or their physicians may feel that AVMRE is an important factor in undertaking more aggressive therapy.

31.4.1 Outcomes of Open Surgery

▶ Table 31.4 contains the percentages of patients who achieve EC1 seizure remission after open surgery for AVM across studies published between 1972 and 2015. Although mean follow-up durations after surgery are sufficiently long, some studies include only minimal follow-up far shorter than the 2 years specified in the Engel's classification. With that limitation in mind, seizure remission rates are between 4 and 93% with a trend of improvement over time. A close look at the earliest study in ▶ Table 31.4, Forster et al, gives a snapshot of outcomes regarding epilepsy before the widespread use of presurgical embolization and microsurgical techniques.[50] In this study, patients with AVM who presented with either hemorrhage or epilepsy were followed long term (mean > 15 years) after partial or total removal of AVMs. Of the 104 patients with AVMRE, only 4% achieved complete seizure remission after surgery. Subanalyses to evaluate factors in favor of seizure remission were not evaluated. Later studies that presumably benefit from modern techniques show marked improvements in seizures outcomes over the 40-year span represented in ▶ Table 31.4. Englot et al

established in their cohort that EC1 outcome was achieved by 117 of the 126 patients (93%) who had preoperative seizures.[19]

The majority of studies of open surgery for AVMRE did not report the full scope of presurgical evaluation, that is, most concentrated on aspects important in visualizing and removing the AVM itself. However, one group detailed their results approaching AVM surgery from the standpoint of the removal of epileptic focus around the AVM, that is, an epilepsy surgery approach. The series by Yeh et al described their experience of 54 patients with both unruptured AVMs and intractable AVMRE and noted a 70% rate of seizure remission sustained for a mean follow-up period of 4.8 years.[43] All patients had some degree of long-term EEG and intraoperative ECoG to delineate cortical epileptogenic regions. Since other studies do not provide much information on the extent of presurgical workup, comparing results of a structurally based extirpation versus a more physiologically based approach is not possible.

Factors that predict seizure remission among surgical studies remained as variable as those factors thought important in emergence of preoperative seizures in AVMs. In fact, in the recent study by Englot et al, none of the factors associated with preoperative AVMRE remained significant postoperately.[19]

Patient-related factors associated with poor seizure control after surgery include older age,[43] longer duration epilepsy,[24,43] and generalized seizures.[24] Previous hemorrhage was one consistent factor associated with presurgical AVMRE. In contrast, prior hemorrhage (in the studies that included both unruptured and ruptured AVMs) was not a factor predicting postoperative seizure remission except in the study by Hoh et al.[24] AVM characteristics associated with absence of seizure-remission include larger AVM size,[25] locations outside frontoparietal regions,[43] and presence of deep perforators.[19] Complete removal of the AVM was noted to be associated with postoperative seizure remission by the majority of studies.[19,24,47]

31.4.2 Outcomes of Embolization

Studies of the antiepileptic effects of pure embolization of AVM are rare (▶ Table 31.5). Embolization does not appear to have any acute anticonvulsant effects, and, in fact, may acutely exacerbate seizures. Kurita et al noted that embolization did not reduce seizures in the interval (mean duration: 3.3 months) between embolization and subsequent SRS.[35] de Los Reyes et al noted that

Table 31.4 Summary of surgery series for arteriovenous malformation–related epilepsy

First author (year)	Min F/U (y)	Mean F/U (y)	Epilepsy with follow-up (N)	EC1 (N [%])	EC1 outcome off AED (%)	Post-op new-onset seizures (%)
Forster (1972)[50]	5	15	104	4 (4)	0	22
Murphy (1985)[22]	2	8.9	46	23 (50)	–	–
Heros (1990)[52]	0.5	3.8	55	28 (51)	0	8
Piepgras (1993)[25]	2	–	117	85 (73)	48	6
Yeh (1993)[43]	2	4.8	54	38 (70)	0	–
Hoh (2002)[24]	0.5	2.9	67	54 (81)	–	–
Englot (2012)[19]	0.5	–	126	117 (93)	–	3
Hyun (2012)[47]	3	3.6	32	25 (78)	–	3
Wang (2103)[51]	0.1	3.2	17	7 (41)	–	18
		Totals	618	381 (62)		

Abbreviations: AED, antiepileptic drug; EC1, Engel class 1.

Table 31.5 Summary of embolization series for arteriovenous malformation–related epilepsy

First author (year)	Min F/U (y)	Mean F/U (y)	Epilepsy with follow–up (N)	EC1 (N [%])	EC1 outcome off AED (%)	Postop new–onset seizures (%)
Fournier (1991)[54]	2	–	21	5 (24)	–	8.2
Osipov (1997)[26]	–	2.2	92	69 (75)	–	–
Hoh (2002)[24]	0.5	2.9	6	3 (50)	–	–
De Los Reye (2011)[53]	0.01	0.25	10	5 (50)	–	20
Englot (2012)[19]	0.5	–	193	161 (83)	–	–
Wang (2013)[51]	0.1	3.2	26	16 (62)	–	–
		Totals	348	259 (74)		

Abbreviations: AED, antiepileptic drug; EC1, Engel class 1.

in their series, 50% of those with AVMRE were seizure free after 3 months. However, 40% of patients without AVMRE experienced de novo seizures within 3 months.[53] The authors note that all patients, regardless of epilepsy status, received postoperative prophylactic AED and speculate that the emergence of de novo seizures after embolization may even be higher. The authors note that those with continuing or new-onset seizures tended to have incomplete obliteration of the nidus.

Three studies featured longer follow-up and demonstrate better outcomes for seizures. Fournier et al presented a series of patients with AVM treated solely with embolization and followed for at least 2 years. Of the 21 patients who presented with seizures, 5 (24%) experienced a "significant reduction" in the frequency of their attacks, and 4 (19%) became "more easily controlled" on AED.[54] Osipov et al followed 69 patients for a mean period of 2.2 years; 75% experienced cessation of seizures.[26] Hoh et al reported that in a mean follow-up period of 2.9 years, of six patients treated with embolization, three (50%)

achieved EC1 outcome. The mean seizure-remission rate among combined embolization studies was 74%.

31.4.3 Outcomes of Stereotactic Radiosurgery

Studies of the responses of seizures for treatment of AVM with SRS began to be reported in the early 1990s, and since then many single-center case series are available (▶ Table 31.6). One clear difference between SRS and other modalities is the clear latency—usually 3 to 6 months—before effects of SRS "kick in" to affect seizures.[19,35] Hyun et al calculated the median time to seizure remission (but without the minimum duration of "seizure remission" defined).[47] Although the median times to seizure remission for open surgery was 1 month and embolization 8 months, the duration of SRS seizure remission was 20 months. The latency to effect is an important consideration comparing case series, since the period of minimum follow-up

Table 31.6 Summary of stereotactic radiosurgery (SRS) for arteriovenous malformation–related epilepsy

First author (year)	SRS method	Min F/U (y)	Mean F/U (y)	Epilepsy with follow–up (N)	EC1 (N [%])	EC1 outcome off AED (%)	Postop new–onset seizures (%)
Lunsford (1992)[58]	GK	1	2	43	0 (0)	–	0
Steiner (1992)[29]	GK	2	–	59	11 (19)	100	6
Sutcliffe (1992)[30]	GK	2	2	48	18 (38)	–	0
Gerszten (1996)[31]	GK	–	3.9	13	11 (85)	100	3
Eisenschenk (1998)[24]	LINAC	0.9	2.2	32	19 (59)	26	–
Kurita (1998)[35]	GK	1.5	3.6	35	28 (80)	31	–
Kida/1998	GK	–	2	79	49 (62)	–	–
Hoh (2002)[24]	PBT	0.5	2.9	110	73 (66)	–	–
Nataf (2003)[60]	LINAC	0.4	3.3	6	4 (67)	–	–
Schäuble (2004)[27]	GK	1	3	51	26 (51)	15	–
Andrade-Souza (2006)[61]	LINAC	2.5	3.5	27	14 (52)	–	–
Lim (2006)[57]	GK	0.7	3.8	43	23 (53)	13	–
Hyun (2012)[47]	GK	3	3.6	50	33 (66)	–	3
Yang (2012)[36]	GK	4	7.5	78	62 (79)	77	–
Wang (2013)[51]	GK/LINAC	0.1	3.2	37	24 (65)	33	18
Ding (2015)[56]	GK	2	7.2	229	45.8 (20)	–	2
Totals				940	437 (47)		

Abbreviations: AED, antiepileptic drug; EC1, Engel class 1; GK, Gamma Knife; LINAC, linear accelerator; PBT, proton beam therapy; SRS, stereotactic radiosurgery.

Table 31.7 Factors associated with seizure remission after stereotactic radiosurgery for arteriovenous malformation

Sex	Male	Not significant	Female
		Kurita (1998)[35] Hoh (2002)[24] Ding (2015)[56]	
Age	Younger	Not significant	Older
		Kurita (1998)[35] Hoh (2002)[24] Schäuble (2004)[27] Ding (2015)[56]	
Neuro deficit	Present	Not significant	Not present
		Kurita (1998)[35]	Hyun (2012)[47]
Prior surgery	Present	Not significant	Not present
	Hoh (2002)[24]	Schäuble (2004)[27] Ding (2015)[56]	
Prior embolization	Present	Not significant	Not present
		Schäuble (2004)[27] Ding (2015)[56]	
Prior hemorrhage	Present	Not significant	Not present
	Hoh (2002)[24] Hyun (2012)[47] Ding (2015)[56]	Schäuble (2004)[27]	
Preoperative seizure frequency	Many	Not significant	Few
			Kurita (1998)[35] Schäuble (2004)[27] Yang (2012)[36]
Seizure type	Simple partial	Not significant	Generalized
	Eisenschenk (1998)[24]/least effective	Kurita (1998)[35] Schäuble (2004)[27] Ding (2015)[56]	Hoh (2002)[24] Hyun (2012)[47]
Seizure history duration	Short	Not significant	Long
	Hoh (2022)[24] Hyun (2012)[47]	Schäuble (2004)[27]	
Size/volume	Larger	Not significant	Smaller
	Eisenschenk (1998)[24] Kurita (1998)[35] Hoh (2002)[24] Ding (2015)[56]		Schäuble (2004)[27]
	More likely	Not significant	Less likely
Frontal	Eisenschenk (1998)[24]	Kurita (1998)[35] Yang (2012)[36] Ding/2015	Wang (2013)[51]
Temporal	Hyun (2012)[47]		Eisenschenk (1998)[24]
Parietal			
Occipital			
Pseudoaneurysm	Present	Not significant	Not present
		Ding (2015)[56]	

Table 31.7 continued

Sex	Male	Not significant	Female
Single draining vein	Present	Not significant	Not present
		Ding (2015)[56]	
Venous drain	Deep	Not significant	Superficial
		Ding (2015)[56]	
Spetzler–Martin grade	More severe	Not significant	Less severe
		Schäuble (2004)[27] Ding (2015)[56]	
Obliteration	Yes	Not significant	No
	Kurita (1998)[35] Hoh (2002)[24] Lim/2006 Hyun (2012)[47] Yang (2012)[36] Wang (2013)[51]	Schäuble (2004)[27] Ding (2015)[56]	Steiner (1992)[29] Kida (2000)[59]

Note: Studies are listed by first author and year of publication.

in some studies is clearly under the observed latency for the anticonvulsant effect of SRS. As seen with radiosurgery for medial temporal lobe epilepsy, the antiepileptic effect of radiosurgery is not immediate.[55] Ding et al noted that seizure outcomes improved over time, as demonstrated by the independent association of longer follow-up with seizure improvement.[56] Keeping in mind the limitation of follow-up time of the studies summarized in ▶ Table 31.6, the mean seizure remission rate for combined studies is 47% (range: 0–80%).

Factors favorable to seizure remission are compared in ▶ Table 31.7. Demographic factors are not associated with seizure remission. Studies differ—but not necessarily in contradiction to each other—in the importance of predominant seizure type. Generalized seizures were found to predict seizure remission[24,47] after SRS; simple partial seizures, on the other hand, were associated with poor outcome and were the type found to be most persistent after SRS.[44] Some studies noted that the fewer preoperative seizures[27,36] or shorter preoperative duration[24,47] were predictors of remission. Whereas prior hemorrhage was found to be a predictor in the development of AVMRE,[19,21,46] the converse is true postoperatively in that hemorrhage was associated with remission in most studies.[24,45,47]

The cortical location of AVM remains an inconsistent variable, with the majority of studies finding no significant effect of location. However, Eisenschenk et al and Hyun et al determined that frontotemporal location (found preoperatively as a promoter of AVMRE preoperatively) was associated with postoperative seizure remission.[44,47] Ding et al evaluated whether AVMRE associated with a temporal lobe AVM was more resistant to SRS than other cortical locations.[48] The rate of seizure remission in those with temporal AVM (18%) and extratemporal AVM (15%) did not differ.

Most other AVM-related factors such as the nature of venous drainage, Spetzler–Martin grade, or pseudoaneurysms did not play consistent roles in seizure outcomes (▶ Table 31.7). The dose/volume of SRS treatment has not had consistent associations with seizure remission. Although the radiosurgery margin dose affected AVM obliteration rates in two of the three studies that evaluated dose, it did not seem to significantly influence seizure outcome.[27,35,56]

The requirement for obliteration of the AVM nidus via SRS remains a controversial factor in prediction of seizure remission. However, the majority of studies summarized in ▶ Table 31.7 found that obliteration of the nidus correlated with seizure remission.[24,35,36,47,51,57] Chen et al performed a meta-analysis of available studies prior to 2013 and calculated corrected odds ratios in the contribution of obliteration in prediction of seizure remission. They found that complete obliteration offered a sixfold chance of seizure remission versus incomplete obliteration (odds ratio of 6.13 95%; confidence interval: 2.16–17.44)[62].

31.4.4 Appearance of AVM-Related Epilepsy after Intervention

The summary tables for open surgery, embolization, and SRS also include the rates of de novo emergence of AVMRE in patients who have been otherwise seizure free. Postoperative seizures can be divided into two groups: acute perioperative seizures, confined to a short period after intervention, and de novo chronic AVMRE.

Regarding acute seizures, as noted earlier, some studies of embolization emphasize the appearance of seizures confined to immediate postoperative period.[53,54] Some studies of open surgery[19,51] or SRS[35,44,58] reported both that some patients experienced a brief exacerbation or single seizure after treatment and that these limited seizures did not appear to predict subsequent AVMRE.

Chronic AVMRE arising after intervention is more common. Reports of de novo AVMRE after open surgery range from 3 to 22% (▶ Table 31.4) and after SRS or multimodal treatment from 2 to 18% (▶ Table 31.6). Although this phenomenon appears across many studies, the relative rarity of de novo AVMRE makes evaluation of risk factors difficult. Wang et al found that frontal lobe location predicted postprocedure AVMRE in those patients who underwent surgery.[51] Ding et al, from their large database, reported that from 778 patients without seizures at presentation, the overall rate of de novo AVMRE was 1.7%. Prior AVM hemorrhage and higher Spetzler–Martin grade were independent predictors of the absence of de novo seizures in the multivariate analysis.[56]

31.4.5 Comparisons with Conservative Therapy and among Interventions

No studies have been able to randomize patients to compare the risks and benefits among available treatment modalities; therefore, judging the issues specific to AVMRE among interventions and between interventions and conservative therapy is limited to accumulated experiences reported in single-center case series.

Conservative Therapy versus Intervention

Several studies have evaluated intervention against "best medical management." Murphy et al compared two groups (20 open surgery and 26 medical management) of patients with and without prior hemorrhage.[22] They found no statistical differences in rates of seizure remission (46% medical and 55% surgical) between the two groups. Josephson et al, as part of their prospective comparison of intervention (154 various combinations of intervention vs. 75 medical management), followed patients for a combined 1,862 person-years with a median completeness of follow-up of 97%.[46] There was no significant difference in the proportions with a first or recurrent seizure over 5 years following AVM treatment, compared to the first 5 years following clinical presentation in conservatively managed adults, in analyses stratified by presentation (hemorrhage, seizure, or incidental). For patients with AVMRE, the chances of achieving 2-year seizure freedom during 5-year follow-up were similar following AVM intervention (seizure free: 52%) or conservative management (seizure free: 57%).

Comparisons among Interventions

▶ Fig. 31.1 shows the proportion of patients reported as seizure free as a function of publication year divided by intervention modality. Overall, most studies of open surgery show higher rates of seizure remission than with embolization or SRS.

Studies of multimodal therapy (various combinations of open surgery, embolization, and SRS) have enabled investigators to compare outcomes by modality in those patients who were treated with a single method.[24,47,51] Each study showed that

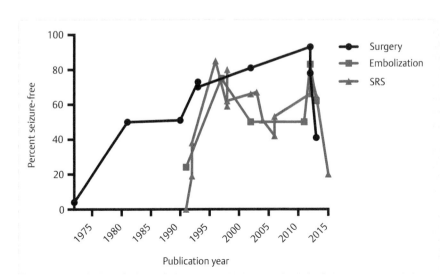

Fig. 31.1 Percentage of seizure-free patients after studies on open surgery, embolization, or stereotactic radiosurgery for arteriovenous malformation by year of publication.

Surgery
Embolization
SRS

open surgery patients tended to have higher rates of seizure remission, and each concluded that the differences were not statistically significant. Each study confirmed that obliteration of the nidus, regardless of intervention method, was the factor most clearly associated with seizure remission. For example, Hoh et al concluded that seizure remission rates among the three modalities were similar in the subgroup with complete AVM obliteration.[24]

Wang et al, the most recent available comparison study, also compared results of those with preoperative AVMRE and those with new-onset AVMRE after intervention.[51] In those with preoperative AVMRE, 57% were seizure free after surgery and 41% after SRS. In those without preoperative AVMRE, de novo AVMRE arose in 36% of those after surgery and 10% of those after SRS. The authors concluded that surgical therapy may result in improved seizure control compared with SRS for patients with AVMRE. Conversely, in patients without AVMRE, surgical resection increases the risk of new-onset seizures compared with SRS.

31.4.6 AED Prophylaxis, Treatment, and Discontinuation in AVMRE

Prophylaxis

The use of AED in patients who have a presumptive epileptic lesion but who are yet to present with seizures is called AED prophylaxis. Studies of febrile convulsions, ischemic stroke, subarachnoid hemorrhage, and head trauma have shown no consistent efficacy in the prevention of epileptogenesis or in neuroprotective aspects of chronic preseizure AED use.[63] Thus, use of chronic AED in prophylaxis in AVM patients without epilepsy is not recommended.

Temporary prophylaxis, on the other hand, in the perioperative period during either intracranial surgery or even SRS is a common procedure intended to minimize the chance of seizure while the patient, for example, is placed in a stereotactic frame. Although use of phenytoin for this purpose was once common, levetiracetam by virtue of intravenous administration, simple kinetics, lack of drug–drug interactions, and no requirements for monitoring during intravenous administration largely has taken its place. At the present, with patients who are not on AED for documented AVMRE, we start levetiracetam at doses of 1,000 to 1,500 mg/d several days before surgery. For those with AVMRE, we maintain ongoing AED after confirming adherence with AED blood levels.

Use of AED in the acute, inpatient setting for patients with hemorrhage from AVM but without seizures is debatable, especially in patients whose seizures may have occurred after injury but before admission and whose history have been confused by absent or unreliable witnesses. However, a study on the use of phenytoin as a neuroprotective agent after acute intracranial hemorrhage demonstrated that those without seizures placed on phenytoin were significantly more likely to have died or experienced worse outcome than those not receiving prophylaxis.[64]

Antiepileptic Drug Treatment of AVM-Related Epilepsy

No studies exist to compare what AED are particularly suited for patients with AVMRE. In addition, there is a paucity of comparative AED trials for focal epilepsy, so most physicians follow general practices for treatment of focal epilepsy[65]; therefore, practical considerations—namely tolerability, side effects, and cost—rule AED selection and maintenance. For AVMRE, we find that a first trial of levetiracetam is helpful because of its low rates of side effects, a wide range of well-tolerated therapeutic doses and predictable kinetics, lack of drug–drug interactions, easy initial titration, and the availability of intravenous and long-acting, 24-hour once-a-day dosing formulations.

Antiepileptic Drug Withdrawal after Seizure Remission

Studies of AVM interventions are uneven in evaluating the proportion of patients who, once achieving postoperative seizure remission, discontinued AED. The percentage of seizure-free patients for whom AED were discontinued are summarized in ▶ Table 31.4, ▶ Table 31.5, ▶ Table 31.6. In general, the ranges of 0 to 100% across the three modalities reflect differences in local practice and are out of control of the authors. Certainly, AED all have both idiosyncratic and dose-related side effects and can contribute to cognitive impairment, mood problems, and medical costs. However, three factors contribute to continuing the use of AED in patients who are seizure free following intervention for AVM. First, the evidence supporting withdrawal of AED is neither specific nor sensitive. Second, the consequences of a wrong guess—relapse after AED discontinuation—carry consequences beyond seizures including loss of driving privileges and employment status. Third, in absence of obvious AED-related side effects, a state not unusual with modern AED, it is difficult for physicians and patients to "fix something that isn't broken" and risk withdrawal.

There are no specific guidelines for withdrawal of AED in successfully treated AVMRE. In general, discontinuation of AED is an option for patients who are seizure free for greater than 2 years. A meta-analysis of 28 studies comprising 4,615 patients who underwent AED withdrawal after at least 2 years' seizure freedom showed that the range of relapse was from 12 to 66%.[66] The cumulative lifetime probability of remaining seizure free at 1 year after withdrawal was 39 to 74% and after 2 years was 35 to 57%. The relapse rate is highest within the first year. Only one randomized trial has been conducted on seizure relapse after AED withdrawal. Whereas 22% of those continuing AED relapsed in 2 years, 41% randomized to withdrawal relapsed.[67] Predictors of relapse in these studies include abnormal EEG, young age at onset, and symptomatic focal seizures.

31.4.7 Secondary Outcomes

Secondary outcomes—psychosocial function beyond the primary outcome of seizures—are not frequently assessed in patients with AVMRE. Assessment of such factors of QOL, employment, driving, mood, and neurocognition are important because these factors determine actual function and achievement. From a prospective study of epilepsy surgery for lesionless surgery, we know that QOL measurements improve quickly after surgery regardless of seizure status, but continued, smaller increments of improvement follow seizure status.[9] Mood, cognition, and health care costs, in general, also follow this pattern, with the limitation that cognitive outcomes vary with the location of epilepsy surgery.[68,69]

Secondary outcomes are commonly assessed after AVM intervention, but AVM and hemorrhage (or for some patients, the expectation of hemorrhage) are the usual focus; AVMRE is mentioned in passing or not at all. Only two studies with a focus on AVMRE have been performed. In one cohort of 78 patients treated with SRS, QOL and employment status were measured along with seizure status.[70] QOL scores were significantly higher for those patients whose SRS resulted in either seizure freedom, discontinuation of AED, or AVM obliteration. Patients who achieved obliteration of the AVM nidus or who were seizure free after SRS had higher rates of employment. Hyun et al measured QOL in a cohort treated in a multimodal comparison. They reported that QOL scores for those with good outcomes (AVM obliteration, seizure remission, or discontinuation of AED) were higher than for those lacking those outcomes.[47] Seizure frequency scores from those patients who failed to achieve obliteration correlated inversely with the QOL measures. Employment status correlated with good outcomes as well.

31.5 Mechanisms

AVM may lead to epilepsy via the mechanisms discussed below, none of which form mutually exclusive hypotheses.

31.5.1 Steal and Ischemia

A high volume of blood flow through the nidus may shunt blood from surrounding the brain, leading to focal hypoperfusion and ischemia of the affected cortex. Focal ischemic brain, with attendant gliosis, neuronal loss, and local changes in excitatory and inhibitory cortical regulation, may undergo epileptogenic changes.[71] Finally, chronic hypoxia could stimulate release of vascular growth factors and neoangiogenesis. This consequent vascular and structural rearrangement could potentiate alter the local balance of excitation and inhibition, providing another pathway to epileptogenesis.[72]

31.5.2 Hemosiderin Deposition

Hemosiderin deposition is another mechanism commonly evoked. Hemosiderin is thought to be an important component of epileptogenesis following head trauma and stroke. As discussed earlier, previous hemorrhage may be a risk factor in development of AVMRE, but, as some studies have demonstrated, is not mandatory. Microbleeding, either from occult bleeding of fragile vessels or from ischemia, can result in hemosiderin deposition that does not require frank intracerebral hemorrhage.[71]

31.5.3 Kindling

Kindling is the process of recurrent epileptic stimulations that eventually alter brain circuits to enable emergence of independent, spontaneous seizures.[73] Secondary epileptogenesis is the phenomenon of a primary epileptic lesion—in this case an AVM—producing one or more secondary epileptic foci remote from the primary lesion. Such a process was hypothesized by Yeh et al during their observations of temporal lobe seizures recorded by EEG/ECoG in the setting of extratemporal AVM.[43]

References

[1] Fisher RS, Acevedo C, Arzimanoglou A, et al. ILAE official report: a practical clinical definition of epilepsy. Epilepsia. 2014; 55(4):475–482

[2] Kwan P, Arzimanoglou A, Berg AT, et al. Definition of drug resistant epilepsy: consensus proposal by the ad hoc Task Force of the ILAE Commission on Therapeutic Strategies. Epilepsia. 2010; 51(6):1069–1077

[3] Shorvon SD, Reynolds EH. Reduction in polypharmacy for epilepsy. BMJ. 1979; 2(6197):1023–1025

[4] Laxer KD, Trinka E, Hirsch LJ, et al. The consequences of refractory epilepsy and its treatment. Epilepsy Behav. 2014; 37:59–70

[5] Kwan P, Brodie MJ. Early identification of refractory epilepsy. N Engl J Med. 2000; 342(5):314–319

[6] Engel J , Jr. Update on surgical treatment of the epilepsies. Summary of the Second International Palm Desert Conference on the Surgical Treatment of the Epilepsies (1992). Neurology. 1993; 43(8):1612–1617

[7] Spencer SS, Berg AT, Vickrey BG, et al. Multicenter Study of Epilepsy Surgery. Initial outcomes in the Multicenter Study of Epilepsy Surgery. Neurology. 2003; 61(12):1680–1685

[8] Langfitt JT, Westerveld M, Hamberger MJ, et al. Worsening of quality of life after epilepsy surgery: effect of seizures and memory decline. Neurology. 2007; 68(23):1988–1994

[9] Spencer SS, Berg AT, Vickrey BG, et al. Multicenter Study of Epilepsy Surgery. Health-related quality of life over time since resective epilepsy surgery. Ann Neurol. 2007; 62(4):327–334

[10] WHO. Disease Burden: Regional Estimates for 2000–2011. Available at: http://www.who.int/healthinfo/global_burden_disease/estimates_regional/en/index1.html. Accessed January 7, 2014

[11] Fisher RS, Vickrey BG, Gibson P, et al. The impact of epilepsy from the patient's perspective I. Descriptions and subjective perceptions. Epilepsy Res. 2000; 41(1):39–51

[12] Quigg M. Fertility in Epilepsy. In: Bui E, Klein A, eds. Women with Epilepsy: A Practical Management Handbook. Cambridge University Press: Cambridge; 2014

[13] Hesdorffer DC. Risk factors for mortality in epilepsy: which ones are correctible? In: Partners against Mortality in Epilepsy Conference Summary. Epilepsy Curr. 2013; 13:6

[14] Ryvlin P, Cucherat M, Rheims S. Risk of sudden unexpected death in epilepsy in patients given adjunctive antiepileptic treatment for refractory seizures: a meta-analysis of placebo-controlled randomised trials. Lancet Neurol. 2011; 10(11):961–968

[15] Tomson T, Nashef L, Ryvlin P. Sudden unexpected death in epilepsy: current knowledge and future directions. Lancet Neurol. 2008; 7(11):1021–1031

[16] Hofmeister C, Stapf C, Hartmann A, et al. Demographic, morphological, and clinical characteristics of 1289 patients with brain arteriovenous malformation. Stroke. 2000; 31(6):1307–1310

[17] Al-Shahi Salman R, White PM, Counsell CE, et al. Scottish Audit of Intracranial Vascular Malformations Collaborators. Outcome after conservative management or intervention for unruptured brain arteriovenous malformations. JAMA. 2014; 311(16):1661–1669

[18] Garcin B, Houdart E, Porcher R, et al. Epileptic seizures at initial presentation in patients with brain arteriovenous malformation. Neurology. 2012; 78(9):626–631

[19] Englot DJ, Young WL, Han SJ, McCulloch CE, Chang EF, Lawton MT. Seizure predictors and control after microsurgical resection of supratentorial arteriovenous malformations in 440 patients. Neurosurgery. 2012; 71(3):572–580, discussion 580

[20] Galletti F, Costa C, Cupini LM, et al. Brain arteriovenous malformations and seizures: an Italian study. J Neurol Neurosurg Psychiatry. 2014; 85(3):284–288

[21] Crawford PM, West CR, Shaw MD, Chadwick DW. Cerebral arteriovenous malformations and epilepsy: factors in the development of epilepsy. Epilepsia. 1986; 27(3):270–275

[22] Murphy MJ. Long-term follow-up of seizures associated with cerebral arteriovenous malformations. Results of therapy. Arch Neurol. 1985; 42(5):477–479

[23] Turjman F, Massoud TF, Sayre JW, Viñuela F, Guglielmi G, Duckwiler G. Epilepsy associated with cerebral arteriovenous malformations: a multivariate analysis of angioarchitectural characteristics. AJNR Am J Neuroradiol. 1995; 16(2):345–350

[24] Hoh BL, Chapman PH, Loeffler JS, Carter BS, Ogilvy CS. Results of multimodality treatment for 141 patients with brain arteriovenous malformations and seizures: factors associated with seizure incidence and seizure outcomes. Neurosurgery. 2002; 51(2):303–309, discussion 309–311

[25] Piepgras DG, Sundt TM , Jr, Ragoowansi AT, Stevens L. Seizure outcome in patients with surgically treated cerebral arteriovenous malformations. J Neurosurg. 1993; 78(1):5–11

[26] Osipov A, Koennecke HC, Hartmann A, et al. Seizures in cerebral arteriovenous malformations: type, clinical course, and medical management. Interv Neuroradiol. 1997; 3(1):37–41

[27] Schäuble B, Cascino GD, Pollock BE, et al. Seizure outcomes after stereotactic radiosurgery for cerebral arteriovenous malformations. Neurology. 2004; 63 (4):683–687

[28] Heikkinen ER, Konnov B, Melnikov L, et al. Relief of epilepsy by radiosurgery of cerebral arteriovenous malformations. Stereotact Funct Neurosurg. 1989; 53(3):157–166

[29] Steiner L, Lindquist C, Adler JR, Torner JC, Alves W, Steiner M. Clinical outcome of radiosurgery for cerebral arteriovenous malformations. J Neurosurg. 1992; 77(1):1–8

[30] Sutcliffe JC, Forster DM, Walton L, Dias PS, Kemeny AA. Untoward clinical effects after stereotactic radiosurgery for intracranial arteriovenous malformations. Br J Neurosurg. 1992; 6(3):177–185

[31] Gerszten PC, Adelson PD, Kondziolka D, Flickinger JC, Lunsford LD. Seizure outcome in children treated for arteriovenous malformations using gamma knife radiosurgery. Pediatr Neurosurg. 1996; 24(3):139–144

[32] Falkson CB, Chakrabarti KB, Doughty D, Plowman PN. Stereotactic multiple arc radiotherapy. III-Influence of treatment of arteriovenous malformations on associated epilepsy. Br J Neurosurg. 1997; 11(1):12–15

[33] Josephson CB, Leach JP, Duncan R, Roberts RC, Counsell CE, Al-Shahi Salman R, Scottish Audit of Intracranial Vascular Malformations (SAIVMs) steering committee and collaborators. Seizure risk from cavernous or arteriovenous malformations: prospective population-based study. Neurology. 2011; 76 (18):1548–1554

[34] Shetty PH, Naik RK, Saroja A, Punith K. Quality of life in patients with epilepsy in India. J Neurosci Rural Pract. 2011; 2(1):33–38

[35] Kurita H, Kawamoto S, Suzuki I, et al. Control of epilepsy associated with cerebral arteriovenous malformations after radiosurgery. J Neurol Neurosurg Psychiatry. 1998; 65(5):648–655

[36] Yang SY, Kim DG, Chung HT, Paek SH. Radiosurgery for unruptured cerebral arteriovenous malformations: long-term seizure outcome. Neurology. 2012; 78(17):1292–1298

[37] Yeh HS, Kashiwagi S, Tew JM , Jr, Berger TS. Surgical management of epilepsy associated with cerebral arteriovenous malformations. J Neurosurg. 1990; 72 (2):216–223

[38] Leblanc R, Feindel W, Ethier R. Epilepsy from cerebral arteriovenous malformations. Can J Neurol Sci. 1983; 10(2):91–95

[39] Thajeb P, Hsi MS. Cerebral arteriovenous malformation: report of 136 Chinese patients in Taiwan. Angiology. 1987; 38(11):851–858

[40] Goodin DS, Aminoff MJ, Laxer KD. Detection of epileptiform activity by different noninvasive EEG methods in complex partial epilepsy. Ann Neurol. 1990; 27(3):330–334

[41] Marsan CA, Zivin LS. Factors related to the occurrence of typical paroxysmal abnormalities in the EEG records of epileptic patients. Epilepsia. 1970; 11(4): 361–381

[42] Salinsky M, Kanter R, Dasheiff RM. Effectiveness of multiple EEGs in supporting the diagnosis of epilepsy: an operational curve. Epilepsia. 1987; 28(4): 331–334

[43] Yeh HS, Tew JM , Jr, Gartner M. Seizure control after surgery on cerebral arteriovenous malformations. J Neurosurg. 1993; 78(1):12–18

[44] Eisenschenk S, Gilmore RL, Friedman WA, Henchey RA. The effect of LINAC stereotactic radiosurgery on epilepsy associated with arteriovenous malformations. Stereotact Funct Neurosurg. 1998; 71(2):51–61

[45] Ding D, Starke RM, Quigg M, et al. Cerebral arteriovenous malformations and epilepsy, Part 1: predictors of seizure presentation. World Neurosurg. 2015; 84(3):645–652

[46] Josephson CB, Bhattacharya JJ, Counsell CE, et al. Scottish Audit of Intracranial Vascular, Malformations (SAIVMs) steering committee and collaborators. Seizure risk with AVM treatment or conservative management: prospective, population-based study. Neurology. 2012; 79(6):500–507

[47] Hyun SJ, Kong DS, Lee JI, Kim JS, Hong SC. Cerebral arteriovenous malformations and seizures: differential impact on the time to seizure-free state according to the treatment modalities. Acta Neurochir (Wien). 2012; 154(6): 1003–1010

[48] Ding D, Quigg M, Starke RM, et al. Radiosurgery for temporal lobe arteriovenous malformations: effect of temporal location on seizure outcomes. J Neurosurg. 2015; 123(4):924–934

[49] Lai EH, Lun SL. Impact on the quality of life of patients with arteriovenous malformations during the latent interval between gamma knife radiosurgery and lesion obliteration. J Neurosurg. 2002; 97(5) Suppl:471–473

[50] Forster DM, Steiner L, Håkanson S. Arteriovenous malformations of the brain. A long-term clinical study. J Neurosurg. 1972; 37(5):562–570

[51] Wang JY, Yang W, Ye X, et al. Impact on seizure control of surgical resection or radiosurgery for cerebral arteriovenous malformations. Neurosurgery. 2013; 73(4):648–655, discussion 655–656

[52] Heros RC, Korosue K, Diebold PM. Surgical excision of cerebral arteriovenous malformations: late results. Neurosurgery. 1990; 26(4):570–577, discussion 577–578

[53] de Los Reyes K, Patel A, Doshi A, et al. Seizures after Onyx embolization for the treatment of cerebral arteriovenous malformation. Interv Neuroradiol. 2011; 17(3):331–338

[54] Fournier D, TerBrugge KG, Willinsky R, Lasjaunias P, Montanera W. Endovascular treatment of intracerebral arteriovenous malformations: experience in 49 cases. J Neurosurg. 1991; 75(2):228–233

[55] Barbaro NM, Quigg M, Broshek DK, et al. A multicenter, prospective pilot study of gamma knife radiosurgery for mesial temporal lobe epilepsy: seizure response, adverse events, and verbal memory. Ann Neurol. 2009; 65(2):167–175

[56] Ding D, Quigg M, Starke RM, et al. Cerebral arteriovenous malformations and epilepsy, part 2: predictors of seizure outcomes following radiosurgery. World Neurosurg. 2015; 84(3):653–662

[57] Lim YJ, Lee CY, Koh JS, Kim TS, Kim GK, Rhee BA. Seizure control of Gamma Knife radiosurgery for non-hemorrhagic arteriovenous malformations. Acta Neurochir Suppl (Wien). 2006; 99:97–101

[58] Lunsford LD, Kondziolka D, Bissonette DJ, Maitz AH, Flickinger JC. Stereotactic radiosurgery of brain vascular malformations. Neurosurg Clin N Am. 1992; 3 (1):79–98

[59] Kida Y, Kobayashi T, Tanaka T, Mori Y, Hasegawa T, Kondoh T. Seizure control after radiosurgery on cerebral arteriovenous malformations. J Clin Neurosci. 2000; 7 Suppl 1:6–9

[60] Nataf F, Schlienger M, Lefkopoulos D, et al. Radiosurgery of cerebral arteriovenous malformations in children: a series of 57 cases. Int J Radiat Oncol Biol Phys. 2003; 57(1):184–195

[61] Andrade-Souza YM, Ramani M, Scora D, Tsao MN, TerBrugge K, Schwartz ML. Radiosurgical treatment for rolandic arteriovenous malformations. J Neurosurg. 2006; 105(5):689–697

[62] Chen CJ, Chivukula S, Ding D, et al. Seizure outcomes following radiosurgery for cerebral arteriovenous malformations. Neurosurg Focus. 2014; 37(3):E17

[63] Wilmore LJ. Prophylactic treatment. In: Engel JJ, Pedley TA, eds. Epilepsy: A Comprehensive Textbook. New York, NY: Lippincott-Raven Publishers; 2008:1371–1375

[64] Messé SR, Sansing LH, Cucchiara BL, Herman ST, Lyden PD, Kasner SE, CHANT investigators. Prophylactic antiepileptic drug use is associated with poor outcome following ICH. Neurocrit Care. 2009; 11(1):38–44

[65] French JA, Kanner AM, Bautista J, et al. American Academy of Neurology Therapeutics and Technology Assessment Subcommittee, American Academy of Neurology Quality Standards Subcommittee, American Epilepsy Society Quality Standards Subcommittee, American Epilepsy Society Therapeutics and Technology Assessment Subcommittee. Efficacy and tolerability of the new antiepileptic drugs, I: Treatment of new-onset epilepsy: report of the TTA and QSS Subcommittees of the American Academy of Neurology and the American Epilepsy Society. Epilepsia. 2004; 45(5):401–409

[66] Specchio LM, Beghi E. Should antiepileptic drugs be withdrawn in seizure-free patients? CNS Drugs. 2004; 18(4):201–212

[67] Chadwick D, Taylor J, Johnson T, The MRC Antiepileptic Drug Withdrawal Group. Outcomes after seizure recurrence in people with well-controlled epilepsy and the factors that influence it. Epilepsia. 1996; 37(11):1043–1050

[68] Devinsky O, Barr WB, Vickrey BG, et al. Changes in depression and anxiety after resective surgery for epilepsy. Neurology. 2005; 65(11):1744–1749

[69] Langfitt JT, Holloway RG, McDermott MP, et al. Health care costs decline after successful epilepsy surgery. Neurology. 2007; 68(16):1290–1298

[70] Yang SY, Paek SH, Kim DG, Chung HT. Quality of life after radiosurgery for cerebral arteriovenous malformation patients who present with seizure. Eur J Neurol. 2012; 19(7):984–991

[71] Kraemer DL, Awad IA. Vascular malformations and epilepsy: clinical considerations and basic mechanisms. Epilepsia. 1994; 35 Suppl 6:S30–S43

[72] Ndode-Ekane XF, Hayward N, Gröhn O, Pitkänen A. Vascular changes in epilepsy: functional consequences and association with network plasticity in pilocarpine-induced experimental epilepsy. Neuroscience. 2010; 166(1):312–332

[73] Morrell F. Varieties of human secondary epileptogenesis. J Clin Neurophysiol. 1989; 6(3):227–275

Index